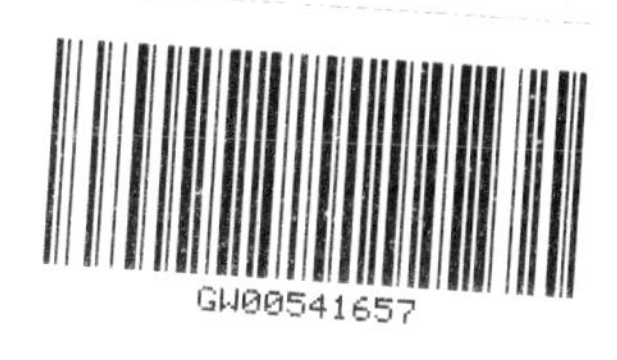
GW00541657

Healthy Plants

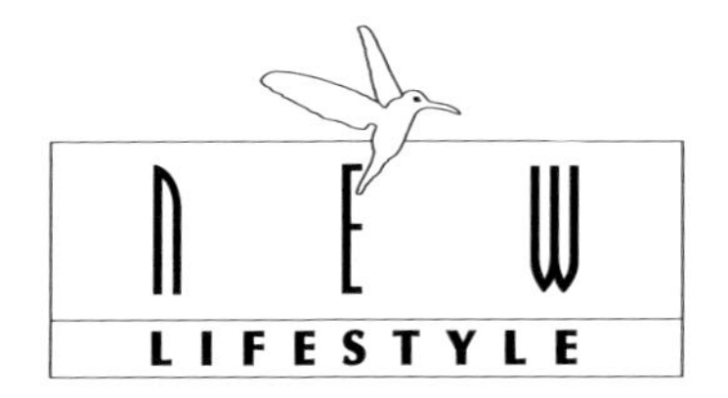

HEALTHY PLANTS

George D. Pamplona-Roger

Doctor of Medicine and Surgery (University of Granada, Spain)
Board-certified general and digestive surgeon
Specialist in Health Education (UNED University, Spain)
Master of Public Health (Loma Linda University, California, USA)

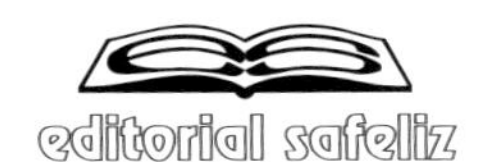

Disclaimer

It is the wish of the author and of the publishers that this book is useful to orientate and to inform our readers regarding the value of medicinal plants. Although the recommendations and information given are appropriate in most cases, they are of a general nature and cannot take into account the specific circumstances of individual situations. Any plant substance, used externally or internally, can cause allergic reactions in some persons. The information given in this book is not intended to take the place of professional medical care either in diagnosing or treating medical conditions. Do not attempt self-diagnosis or self-treatment for serious or long-term problems without consulting a qualified medical professional. Always seek a physician's advice before undertaking any self-treatment or if symptoms persist. Neither the publisher nor the author can assume responsibility for problems arising from the mistaken identity of any plant or from the inappropriate use made of it by readers. Advice is given in page 50 on the safe use of medical herbs.

Collection: **New Lifestyle**
Title: **Healthy Plants**
Original title in Spanish edition: *Salud por las plantas medicinales*

Author: George D. Pamplona-Roger
Illustration credits: See page 382
Design and project development: Editorial Safeliz team

Pradillo, 6 · Pol. Ind. La Mina
E-28770 · Colmenar Viejo, Madrid, Spain
Tel.: [+34] 91 845 98 77 · Fax: [+34] 91 845 98 65
admin@safeliz.com · www.safeliz.com

April 2007: 2nd print of the 1st edition in English language

ISBN: 978-84-7208-120-8
Legal Deposit: M-10267-2007

Printing: Ibergraphi 2002 · E-28830 San Fernando de Henares, Madrid, Spain
PRINTED IN THE EUROPEAN UNION

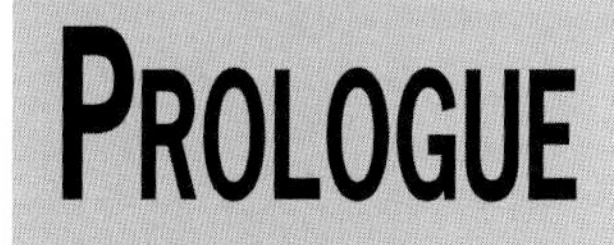

Throughout the ages, plants have been used by humans as a source of food, cosmetics and medicines, and have provided raw materials for the construction of shelters and the manufacture of clothing. The significance of tropical forests in the maintenance of the earth's ecological balance is only now being fully appreciated and understood. There is an urgent need to conserve and use these resources in an environmentally sustainable and economically beneficial manner.

Plants have served as the basis of sophisticated traditional medicine systems for thousands of years in countries such as China and India. These plant-based systems continue to play an essential role in health care. It has been estimated by the World Health Organization that about 80% of the world's inhabitants rely mainly on traditional medicines for their primary health care.

Plant products also play an important role in the health care systems of the remaining 20 percent of the population who mainly reside in developed countries. Analysis of data on prescriptions dispensed from community pharmacies in the United States from 1959 to 1980 indicates that about 25 percent contained plant extracts or active components derived from higher plants. At least 119 chemical substances, derived from 90 plant species, can be considered as important drugs currently in use in one or more countries.

The United States National Cancer Institute (NCI) was established in 1937, its mission being "to provide for, foster, and aid in coordinating research related to cancer." The NCI has screened well over 100,000 plant extracts for anticancer activity and over 30,000 for anti-AIDS activity.

The development of clinically effective anticancer agents such as taxol, and the discovery of potential anti-AIDS agents such as michellamine B, demonstrate the value of plants as sources of potential new drugs, and highlight the importance of conserving these valuable resources.

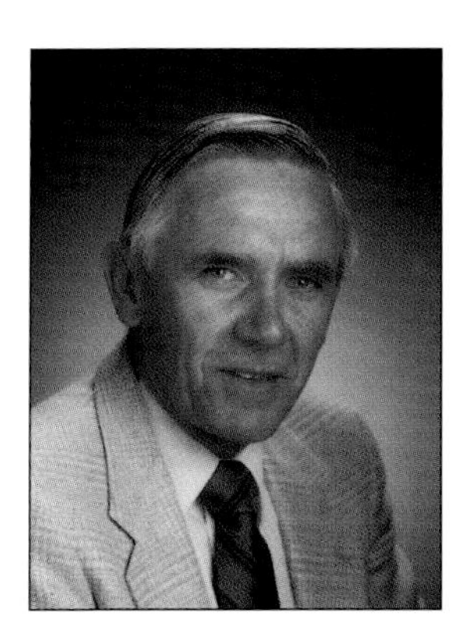

DR. GORDON M. CRAGG
Natural Products Branch,
U. S. National Cancer Institute

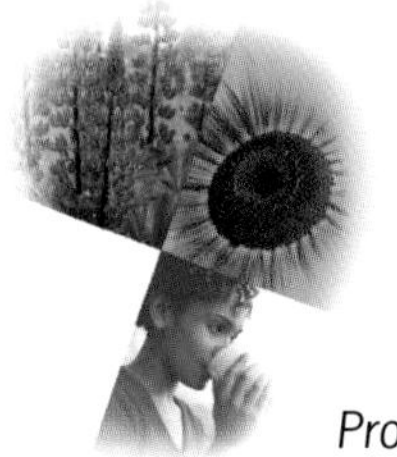

GENERAL PLAN

Prologue 5
General Plan of the Work 6
Index of Diseases 8
Index of Plants 12
Meaning of the Icons of Botanical Parts 16
Meaning of the Icons of Anatomical Parts 17
Plant Pages: Description and Format 18
Description of Boxes and Tables 19

1 The Vegetal World **21**

2 Methods for Preparing and Using Plants **35**

3 Plants for the Eyes **57**

4 Plants for the Nervous System **65**

5 Plants for the Mouth, Nose and Throat **87**

6 Plants for the Heart **105**

7 Plants for the Arteries **115**

8 Plants for the Veins **127**

9 Plants for the Blood **135**

10 Plants for the Respiratory System **145**

OF THE WORK

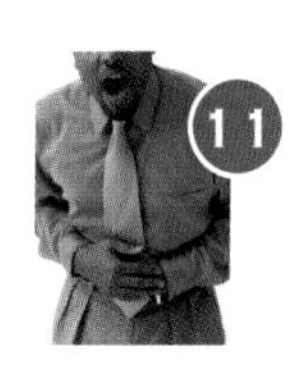

11 Plants for the Digestive System 171

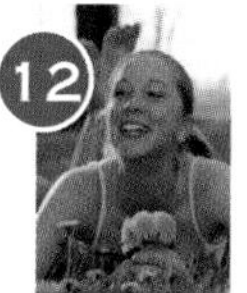

12 Plants for the Liver 191

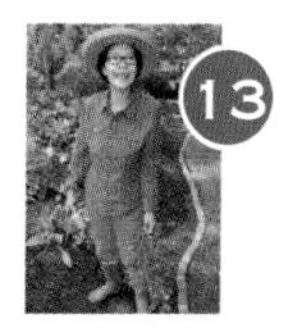

13 Plants for the Stomach 205

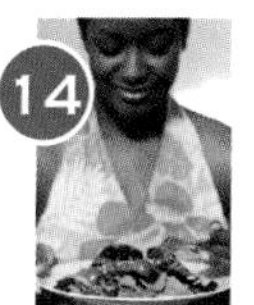

14 Plants for the Intestine 237

15 Plants for the Urinary System 267

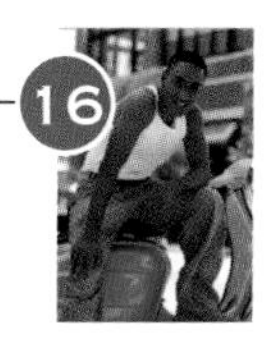

16 Plants for the Sexual Organs 289

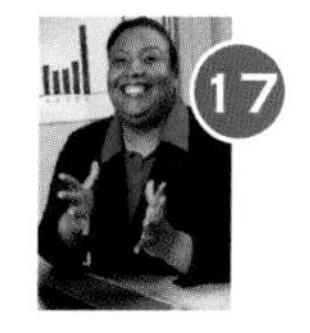

17 Plants for the Metabolism 309

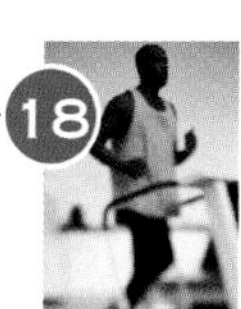

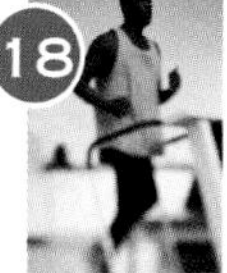

18 Plants for the Locomotive System 317

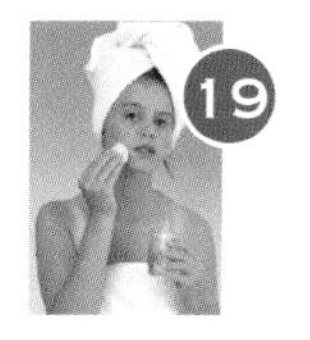

19 Plants for the Skin 335

20 Plants for Infectious Diseases 357

Index of Scientific Names *380*
Units of Measure *383*

Index of Diseases

Abscesses 341
Ache, kidney, see Lumbago 319
Ache, rheumatic, see Rheumatic pain . . 319
Ache, stomach 208
Aches and Neuralgia 69
Acid, uric, excess of, see Gout 311
Acidity, stomach 206
Acne 339
Affections, heart 106
AIDS 361
Alimentary intoxication, see Salmonellosis 358
Alteration, heartbeat rate, see Arrhythmia 107
Amebiasis 360
Amebic dysentery, see Amebiasis 360
Analgesic plants, see Aches and neuralgia 69
Anemia 136
Angina pectoris 107
Anorexia, see Appetite, lack of 172
Anxiety 67
Anxiolytics, see Nervousness and anxiety 67
Aphonia 92
Appetite, excess of, see Bulimia 310
Appetite, lack of 172
Arrhythmia 107
Arteriosclerosis 117
Arthritis, uric, see Gouty arthritis 319
Arthritism, see Gouty arthritis 319
Arthrosis 320
Ascaris, intestinal, see Intestinal parasites 241
Ascitis, see Fluid in the abdomen 192
Asthenia 67
Asthma 148
Attack, heart 107

Back ache, see Lumbago 319
Bad breath 172
Bad taste in mouth 89
Beauty, skin 340
Belches, see Stomach gas 207
Biliary colic 193
Blepharitis 59
Bloated stomach 207
Blood flow, lack of 117
Bones, weakness, see Osteoporosis . . . 318
Brain circulatory insufficiency, see Lack of blood flow 117
Bronchitis 147
Bruises, see Contusion 318
Bulimia 310

Calculi, urine, see Urinary lithiasis 268
Callus 336
Cardiopathy, see Heart affections 106
Cellulitis 339
Cephalalgia, see Headaches 69
Cervicitis 293
Chilblains 117
Cholelithiasis, see Gall bladder dysfunction 193
Cholera 359
Cholesterol, plants against high 117
Chronic gastritis 208
Cirrhosis, see Hepatitis 192
Climateric stage, see Menopause 292
Cold, chilblains 117
Colic, kidney 269
Colitis 240
Conjunctivitis and blepharitis 59
Constipation 241
Contusion 318
Convalescence 359
Corns, see Callus 336
Coronary heart disease, see Angina pectoris 107
Cough 148
Cracks, skin 336
Cystitis 271

Depression, immune system, see Low defenses 358
Depression, nervousness 66
Diabetes 311
Diarrhea, see Gastroenteritis 240
Difficult digestion, see Dyspepsia 207

Digestion, disorders, see Dyspepsia . . . 207
Diseases, febrile, see Febrile diseases . 359
Diseases, psychosomatic 68
Dropsy 269
Dry skin 339
Dysmenorrhea 292
Dyspepsia. 207

Eczema 338
Edema 269
Enuresis 270
Epilepsy 69
Epistaxis, see Nose, bleeding. 92
Erythema pernio, see Chilblains 117
Excess of appetite, see Bulimia 310
Excessive menstruation 293
Excessive perspiration of feet,
see Foot, disorders 320
Excessive sexual excitation 290
Eyelids, inflammation,
see Conjunctivitis and blepharitis 59

Fainting 117
Fatigue and asthenia 67
Febrile diseases 359
Feet blisters, see Foot, disorders 320
Female sterility 291
Fermentation, intestinal 239
Fever, typhoid 359
Fluid in the abdomen 192
Fluid, retention, see Edema 269
Foot bruises, see Foot disorders 320
Foot disorders 320
Fungi, skin, see Skin mycosis. 338
Furuncles and abscesses. 341

Gall bladder, dysfunction. 193
Gas, intestinal 238
Gas, stomach 207
Gastric hypotonia,
see Bloated stomach 207
Gastric juice, lack of 206
Gastric ptosis, see Bloated stomach. . . 207
Gastritis 209
Gastritis, chronic 208
Gastroenteritis 240
Gingivitis. 89
Gout. 311
Gouty arthritis 319
Growth, tooth 89
Gums, disorders, see Pyorrhea,
gingivitis, and parodontosis. 89

Hair loss 340
Halitosis, see Bad breath 172
Headaches 69
Heart affections 106
Heart diseases 106
Heart, coronary, see Angina pectoris . . 107
Heartbeat rate alteration,
see Arrhythmia. 107
Hemorrhage 136
Hepatic colic, see Biliary colic 193
Hepatitis. 192
Herpes 341
High blood pressure 116
Hoarseness, see Aphonia. 92
Hypermenorrhea,
see Excessive menstruation 293
Hypertension,
see High blood pressure 116
Hyperuricemia, see Gout 311
Hypochlorhydria,
see Lack of gastric juice. 206
Hypotension, see Low blood pressure. . 116

Immune system depression,
see Low defenses 358
Incontinence, urinary 271
Infection, kidney, see Pyelonephritis . . . 270
Infection, urinary 270
Infection, urine bladder, see Cystitis . . . 271
Infection, urine, see Urinary infection . . 270
Influenza. 361
Insomnia. 68
Insufficiency, kidney,
see Nephritis and nephrosis 270
Insufficient intellectual performance . . . 66
Intellectual, insufficient performance . . . 66
Intestinal atony 240
Intestinal colic. 240
Intestinal dysbacteriosis. 239
Intestinal fermentation 239
Intestinal flora, alterations,
see Intestinal dysbacteriosis 239
Intestinal gas 238
Intestinal parasites 241
Intestinal spasm, see Intestinal colic . . . 240
Intestinal worms,
see Intestinal parasites 241

Intestine, alterations of the flora,
see Intestinal dysbacteriosis 239
Intestine, atony 240
Intestine, colic. 240
Invigorant plants,
see Fatigue and asthenia 67
Irregular menstruation 293
Irritable bowel syndrome 239
Irritation, skin 339
Itching, throat, see Throat irritation 90

Joint sprain, see Sprain 318

Keratitis 58
Kidney ache, see Lumbago 319
Kidney colic 269
Kidney insufficiency,
see Nephritis and nephrosis 270

Lack of appetite, see Appetite, lack of . 172
Lack of blood flow. 117
Lack of gastric juice 206
Laringitis 91
Leukorrhea 293
Lip sores 88
Lithiasis, renal, see Urinary lithiasis. . . . 268
Lithiasis, urinary 268
Liver insufficiency,
see Liver, dysfunction. 192
Liver stones,
see Gall bladder dysfunction 193
Liver, dysfunction 192
Liver, toxicity 193
Loss of hair 340
Loss of memory 67
Low blood pressure. 116
Low defenses 358
Lumbago 319
Lung emphysema 149

Malaria 360
Male sterility 291
Malnutrition. 311
Memory, loss of 67
Menopause. 292
Menstruation, excessive. 293
Menstruation, irregular. 293
Menstruation, pain, see Dysmenorrhea . 292
Menstruation, retention of fluids 291
Migraine 68
Mouth ulcers. 88
Mouth, bad taste in 89
Multiple sclerosis, see Organic
diseases of the nervous system 69
Mycosis, skin 338
Myocardial infarction 107

Nails, fragile 341
Neck of the uterus, infection,
see Cervicitis 293
Nephritis and nephrosis 270
Nephrosis 270
Nervous system,
organic diseases of the. 69
Nervous tension, see Stress. 68
Nervousness and anxiety 67
Nervousness, stomach 208
Neuralgia 69
Neurasthenia,
see Nervousness and anxiety 67
Nipple sores 291
Nose, bleeding 92
Nose, inflammation, see Rhinitis 91

Obesity 310
Organic diseases
of the nervous system 69
Osteoporosis 318
Ovary, insufficiency 291

Pain, rheumatic 319
Palpitations. 106
Pancreatic, insufficiency. 193
Parasites, intestinal 241
Parkinson disease, see Organic
diseases of the nervous system 69
Parodontosis. 89
Pharyngitis 90
Phlebitis 128
Plants, sedatives,
see Nervousness and anxiety 67
Pneumonia 147
Portal hypertension,
see Fluid in the abdomen 192
Pregnancy 291
Premature ejaculation 291
Prostate hypertrophy,
see Prostate, afflictions 290
Prostate, afflictions 290
Prostatitis, see Prostate, afflictions. . . . 290
Psoriasis 340
Psychosomatic diseases 68

Pyelonephritis 270
Pyorrhea, gingivitis, and parodontosis . . 89
Pyrosis, see Stomach acidity 206

Retention of liquids before menstruation, see Menstruation, retention of fluids . 291
Retention of liquids, see Edema 269
Rheumatic pain 319
Rhinitis 91
Rickets 318
Ringworm 341
Roughness, see Callus 336
Roundworms, intestine, see Intestinal parasites 241

Salmonellosis 358
Sand in the urine, see Urinary lithiasis . . 268
Scabies 341
Sciatica 320
Sexual hyperexcitation, see Excessive sexual excitation 290
Sexual impotence 290
Sexual, excessive excitation, see Excessive sexual excitation 290
Sinusitis 91
Skin beauty 340
Skin cracks 336
Skin dryness 339
Skin fungi, see Skin mycosis 338
Skin irritation 339
Skin mycosis 338
Skin sores 337
Skin stretch marks 338
Sleeplessness, see Insomnia 68
Sore throat, see Tonsillitis and pharyngitis 90
Sores, lips 88
Sores, nipple 291
Spasm, intestinal, see Intestinal colic . . 240
Sports 320
Sprain 318
Stomach ache 208
Stomach acidity 206
Stomach gas 207
Stomach nervousness 208
Stomach ulcer 209
Stomach, lack of juice, see Lack of gastric juice 206
Stones in the urine, see Urinary lithiasis 268
Stress 68
Stretch marks, skin 338
Students, see Insufficient intellectual performance 66
Sty 58
Sugar in the blood, excess, see Diabetes 311
Swelling before menstruation, see Menstruation, retention of fluids . 291

Tachycardia 106
Taste in mouth, bad 89
Teething 89
Throat itching, see Throat, irritation . . . 90
Throat, irritation 90
Throat, sore, see Tonsillitis and pharyngitis 90
Thrombosis 136
Tonsillitis, see Tonsillitis and pharyngitis 90
Toothache 89
Toxoinfection, alimentary, see Salmonellosis 358
Tuberculosis 360
Typhoid fever 359

Ulcer, stomach 209
Ulcers, mouth, see Mouth ulcers 88
Urethritis 271
Uric acid, excess of, see Gout 311
Uric arthritis, see Gouty arthritis 319
Urinary calculi, see Urinary lithiasis 268
Urinary incontinence 271
Urinary infection 270
Urinary lithiasis 268
Urine calculi, see Urinary lithiasis 268

Vaginal flow, see Leukorrhea 293
Vaginitis, see Leukorrhea 293
Varicose ulceration 128
Varicose veins 128
Veins, inflammation, see Phlebitis 128
Vomiting 208

Warts 336
Weight loss 310
Whooping cough 360
Worms, intestinal, see Intestinal parasites 241
Wounds and sores 337

Index of Plants

Abelmosk *(Hibiscus abelmoschus)*, 176
Achillea, see Milfoil, 342
Agave *(Agave americana)*, 272
Agrimony, see Sticklewort, 99
Alder buckthorn *(Rhamnus frangula)*, 258
Alfalfa *(Medicago sativa)*, 137
Aloe *(Aloe vera)*, 344
Althea *(Althaea officinalis)*, 94
American pennyroyal *(Hedeoma pulegioides)*, 227
Anise *(Pimpinela anisum)*, 230
Annatto tree *(Bixa orellana)*, 347
Arnica *(Arnica montana)*, 321
Artemisia, see Mugwort, 294
Artichoke *(Cynara scolymus)*, 197

Balm *(Melissa officinalis)*, 76
Barberry *(Berberis vulgaris)*, 194
Bardana, see Burdock, 346
Basil *(Ocimum basilicum)*, 182
Bearberry *(Arctostaphylos uva-ursi)*, 274
Beech tree *(Fagus silvatica)*, 247
Bistort *(Polygonum bistortum)*, 93
Bird's tongue, see Common Ash Tree, 326
Bitterwort, see Gentian, 220
Black elder *(Sambucus nigra)*, 374
Black mustard *(Brassica nigra)*, 322
Blackthorn *(Prunus spinosa)*, 184
Blue centaury, see Cornflower, 60
Blue vervain *(Verbena hastata)*, 84
Boldo *(Peumus boldus)*, 198
Bramble *(Rubus fruticosus)*, 264
Brier hip *(Rosa canina)*, 372
Buchu *(Barosma betulina)*, 277
Burdock *(Arctium lappa)*, 346

Cactus *(Cereus grandiflorus)*, 108
Caimito *(Chrysophyllum caimito)*, 154
Calendula *(Calendula officinalis)*, 296
Camphor tree *(Cinnamomum camphora)*, 109
Canadian fir tree *(Abies balsamea)*, 151
Cane *(Arundo donax)*, 276
Cannafistula tree, see Purging cassia, 244
Caraway *(Carum carvi)*, 174
Carob tree *(Ceratonia siliqua)*, 245
Carrageen, see Irish moss, 153
Cascara sagrada *(Rhamnus purshiana)*, 260
Castor bean *(Ricinus communis)*, 262
Catnip *(Nepeta cataria)*, 181
Chenopodium, see Wormseed, 211
Chicory *(Cichorium intybus)*, 212
Chinese anise, see Star anise, 222
Chinese cinnamon *(Cinnamomum aromaticum)*, 215
Cinchona tree *(Cinchona officinalis)*, 364

Cinnamon tree
(*Cinnamomum zeylanicum*), 214
Clove tree (*Eugenia caryophyllata*), 96
Cocowort, see Shepherd's purse, 298
Comfrey (*Symphytum officinalis*), 354
Common ash tree (*Fraxinus excelsior*), 326
Common plantain (*Plantago major*), 162
Copaiba (*Copaifera officinalis*), 280
Coriander (*Coriandrum sativum*), 216
Cornflower (*Centaurea cyanus*), 60
Cumin (*Cuminum cyminum*), 218
Cypress (*Cupressus sempervirens*), 132

Daisy, see Wild daisy, 362
Damiana (*Turnera diffusa*), 307
Dandelion (*Taraxacum officinale*), 202
Desert tea (*Ephedra distachya*), 155
Devil's claw
(*Harpagophytum procumbens*), 328
Digitalis, see Foxglove, 112
Dill (*Anethum graveolens*), 173

Early purple orchid (*Orchis mascula*), 253
Echinacea (*Echinacea angustifolia*), 366
Elder, see Black elder, 374
English walnut, see Walnut tree, 248
English watercress, see Hedge mustard, 101
Ephedra, see Desert tea, 155
Eryngo (*Eryngium campestre*), 281
Eucalyptus (*Eucalyptus globulus*), 156
Euphrasy, see Red eyebright, 62
European blackberry, see Bramble, 264
European pennyroyal
(*Mentha pulegium*), 226
Evening primrose (*Oenothera biennis*), 124

False acacia (*Robinia pseudoacacia*), 232
Fennel (*Foeniculum vulgare*), 175
Fenugreek
(*Trigonella foenum-graecum*), 234
Fever plant, see Evening primrose, 124
Flax (*Linum usitatissimum*), 250
Fleawort, see Psyllium, 254
Foxglove (*Digitalis purpurea*), 112
Fucus (*Fucus vesiculosus*), 312
Fumitory (*Fumaria officinalis*), 196

Garden Violet (*Viola odorata*), 168
Garlic (*Allium sativum*), 118
Gentian (*Gentiana lutea*), 220
German camomile
(*Matricaria chamomilla*), 178
Giant reed, see Cane, 276
Ginger (*Zingiber officinale*), 189
Ginkgo (*Ginkgo biloba*), 122
Ginseng (*Panax ginseng*), 300
Golden rod (*Solidago virga-aurea*), 286
Goldenseal (*Hydrastis canadensis*), 100
Ground cherry (*Physalis viscosa*), 353
Guinea sorrel (*Hibiscus sabdariffa*), 177

Hawthorn (*Crataegus monogyna*), 110
Hazel nut, see Witch hazel, 129
Hedge mustard
(*Sisymbrium officinale*), 101
Herb louise, see Lemon verbena, 225
Herb Robert (*Geranium robertianum*), 63
Hibiscus, see Abelmosk, 176
High mallow (*Malva silvestris*), 252
Hops (*Humulus lupulus*), 72
Horse chestnut
(*Aesculus hippocastanum*), 130
Horsetail (*Equisetum arvense*), 348

Iceland moss (*Cetraria islandica*), 152

Indian fig *(Opuntia ficus-indica),*
see Prickly pear, 352
Indian senna, see Tinnevelly senna, 242
Ipecac *(Cephaelis ipecacuana),* 210
Irish moss *(Chondrus crispus),* 153

Javan tea *(Ortosiphon stamineus),* 315
Juniper *(Juniperus communis),* 282

Kelp *(Laminaria saccharina),* 314
Kidney vetch *(Anthyllis vulneraria),* 327

Laurel *(Laurus nobilis),* 224
Lavender *(Lavandula angustifolia),* 74
Lavender cotton
(Santolina chamaecyparissus), 233
Lemon balm, see Balm, 76
Lemon verbena *(Lippia triphylla),* 225
Lentiscus, see Mastic tree, 98
Licorice *(Glycyrrhiza glabra),* 158
Linden *(Tilia europaea),* 80
Lion's tooth, see Dandelion, 202
Luceme, see Alfalfa, 137
Lungwort *(Pulmonaria officinalis),* 164

Madder *(Rubia tinctorum),* 284
Mallow, see High mallow, 252
Marigold, see Calendula, 296
Marjoram *(Origanum majorana),* 183
Marshmallow, see Althea, 94
Mastic tree *(Pistacia lentiscus),* 98
Maypops, see Passion flower, 78
Meadow-sweet *(Filipendula ulmaria),* 324
Mexican damiana, see Damiana, 307
Milfoil *(Achillea millefolium),* 342
Milk thistle *(Silybum marianum),* 200
Mother of thyme *(Thymus serpyllum),* 166
Mugwort *(Artemisia vulgaris),* 294

Nasturtium *(Tropaeolum majus),* 378
Nettle *(Urtica dioica),* 142
New Jersey tea
(Ceanothus americanus), 95
Noni *(Morinda citrifolia),* 368

Oak tree *(Quercus robur),* 102
Orange tree *(Citrus aurantium),* 70
Orchid, see Early purple orchid, 253
Orthosiphon, see Javan tea, 315

Passion flower *(Passiflora incarnata),* 78
Pellitory of the wall
(Parietaria officinalis), 283
Peppermint *(Mentha piperita),* 180
Peruvian bark, see Cinchona, 364
Pine tree *(Pinus pinaster),* 160
Plantain, see Common plantain, 162
Prickly lettuce *(Lactuca virosa),* 73
Prickly Pear *(Opuntia ficus-indica),* 352
Psyllium *(Plantago psyllium),* 254
Purging cassia *(Cassia fistula),* 244
Purple passion flower *(Passiflora edulis),* 79
Purslane *(Portulaca oleracea),* 256

Quassia *(Quassia amara),* 229

Red eyebright *(Euphrasia officinalis),* 62
Rhatany *(Krameria triandra),* 97
Rhubarb *(Rheum officinale),* 261
Robinia, see False acacia, 232
Rock's tea *(Jasonia glutinosa),* 223
Rose *(Rosa gallica),* 302
Rose bay, see Willowherb, 246
Rosemary *(Rosmarinus officinalis),* 330
Rue *(Ruta graveolens),* 303

Sacred bark, see Cascara sagrada, 260
Saffron *(Crocus sativus),* 217

Sage *(Salvia officinalis)*, 304
Saxifrage *(Saxifraga granulata)*, 285
Saw palmetto, see Shrub palmetto, 306
Scurvy grass, see Watercress, 138
Shepherd's purse *(Capsella bursa-pastoris)*, 298
Shrub palmetto *(Serenoa repens)*, 306
Silver birch, see White birch, 278
Silver fir *(Abies alba)*, 150
Speedwell *(Veronica officinalis)*, 235
Spirulina *(Spirulina maxima)*, 140
St. Johnswort *(Hypericum perforatum)*, 350
Star anise *(Illicium verum)*, 222
Sticklewort *(Agrimonia eupatoria)*, 99
Stinging nettle, see Nettle, 142
Sugar cane *(Saccharum officinarum)*, 165
Summer savory *(Satureja hortensis)*, 187
Sweet root, see Licorice, 158

Tamarind *(Tamarindus indica)*, 263
Thyme *(Thymus vulgaris)*, 376
Tinnevelly senna *(Cassia angustifolia)*, 242
Tiny savory *(Satureja obovata)*, 187
Tormentil *(Potentilla erecta)*, 257
Turmeric *(Curcuma longa)*, 219

Valerian *(Valeriana officinalis)*, 82
Vanilla *(Vanilla planifolia)*, 188
Vervain *(Verbena officinalis)*, 84

Walnut tree *(Juglans regia)*, 248
Watercress *(Nasturtium officinalis)*, 138
White birch *(Betula alba)*, 278
White savory *(Satureja fruticosa)*, 187
White willow *(Salix alba)*, 332
Wild daisy *(Bellis perennis)*, 362
Wild marjoram *(Origanum vulgare)*, 228
Willow, see White willow, 332
Willowherb *(Epilobium angustifolium)*, 246
Winter savory *(Satureja montana)*, 186
Witch grass *(Agropyrum repens)*, 273
Witch hazel *(Hamamelis virginiana)*, 129
Wormseed *(Chenopodium ambrosioides)*, 211
Woundwort, see Kidney vetch, 327

Meaning of the Icons of Botanical Parts

In this encyclopedia there are a number of icons, symbols, and tables which describe plants, body organs, and ailments. We describe these icons on the following four pages so the reader can be familiar with them and interpret their meaning more easily.

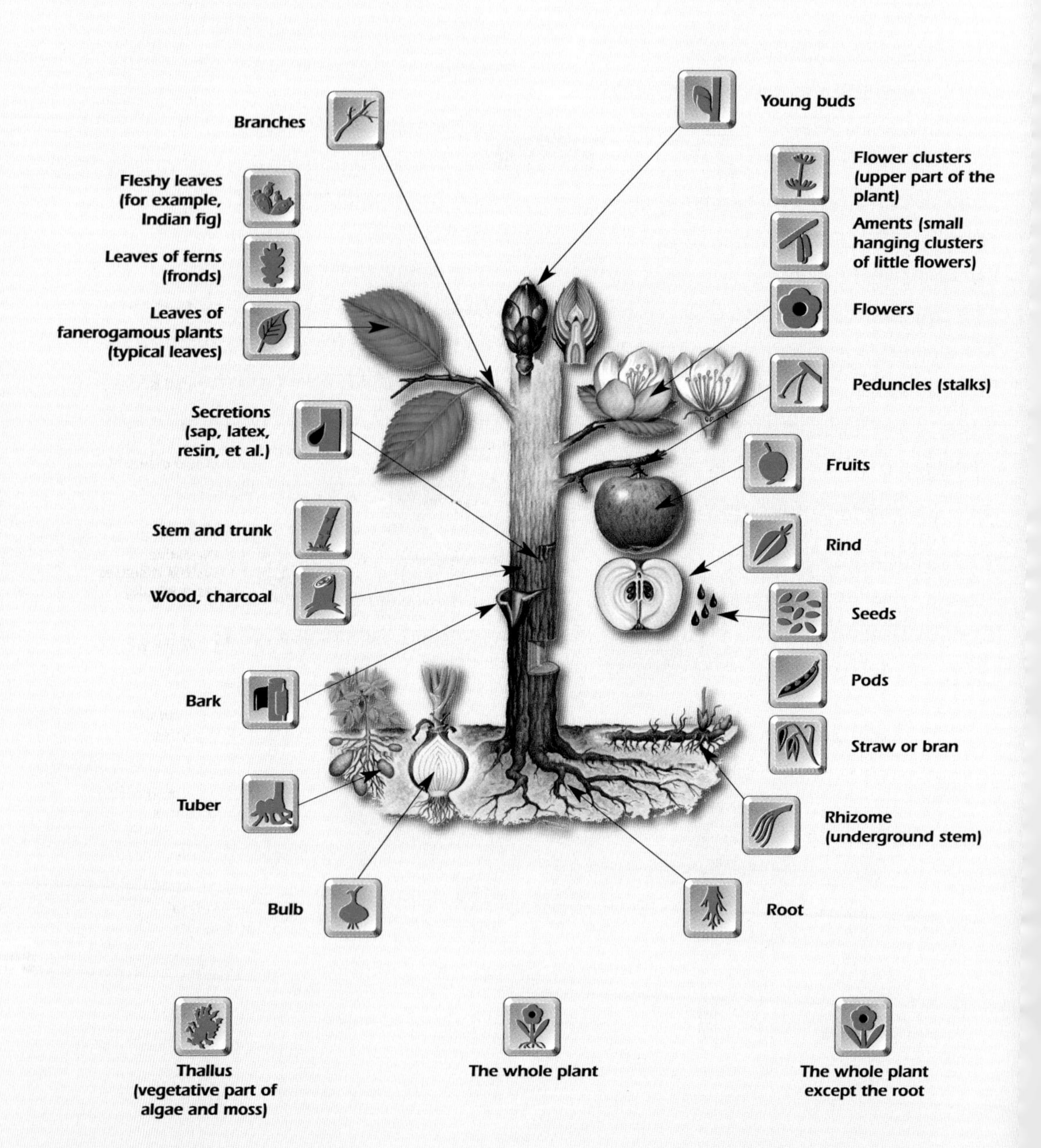

Meaning of the Icons of Anatomical Parts

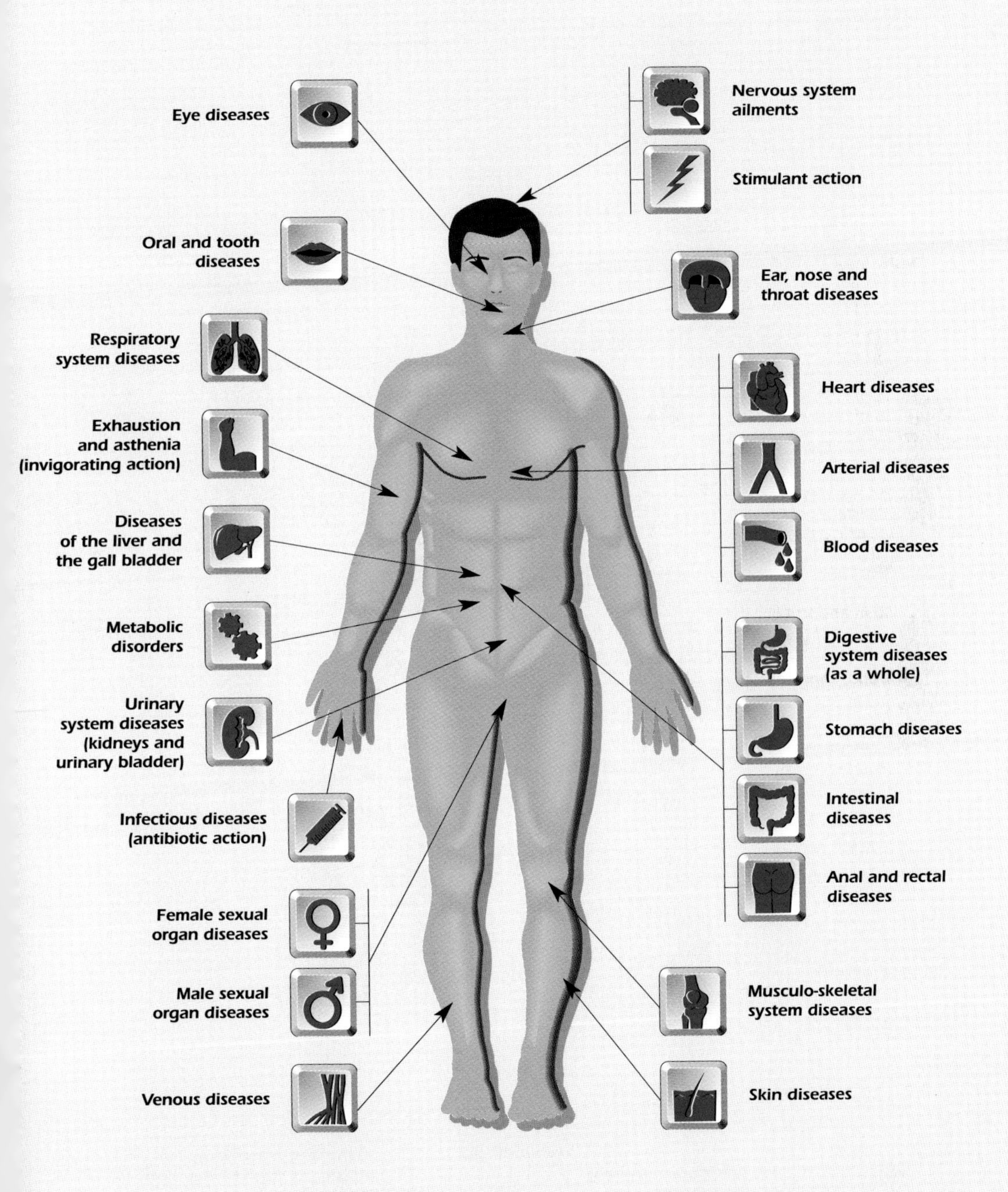
Eye diseases
Nervous system ailments
Stimulant action
Oral and tooth diseases
Ear, nose and throat diseases
Respiratory system diseases
Heart diseases
Exhaustion and asthenia (invigorating action)
Arterial diseases
Diseases of the liver and the gall bladder
Blood diseases
Metabolic disorders
Digestive system diseases (as a whole)
Urinary system diseases (kidneys and urinary bladder)
Stomach diseases
Infectious diseases (antibiotic action)
Intestinal diseases
Anal and rectal diseases
Female sexual organ diseases
Male sexual organ diseases
Musculo-skeletal system diseases
Venous diseases
Skin diseases

Plant Pages: Description and Format

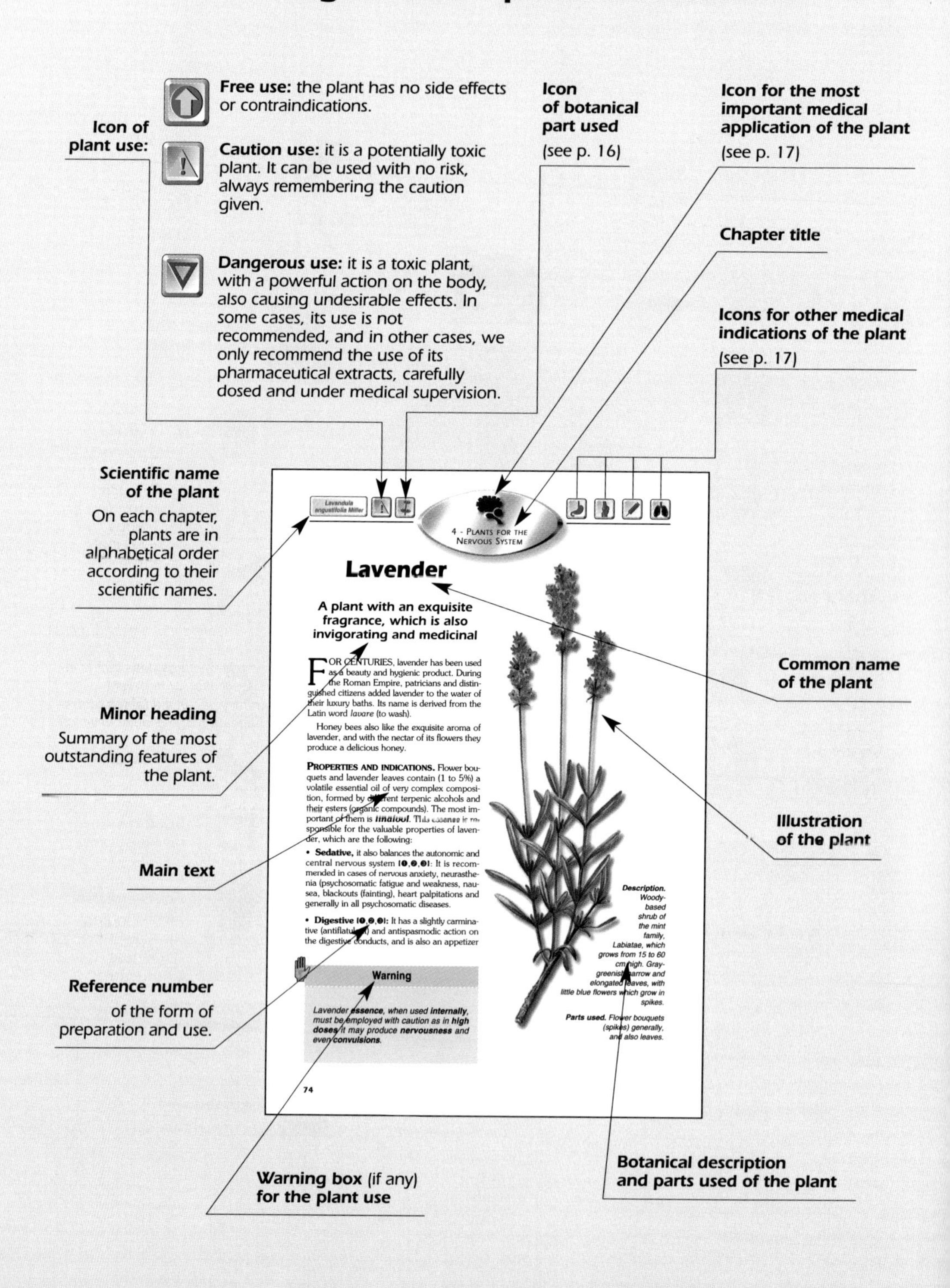

Icon of plant use:
Free use: the plant has no side effects or contraindications.
Caution use: it is a potentially toxic plant. It can be used with no risk, always remembering the caution given.
Dangerous use: it is a toxic plant, with a powerful action on the body, also causing undesirable effects. In some cases, its use is not recommended, and in other cases, we only recommend the use of its pharmaceutical extracts, carefully dosed and under medical supervision.
Icon of botanical part used
(see p. 16)
Icon for the most important medical application of the plant
(see p. 17)
Chapter title
Icons for other medical indications of the plant
(see p. 17)
Scientific name of the plant
On each chapter, plants are in alphabetical order according to their scientific names.
Minor heading
Summary of the most outstanding features of the plant.
Main text
Reference number of the form of preparation and use.
Warning box (if any) for the plant use
Common name of the plant
Illustration of the plant
Botanical description and parts used of the plant
Lavandula angustifolia Miller
4 - Plants for the Nervous System
Lavender
A plant with an exquisite fragrance, which is also invigorating and medicinal
Warning
74

Description of Boxes and Tables

Preparation and Use

Internal use

❶ **Infusion** with 30-40 g of flower bouquets and leaves per liter of water. Drink three cups daily, sweetened with honey, after meals.

❷ **Fluid extract.** Take 30 drops, three times a day.

❸ **Essence.** The usual dose is 3-5 drops, two or three times a day.

External use

❹ **Lavender essence.** A few drops, inhaled or rubbed on the skin, are enough to produce the desired effect.

❺ **Cleansing and compresses.** The same infusion method as for internal use is valid, though it may be prepared with a higher concentration of plant. Wash wounds and ulcers directly with this infusion, after which a soaked compress may be applied on the affected area for 15 to 20 minutes.

❻ **Warm fomentations.** These are prepared with lavender infusion, or by adding some drops of lavender essence to water. Apply on the neck, back and knees.

❼ **Lotions and frictions.** These may be applied using a few drops of essence, with oil, or with lavender water.

Preparation and use box

Reference number

Each of the different forms of preparation and use is given a reference number. In the main text, these forms of preparation and use are implied by using this number.

How To Obtain Lavender Oil

Lavender oil. *Dissolve 10 g of essence in 100 g of olive oil. It may also be prepared by mixing 250 g of dried plant with one liter of oil, steep in cold extract for two weeks and filter after this time. It is used as a lotion applied to the aching area.*

Information box

With detailed information concerning the plant which is being described.

Purple Passion Flower

In Brazil and the West Indies another species of Passiflora *grows, the* Passiflora edulis *Sims. (=* Passiflora laurifolia *F. Vill.), which is a purple passion flower, with purple flowers (as its name indicates), also known as passionfruit. It is the best known species of the genus* Passiflora *in America.*

Purple passion flower renders a sweet, somewhat acid fruit, whose truly "tropical" flavor is present in soft drinks made with its gelatinous flesh. The oil obtained from its seeds is edible. However, ***it is not considered*** *to be* ***a true medicinal herb.***

Related botanical species box

It describes other species similar to the main plant related to morphology and medicinal properties.

Each chapter includes the most important plants for the treatment of a given organ or system diseases.
When a plant has ***several applications****, which frequently happens, the plant is included in the chapter dealing with its most important application of that plant.*
In order to compensate for this fact, and to make search easier, in the ***tables of diseases*** *we list all plants useful for each ailment, independent of the chapter in which they are described.*

Disease

Some diseases or disorders, of the organ or system being described in each chapter, are listed here. For obvious reasons, the list of disorders and ailments **is not exhaustive**. We have only selected the most representative ailments of each organ, and those which will be more easily healed or eased with a phytotherapeutical treatment.

Depression, Nervousness

Definition

It is a psychological state of melancholy and deep sadness, with or without any evident cause, as well as a loss of appetite, insomnia, and a propensity to inactivity.

Phytotherapy

We recommend those plants with **an invigorating and balancing** action on the nervous system, as well as those which add nutritive substances such as vitamin B or lecithin. **Stimulant or excitant** plants or substances **must not be used** in the treatment of depression.

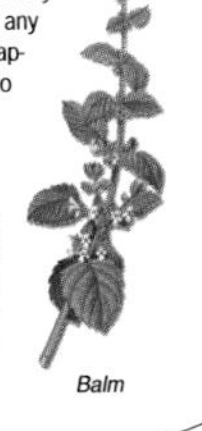

Balm

Balm	Balances the nervous system
Valerian	Mild sedative, decreases anxiety
Mother of thyme	Invigorating and revitalizing
Ginseng	Antidepressant and anxiolytic
Sage	Stimulates suprarenal gland function
St. Johnswort	Invigorator and nervous system stabilizer
Thyme	General invigorator. Stimulates intellectual performance

Action

The most outstanding action of the plant toward the disease whose treatment is being described.

Plant

Common name of the plants most appropriate for each disease. Each plant can be taken or applied alone, or in combination with any other of the plants recommended for that disease.

1

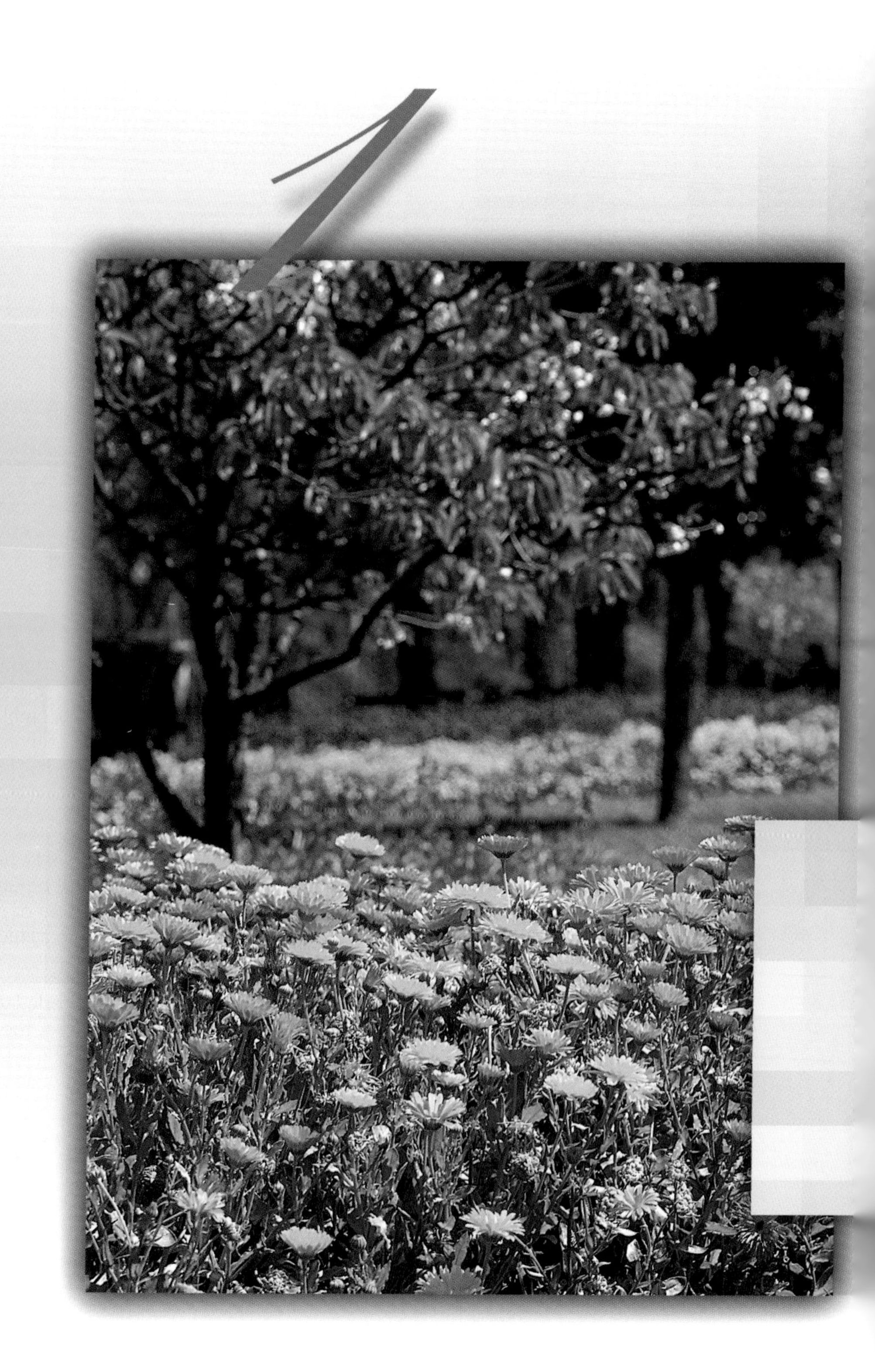

The Vegetal World

SUMMARY **PAGES**

Anatomy of a Flower 30
Anatomy of Leaves. 26
Guardians or Killers? 32
Types of Inflorescences. 29
Types of Leaves 24
Types of Roots 27
Types of Stems 28

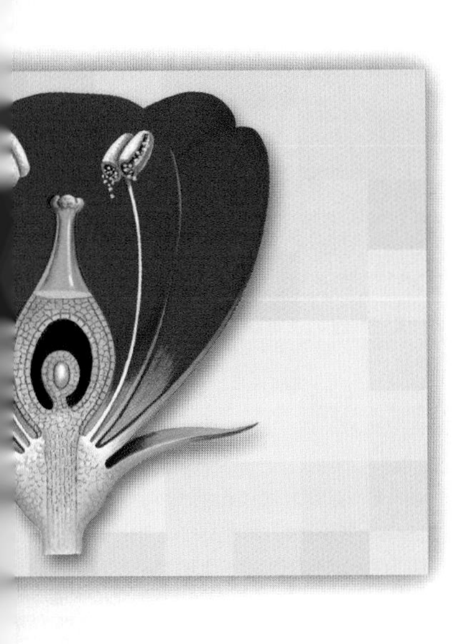

"WHAT A SURPRISE! This piece of cork is formed by thousands of tiny cells, joined together. It resembles a honeycomb!" said Robert Hooke, a famous seventeenth century English physicist, astonished by what he saw through his microscope.

His scientific spirit surprised him at what others would not even have noticed. Hooke had just discovered that living tissues are not a uniform and continuous mass, such as stones or minerals, but a mass made of innumerable little independent units.

"Since these little cavities form cork, I will call them cells," Hooke said. "Besides, the Latin word *cellula* means little cavity."

Cells: The Units of Life

When studying other plants under the microscope, scientists noticed that not only the bark of cork oak trees was formed by cells. All living

The Vegetal Cell

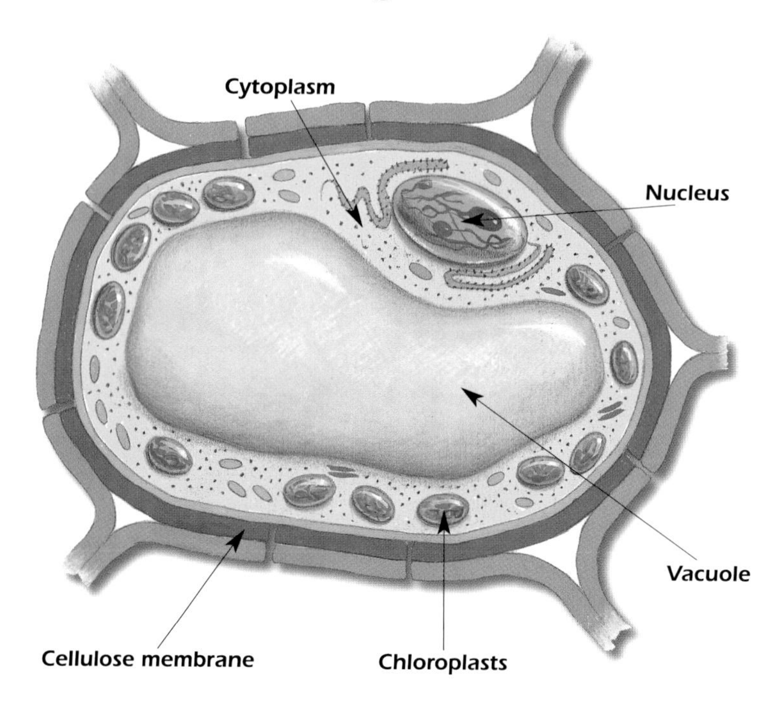

beings, vegetals and animals, are formed by one or many grouped cells.

Each cell is a life unit. It is the smallest part of a living being that has its own life, that is to say, cells are born, get fed, grow, reproduce themselves and die.

The size of cells generally varies in a range between five and 50 microns (a thousandth of millimeter), which means that in one millimeter there may be from 20 to 200 cells, depending on their size.

Some cells will only live for a few minutes, continually being renewed, while others live as long as the living being of which they are part.

Features of Vegetal Cells

Vegetal cells present two basic features which cannot be found in animal cells:

1. A Cellulose Membrane

It is a thick cell wall, located outside and around the cytoplasmic membrane and is made of cellulose. It is like a porous case which isolates and protects the cell, and remains when it dies, becoming a kind of sarcophagus. Animal cells do not have any such thick cellulose membrane, therefore when they die they rot and leave no remains.

Thus, what Hooke observed through the microscope—cork—were not bark cells of the cork oak tree, but their cases or cell membranes, which remain after the cell dies. Wood is also formed by the thick cellulose and lignin walls which once covered the now-already-dead stem cells.

2. Plasts

This is another peculiar feature of vegetal cells. Plasts are corpuscles located inside the cytoplasm, which contain diverse coloring substances. The most common ones are **chloroplasts,** green-colored because of their chlorophyll content.

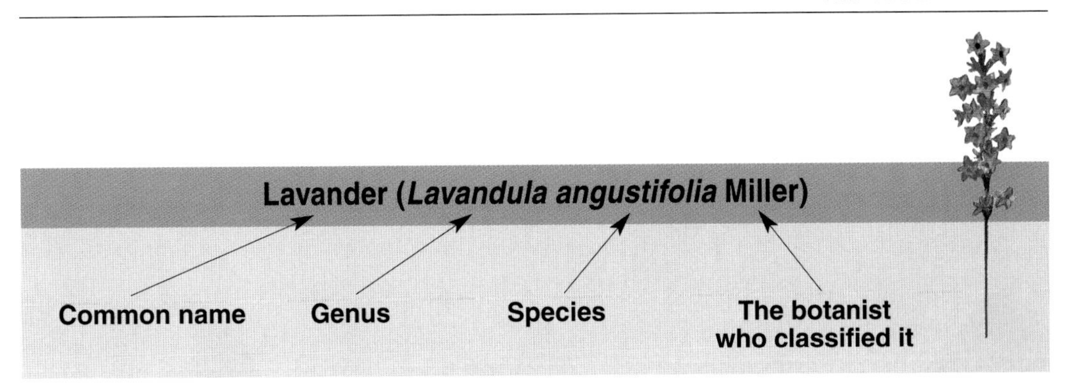

Photosynthesis takes place inside the chloroplasts. This is an extraordinary chemical reaction where the inorganic mineral substances of air and soil turn into starch and other organic substances, thanks to sunlight energy.

Cells are fantastic chemical laboratories. In each of them, despite their tiny size, thousands of chemical reactions take place, and their result is the synthesis of sugars (carbohydrates), lipids (fats), and proteins, which either accumulate inside the cell or flow outside it.

Diversity of the Vegetal Kingdom

"These bricks are for building the outer walls, those for covering the inner rooms, those tiles are for the kitchen floor...."

An architect gives appropriate orders so that each and every one of the hundreds and even thousands of elements that form the house goes to its appropriate place. When the building is finished, everyone will acknowledge the work of the man who designed the house and supervised the work.

However, very few people are conscious of the admirable fact that the billions of "bricks," that is to say, cells, that form a plant or any other living being are perfectly disposed each one in its place, and all of them in good working order. Who was the architect or engineer that designed this? Who directed the work? Why do epidermic cells always gather in order to cover leaves and stems? Why do hollow and elongated cells join each other to form the vessels through which sap flows?

Are we conscious of the merit of our house's architect? Order cannot ever be born from chaos, even after millions of years. Pure chaos just gives birth to increasing disorder.

In order to cause and keep harmony, the direct action of a Superior Intellect is needed. When penetrating deeper into the study of the vegetal world, we cannot help but acknowledge the action of the universe's Creator, who designed the "buildings" (living entities) and distributed their "bricks" (cells) in perfect order.

The Names of the Plants

How can the great variety of plants in the vegetal world be named in an orderly manner? And, how can they be classified? According to the color of their flowers, to the shape of their leaves, or maybe to the chemical substances they produce?

In order to overcome this chaos, in 1753 the great Swedish naturalist and botanist Carolus Linnaeus, introduced a name and classification system for plants which has obtained worldwide recognition and success. It is called the **binomial system,** because it gives each species two names: the first is the **genus** name, while the second is the name of the **species.** Linnaeus had, like Adam in Eden, the privilege of giving names to all known plants. He used the Latin language, which, being a dead language, would not allow any deformation in names.

Types

According to Their Shape

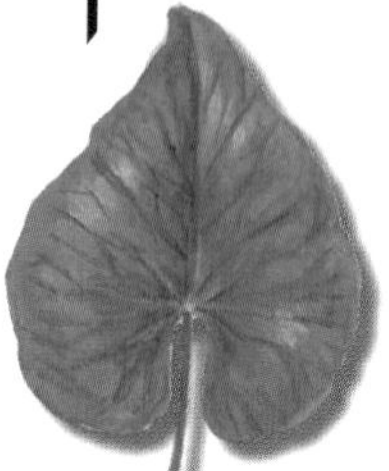

Heart-shaped
Its shape resembles a heart; for example, black briony.

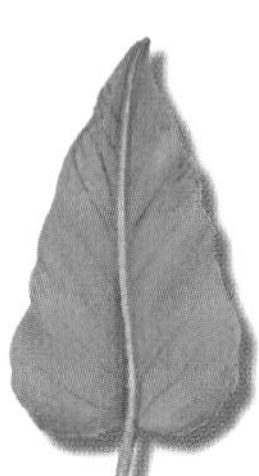

Lanceolated
Its shape resembles a spear; for example, bistort.

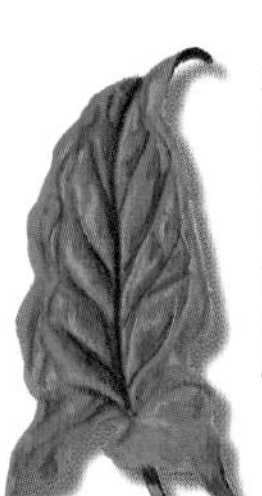

Arrow-shaped
For example, red bindweed. The shape of these leaves resembles an arrow.

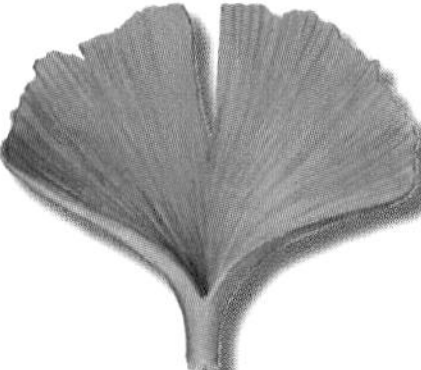

Bilobulated
This type of leaf is cut into two lobules; for example, ginkgo.

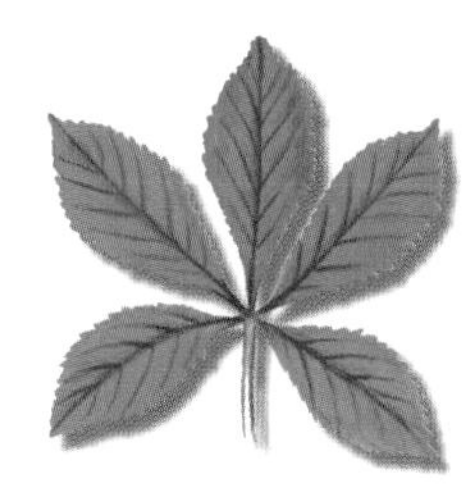

Hand-shaped
This is a compound leaf, in which the divisions are shaped like the fingers of a hand; for example, the horse chestnut.

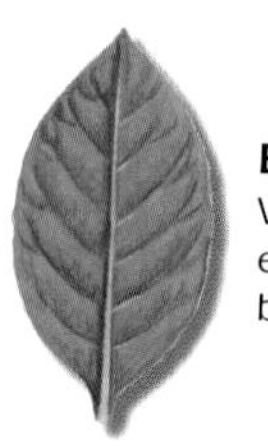

Ellipsoidal
With shape of ellipse; for example, belladonna.

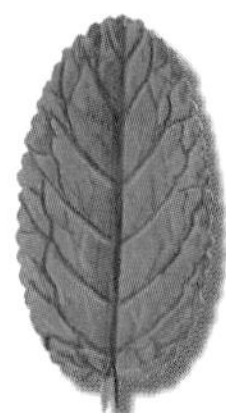

Oval
Shaped as an oval; for example, figwort.

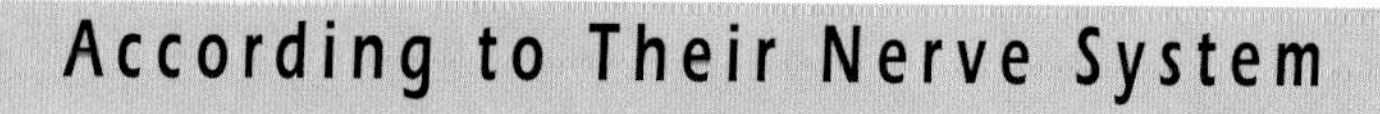

According to Their Nerve System

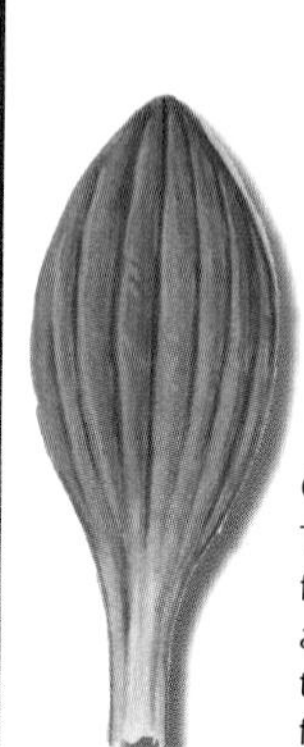

Curvinerve
The nerves form a curve along the leaf; for example, the common plantain.

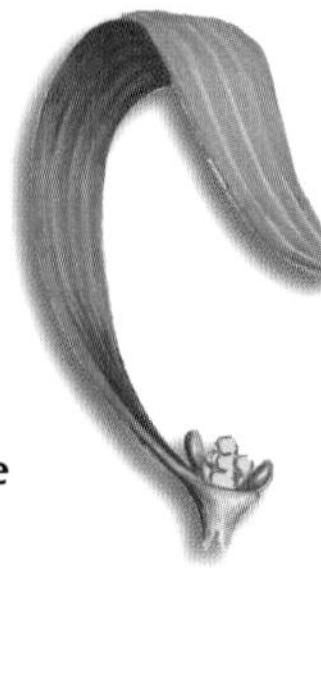

Parallelinerve
The nerves run parallel along the leaf; for example, mistletoe.

Pennínerve
The nerves stem from a central axis; for example, the hazelnut.

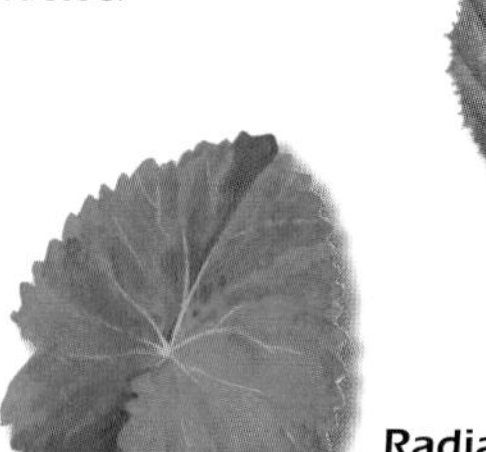

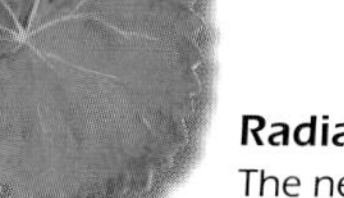

Radial
The nerves stem as a radius from a common center; for example, the cowslip.

# of Leaves

According to the Edges

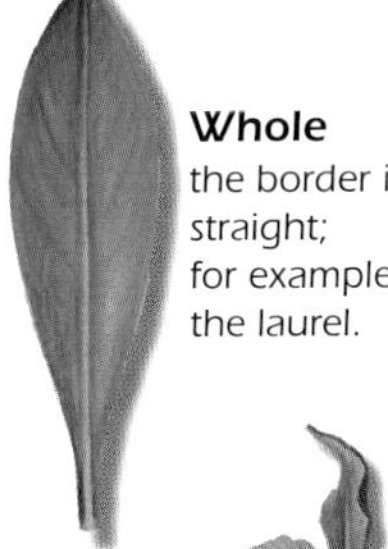

Whole
the border is straight; for example, the laurel.

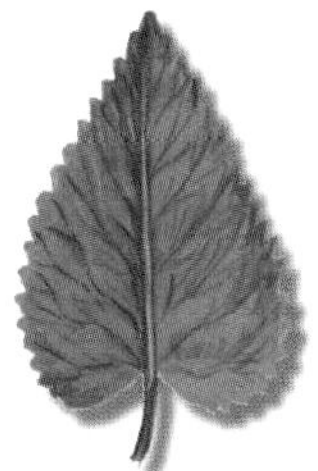

Toothed
the border has tiny teeth; for example, the nettle.

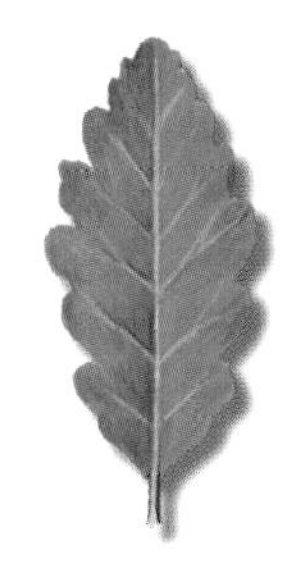

Lobulated
the border has cracks which form lobules; for example, the oak tree.

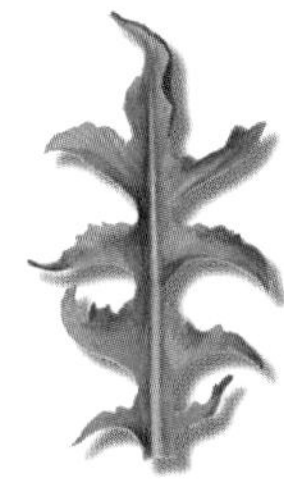

Divided
The cracks of the border reach the central nerve; for example, chicory.

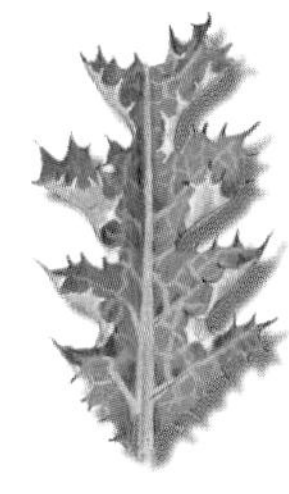

Split
The cracks of the border almost touch the central nerve; for example, the milk thistle.

According to the Position on the Stem

Petioled
These leaves join the stem by means of a petiole.

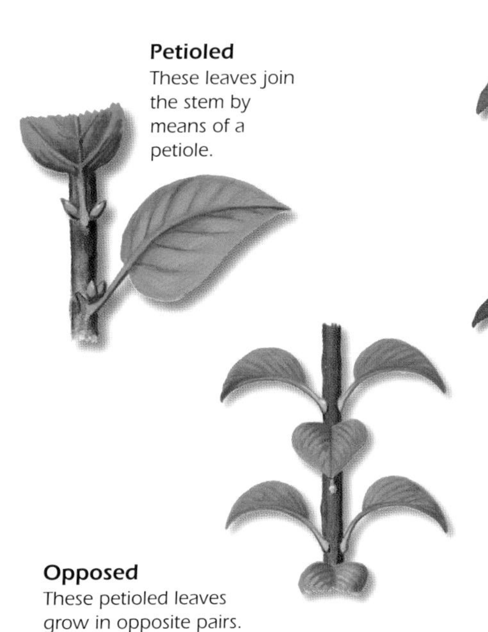

Opposed
These petioled leaves grow in opposite pairs.

Alternated
These are petioled leaves which grow one at a time along the stem.

Sessile
These leaves do not have petiole. When they grow embracing the stem their are called decurrent leaves.

Anatomy of Leaves

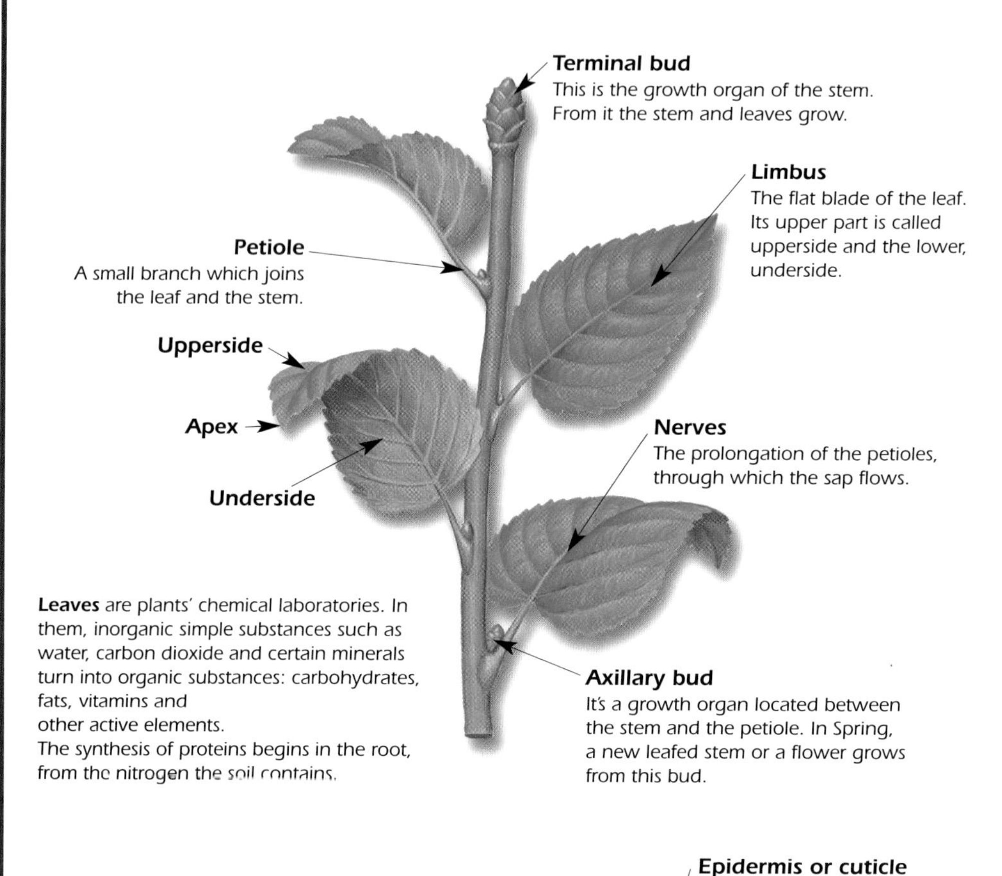
Terminal bud
This is the growth organ of the stem. From it the stem and leaves grow.
Limbus
The flat blade of the leaf. Its upper part is called upperside and the lower, underside.
Petiole
A small branch which joins the leaf and the stem.
Upperside
Apex
Underside
Nerves
The prolongation of the petioles, through which the sap flows.
Axillary bud
It's a growth organ located between the stem and the petiole. In Spring, a new leafed stem or a flower grows from this bud.

Leaves are plants' chemical laboratories. In them, inorganic simple substances such as water, carbon dioxide and certain minerals turn into organic substances: carbohydrates, fats, vitamins and other active elements.
The synthesis of proteins begins in the root, from the nitrogen the soil contains.

Microscopic Section of a Leaf

Epidermis or cuticle
A layer which covers leaves to keep them moist.

Parenchyma
Formed by cells containing abundant chlorophyll, which give leaves their green color.

Nerves
They are sap-conductive vessels.

Stomas
Little holes located in the underside of the leaf, through which carbon dioxide is absorbed and water vapor and oxygen eliminated.
Stomas are surrounded by lips which act as valves, opening and closing to control the flow of gas, according to the plant's needs.

Types of Roots

Besides attaching the plant to the ground, the root absorbs nutrients and water from the earth through tiny absorbent hairs located at the tips of its branches.

Common root

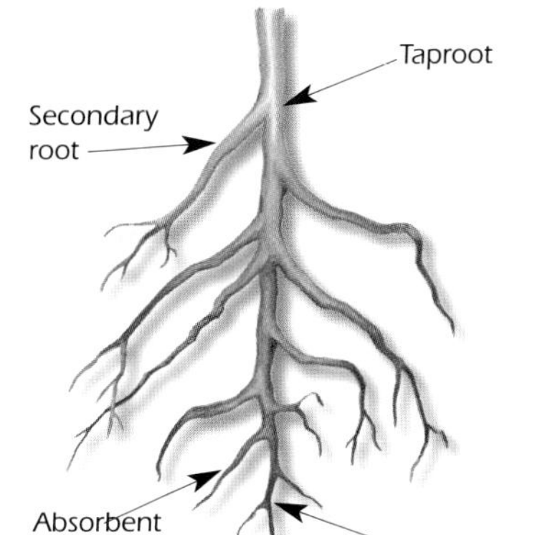

Tuber root

It produces swellings called tubers, in which carbohydrates, proteins and other reserve nutrients are stored.

Turnip-shaped root

With a conic shape, it also stores reserve nutrients. Example: the carrot.

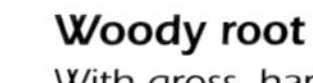

Fasciculated root

The secondary roots grow together at the base of the stem and are all similarly sized; for example, the onion.

Woody root

With gross, hard ramifications. For example, the oak tree.

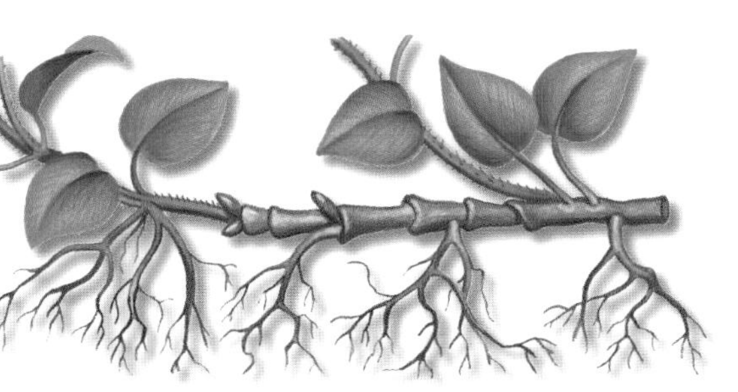

Adventitious roots

Those which grow directly from an air stem or an underground stem or rhizome; for example, veronica.

Bulb

The bulb is not actually a root, but an underground bud which consists of fleshy leaves arranged in superimposed layers, for example, the onion.

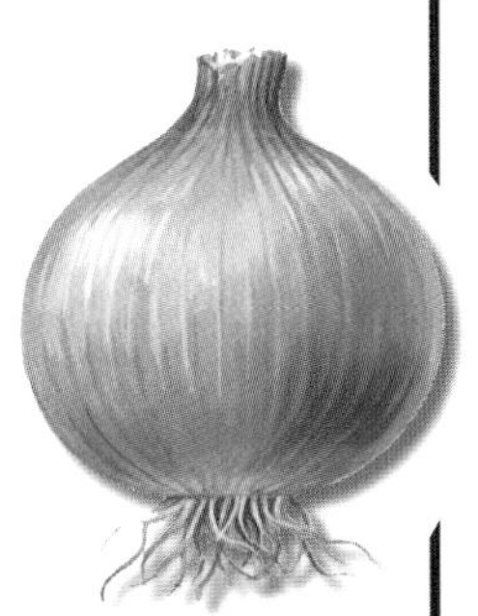

Types of Stems

The stem connects the root and the leaves, and contains conductive vessels through which the sap flows.

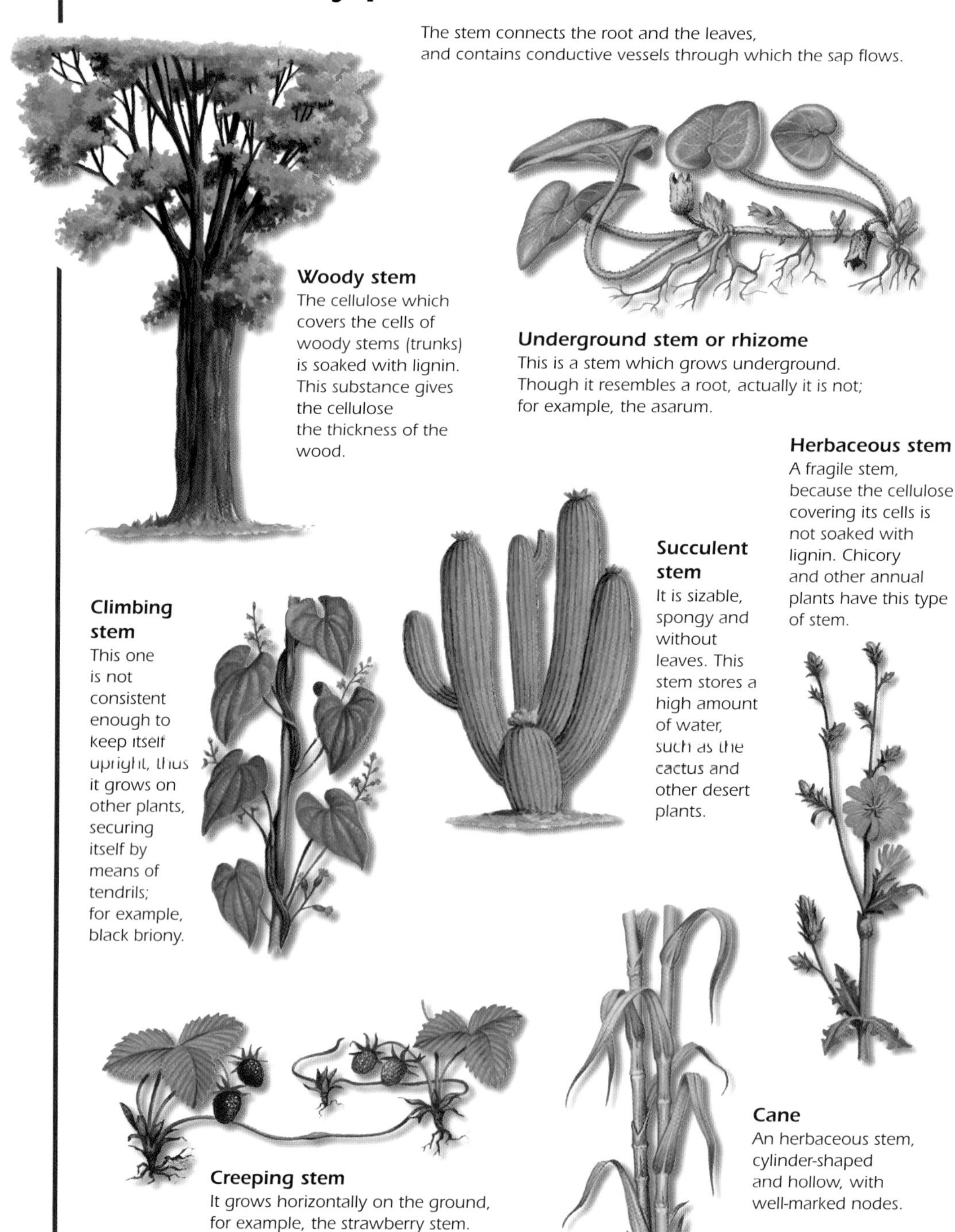

Woody stem
The cellulose which covers the cells of woody stems (trunks) is soaked with lignin. This substance gives the cellulose the thickness of the wood.

Underground stem or rhizome
This is a stem which grows underground. Though it resembles a root, actually it is not; for example, the asarum.

Herbaceous stem
A fragile stem, because the cellulose covering its cells is not soaked with lignin. Chicory and other annual plants have this type of stem.

Succulent stem
It is sizable, spongy and without leaves. This stem stores a high amount of water, such as the cactus and other desert plants.

Climbing stem
This one is not consistent enough to keep itself upright, thus it grows on other plants, securing itself by means of tendrils; for example, black briony.

Creeping stem
It grows horizontally on the ground, for example, the strawberry stem.

Cane
An herbaceous stem, cylinder-shaped and hollow, with well-marked nodes.

Types of Inflorescences

Inflorescences are groups of flowers which grow from a common peduncle.

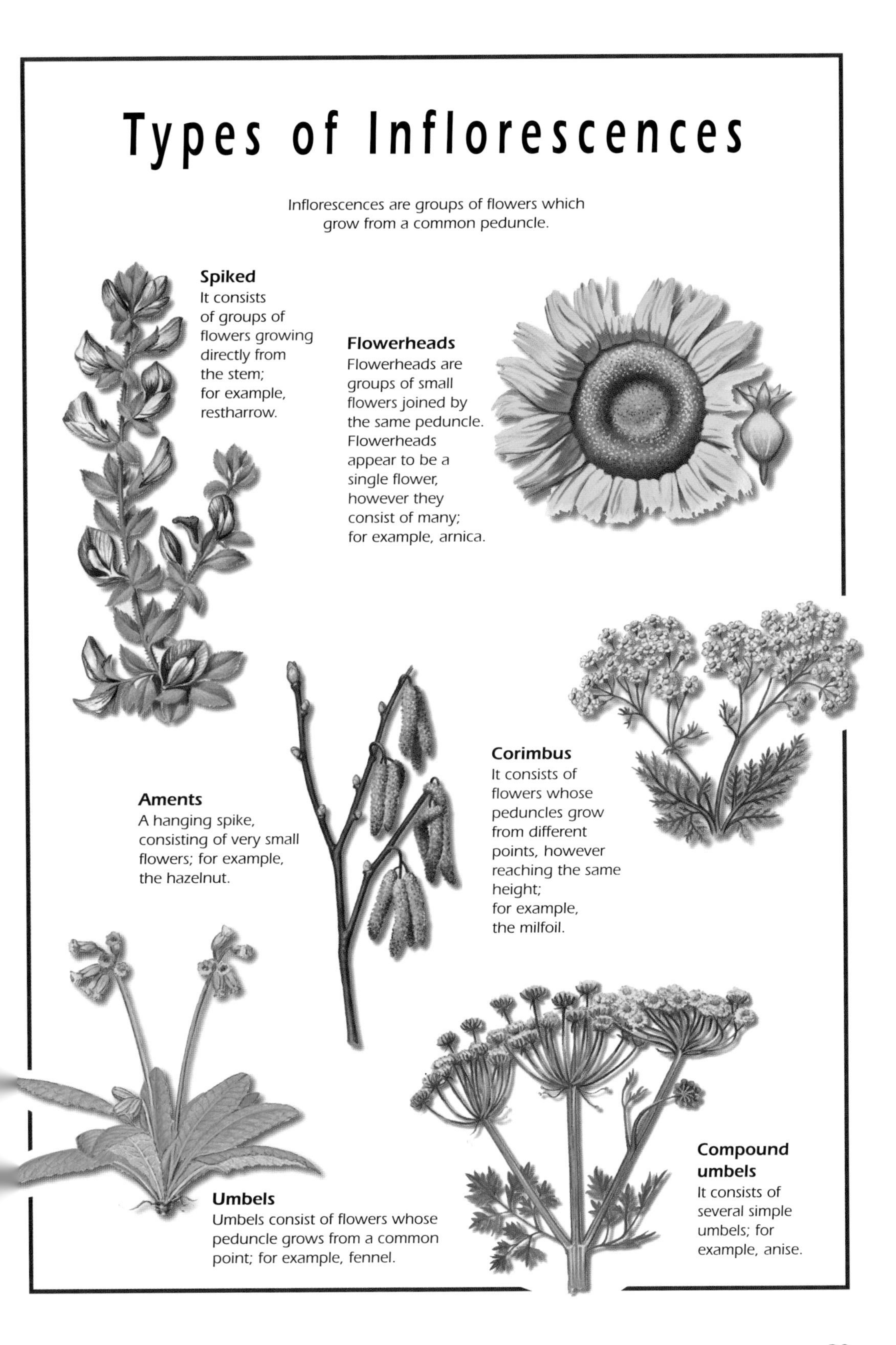

Spiked
It consists of groups of flowers growing directly from the stem; for example, restharrow.

Flowerheads
Flowerheads are groups of small flowers joined by the same peduncle. Flowerheads appear to be a single flower, however they consist of many; for example, arnica.

Aments
A hanging spike, consisting of very small flowers; for example, the hazelnut.

Corimbus
It consists of flowers whose peduncles grow from different points, however reaching the same height; for example, the milfoil.

Umbels
Umbels consist of flowers whose peduncle grows from a common point; for example, fennel.

Compound umbels
It consists of several simple umbels; for example, anise.

Anatomy

The flower is the reproductive organ of **fanerogamous** plants (with flowers). These plants are divided into two groups: **gymnosperms,** whose seeds are uncovered (with no fruit, such as the pine tree and other Coniferae) and **angiosperms,** whose seeds are covered by a more or less fleshy fruit. The flowers of angiosperm plants are the largest and most beautiful.

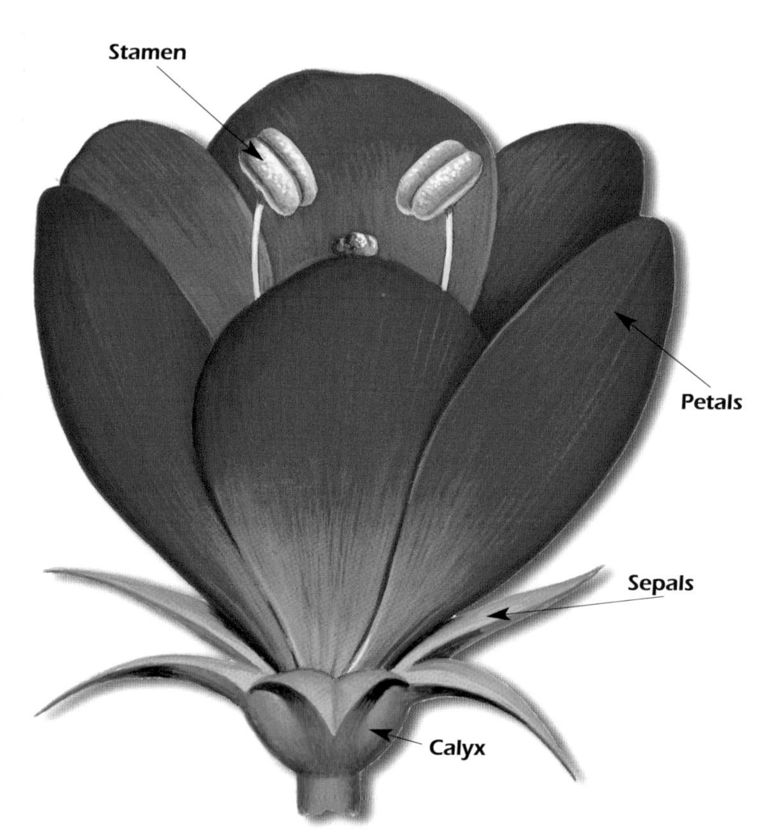

Types of Flowers

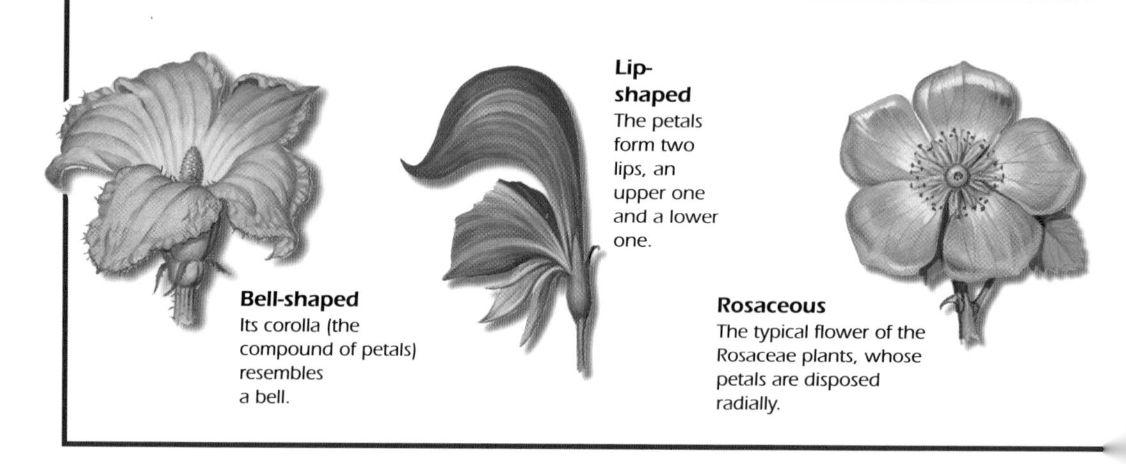

Lip-shaped
The petals form two lips, an upper one and a lower one.

Bell-shaped
Its corolla (the compound of petals) resembles a bell.

Rosaceous
The typical flower of the Rosaceae plants, whose petals are disposed radially.

# of a Flower

Pistil or gyneceum
The female organ of the flower. It consists of the stigma (an ovary-surface that receives pollen), the style (the conduct through which the pollen is channelled) and the ovary with one or several ovules (germinative cells).

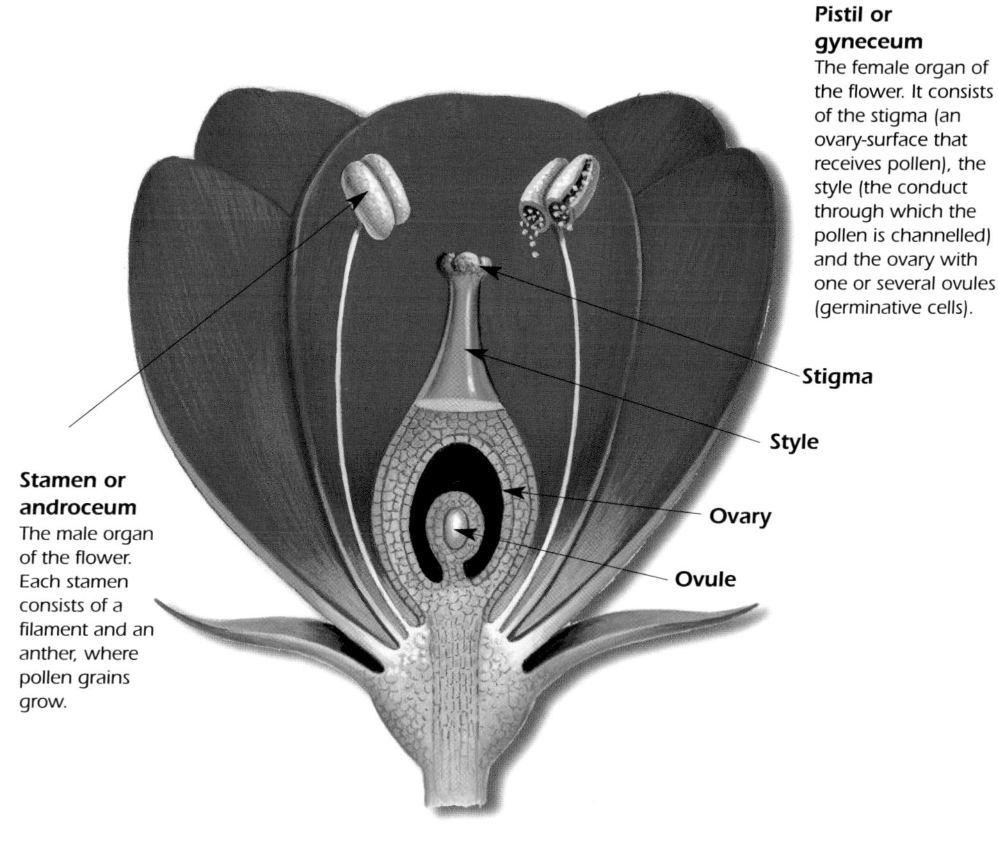

Stamen or androceum
The male organ of the flower. Each stamen consists of a filament and an anther, where pollen grains grow.

A Grain of Pollen

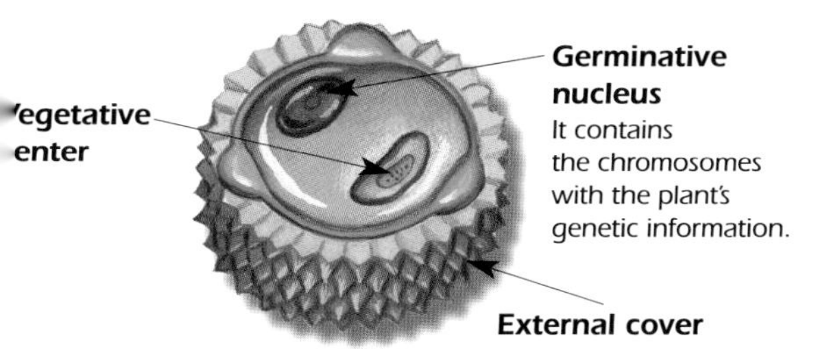

Germinative nucleus
It contains the chromosomes with the plant's genetic information.

The fecundation of flowers
In order for fecundation (fertilization) to take place, to form the seed and then the fruit,
a grain of pollen must Fall on the stigma of the flower. When the pollen and the flower belong to the same species, the pollen produces an elongation which goes down the style to the ovary. There, the male pollen chromosomes join the female ovule chromosomes, thus forming the seed and the fruit.
Plants with flowers reproduce sexually. This means that there are two parts, male or female, which must join to give birth to a new plant.

Guardians or Killers?

Endangered Plants

Plants are ***indispensable*** life agents of the Earth. All animals and human beings depend on green plants for food, because plants are ***the only*** living beings able to take advantage of solar energy and which produce carbohydrates, proteins, fats, vitamins and other organic substances.

Plants make decisive contributions to the ***ecological balance*** and to the preservation of the ***environment.*** They prevent soil erosion, store water and fertilize the ground.

Plants are a very important source of medicinal substances.

Human beings, who should be the guardians of this biodiverse legacy conferred upon us by the Creator, often become its killers. According to the International Union for Nature Preservation, 20% of the 390,000 species all over the world (some 78,000) are endangered and may disappear.

What are the causes of such vegetal species disappearing? These are some of them:

- Forest **fires.**
- **Tourist development** of coasts and mountain lands.
- Water, soil and air **pollution** (because of farm herbicides).
- Amateurs **gathering** rare species.
- **Building** of dams, highways and roads.

"Forests appear before civilizations. Deserts follow civilizations."
François-René Chateaubriand (1768-1848), French author and politician.

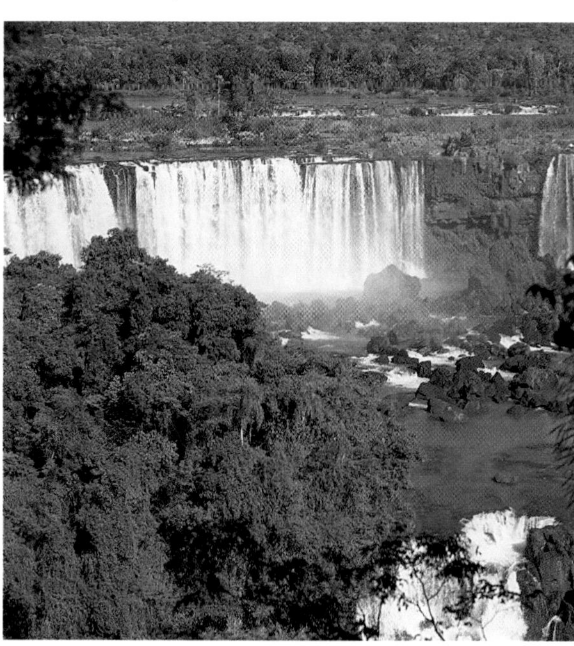

Gathering, not Plundering

- *Gather only in those **places** where this practice is **allowed,** never in natural or national parks, nor in biological reserves.*
- ***Respect protected species,** for they are endangered (get information from the agriculture authorities of the area first).*
- *Gather only **small amounts** of plants, especially when they are not abundant.*
- *Gather, but do **not kill or uproot** the plants if possible.*

Could we imagine how significant the loss of the *Cinchona* trees in South American forests would have been, if they had been razed by bulldozers before quinine, which prevents malaria, was discovered? What if those beautiful flowers of the foxglove family had been prematurely gathered before the heart-stimulant glycosides which have healed so many people with heart disease had been discovered?

Let us ***all*** do our part to preserve vegetal species in the best way. And if we go out gathering plants, let us bear in mind the advice for gathering, not plundering.

The picture on the left shows the fantastic Iguazu Falls, on the border between Brazil and Argentina. South America houses the largest forests on the planet, a true vegetal reserve which hides many botanical-medicinal secrets. This is why the Amazon forest has been called "the largest pharmacy in the world."

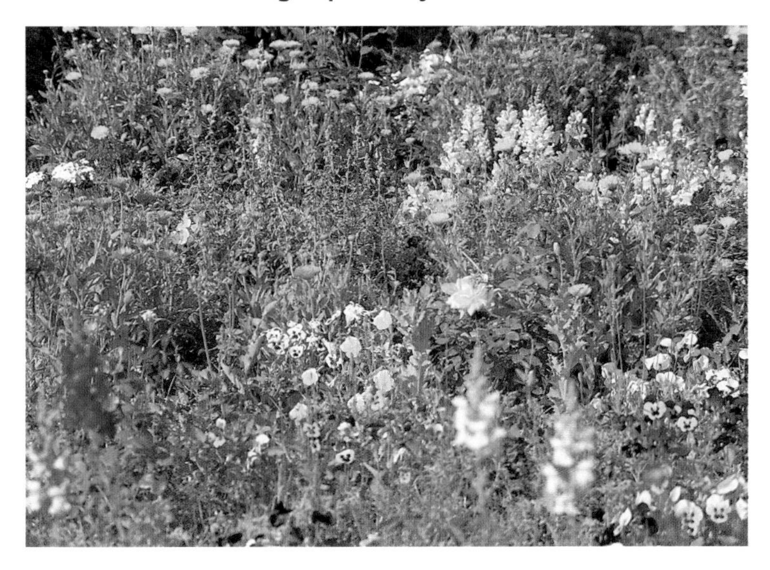

According to the Holy Bible, plants were the first to be created and could thus exist without animals and human beings. However, animals and human beings could never survive without plants. To respect and protect them is one of our duties as inhabitants of the Earth.

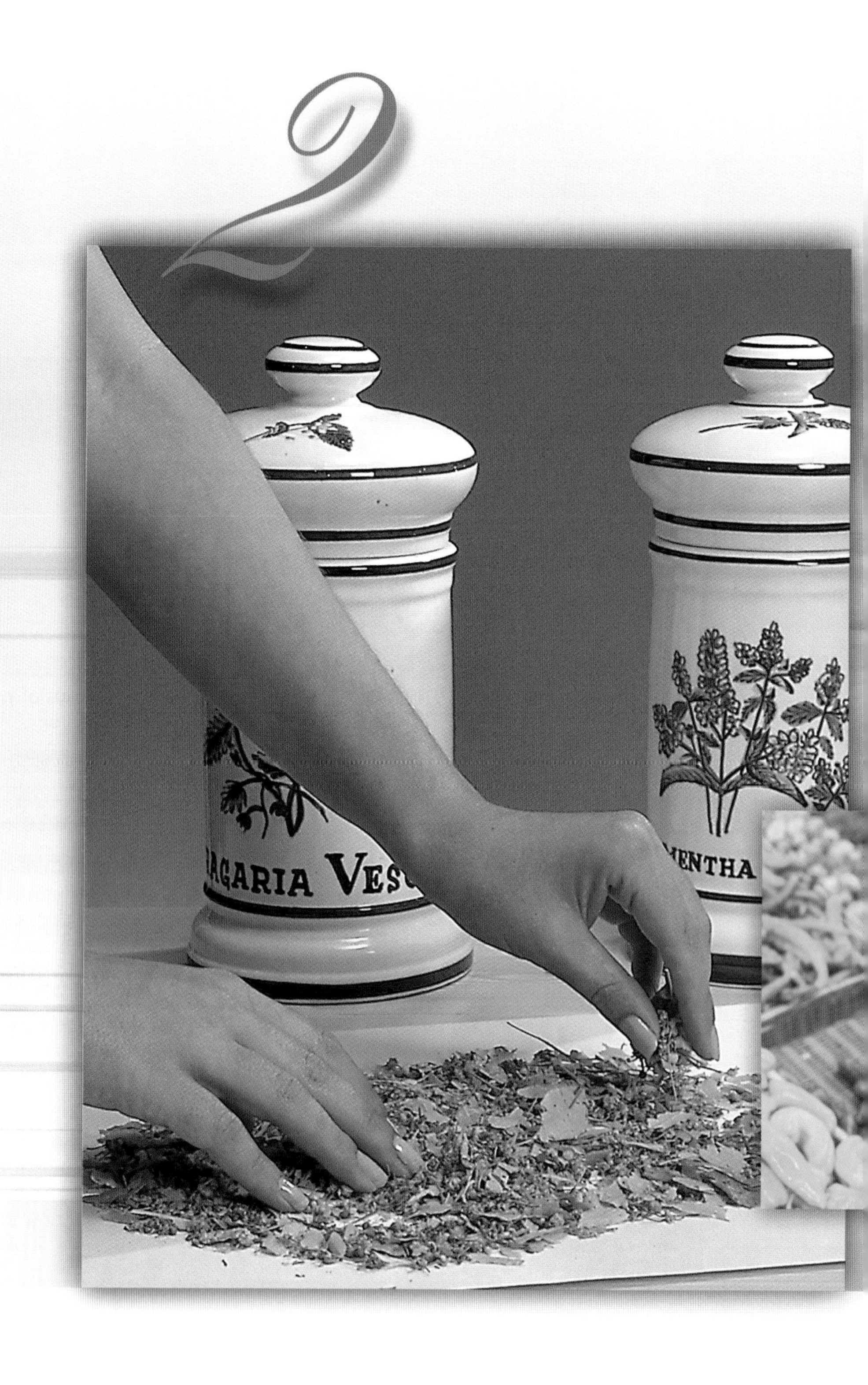

Methods for Preparing and Using Plants

SUMMARY PAGES

A Pioneer of Modern Phytotherapy . . . 55
Aromatherapy 52
Fomentations. 47
Ways to Apply Essential Oils 53
Hip Baths or Sitz Baths 46
How To Obtain
the Best Results From Plants 54
Juices, Tinctures, Syrups and Extracts . . 48
Safe Use of Medicinal Herbs 50
The Art of Preparing Herbal Teas 37

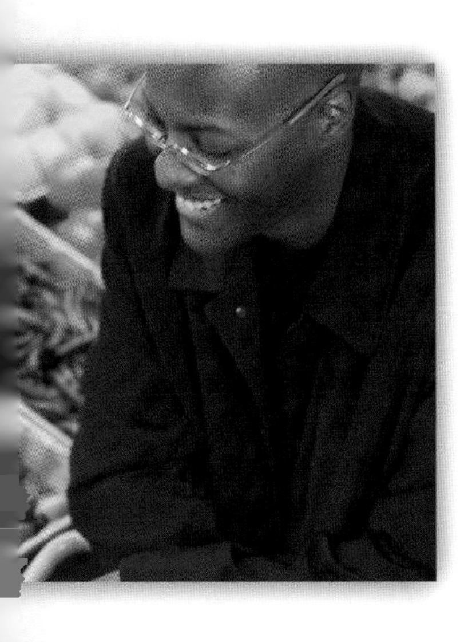

THERE ARE different ways of preparing medicinal herbs for use. All these methods aim:

• **To make the administration** of the plant **easier.**

• **To increase the concentration** of any **active component** of the plant that, due to its physical-chemical properties, dissolves easier by means of a specific preparation method. For instance, steam distillation is used to extract and concentrate essential oils.

• **To favor the preservation** of the plant or its preparations. For instance, decoctions (extracts from boiling) are more stable than fresh juices, and even than infusions, given that during decoctions the liquid boils and sterilizes.

For each medicinal plant there are certain optimum methods of preparation and use. It is worth knowing what they are and how to apply them, so that the properties of each plant are properly applied.

Herbal Teas

Herbal teas are obtained by treating vegetable products with water. This is the most popular method used to prepare medicinal herbs. Water is an ideal means of extracting most of the chemical substances produced by plants, because it is a universal dissolvent *par excellence.*

Herbal teas are mostly used for oral intake, however some other uses include compresses, eyedrops, lotions, etc., as we shall see in the section entitled "Methods of use" (p. 64).

Herbal teas are the result of the action of water on vegetable products. Depending on the method used, we will find three ways to obtain a herbal tea: infusion, decoction and cold extract.

Infusion

Infusion is the ideal procedure to obtain herbal teas from the **delicate parts** of plants: flowers, leaves, clusters and stem buds. With infusions, many active substances are extracted with almost no alteration of their chemical structure, thus preserving almost all of their properties.

Conservation of Infusions

As a rule, infusions may be preserved for about twelve hours. Prepare them in the morning, and drink them during the course of the day. If the weather is hot, keep infusions in the refrigerator. They may be warmed, but not boiled again. Infusions prepared 24 hours before should not be consumed.

Decoction

Decoction is mainly used to prepare herbal teas from the **hard parts** of plants (roots, rhizome, seeds) which require sustained boiling to liberate their active principles. Decoction has a disadvantage: some of the active principles may degrade because of the prolonged action of the heat.

Conservation of Decoctions

After boiling, decoctions may be preserved longer than infusions, especially when kept in the refrigerator. They may be used for several days, though it is better not to keep them for more than one week.

Cold extract

The cold extract method is used to extract the active principles of a plant or part of it, by using water at room temperature as a dissolvent (other applicable dissolvents are alcohol or oil). Cold extract consists of soaking the parts of the plant after it has been ground.

This method is the most suitable for plants whose active principles **degrade with heat.**

Preservation of Cold Extracts

Cold extracts may be preserved up to one month, especially when the dissolvent is alcohol or oil instead of water.

Dosage of Herbal Teas

As a rule, medicinal herbs do not require as strict a dosage as medicines. Due to the wide tolerance range for most of them, there is no need to measure with absolute precision the weight of plant for a herbal tea, nor the volume of it to be drunk.

In the particular analysis of each plant we detail its doses. However, the usual rule establishes that for an adult person the doses are as follows:

- **Infusions**. 20 to 30 grams of dry plant per liter of water, which is approximately equal to a teaspoon (2 g) per cup of water (150 ml).
- **Decoctions and cold extracts**. 30 to 50 grams per liter of water.

For an adult, it is usual to drink from three to five teacups daily (150 ml each).

In this work, unless indicating another rule, the amounts we give always refer to dry plants. When fresh plants are used, the amounts must be three or four times more in order to obtain the same effects as with the dry plant.

Child Dosage

Herbal teas for children are less concentrated (with less amount of herbs), or are prepared

The Art of Preparing Herbal Teas

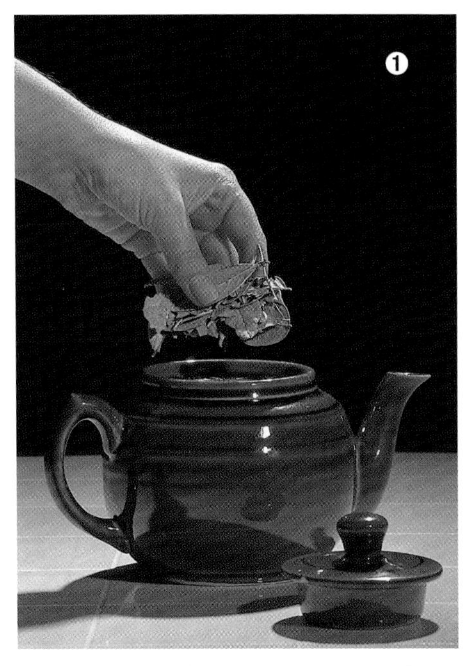

1. Put the part of the plant to be used in an suitable container. The plants may be loose or placed into a tea strainer or a small bag.

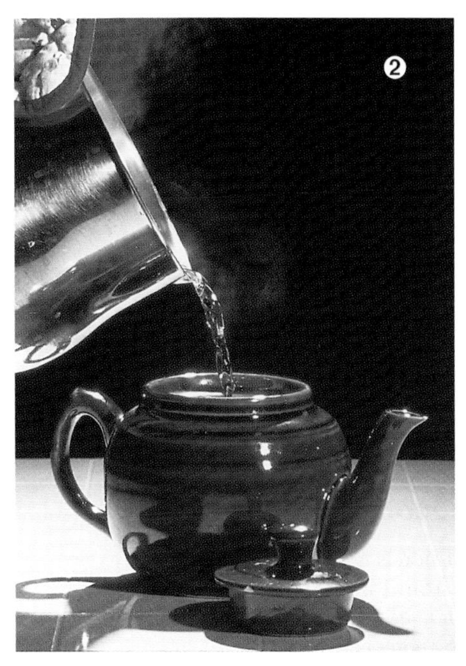

2. Blanch the plants with almost boiling water.
The usual method is to first introduce the plants, and then pour water over them, but this can also be done the other way round.

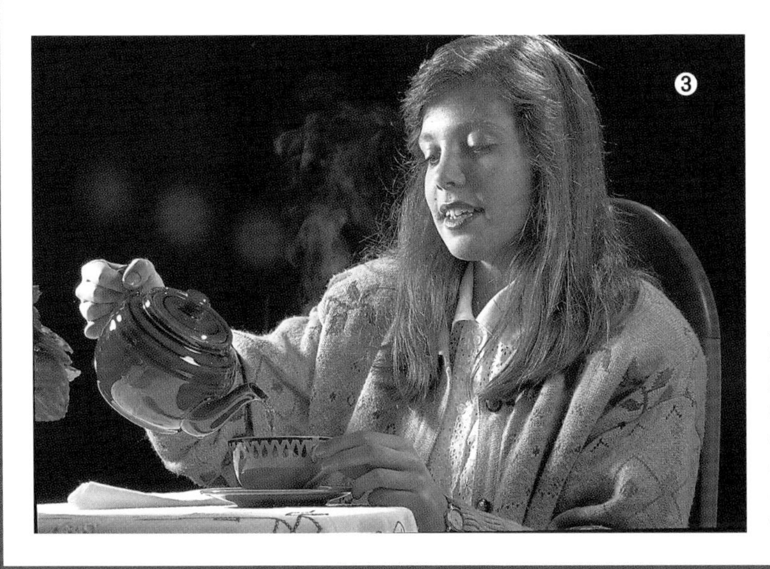

3. Drink the infusion after letting it steep and cool in a covered container to avoid loss of active ingredients through evaporation.

Infusion Bags

There are many products made from plants which are sold commercially in little bags to be consumed as infusions. The plants are ground up and already measured out in a bag which serves as a strainer. Its use is quite simple:

1. Place the bag inside a cup or glass.

2. Pour boiling water on.

3. Steep for some five minutes, covering the container with a plate lid or other kind of cover.

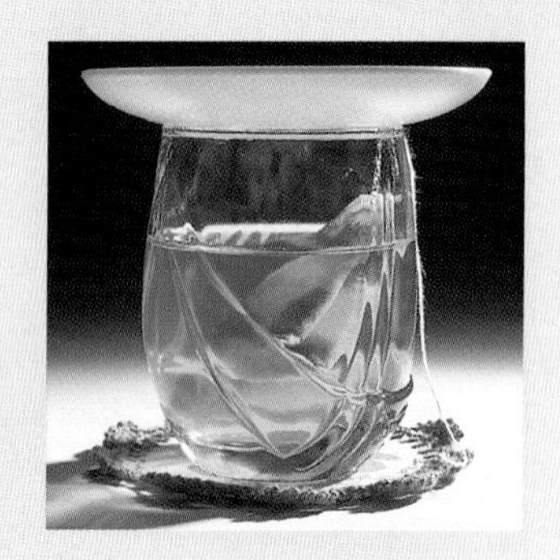

with the same concentration, but the children are given a smaller quantity of herbal tea. Child dosage is reduced proportionally, depending on the child's age.

- **School-age** (six to 12 years): **half** an adult dose.
- **pre-school age** (two to six years) **a third** of an adult dose.
- **children up to two years old:** from **a quarter** to **one eighth** of an adult dose.

Only plants devoid of any toxic effect should be administered to children.

Dosage of Herbal Teas

Volume	Dry flowers or leaves*	Dry roots or rhizome*
One teaspoon = 5 ml	1 g	3 g
Two teaspoons = 10 ml	2 g	5 g
One tablespoonful = 15 ml	4 g	10 g
A pinch = 2 ml	0.5 g	1.5 g
A handful = 20 ml	5 g	12 g

* Approximate amounts

When and How To Sweeten Herbal Teas

It is **better** to drink herbal teas **unsweetened.** However, there are some cases which may require the drink to be sweetened.

- When plants have an **unpleasant flavor.**
- When **children** drink herbal teas, with the exception made for those with vermifuge effects (expulsion of intestinal parasites). In this case, sweetening of the herbal tea is not recommended, because sugar and honey promote the growth of parasites.
- When herbal teas are administered to **convalescent or weak** patients.

Those herbal teas with an **appetizing** effect **should not** be sweetened, because sugars may diminish the sensation of hunger. Also, **diabetic persons** should abstain from adding sugar to herbal teas, and use artificial sweeteners instead.

Honey is the ***ideal product*** to sweeten

Cold Extract with Oil

Fill a jar with the part of the plant to be used for cold extract, then cover with oil, preferably olive oil. Steep for several days or weeks, depending on the plant.

Through this method, St. Johnswort, English lavender, annatto, Madonna lily, arnica and laurel oils, among others, are obtained.

The oils obtained are used over all in local application on the skin. Hence, the emollient (soothing) properties of oil are combined with the specific action of the plant used.

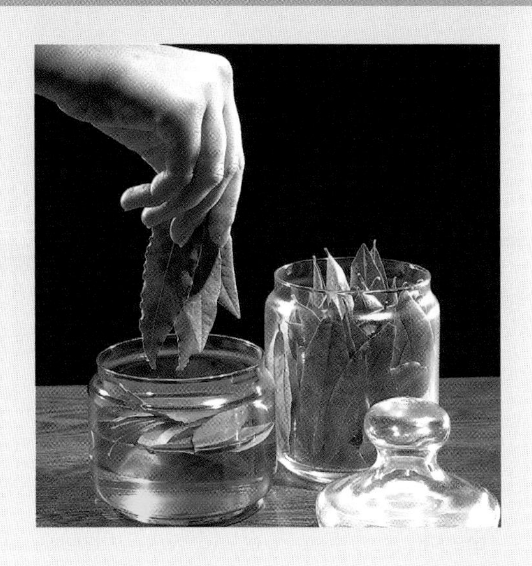

herbal teas. It comes from flowers, and besides sugars, it contains minerals and vitamins with a high nutritive value. Honey may be substituted by **brown sugar, molasses** (sugar cane honey), or **maple syrup,** which are all also rich in minerals and vitamins, and have better properties than refined sugar.

One Plant or Several Plants in Our Herbal Teas?

A mixture of several kinds of plants in the same herbal tea may have positive effects if the plants are well combined, according to their chemical composition and their properties.

However, when the mixture is not well combined, medicinal effects may disappear. In part two of this work we offer lists of plants that may be mixed to treat several ailments.

With the mixture of several plants, possible undesirable effects of each of them can occur (bad taste, digestive intolerance). However, it is not always necessary to mix plants. One plant, when well applied, may exert better effects than the mixture of several, poorly combined ones.

Methods of Use

When applying a plant or any plant-based preparations, there are two methods to consider:

- **Internal use.** The substance is taken through the mouth, entering the stomach and then the digestive system. From there, these substances exert their action, whether absorbed and passing into the blood system or by acting directly on the digestive system (such as bran or the mucilaginous substances of some plants).

Herbal teas (infusions, decoctions, cold extracts), and oils, syrups, juices, powders, tinctures, and other gallenic pharmaceutical preparations are employed internally.

- **External use.** The plant or its preparations

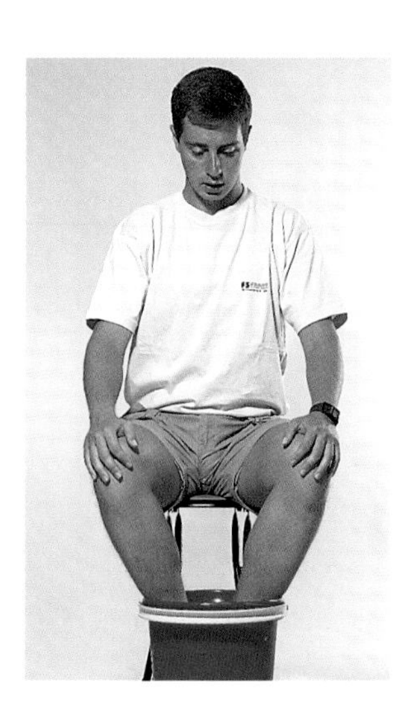

Hot foot baths are very effective in relieving head congestion, colds or flu.

are applied on the skin or in the orifices of the person (mouth, ears, vagina, etc.), not entering the digestive system.

The same herbal teas, juices, oils and other preparations used internally may also be used externally, though it is better if they are more concentrated.

Baths

A bath is the complete or partial immersion of the body in water, to which preparations of medicinal plants may be added. Examples are:

• **Concentrated infusions or decoctions**. An infusion or decoction to be added in bath water may be prepared with 40 to 80 g of plant (two or three big handfuls) per liter of water. For a normal bathtub, two or three liters of infusion or decoction are usually enough. Once strained, they are added to the water in the bathtub.

• **Essences**. Five to ten drops of essence, dissolved in the bath water, are usually enough.

Baths are especially used because of their antirheumatic, relaxing and sedative effects (for example, with lavender cotton, sweet flag, lavender, marjoram, or wild clover). A bath with sweet flag is especially effective against insomnia.

Foot Baths

Foot baths, taken with hot water, are quite useful to alleviate headaches (especially when mustard flour is added to the water), and to improve the blood flow in the legs (with grapevine or blind nettle leaves, for instance). They are usually taken by adding one liter of the same infusion or decoction employed for internal use, to 3 or 5 liters of water.

Hand Baths

Hand baths are successfully used to improve blood circulation in the upper limbs. They must be taken with warm or slightly hot water. In order to prevent itching, swelling, and cold and blue hands caused by arterial spasms, hand baths with ginkgo are recommended.

Cataplasms or Poultices

Poultices are prepared in several ways:

• With **seed flours** (flax, mustard, fenugreek).

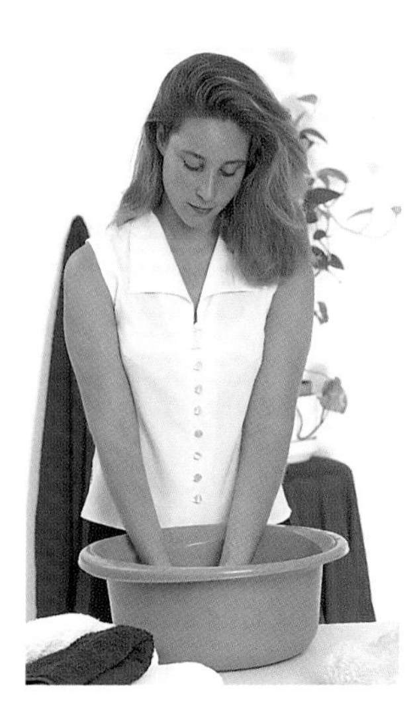

Hand baths are very effective against chilblains (itching, swelling, cold).

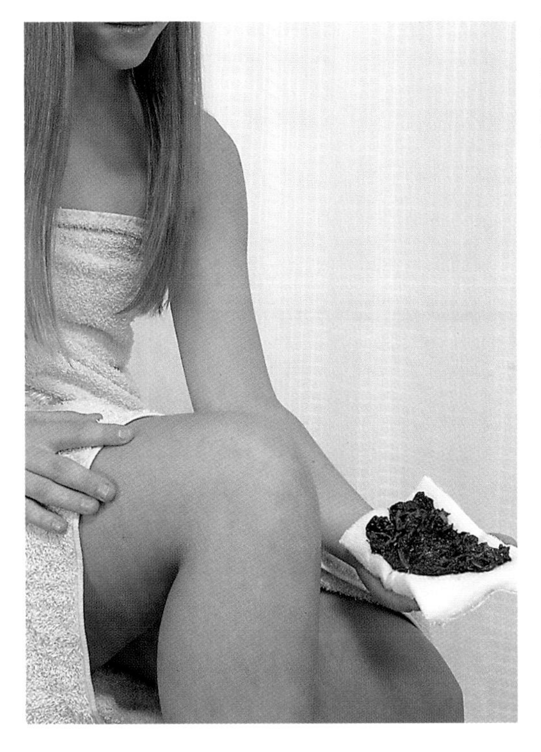

Medicinal herb poultices have a strong anti-inflammatory effect on the skin and deep tissues.

Knead flour with water until a fluid, uniform paste is formed. This done, warm it in a container, continuously stirring, until it acquires a pasty consistency. Apply a coat, one or two centimeters thick, on the skin, and cover with a cotton or flannel cloth.

• With ground **leaves or roots** from fresh plants (burdock, watercress, onion, cabbage, comfrey). They are ground until a uniform paste is obtained, then spread on a cloth and applied hot or cold as required.

• With **fruits** (strawberries, figs), mashed and wrapped with a cloth.

Use of Poultices

Cataplasms or poultices, in contact with the skin for long periods, reinforce several properties of the plant, such as the following:

• **Cicatrizant,** to promote healing (sorrel, burdock, cabbage, comfrey, figs, common plantain).

• **Resolvent,** to soften and promote drainage of abscesses and furuncles (avocado, fenugreek, borage, flax, cassava).

• **Analgesic and sedatives,** against abdominal pain, cystitis, menstrual pain, etc. (corn grains, flax, thyme).

• **Pectoral and anti-inflammatory.** The best compresses are those prepared with linseed flour (flax seeds). Some mustard may be added to these in order to produce a revulsive effect.

• **Revulsive.** Those which attract blood to the skin, relieving the congestion of internal organs. These are usually prescribed for rheumatic affections, and prepared with cowslip, nettles, mustard or rue.

Methods of Application of Poultices

When applying poultices some points should be considered:

• **Temperature.** Poultices are applied warm or hot, between 40° and 50° C (100-120° F). A practical method to warm them is to put them under an iron for some minutes, wrapped in a cloth.

• **Skin protection.** Poultices with a revulsive effect, especially those containing mustard flour, called **sinapisms,** may provoke skin irritation. They must thus be carefully wrapped in a flannel cloth. It is sufficient to wrap other poultices in a gauze.

• **Duration.** From five to ten minutes. It is best to apply a poultice several times a day instead of once for long periods.

Compresses

Compresses are easier to use than cataplasms, though their effects are less intense.

Application of Compresses

Compresses are applied in the following way.

• **Soak** a gauze or flannel cloth in herbal tea, juice, tincture, or other liquid preparation.

• **Apply** it on the affected skin area for some time, depending on the plant used (generally from five to 10 minutes).

• If the gauze or cloth dries, **soak it again.** It is better to frequently change compresses and apply them several times a day rather than use the same one for a long time.

Some plants may stain the skin when applied in compresses, especially those plants which contain tannins (English oak, English walnut, black alder). Rubbing with lemon juice will help to recover the normal skin color.

Use of Compresses

Compresses are used as **cicatrizants and antiseptics** on wounds and skin ulcers (sticklewort, black alder, hazelnut, calendula, nasturtium, onion, cabbage, horsetail, ivy, English walnut, licorice, English oak), to **make skin more beautiful** (strawberry, witch hazel, rose, linden), for the **eyes** (cornflower, camomile), or as **analgesics and sedatives** (oats, European mistletoe).

Fomentations

Fomentations are applied in the same way as compresses, but the liquid must be as hot as the skin can resist. Two more cloths are used apart from the one soaked in the medicinal infusion or decoction: a dry one under it, to protect skin, and another over it to maintain the heat.

Fomentations are mainly used in **respiratory diseases** (catarrhs and bronchitis), **throat** and **trachea** inflammations, **colic spasms** (of kidneys, liver and intestine) and **sciatica.** In these cases they are applied using the same herbal tea used internally, which reinforces its action.

Compresses are applied by soaking a cloth in the liquid obtained from the medicinal herbs (herbal tea, juice, etc.).

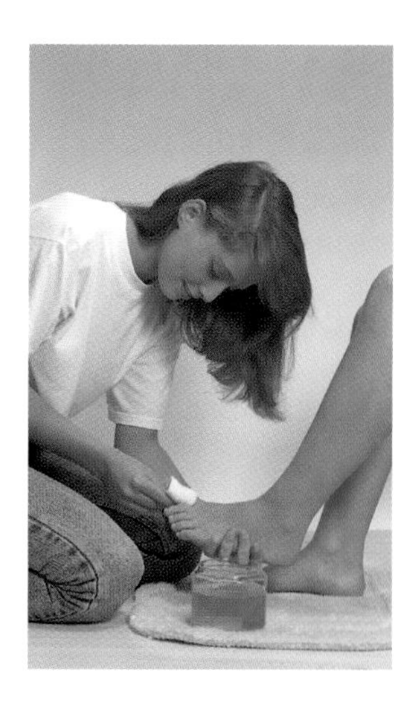

Lotions and Friction

Lotions are applied using an infusion, decoction, cold extract or juice which is applied through a gentle massage over the skin.

Friction are applied in the same way, usually employing essential oils and with a more vigorous massage.

They can be applied with bare hands or with a soft cloth soaked in the liquid.

Use of Lotions and Frictions

Lotions and frictions may be used for the following:

• **Skin afflictions** in general (for example, bilberries, calendula, bennet, echinacea, olive leaves, nettle, pansy, soapwort, thyme or coltsfoot).

• **Pruritus,** itching (borage, black nightshade, speedwell).

• **Beauty:** elimination of cellulitis, making skin more beautiful or encouraging weight loss (strawberry, echinacea, rose, kneeholly).

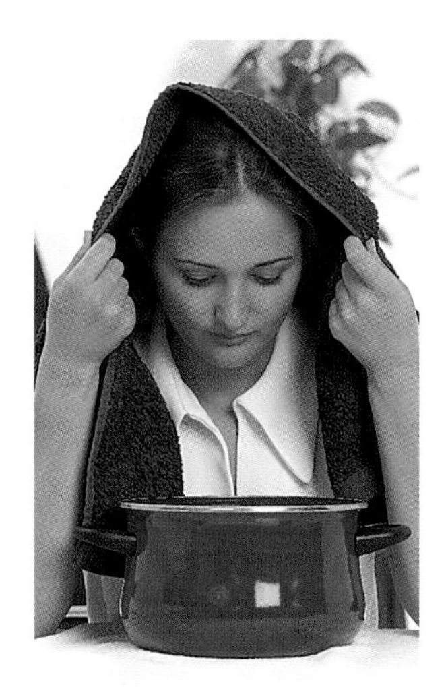

Steam inhalations with linden leaves clean, soothe and make facial skin more beautiful.

- **Rheumatism** (lavender, laurel).
- **Mosquito** repellent (wormwood).

Steam Baths

Steam baths are applied to the head, torso or even to the whole body.

Application of Steam Baths

Steam baths are applied in the following way:

1. Place a **bowl of boiling water** containing the plants to be used on a stool. The bowl must be covered. Instead of plants, two or three drops of an essential oil may be added to the water.

2. The patient **sits** on a chair with his head over the bowl and **covers** his head with a large towel or a sheet, so as to keep the steam from escaping.

3. Partially uncover the bowl in order to let steam out.

4. The application takes from **10 to 15 minutes,** or until there is no steam left.

5. Finish with a **friction** of cold water or alcohol on the area being exposed to the steam.

Use of Steam Baths

Steam baths are very useful for **respiratory diseases:** sinusitis, pharyngitis, laryngitis, tracheitis, bronchial catarrhs and bronchitis, as well as for **otitis** (infection or inflammation of the ear). They facilitate the elimination of mucus, germs and cellular waste from the respiratory mucosa, thus accelerating the regeneration and healing process.

Gargles

Gargles are an easy way to apply medicinal plants to the throat.

Gargling Instructions

Gargles are done this way:

1. Sip (but do not swallow) some warm herbal tea (generally an infusion). Very hot, or very concentrated liquids must not be taken.

2. Lean your **head backwards.**

3. Try to pronounce **the letter "o"** for **half to one minute.**

4. Spit out the liquid. It must *never* be swallowed, as it is supposed to absorb the waste substances.

5. Repeat the whole process for five to ten minutes.

Gargles and mouth washing with pomegranate fruits, rind or flowers are useful in the cases of pharyngitis, gingivitis (inflammation of the gums) and parodontosis (falling and loosening of the teeth).

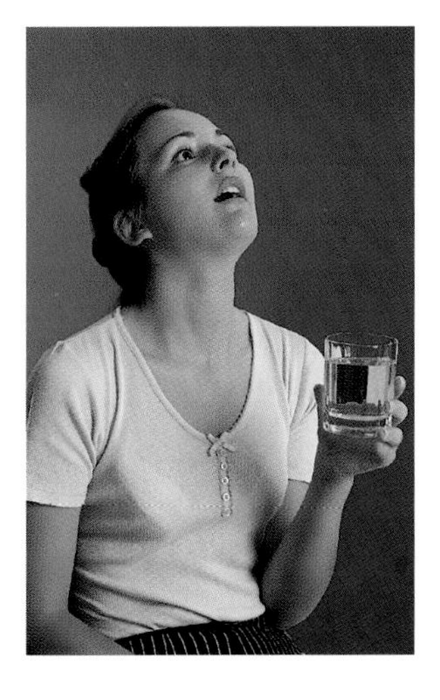

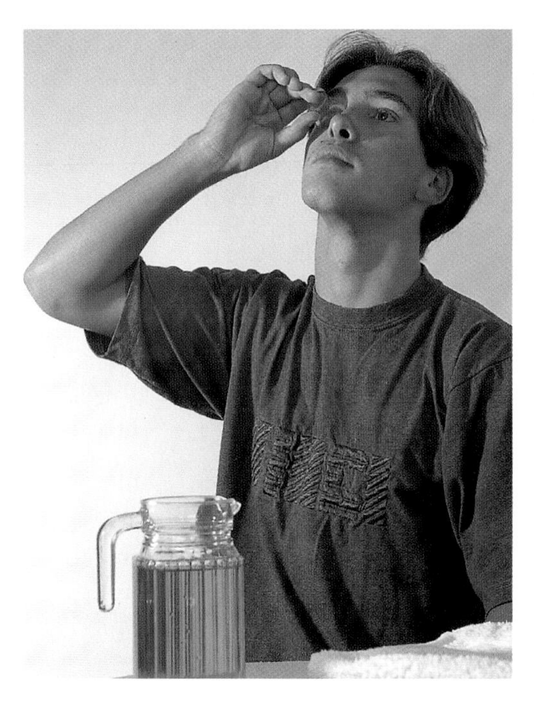

Eye baths must be done by dripping the liquid from the temple to the nose, as this is the directions tears flow.

Use of Gargles

Gargles act on the mucus which covers the rear part of the mouth, the pharynx (throat) and the tonsils. They remove mucous, germs, dead cells and toxins in these areas in the case of irritation, inflammation or infection. They have emollient (soothing), antiseptic and astringent (dry, reduce inflammation and healing effects.

The plants most used for gargles are black alder, bistort, bennet, chestnut bark and leaves, onion, five-finger grass, white dryas, blackthorn, willowherb, strawberry, restharrow, pomegranate, goldenseal, common plantain, English walnut, rhatany, rosemary, black elder, tormentil, and vervain.

Mouth washing

Mouth washing is done by **taking a sip of liquid** (generally an infusion or decoction) and **rinsing** the mouth. It is very useful in cases of stomatitis, gingivitis, pyorrhea, and other **mouth-tooth afflictions.** It is done with the same plants as those used for gargles.

Eyedrops

Eyedrops are liquids employed to heal eyes or eyelid affections.

They **must not be too concentrated, nor irritating,** and should be applied **warm.** It is recommended that they come from infusions made with water previously boiled for five minutes, or with decoctions in order to achieve better sterilization. Eyedrops made with cornflower, motherwort, red eyebright, camomile, and grape leaves are frequently used.

Eye Baths

Eye bathing is done by soaking a **compress** in a plant decoction and gently dripping the liquid from the temple to the nose.

As with eyedrops, it is recommended to ensure good sterilization of the liquid to be used to wash the eyes, preferably decoctions. Five minutes of boiling are enough to obtain adequate sterilization for decoctions, as well as for infusions.

Enemas

Enemas are the introduction of a liquid into the large intestine through the anus, by means of a rubber irrigator. The liquid may be a low-concentrated infusion or decoction warmed to body temperature (37° C).

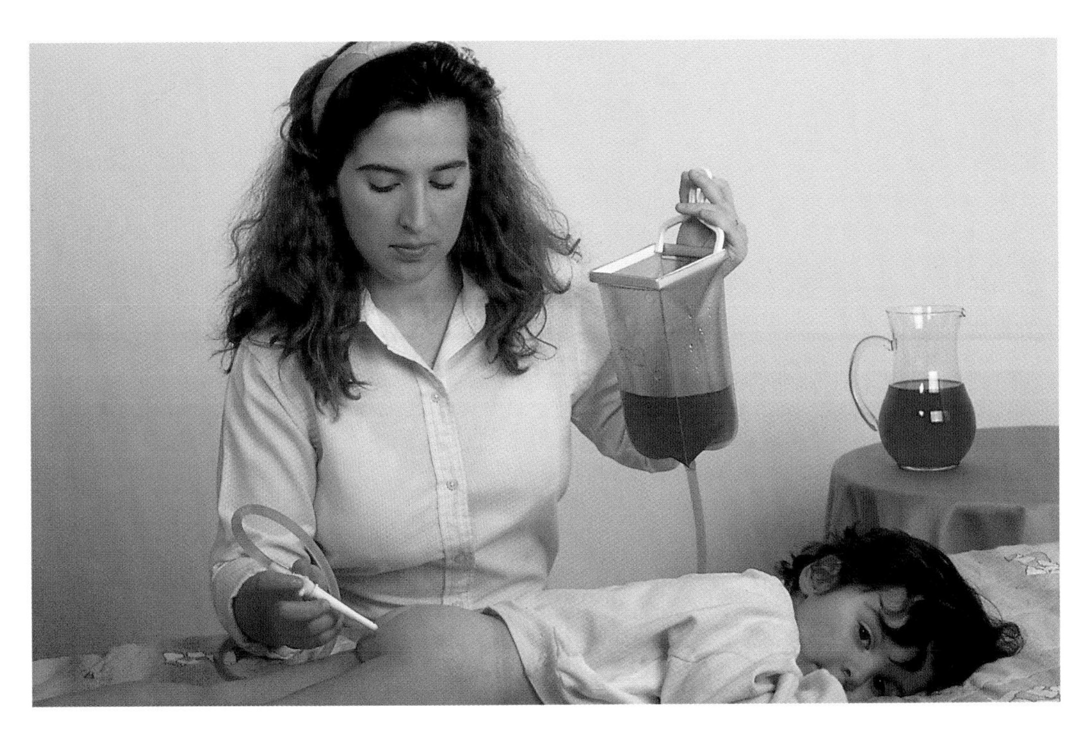

Enemas made using medicinal herb infusions or decoctions combine the cleansing action of water with the therapeutic effects of plants.

Caution in the Use of Enemas

When giving an enema, some points should be remembered:

1. Lay the patient down on his **right side,** with his **legs bent inwards.**

2. Introduce the tip of the irrigator with the help of **oil** or **Vaseline.**

3. Avoid the liquid entering with **excessive pressure.** The recipient containing the liquid must not be held more than one meter above the body of the patient.

4. Three hundred to 500 ml of liquid are enough for adults. For **children, 100-200 ml** suffice.

5. The patient must **retain** the liquid for **five to ten minutes.**

6. Do not apply more than three enemas daily, which should be administered **after meals.**

7. In many cases, a prescription and the supervision of a physician are required.

Aims of Enemas

The aims of enemas are:

- **To evacuate** the rectum and the large intestine in cases of **constipation,** especially due to fever or infectious afflictions (for example, with olive leaves, high mallow or tinnevelly senna).
- **To reduce inflammation** of the anus and rectum in the case of **fissures, hemorrhoids** and **anal inflammation** (with common plantain, English oak or psyllium).
- **To reduce inflammation** of the large intestine in cases of **colitis** or **diarrhea** (horseweed, high mallow), **digestive spasms** (asafetida) or **breast-feeding babies diarrhea** (loosestrife).
- To eliminate **intestinal parasites** (garlic, quassia, tansy).

Hip Baths or Sitz Baths

For Sitz baths with medicinal plants, one or two liters of infusion or decoction are prepared (generally more concentrated than those employed in internal use), and poured into the bathtub, adding the required amount of water to reach the hips, under the navel.

Hip baths produce a circulatory stimulation in the lower part of the abdomen, and have favorable effects on the organs of the area: large intestine, bladder and internal genital organs. Moreover, hip baths act directly on the skin and the external tissues of the genital organs and the anus. They are quite effective in the following cases:

- **Anal and rectal dysfunctions**, such as hemorrhoids or anal fissure.
- **Cystitis and urinary dysfunctions**.
- **Prostate dysfunctions**.
- **Gynecological dysfunctions**, especially painful menstruations and female genital infections.

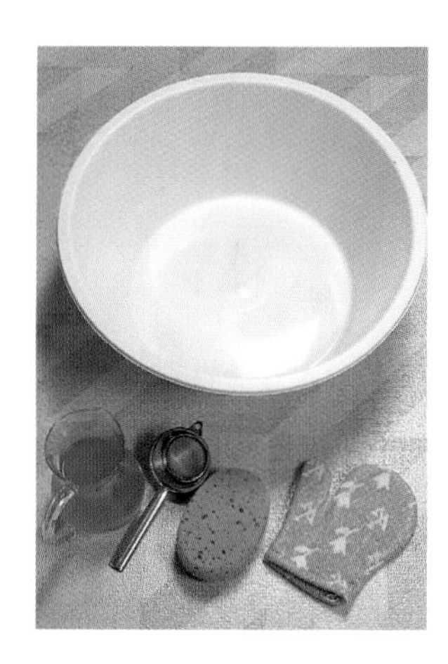

The elements required to prepare a hip bath: a bowl, the infusion to add to the water, a strainer and a sponge or bathglove.

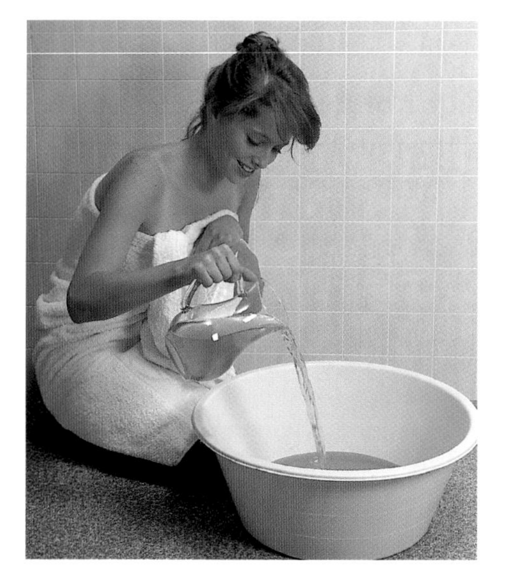

Hip baths are taken with **warm or cold water,** unless contraindicated, so as to achieve a more invigorating effect. Nevertheless, in some cases the **water should be hot:**

- **Abdominal spasms** caused for instance by digestive colics, cystitis or dysmenorrhea (painful menstruation).
- **Anal fissure:** An affliction whose symptoms are small tears or ulcerations in the anal tissues which causes painful defecation along with minor bleeding. This should not be confused with **hemorrhoids**. When there is a fissure, hot hip baths should be taken, while hemorrhoids require cold hip baths.

A hip bath **must not last** for more than three minutes if taken with cold water, while when taken with warm or hot water it may last 10 minutes. It is usual to have one or two baths daily, and even three, changing the water each time.

Fomentations

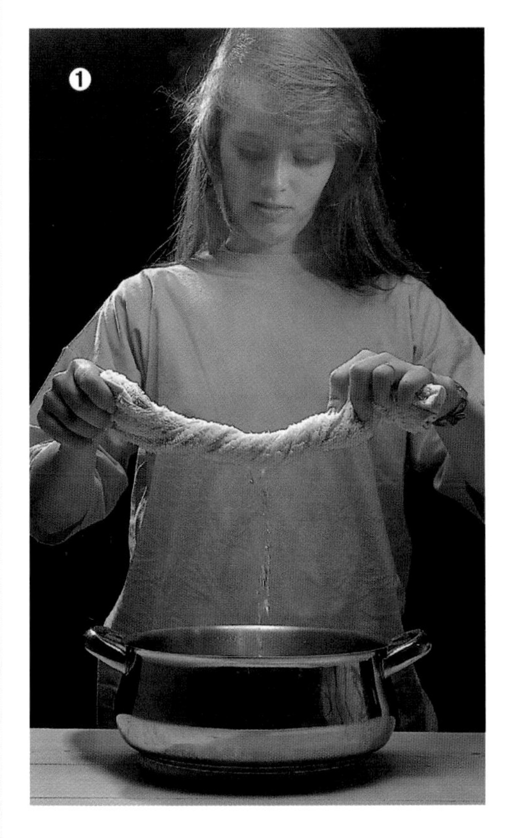

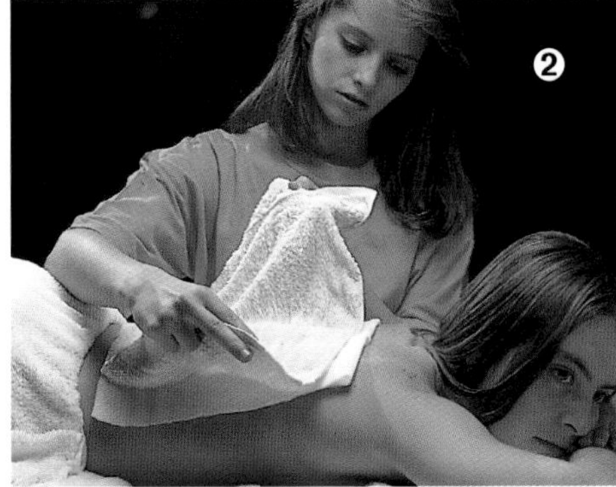

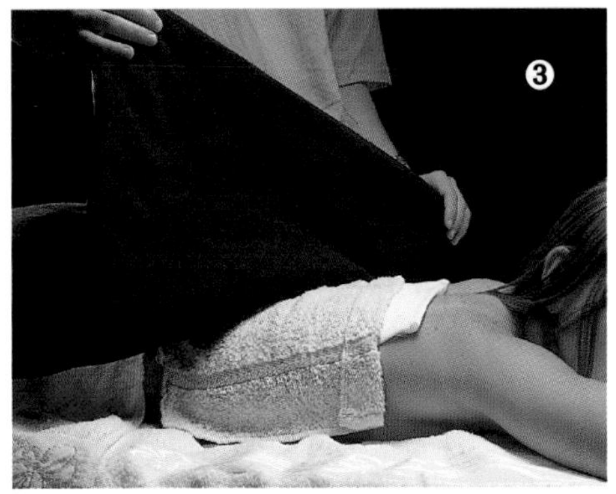

1. Prepare one or two liters of **infusion or decoction** of the plant. It is usually better if they are slightly **more concentrated** than usual (50 to 100 g per liter of water). From five to ten drops of **essence** of the plant may be also added to one or two liters of hot water.

2. When the liquid is **hot,** soak a **cotton cloth or towel** (picture ❶).

3. **Wring** out the cloth, then apply it to the affected area, protecting the skin with **another dry cloth** (picture ❷).

4. **Cover** these two cloths with a **woollen-blanket** to maintain the heat. Wool preserves heat better, even when wet or soaked (picture ❸). Care should be taken that the person is not burned.

5. After **three minutes**, when the cloth begins to cool, soak it again in the hot liquid.

6. The application of fomentations must take place for **15 to 20 minutes.** To finish, **rub cold water** on the affected area.

Juices, Tinctures,

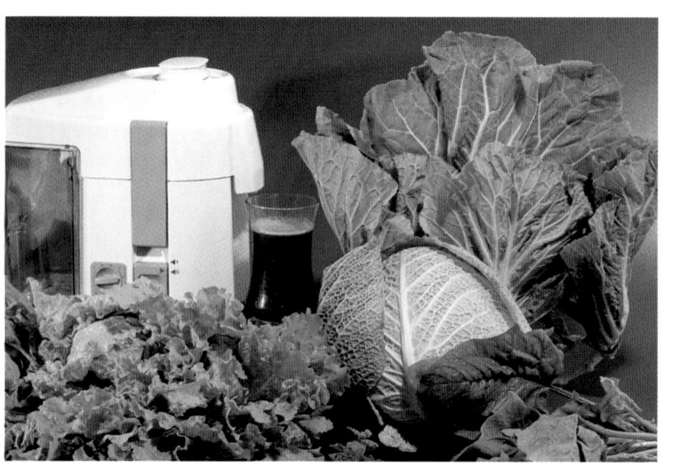

Fresh juices of plants are the best form in which to prepare and ingest them, since it preserves their vitamins, enzymes and active ingredients. However, juices must be taken shortly after being prepared in order to maintain all their nutrients.

Juices

Juices must be made from **fresh plants**, soon after they are picked, by mashing them in a mortar and then filtering them. They may also be made using an electric blender.

Juices may be obtained either from herbaceous plants or from leaves and fruits. The juice of aloe leaves is highly appreciated due to its appetizing and digestive properties.

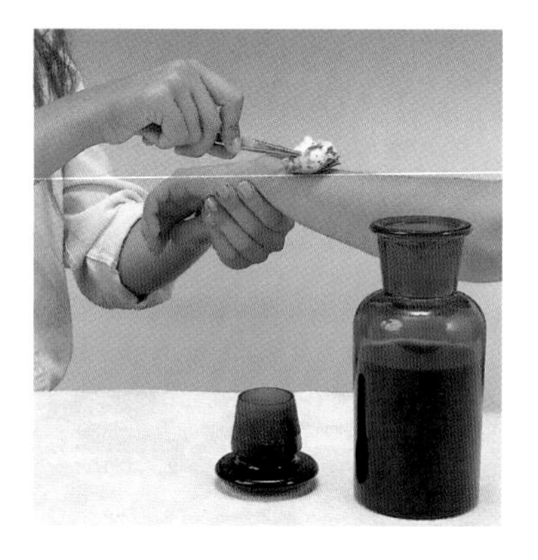

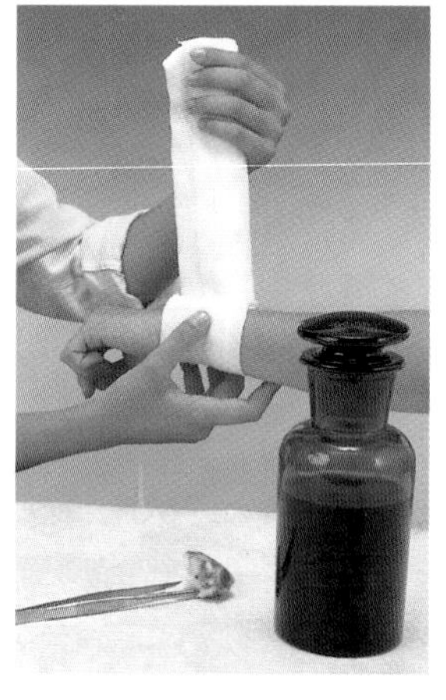

External uses are the most secure way to use tinctures.

When taken orally, caution must be exercised given their alcohol content.

Tinctures

Tinctures are alcoholic solutions which contain a high concentration of certain active components of the plant, precisely those which are alcohol-soluble. Tinctures are prepared by putting a well-dried, ground plant in alcohol at room temperature for two or three days, or even up to 15 days, such as in the case of arnica.

Syrups and Extracts

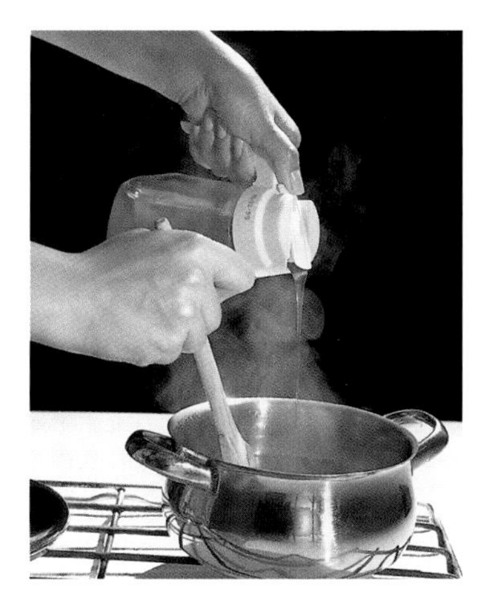

Syrups

Syrups are prepared by adding honey or sugar (preferably non-refined sugar) to a more concentrated than usual infusion or decoction, as well as to fruit juices. As a rule, syrups are made in a proportion of 50%, that is to say, adding the same weight of sugar or honey as infusion or fruit juice.

By heating the mixture, the dissolution of sugar is easier.

The preparation of onion syrup to combat coughs.

Extracts

Advantages:

Higher concentration: This usually makes the extract have a **more powerful effect** than the whole plant.

Greater availability. Extracts are available whenever needed, in any season and at any time, and their **use is** as **simple** as taking **a few drops.**

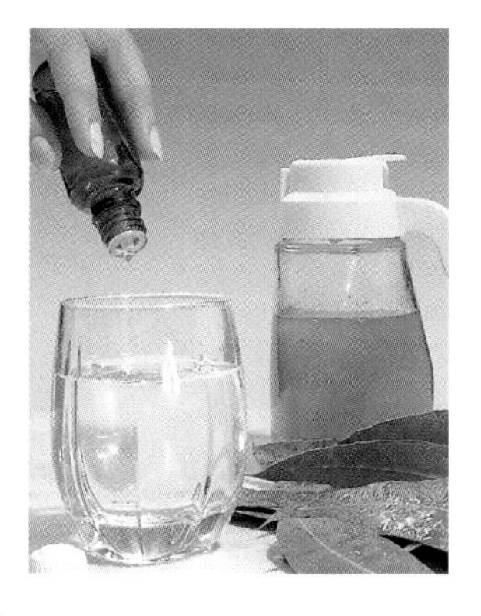

Extracts of medicinal herbs must be always regarded as pharmacological products, both for their advantages as well as their side effects.

Disadvantages:

Higher risk of poisoning: The risk of poisoning rises from the moment the natural balance of plant components is altered through extraction or concentration. Thus, **doses** of extracts must be **carefully respected.**

Higher risk of degradation of the active elements: When the extract has not been obtained in a specialized laboratory through the correct methods, there is the risk of destroying active elements of the plant which may be sensitive to heat or to the dissolvents used.

The presence of dissolvents: The most used dissolvent is **ethyl alcohol.** Remains of it in the extract are harmful to children and to certain people to whom alcohol is noxious, even in small amounts.

Safe Use of Medicinal Herbs

The first step is to adopt a healthy lifestyle

Before applying any plant regularly or continuously (as with any other medicine), one must bear in mind the following points:

1. Look for the causes of the disease, When a strange symptom appears, it is better to ask for a **professional medical diagnosis** to be carried out, with **scientific** means and procedures. Only after that can a medicinal herb based treatment or any other cure be safely applied.

2. Give up bad health habits. The **first step** to restoring health should be the adoption of a **healthy lifestyle,** and the avoidance of bad habits. Taking mucolythic or expectorant plants to heal bronchitis is useless if a person continues smoking or breathing polluted air.

3. Use only well-identified plants. It is recommended and safest to make sure that plants are bottled and correctly labelled under the auspices of a pharmaceutical laboratory or professional.

4. Avoid self-prescriptions. It is best that plants are prescribed or recommended by a competent physician.

Notwithstanding, the health laws of most countries list certain plants which may be freely used without a medical prescription. In this case, we recommend **responsible self-prescription:** one decides which plants are going to be taken, but in a responsible way. First, educate yourself on the properties of the plants as well as the precautions that their use requires.

5. Be cautious when taking a plant for long periods of time. As a rule, avoid the continuous use of any plant for more than two or three months. When the condition seems to require this, it is better to be informed on possible undesirable side effects of the plant. Requesting medical counsel is also advised.

6. Care must be taken with pregnant women and with children. As with all medicines, extreme caution is required when any medicinal herb is to be given to pregnant women and children.

Practical Cases

1. Look for the cause of the illness

John was a robust man, aged 55, who had never suffered serious illness. More than a year ago, he lost his appetite, and certain foods, such as meat, made him nauseous.

He prescribed for himself some plants that a neighbor recommended. He was assured they were quite effective in the recovery of appetite. During the first months he improved. However later, though he had no pain, his appetite did not improve, and he lost weight. Finally he decided to see a doctor.

An endoscopic exam of his intestine revealed that the cause of his lack of appetite was stomach cancer. The tumor was too large for successful surgical results.

This is a typical case of stomach cancer. Had John consulted the cause of his symptoms when they appeared, the prognostic of his disease would have been more favorable.

2. Avoid bad health habits

Steve was a truck-driver, who spent many hours driving. He suffered from hemorrhoids, which quite often became swollen and bled.

Steve liked spicy foods with chili and pepper. He seldom ate fruit. When he ate spicy meals, he noticed that his hemorrhoids worsened. He discovered some plants recommended at a natural remedy store. Using them in hip baths, he obtained much relief. He continued eating spicy meals and taking hip baths.

Nonetheless, the hemorrhoids worsened and one day he felt an intense pain which neither the plants nor any other remedy could alleviate. His doctor sent him to a surgeon: the diagnosis was hemorrhoid thrombosis, a very painful complication of hemorrhoids.

Had Steve adopted healthier eating habits, his hemorrhoids would not have worsened, and the medicinal hip baths he used would have been enough to improve and even heal his ailment.

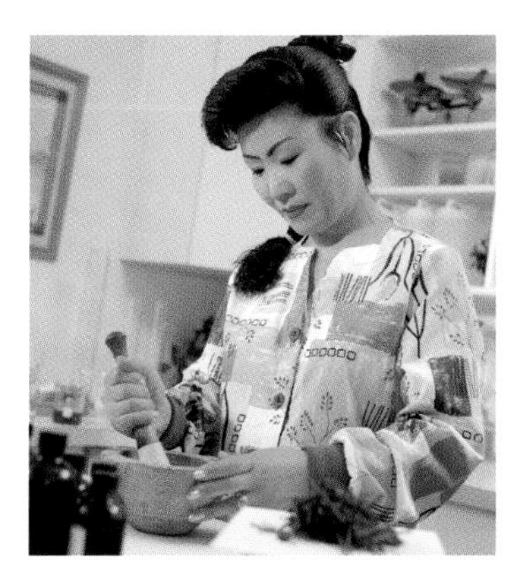

An adequate use of medicinal herbs, as well as the adoption of healthy life style habits may prevent weakness of our bodies from evolving into open diseases.

Aromatherapy

The Therapeutical Use of Essential Oils (Essences)

The Power of Aroma

Before reaching the lungs and passing into the blood, the molecules of the essence stimulate the olfactory (smell) cells in the **nostrils** [1].

These cells are actually neurons, which through the olfactory nerve send electric pulses with the coded smelling message. The **smell nerve** [2] carries the stimulus to different parts of the brain: the amygdala and the hippocampus of the **temporal lobe** [3], where scent memory lies; the **thalamus** [4], where emotions lie, and overall, the **hypothalamus** [5], and, throughout it, the **hypophysis** [6], the regulating center of hormone production for the whole body.

The relationship between the olfactory nerve, the thalamus, the hypothalamus, and the hypophysis could explain the well-known regulative effects of aromas on the neurohormonal system.

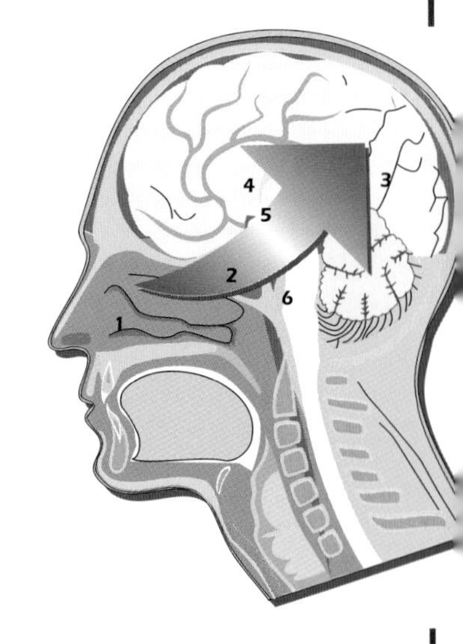

Still for the Distillation of Essential Oils or Essences

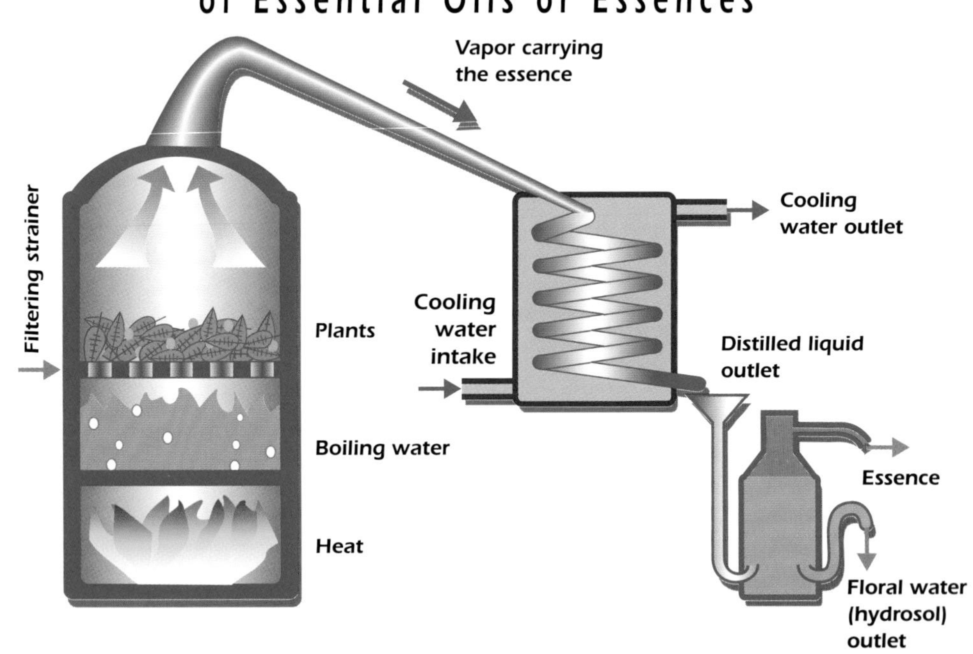

Ways to Apply Essential Oils

Aromatherapy, which literally means "treatment by means of aromas," is actually one of the methods of phytotherapy ("treatment by means of plants"). The healing properties of essential oils were known in ancient times, though only in an empirical way. Today, we know the reason why essential oils produce certain physiological effects on the body. However, there is much research still needed on how certain aromas influence the state of mind and even behavior.

In order to obtain good results, treatment with essential oils must last from one to three weeks, applied in any of the following four ways:

Atmospheric diffusion

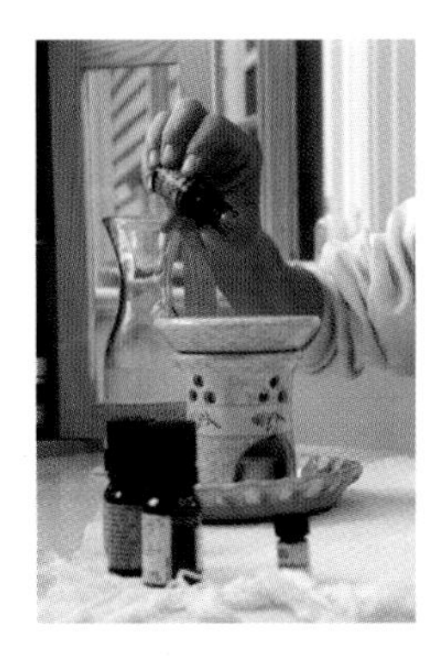

Internal use

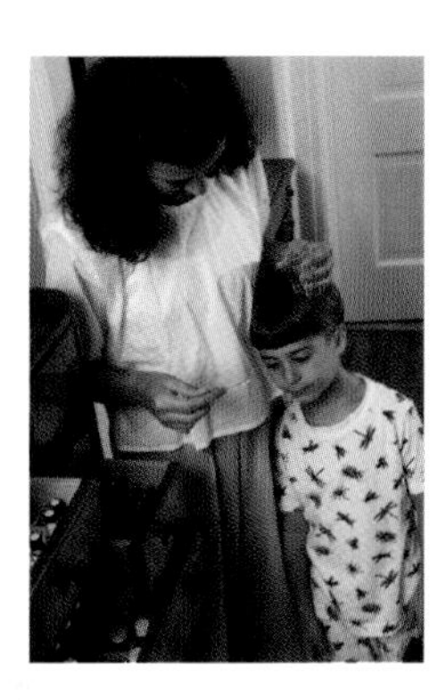

Essence baths

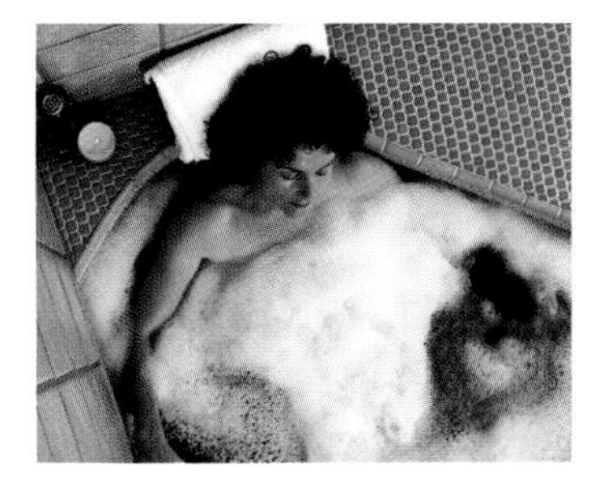

Massaging the skin

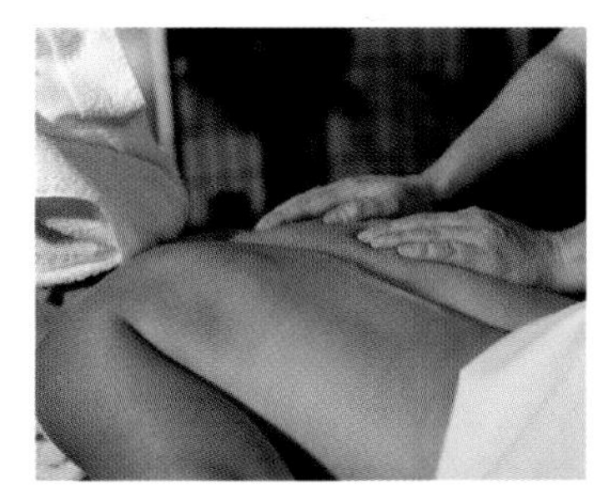

How To Obtain the Best Results From Plants

The best results are obtained by using plants combined with other natural agents that offer medicinal action, such as **water** (hydrotherapy), **the sea** (talasotherapy), **the sun** (heliotherapy), **medicinal soils** (geotherapy), **physical exercise** and **healthy food** based on vegetal products.

Moreover, a healthy lifestyle is required, which means **avoiding tobacco,** alcoholic beverages, and other drugs.

The **combined action** of all these factors is a notable stimulant on the defensive and health mechanisms of the body, which will finally overcome the disease.

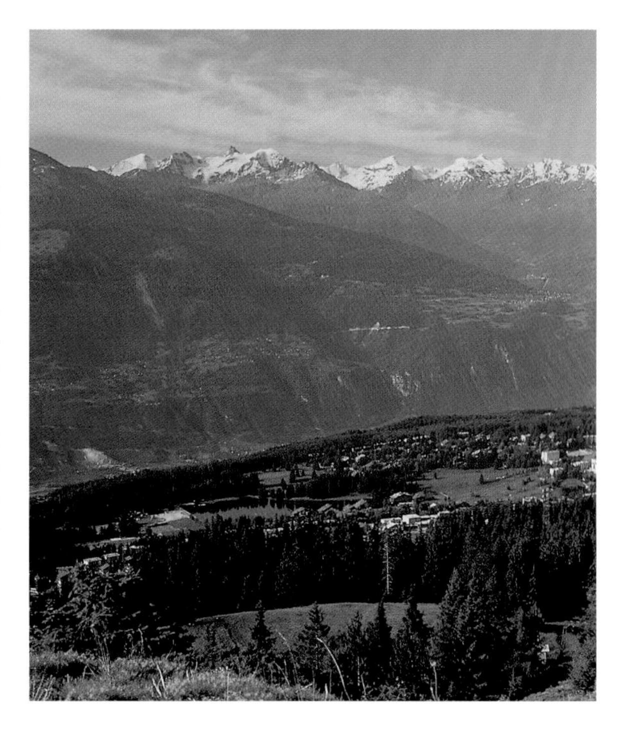

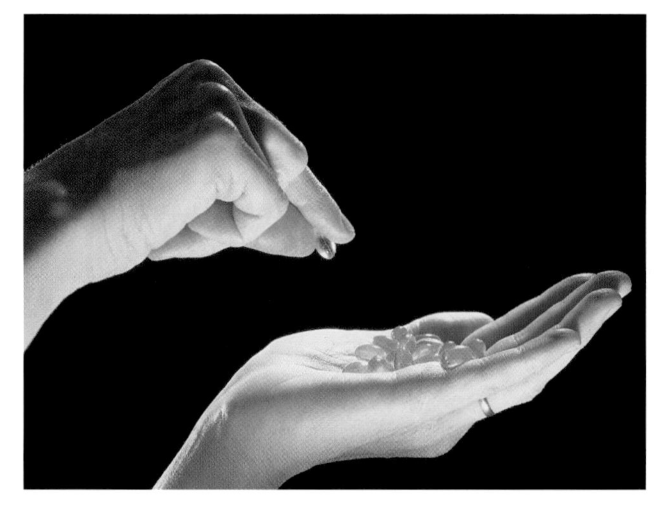

In vegetal remedies, the active components have the advantage of being combined with many other substances that appear to be inactive. However, these complementary components give the plant as a whole a safety and efficiency much superior to that of its isolated and pure active components.

Furthermore, the efficiency of medicinal herbs increases when they are used within the frame of natural revitalizing treatment.

A Pioneer of Modern Phytotherapy

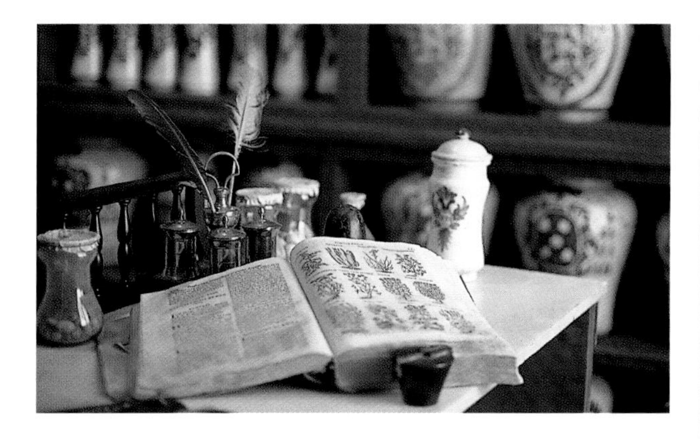

In the late nineteenth and early twentieth centuries, physicians still prescribed medicines based on very energetic chemical substances, some of which were recently discovered and at present are regarded as poisonous: **calomel** or mercuric cyanide (with strongly purgative action), **tartar emetic** (vomitive), **strychnine** (toxic excitant), or **arsenic salts** (against syphilis and other infectious diseases). The developments of the newly-born **chemical and pharmaceutical industry,** both in Europe and in the United States, had brought about great social enthusiasm.

Within that environment of pharmacological euphoria, when all scientific interest was placed on chemically synthesized medicines, Ellen G. White, an outstanding American author with great teaching and preventive ability, wrote: "There are simple herbs that can be used for the recovery of the sick, whose effect upon the system is very different from that of those drugs that poison the blood and endanger life." *

This pioneer of modern phytotherapy recommended the popular use of certain medicinal herbs, such as **hops** infusion (sedative), **foot baths with mustard** (to clear the head), **charcoal** (because of its detoxifying effect), and **pine, cedar,** and **fir trees** (for respiratory diseases).

Besides promoting the rational use of medicinal herbs as an alternative to the aggressive medicinal remedies used at that time, Ellen G. White emphasized a fact currently well-known in medical science, which however was a real novelty a century ago: **Health does not come naturally,** but through a healthy way of life, and especially, from nutrition.

Today, her central idea about health is truer than ever: the intelligent use of **natural agents** such as water, the sun, air, medicinal herbs, healthy food, as well as the adoption of healthy habits (physical exercise, adequate rest, good mental health, and trust in God) may do more for health than all powerful, chemically synthesized medicines or aggressive treatments.

---

* Selected Messages, Book 2, p. 288, Review & Herald Publishing Association, Washington D.C., 1958.

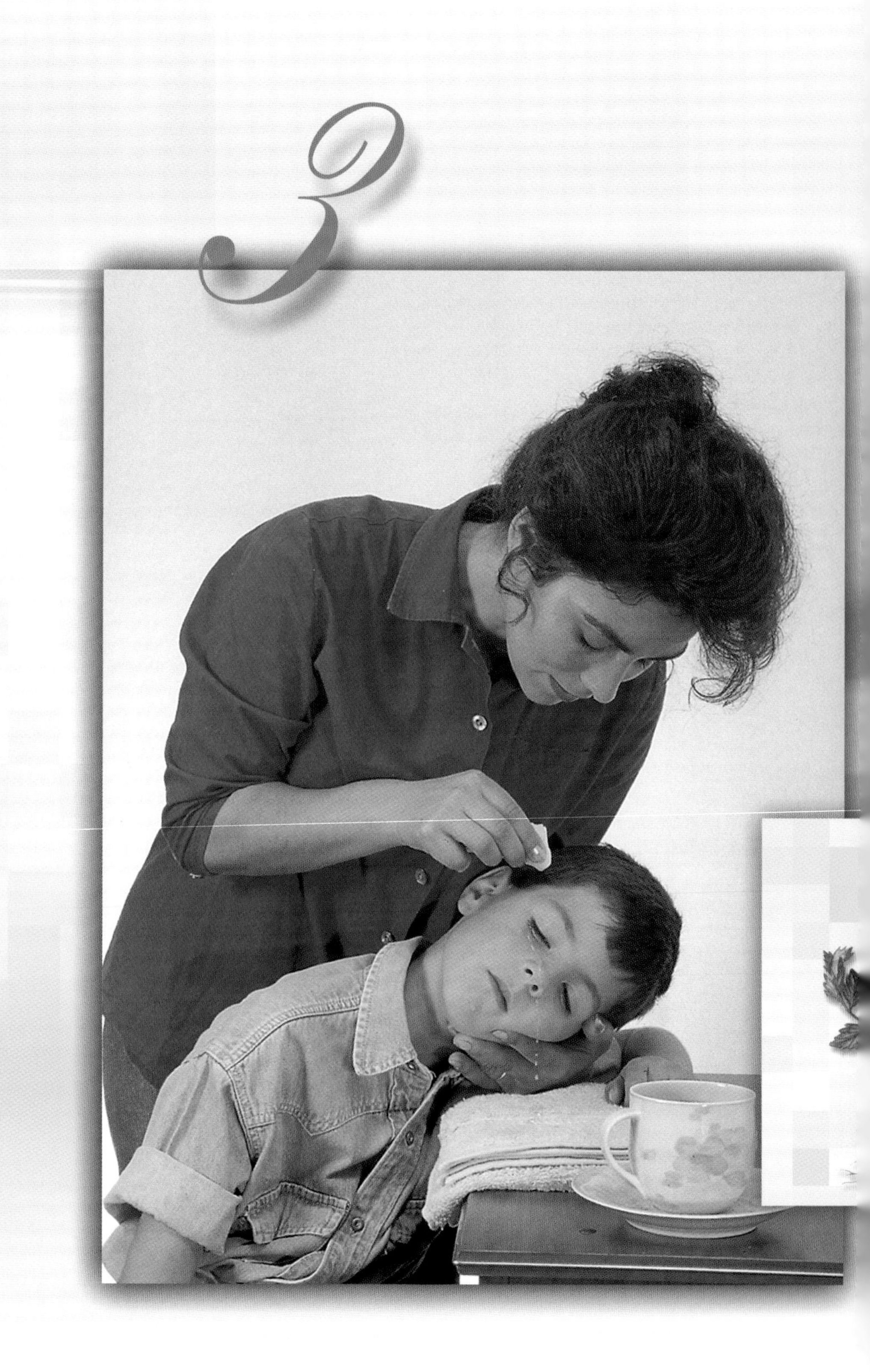

Plants for the Eyes

DISEASES	PAGES
Blepharitis	59
Conjunctivitis and blepharitis	59
Eyelids, inflammation, see Conjunctivitis and blepharitis	59
Keratitis	58
Sty	58

PLANTS	PAGES
Cornflower	60
Herb Robert	63
Red eyebright	62

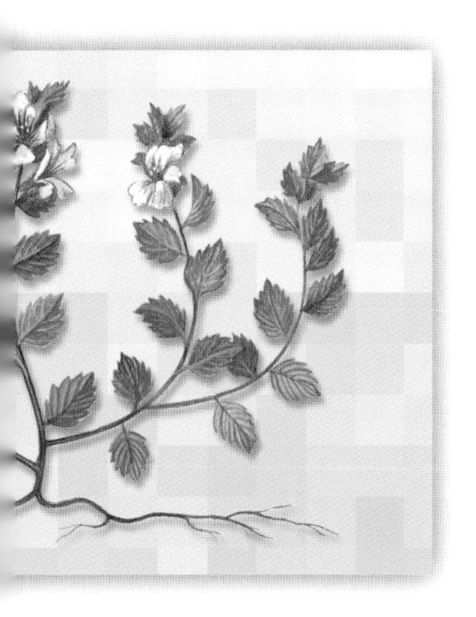

MEDICINAL plants contribute to the proper functioning of the eyes through two mechanisms: ***locally*** applied on the eyes, they have an **antiseptic and anti-inflammatory** effect, which is useful for eye hygiene, and in the case of conjunctivitis or other infectious or inflammatory afflictions of the anterior pole of the eye.

When they are ***consumed orally,*** some medicinal herbs supply **vitamin A and anthocyanines,** which improve visual acuity.

Vitamin A is also needed for the proper functioning of the retinal cells, which are sensitive to light processes.

Anthocyanines are substances of a glycosidic nature which give their typical blue color to some flowers and fruits. They have antiseptic and anti-inflammatory action, and exert a protective action on the capillaries, especially on those of the retina. These substances thus improve blood circulation in the retina. Moreover, anthocyanines favor the production of light-sensitive pigment in the retinal cells.

Therefore, when consumed internally, plants containing vitamin A and anthocyanines improve visual acuity and night vision.

KERATITIS

Keratitis is the inflammation of the cornea, a transparent disc approximately one millimeter thick, which covers the anterior part of the eyeball. Its seriousness depends on the fact that an inflamed cornea may become opaque and make vision more difficult. Apart from ***specialized treatment,*** these plants, as well as those used for **conjunctivitis,** are recommended.

RED EYEBRIGHT	Antiseptic and anti-inflammatory
CAMOMILE	Useful for eye baths
THYME	Disinfectant and antiviral

STY

Sties are little furuncles that appear on the edge of the eyelids. The aim of the treatment is to make them ripe and open. Plants that have been recommended for **conjunctivitis** may be also applied, if possible in compresses over the eyelids.

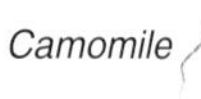

Camomile

CORNFLOWER	Anti-inflammatory
OAK TREE	Anti-inflammatory
CAMOMILE	Useful for eye baths

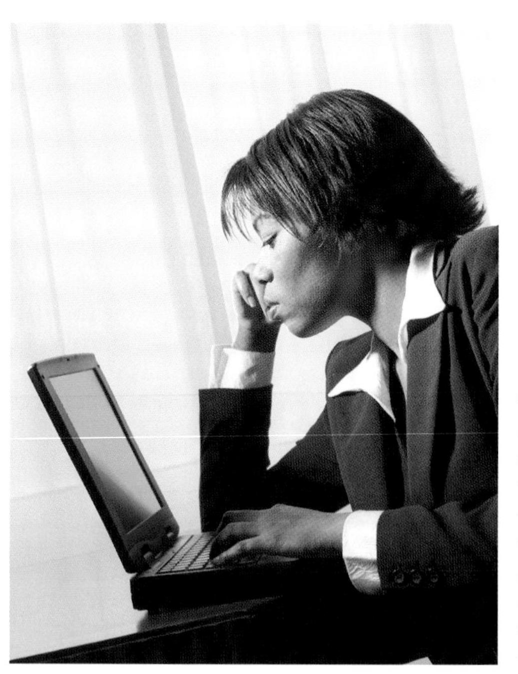

The plants most used to irrigate the eyes in case of irritation, itching, or eye fatigue due to eyestrain (for instance, those persons who work with computers) are the following: cornflower, red eyebright, witch hazel, camomile and rose.

Irrigation and compresses with these plants help make the circles under the eyes disappear, and make the eyes more beautiful, bestowing a clear and shimmering gaze.

CONJUNCTIVITIS AND BLEPHARITIS

Definition

The conjunctiva is a delicate membrane which connects the eyeball and inner eyelid. It is usually transparent, but when it is irritated or inflamed **(conjunctivitis)** it turns a blood-red color.

Causes

In most cases, conjunctivitis is produced by microorganisms (viruses or bacteria), and worsens on being exposed to smoke, dust, polluted water or excessive light. To strain one's eyes may also produce irritation or congestion of the conjunctiva.

Phytotherapy

Phytotherapeutic healing is based on the local application of ***anti-inflammatory, emollient, and antiseptic*** plants. All emollient plants (see chapter 27, page 680) are generally recommended.

In chronic or persistent cases, conjunctivitis may be related to a lack of vitamin A, or to toxicity due to liver or kidney dysfunctions.

Blepharitis

Blepharitis is the technical name for eyelid inflammation. In local application, it is treated with the same plants as conjunctivitis. It is worth paying attention to the lack of nutrients, especially the lack of vitamin A, and of trace elements such as iron.

Witch hazel

CORNFLOWER	Reduces the inflammation of the anterior pole of the eyes
RED EYEBRIGHT	Antiseptic and anti-inflammatory
HERB ROBERT	Astringent (dries the conjunctival mucosa)
OAK TREE	Anti-inflammatory. Very useful for conjunctivitis caused by irritation or allergy
WITCH HAZEL	Sedates and soothes eyes. Alleviates itching caused by dust, smoke, or tiredness
COMMON PLANTAIN	Soothing and anti-inflammatory
GARDEN VIOLET	Soothing. Especially useful for blepharitis
FENNEL	Anti-inflammatory
GERMAN CAMOMILE	Cicatrizant, emollient, and antiseptic
PURSLANE	Emollient and anti-inflammatory
ROSE	Alleviates itching, reduces inflammation, and infection
BRIER HIP	Anti-inflammatory and antiseptic
BLACK ELDER	Soothing and antiseptic

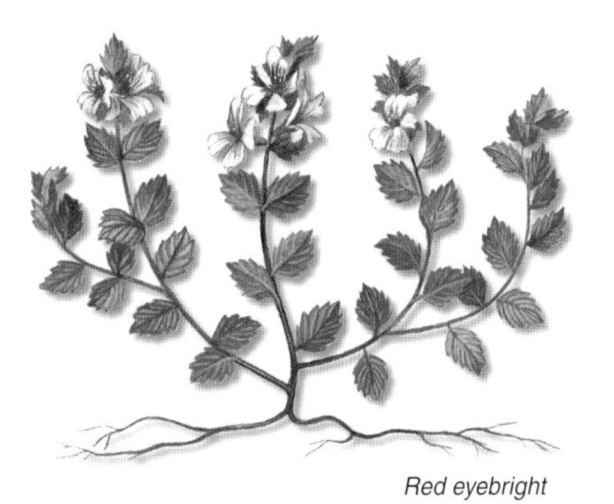

Red eyebright

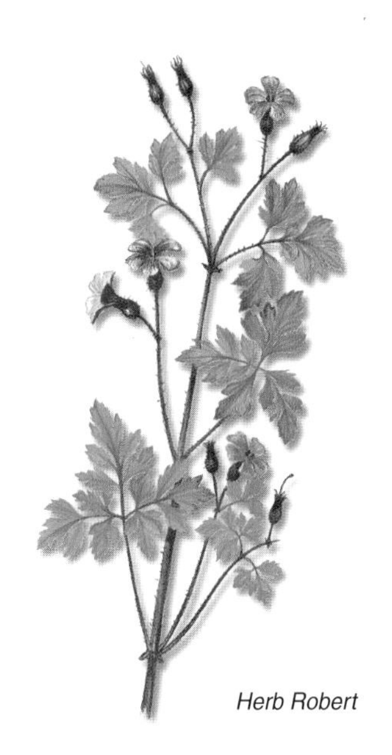

Herb Robert

Cornflower

A good remedy for your eyes

CORNFLOWER covers the golden grain prairies from late Spring onwards with its gracious blue flowers. From ancient times, the seeds of crops have been mixed with cornflower seeds, and have been dispersed all over the world. Pliny the Elder, a first century Roman naturalist, described the cornflower as "an annoying flower for reapers," who surely tried not to cut it with their sickles and scythes. A few other words have reached us from the classical writers about this delicate plant.

Its medicinal virtues were discovered by Mattioli, a sixteenth century botanist who declared that "the blue flowers of the cornflower alleviate reddened eyes." The healing virtues of the plant were due, according to Mattioli, to the combination of opposed colors, blue versus red, in compliance with the theory of signs.

At present, herbicides and selection processes of crops are terminating with cornflower as if it were another weed.

PROPERTIES AND INDICATIONS. ***FLOWERS*** contain anthocyanins and polyines, whose action is **antiseptic** and **anti-inflammatory,** bitter substances which act as **appetizers** and **eupeptics** (that facilitate digestion), and also flavonoids that have a mild **diuretic** effect.

Flowers should be taken in infusions before meals **(❶)**. It is better not to sweeten the infusions.

CORNFLOWER WATER, obtained by the decoction of its flowers, is primarily used in applications on the eyelids, due to its notable **anti-inflammatory** effect.

Eye irrigation and baths with cornflower water ease itching and eye irritation, besides giving a fresh and smooth look to tired eyelids. Thus, in many places this plant is given the name

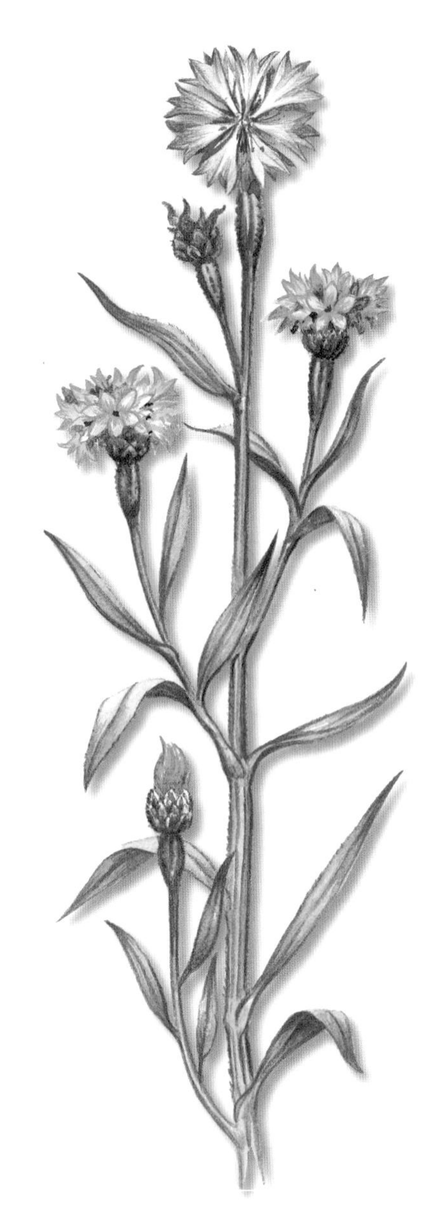

Description. *The plant belongs to the family of the Compositae. It has a thin, stiff stem, which grows up to 50 cm high. It has composite, bright blue-colored flowers, and narrow leaves which appear to be covered with a smooth velvet layer.*

Parts used. *Flowers.*

Preparation and Use

INTERNAL USE

❶ **Infusion.** 20-30 g of young flowers per liter of water. Have one cup before each meal.

EXTERNAL USE

Cornflower water. In order to obtain it, preferably fresh flowers are decocted in a proportion of 30 g (2 tablespoons) per liter of water. Boil for five minutes. It is applied on eyes when warm, in one of the following ways:

❷ **Compresses.** Soak a gauze and maintain it for 15 minutes over the affected eye, twice or three times a day.

❸ **Eye bath.** In an suitable container, or simply wringing out a soaked cloth over the affected eye. Cornflower water must fall from the temple to the nose.

❹ **Eye drops.** A few drops of cornflower water into the eye, three times a day.

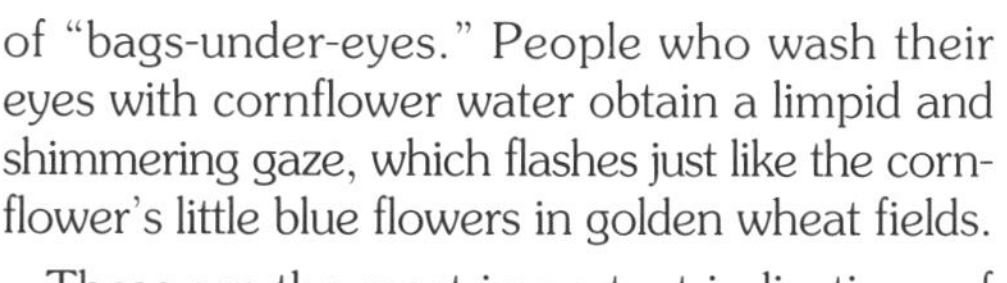

of "bags-under-eyes." People who wash their eyes with cornflower water obtain a limpid and shimmering gaze, which flashes just like the cornflower's little blue flowers in golden wheat fields.

These are the most important indications of cornflower water.

- **Conjunctivitis** (inflammation of the mucous membrane that covers the anterior part of eyes) {❷,❸,❹}. Eye cleansing with cornflower water, as well as eye drops, will help to eliminate eye secretions (sleep) and to make eye congestion disappear.
- **Blepharitis** (inflammation of the eyelids) and **styes** (little furuncles which appear in the edge of the eyelids) {❷,❸}. In this case, the application of cornflower water in compresses or in eye baths is recommended.

In ancient times, the cornflower was supposed to clear and preserve vision, although only that of blue-eyed people. Thus, in French this plant is called *casselunettes* (glasses-breaker). Today we know that this was merely a myth, nevertheless we should remember that cornflower is good for the eyes.

Cornflower flowers contain anthocyanins, which have antiseptic and anti-inflammatory action. Their infusion produces an improvement in the blood circulation in the retinal capillaries, besides having appetizing and eupeptic effects.

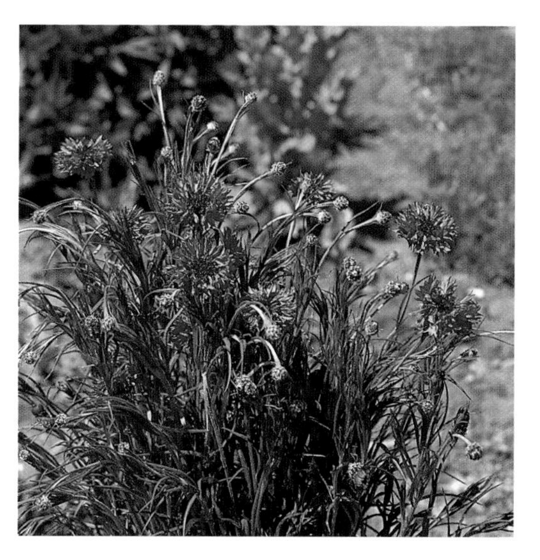

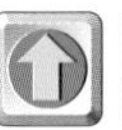
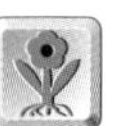
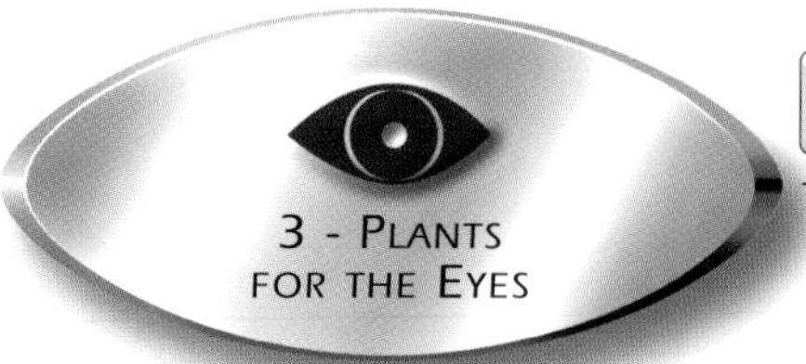

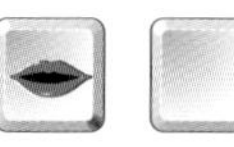
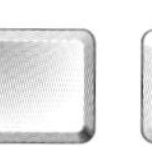

Red Eyebright

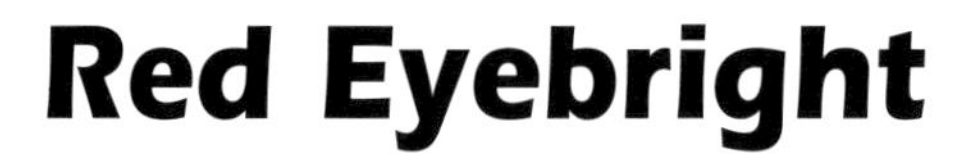

Ideal for eye baths

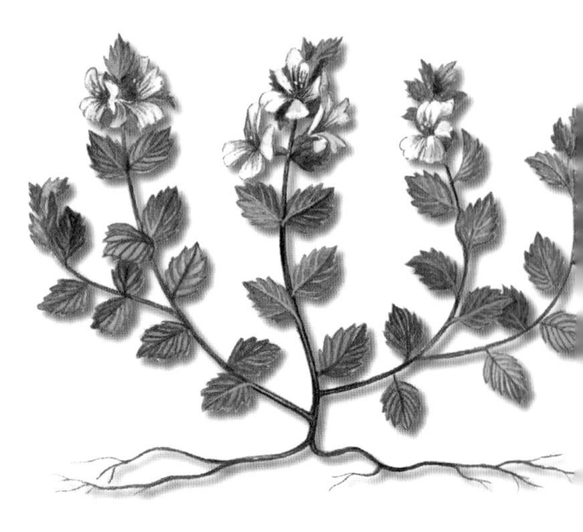

PROPERTIES AND INDICATIONS. The whole plant contains the glycoside substance aucubine, as well as tannins, phenolic acids, flavonoids, vitamins A and C, and traces of essences. It has **antiseptic, anti-inflammatory and astringent** properties, which are especially effective on the conjunctival mucosa.

It has been used since the Middle Ages and onwards to heal **conjunctivitis, blepharitis** (inflammation of the eyelids), superficial **keratitis** (inflammation of the cornea) and eye **tearing [❶,❷]**. Washing **sleepy eyes** with red eyebright renders good results. Besides cleansing secretions, it reduces the inflammation and dries the conjunctiva.

It is also applied as gargles and mouth rinses in cases of **stomatitis** (inflammation of the oral mucosa) and **pharyngitis [❸]**, as well as in nasal irrigations for **rhinitis [❹]** (inner nasal inflammation).

Description. *Annual herb of the family of the Scrophulariaceae, growing from 10 to 30 cm high. Its flowers are white with purple lines and their corolla is formed by two lips. It is a parasite which feeds on the roots of other plants.*

Parts used. *The whole plant.*

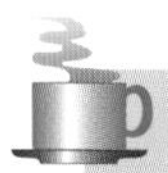

Preparation and Use

EXTERNAL USE

Infusion with 40 g of plant per liter of water. It has diverse applications.

❶ **Eye irrigation.** Let the liquid drop from the outside inwards, that is, from the temple to the nose. Eye baths should be done mainly in the morning.

❷ **Eyedrops.** 5-10 drops in each eye, four times a day.

❸ **Gargles and rinses.** In cases of oral or pharyngeal conditions.

❹ **Nasal irrigations,** in case of rhinitis or coryza.

Red eyebright is found in the mountainous regions of Europe and America.

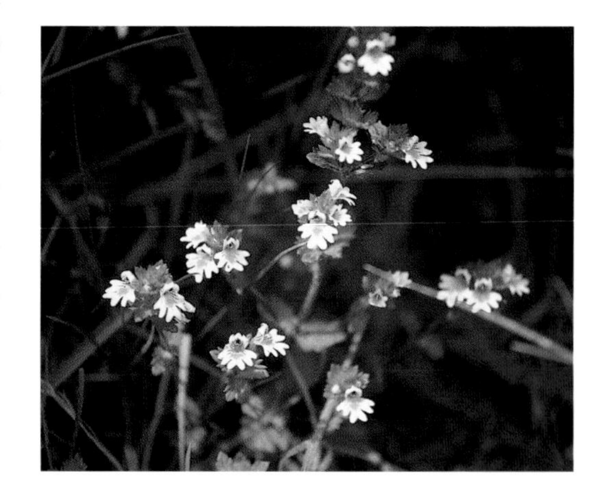

Herb Robert

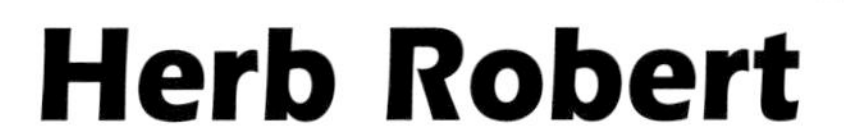

Cleans eyes and reduces mouth inflammation

TAKE CARE with this plant, which may be mistaken for poison hemlock. Both plants have unpleasant smells, and very similar leaves. However, Herb Robert is easy to identify because of its rose-colored flowers, and its dried fruits, which are lamp-shaped.

PROPERTIES AND INDICATIONS. The whole plant contains a bitter substance (geraniine), an essential oil which gives the plant its typical aroma, as well as important amounts of tannin which determine its astringent action. When ***used internally,*** it has **astringent, diuretic, and blood thinning** properties, as well as acting as a mild hypoglycemic. It is used in cases of **diarrhea, edema** (liquid retention), and as a complement in a **diabetic** diet [❶,❷].

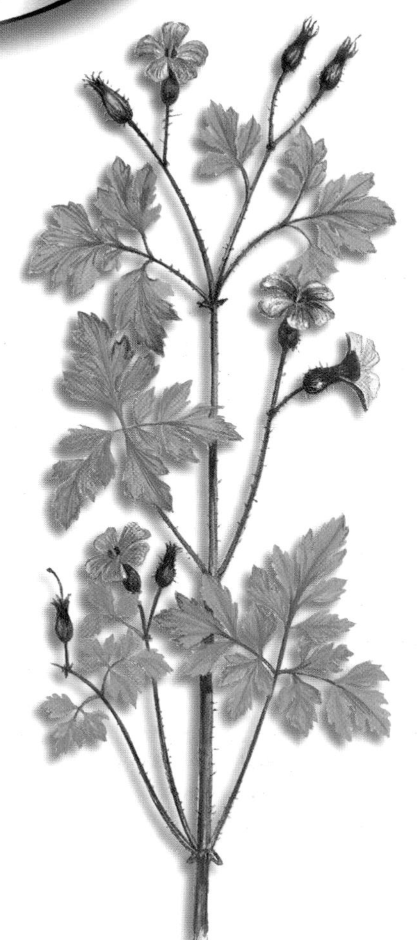

Description. *Herbaceous plant of the family of the Geraniaceae, growing from 20 to 60 cm high. The whole plant has a reddish color, with a typically unpleasant smell. Its flowers are pink, and appear in pairs.*

Parts used. *The whole plant.*

At present it is mainly ***used externally,*** because of its **astringent and vulnerary** (healing) properties, in the following cases:

- **Eye afflictions:** eye irritation, eye drainage, conjunctivitis [❸].
- **Mouth afflictions:** stomatitis, pharyngitis, gingivitis [❸].
- **Skin eruptions:** herpes, shingles, eczemas and skin inflammations [❹].

Preparation and Use

INTERNAL USE

❶ **Decoction** with 20 g of plant per liter of water, drinking three or four cups a day.

❷ **Essence.** The usual dose is two to four drops, three times a day.

EXTERNAL USE

❸ Eye and mouth **rinses,** with a decoction of 40 g of plant per liter of water.

❹ **Compresses,** with the same decoction (40 g per liter).

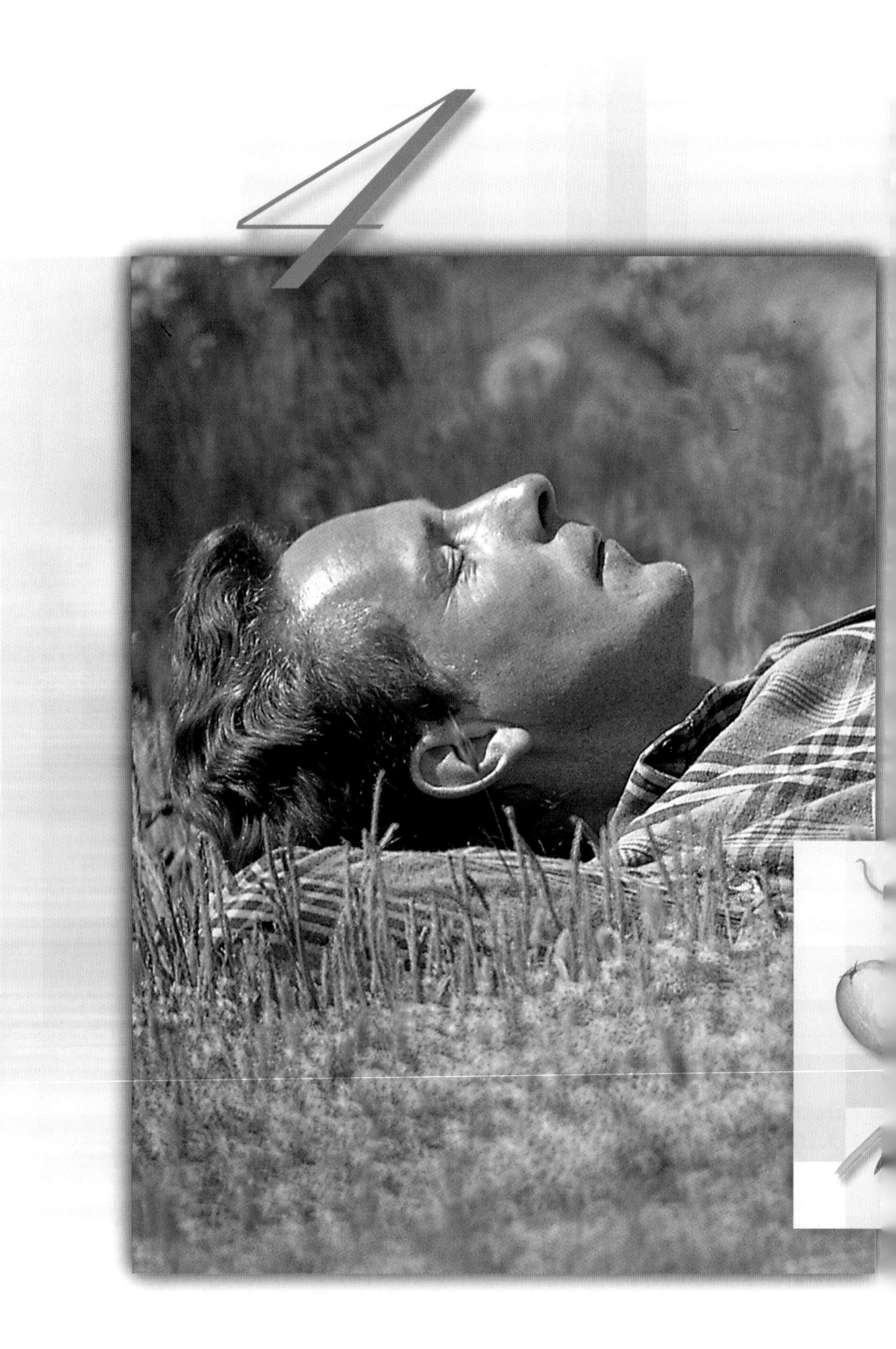

Plants for the Nervous System

DISEASES	PAGES
Aches and Neuralgia	69
Analgesic plants, see Aches and neuralgia	69
Anxiety	67
Cephalalgia, see Headaches	69
Depression, nervousness	66
Epilepsy	69
Fatigue and asthenia	67
Headaches	69
Insomnia	68
Insufficient intellectual performance	66
Memory, loss of	67
Migraine	68
Nervous tension, see Stress	68
Nervousness and anxiety	67
Neuralgia	69
Organic diseases of the nervous system	69
Psychosomatic diseases	68
Stress	68

PLANTS	PAGES
Balm	76
Blue vervain	84
Hops	72
Lavender	74
Linden	80
Orange tree	70
Passion flower	78
Pricky lettuce	73
Purple passion flower	79
Valerian	82
Vervain	84

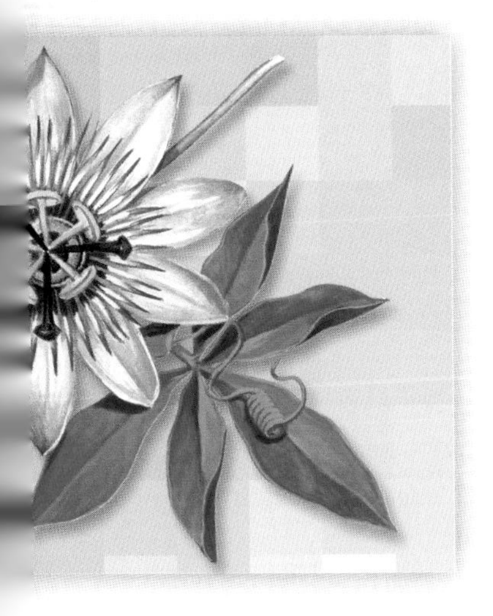

Medicinal herbs exert notable actions both on the central nervous system, on which our mental functions are based, and on the autonomic nervous system, which regulates and coordinates the activity of the diverse organs of the body.

Unlike most psycho-pharmaceutical products (medicines which act on mental functions), plants exert their invigorating and sedative effects on the nervous system in a physiological, mild, and safe way.

Moreover, it is very unlikely that the use of the medicinal herbs we recommend may cause any kind of physical or psychological dependence, unlike stimulants, sedatives, narcotics and other chemically synthesized medicines.

Chemical medicines indeed have a more powerful effect than medicinal herbs, although they present a higher degree of side effects and risks. In the case of acute nervous excitation, for instance, a psycho-pharmacological product with sedative or anxiolytic action (which eliminates anxiety) may produce a quick and even spectacular effect, though it will likely be accompanied by undesirable side effects quite soon after, such as uncoordinated motor skills and drowsiness.

On the other hand, plants act on the body by regulating and balancing its vital processes, rather than stopping or combating certain symptoms. Thus, they have a genuine balancing effect on the complex nervous and mental systems, and prevent disorders and unbalanced mental conditions.

Fatigue and Asthenia

Fatigue and asthenia (excessive tiredness) are two of the most frequent illnesses of Western society, strongly conditioned by concepts such as productivity and work. The nervous system, which acts as the "director" of organic functions, is in charge of maintaining the vital tone which allows us to carry out our daily activities. Enhancing that vital tone is one of the most urgent needs of many persons who suffer from nervous fatigue, asthenia or stress. Therefore, they often take stimulant or excitant substances which, besides producing a momentary effect, also produce further tiredness after their effects have passed.

To treat fatigue and asthenia, two types of medicinal herbs should be administered:

- **Nutritive** plants, which provide basic nutrients that are normally absent in diets, and that nervous cells need for their proper functioning: vitamins and trace elements.
- **Invigorating** plants, which contribute as a physiological, non-irritating stimulus to the nervous system function, as well as to the rest of the bodily functions.

INSUFFICIENT INTELLECTUAL PERFORMANCE

Treatment

Plants rich in essential fatty acids such as linoleic acid, pectin, B vitamins, and minerals such as phosphorus, favor good intellectual performance. Also convenient, though not to be taken continuously, are non-excitant **invigorating** plants such as ginseng or thyme. Students and all people with intense intellectual demands may benefit from their use.

WALNUT	Supplies essential fatty acids, phosphorus and B vitamins
GINSENG	Invigorator, increases the ability to concentrate and improves memory
THYME	Stimulates intellectual performance and mental activity

DEPRESSION, NERVOUSNESS

Definition

It is a psychological state of melancholy and deep sadness, with or without any evident cause, as well as a loss of appetite, insomnia, and a propensity to inactivity.

Phytotherapy

We recommend those plants with **an invigorating and balancing** action on the nervous system, as well as those which add nutritive substances such as vitamin B or lecithin. **Stimulant or excitant** plants or substances **must not be used** in the treatment of depression.

Balm

BALM	Balances the nervous system
VALERIAN	Mild sedative, decreases anxiety
MOTHER OF THYME	Invigorating and revitalizing
GINSENG	Antidepressant and anxiolytic
SAGE	Stimulates suprarenal gland function
ST. JOHNSWORT	Invigorator and nervous system stabilizer
THYME	General invigorator. Stimulates intellectual performance

FATIGUE AND ASTHENIA

Definition

Fatigue is weakness of the body subsequent to excessive effort, which is not accompanied by the necessary recovery of the affected organs or systems.

Causes

Physical fatigue is usually preceded by a high muscular effort or a serious disease. **Nervous tiredness** may appear after a period of sustained high intellectual activity, or prolonged nervous tension.

Physical and nervous fatigue are closely related to one another, one appearing as consequence of the other, and vice-versa.

Asthenia is the lack or loss of strength and energy which appears spontaneously, with no direct relation to any previous effort.

GARLIC	Activates metabolism
WATERCRESS	Increases appetite and activates metabolism
SPIRULA	Nutrient, invigorating, revitalizing
MOTHER OF THYME	Invigorating and revitalizing
PEPPERMINT	Invigorator
BASIL	Invigorator, increases blood pressure
WINTER SAVORY	Invigorator for the nervous system
GINSENG	Improves physical performance
DAMIANA	Nervous system invigorator
ROSEMARY	General invigorator
ALOE	Invigorator, stimulates body defenses
BRIER HIP	Invigorator, antiscorbutic
THYME	General invigorator. Stimulates intellectual performance

LOSS OF MEMORY

Phytotherapy

Besides the two plants with vasodilating action on the cerebral arteries (improving blood circulation to the brain), all plants used for **insufficient intellectual performance** are also recommended.

GINKGO	Improves blood flowing into the brain

NERVOUSNESS AND ANXIETY

Definition

Nervousness is a state of nervous excitation, whether justified or not.

Anxiety is an undesirable and unjustified emotion whose intensity is not in proportion to its likely cause. Anxiety is different than fear. The latter implies the presence of a known actual danger. Anxiety usually manifests itself externally, in a state of nervous hyperexcitation.

Phytotherapy

Medicinal herbs can be highly effective in combating nervousness and anxiety, sedating and balancing the nervous system.

ORANGE TREE	Sedative and mildly narcotic
HOPS	Sedative and narcotic
PRICKLY LETTUCE	Sedative, calms nervous excitation
LAVENDER	Sedative and balancing on the nervous system
BALM	Mild sedative and stabilizer
PASSION FLOWER	Decreases anxiety
LINDEN	Sedative and relaxing
VALERIAN	Mild sedative, decreases anxiety
HAWTHORN	Sedative on the autonomic nervous system, anxiolytic
EVENING PRIMROSE	Helps balancing the nervous system and the hormonal balance
MARJORAM	Sedative, alleviates anxiety
LEMON VERBENA	Alleviates anxiety
WHITE WILLOW	Sedative, mildly narcotic

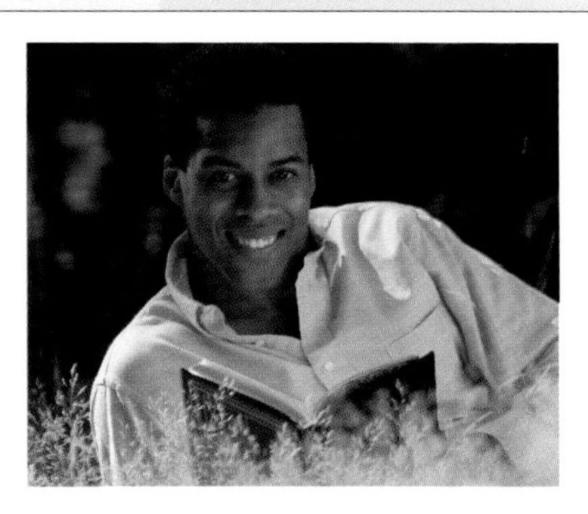

STRESS

Phytotherapy

The phytotherapeutic healing of stress consists of the combination of two kinds of plants, **invigorating** herbs which augment vital energy to confront daily stressful situations, and **balancing or sedative** plants in order to soften the organic response to certain stressful situations.

Besides the aforementioned plants, we recommend invigorating herbs such as Winter savory, peppermint, or rosemary, and balancing ones such as hawthorn.

BALM	Mild sedative and stabilizer
PASSION FLOWER	Decreases anxiety
LINDEN	Relaxing, tranquilizer
GINSENG	Invigorator
DAMIANA	Invigorating and revitalizing
ROSE	Sedative of the autonomic nervous system

MIGRAINE

Definition

An intense headache which usually affects half the head and appears periodically, related to eye dysfunctions.

Phytotherapy

During a migraine crisis there is a spasm of the arteries which feed blood to the head, hence **antispasmodic** plants are useful. In many cases, migraine crises are caused by digestive fermentation or certain foods.

ORANGE TREE	Antispasmodic and sedative
LINDEN	Prevents migraine crises
VERVAIN	Antispasmodic, analgesic, decreases migraine intensity
GARDEN VIOLET	Anti-inflammatory, calms headaches
BASIL	Antispasmodic, calms migraines related to indigestion
MILK THISTLE	Regulates the tone of blood vessels
SPEEDWELL	Digestive, invigorator, alleviates migraine with a digestive cause

INSOMNIA

Definition

Insomnia is chronic sleeplessness, either due to difficulties in falling asleep or continuous awakening.

Treatment

Unlike most chemically synthesized narcotics, the medicinal herbs we recommend are able to induce a natural, restorative sleep, with no residual somnolence the morning after, and no risk of addiction.

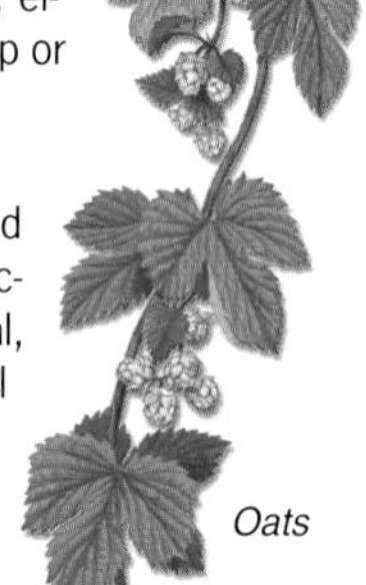

Oats

ORANGE TREE	Sedative and mild narcotic
HOPS	Sedative and narcotic
PRICKLY LETTUCE	Sedative, calms nervous excitation
LAVENDER	Sedative, calms excitation
BALM	Mild sedative and stabilizer
PASSION FLOWER	Sedative, induces a natural sleep
LINDEN	Induces a natural sleep, without sleepiness the morning after
VALERIAN	Mild sedative, decreases anxiety, narcotic
WHITE WILLOW	Sedative, mild narcotic

PSYCHOSOMATIC DISEASES

Definition

The diseases of psychological origin, at least in part, but which manifest themselves as functional alterations in multiple organs. Some of the most frequent psychosomatic diseases are: **gastric ulcer, irritation of the colon, heart attacks,** and certain skin **eczemas.**

Phytotherapy

These plants balance and modify the autonomic nervous system, which is the true pillar of the relationship between mind and body.

LAVENDER	Sedative central and autonomic nervous system stabilizer
VALERIAN	Sedative, decreases anxiety
ROSE	Sedative of the autonomic system

ACHES AND NEURALGIA

Phytotherapy

Orange tree

These analgesic plants act either internally, when taken, or externally, when locally applied to the skin. Their action is not usually as quick and intense as that of chemically synthesized analgesics, or those made from pure substances. However, the effects of these plants are longer and generally lack most undesirable side effects.

Neuralgia

Neuralgia is a special type of ache, whose features are intensity, intermittence and localization in the trajectory of a nerve. The phytotherapeutic treatment especially includes **preventive action.**

ORANGE TREE	Antispasmodic and sedative. Useful against migraine
HOPS	Calms stomach ache and neuralgia
PASSION FLOWER	Antispasmodic, calms muscle tightness and neuralgia
VALERIAN	Analgesic for sciatica and neuralgia
VERVAIN	Analgesic for rheumatic aches and neuralgia
MEADOWSWEET	Analgesic and anti-inflammatory for osteomuscular aches and neuralgia

HEADACHES (cephalalgias)

Causes

Headaches or **cephalalgias** have many sources. The most usual are:

- **Congestion,** that is, excessive accumulation of blood in the head. Thus, **revulsive** plants such as mustard are used. These plants deviate blood to other areas.
- **Lack of blood** in the head, thus the use of **vasodilating** plants is recommended.
- **Bad digestion** or gall **bladder** dysfunctions. **Digestive and cholagogue** plants are used.

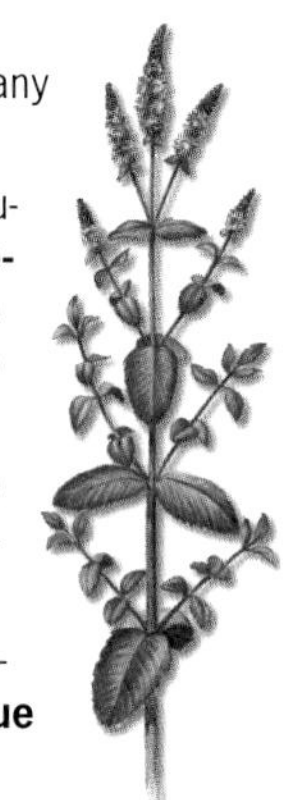

Peppermint

BALM	Antispasmodic and sedative. Calms headaches caused by nervous tension
GINKGO	Vasodilator, enhances blood flow to the brain
PEPPERMINT	Invigorator and digestive
BOLDO	Normalizes the functioning of the gall bladder
EUROPEAN PENNYROYAL	Calms headaches with a digestive cause
BLACK MUSTARD	Revulsive, reduces congestion of the head in the case of nose catarrh or influenza

ORGANIC DISEASES OF THE NERVOUS SYSTEM

The oil of the evening primrose is very rich in linoleic acid, an essential factor in the development and correct functioning of the neurons. Its use is a fine **complement** to the specific treatment of the organic diseases of the nervous system, such as the **Parkinson disease** and the **multiple sclerosis.**

EVENING PRIMROSE	Helps balance the nervous system and the hormonal system

Valerian

EPILEPSY

Though these plants **do not substitute** the medical treatment for epilepsy, they may help to reduce the antiepileptic product dosage, and equilibrate the patient.

PASSION FLOWER	Sedative and antispasmodic. Allows to decrease the frequency and intensity of the epileptic crises
VALERIAN	Sedative, antispasmodic, and anticonvulsive, prevents epileptic attacks to appear

Orange Tree

The flowers are sedative, the fruits are invigorating

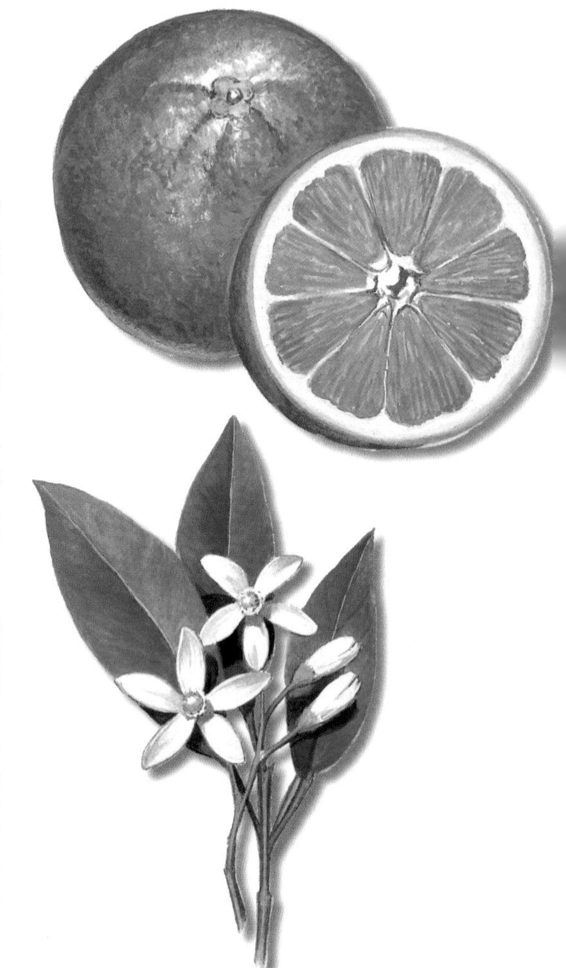

SINCE THE ORANGE tree arrived on the Mediterranean coast of southern Europe, from the Middle East and Asia in Ancient Times, its success has never decreased. Its elegant shape, the rich aroma of its flowers, and over all the excellence of its fruit—as with sweet oranges—made it conquer the fields and tables of the whole world.

A few years after Columbus reached America, Spaniards took the orange tree there, more specifically to Mexico, Florida and California, where we currently find the largest orange orchards in the world.

PROPERTIES AND INDICATIONS. The whole tree is rich in aromatic essences with medicinal effects, though the highest concentration is found in its flowers.

The sweet orange is the most known and cultivated of its varieties. However, the orange tree most often used in phytotherapy is the bitter or sour one, because even though both types of orange trees offer the same properties, the bitter orange has a higher concentration of aromatic substances and active components.

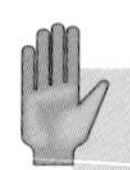

Warning

*Those persons suffering from **gall bladder** dysfunction should avoid **breakfast** oranges. Due to their cholagogue action, they provoke quick emptying of the gall bladder, which may produce slight abdominal upsets such as a feeling of bloatedness in the stomach and a sensation of distension.*

***Description.** A tree with thorns on its branches, of the Rutaceae family, growing up from 2 to 5 m high. Its evergreen leaves bear a small winged heart-shaped petiole. Flowers are white, and grow on the axis of leaves. Its fruits are the well-known oranges.*

***Parts used.** Leaves, flowers and fruits (especially those of the sweet orange tree.*
See table on next page).

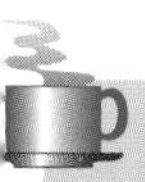

Preparation and Use

INTERNAL USE

❶ **Infusion** of leaves and/or flowers, 10-20 g per liter of water (three leaves or six flowers are enough to prepare a sedative infusion). Drink three or four cups daily, especially before going to bed.

❷ **Decoction.** Boil 30 g of dry rind, cut into pieces, in half a liter of water for 15 minutes. It may be sweetened with honey. Drink a cup after each meal.

The ***LEAVES***, and generally the ***FLOWERS*** of orange tree, known in some countries by the name of *azahar* (from Arabic *az-zahar*, which means white flower) contain an essence composed of limonene and linalol, among other aromatic substances. To these substances it owes its **sedative, antispasmodic and** slightly **somniferous** (producing sleepiness) action. Its use is recommended in the following cases:

- **Insomnia** [❶]: it provides mild sedation, which makes it easier to fall asleep.
- **Nervousness and irritability** [❶]: it renders good results in these cases, without the danger of addiction or other bad side effects. It may be taken even by children, whom it tranquilizes, producing calm sleep.
- **Migraines** caused by arterial spasms [❶].
- **Digestive dysfunction:** stomach spasms and gastric pain of a nervous origin (nerves in stomach), as well as aerophagia and belching [❶].
- **Heart palpitations, fainting and weakness.** Orange blossoms are part, along with the melissa, of the famous Carmel water.
- **Menstrual pain,** caused by uterine spasms [❶].

Orange blossom essence is extracted from the flowers, and the essence called ***petitgrain*** is extracted from the leaves.

The ***RIND*** of the fruits [❷], especially that of bitter oranges, is rich in flavonoid glycosides (naringine, hesperidine and rhutine), whose action is similar to that of vitamin P. Thus, it is used in cases of **capillary and vascular weakness** (edema, varicose veins, blood clotting dysfunction). It is a good **digestive tonic**, with an appetizer effect, and it aids in digestion. It also has a slight **sedative** effect, like the flowers and leaves.

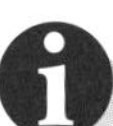

Orange

*The sweet orange is one of the most appreciated fruits, throughout cold countries, since it is a source of **vitamin C** in Winter. It is directly eaten, or its juice drunk, which is delicious. Orange **juice** must be drunk **immediately after being prepared,** in order to take advantage of all its medicinal and nutritive properties. The vitamin C is quickly destroyed when in contact with oxygen, as well as other components which undergo unfavorable changes that notably alter their aspect and flavor. Thus, vitamin C is usually added to industrial orange juices, though this does not recreate all the original properties.*

*Oranges contain vitamins A, B, C, and P, as well as flavonoids, sugars, organic acids and mineral salts. They have **antiscorbutic** (preventing scurvy), **invigorating, appetizing and cholagogue** properties (provoking the emptying of gall bladder). They are recommended in the following cases:*

- ***Infectious diseases or fever.***
- ***Fatigue, asthenia** (sensation of tiredness).*
- ***Malnutrition, anemia, rickets.***
- ***Thrombosis, arteriosclerosis and circulation dysfunctions** in general. Oranges diminish blood viscosity, and produce a protective effect on blood vessels, due to vitamin P, among other substances.*

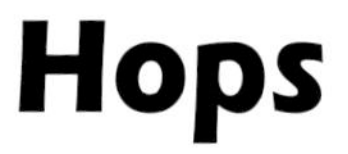

Hops

Calms nerves and tones up the stomach

THE ROMAN NATURALIST Pliny the Elder christened this plant with the name of *Lupulus*, because it overgrows the gardens where it grows, as if it were a *Lupus* (the Latin word for wolf). From the Middle Age on, lupulin has been used to give aroma and preserve beer, and many additional properties have been discovered since then.

PROPERTIES AND INDICATIONS. *LUPULIN*, a powder which falls when the hop cones are shaken, contains an essence that is rich in terpenic hydrocarbons, is what provides this powder with its **sedative** and **narcotic** (which induces sleep) actions. It also contains a resin with bitter ingredients, which explain its tonic, **digestive, and appetizer** action. The cones also contain flavonoids, which are substances with **estrogenic and antiseptic** action. It is used in the following cases:

- **Nervous states, insomnia, migraine.** [❶,❷].
- **Difficult digestion and lack of appetite** [❶].
- **Stomach ache, neuralgic** pain [❸,❹], ***externally*** applied in the form of compresses or poultices.

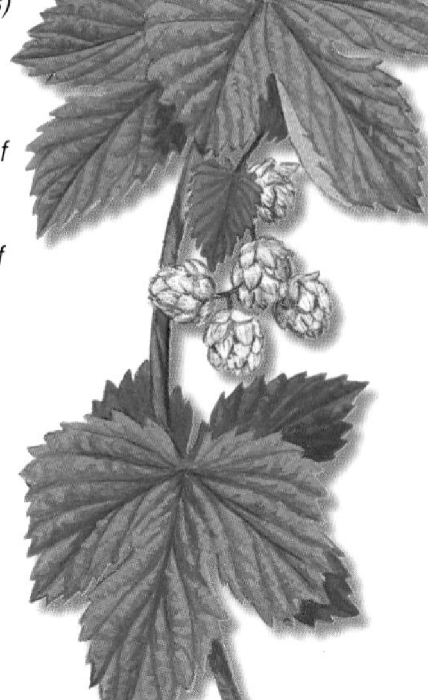

Description. *Vivacious vine, of the Cannabinaceae family, whose stem may reach up to six meters. It is a dioicous plant, whose female plants produce globular flowers that take a conic shape (cones or catkins) when the fruit ripens.*

Parts used. *Cones (flowers of the hops plant) and lupulin (the golden powder of these fruits).*

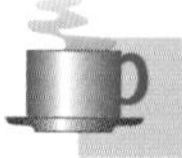

Preparation and Use

INTERNAL USE

❶ **Infusion** with 10-20 g of cones per liter of water, drinking three or four cups daily.

❷ **Dry extract.** Up to 2 daily grams distributed over two or three intakes.

EXTERNAL USE

❸ Warm **compresses** with the same infusion of hop cones as described for internal use. These compresses are applied over the aching area.

❹ **Poultices.** These are prepared by putting a handful of hop cones on a cotton cloth, and wrapping them. Then soak the gauze in warm water, and apply it over the aching area (it is usually employed on the stomach).

Prickly Lettuce

Sedative and sleep inductive

FARMED LETTUCE, when it is green, completely grown and mature (wild lettuce is even better) it is a valuable remedy used since ancient times.

PROPERTIES AND INDICATIONS. Its leaves contain chlorophyll, mineral salts, vitamins and a bitter substance. The active components that act on the nervous system, however, are found in the milky latex which springs from the plant's stems when cut. From this latex, and by means of a process called solidification, ***lactucarium*** is obtained.

Prickly lettuce leaves, and especially latex, have the following properties:

- **Sedative [❶,❷,❸],** similar to opium, though unlike this, lettuce does not have any noxious effect, so it may be used even with children, in whom it calms excessive activity and eases sleep.
- **Anaphrodisiac [❶,❷,❸].** It helps control sexual excitation. Dioscorides said that "represses the disorderly appetite for fornication."
- **Antitussive [❶,❷,❸].** Lettuce is especially recommended for irritant coughs and whooping cough.

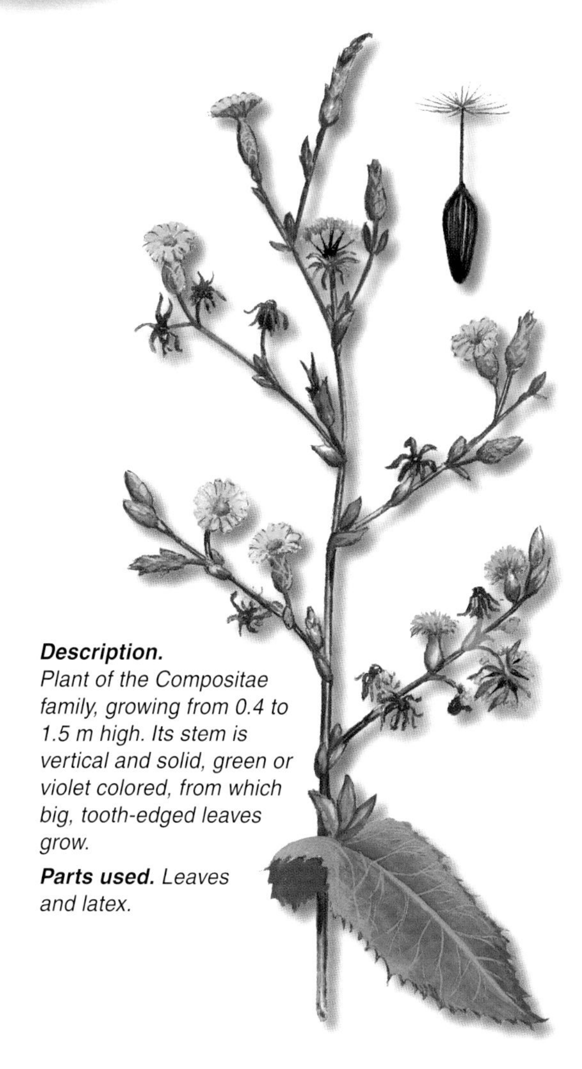

Description. *Plant of the Compositae family, growing from 0.4 to 1.5 m high. Its stem is vertical and solid, green or violet colored, from which big, tooth-edged leaves grow.*

Parts used. *Leaves and latex.*

Preparation and Use

INTERNAL USE

❶ **Decoction,** during ten minutes, with one hundred grams of lettuce per liter of water. Drink three cups, sweetened with honey, every day, and another cup before going to bed. Use wild lettuce, or well grown and blooming, when farmed lettuce.

❷ **Lactucarium.** Usually from 0.1 to 1 g in a daily intake.

❸ **Fresh juice.** Obtained by means of a blender. Drink half a cup two or three times a day, especially before going to bed. It may be mixed with lemon juice.

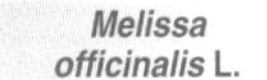

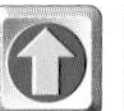
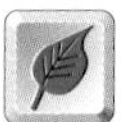
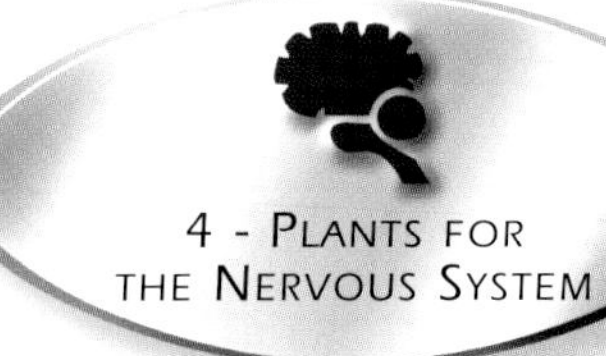

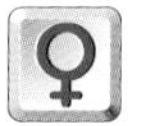
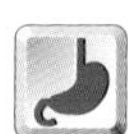
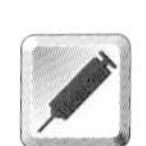
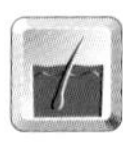

Balm

Balances the nervous system

IBN SINA (*Avicenna*), the great eleventh century Arabic physician, said that balm "has the admirable property of giving comfort and joyfulness." From the early seventeenth century onwards the Barefooted Carmelites prepared the famous "Carmel water" from this plant. This water became a popular remedy for nervous crises, weaknesses and syncopes.

PROPERTIES AND INDICATIONS. The leaves and flowers of the balm contain 0.25% of essential oil that is rich in citral and citronellal aldehydes, to which it owes its **antispasmodic, sedative, carminative** (to reduce flatulence), **digestive, and antiseptic** actions. It is useful in the following cases:

- **Nervous problems [❶,❷]**. Excitation, anxiety, tension headaches (headaches of nervous origin).
- **Stress and depression [❶,❷]**. Balm is often recommended in cases of stress and nervous depression because of its gentle sedative and balancing effects on the nervous system.

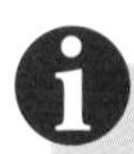

Carmel Water

*Carmel water is **not recommended,** due to its high alcohol content. The author met an old woman who managed to obtain her dose of alcohol in pharmacies by buying several bottles of Carmel water which she frantically drank.*

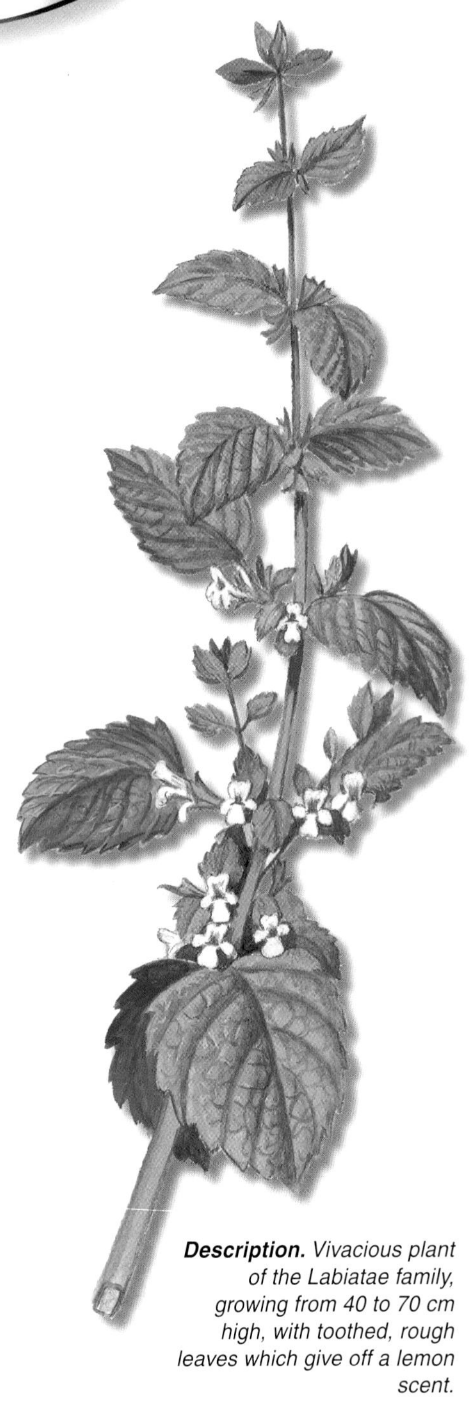

Description. *Vivacious plant of the Labiatae family, growing from 40 to 70 cm high, with toothed, rough leaves which give off a lemon scent.*

Parts used. *Leaves and flowers.*

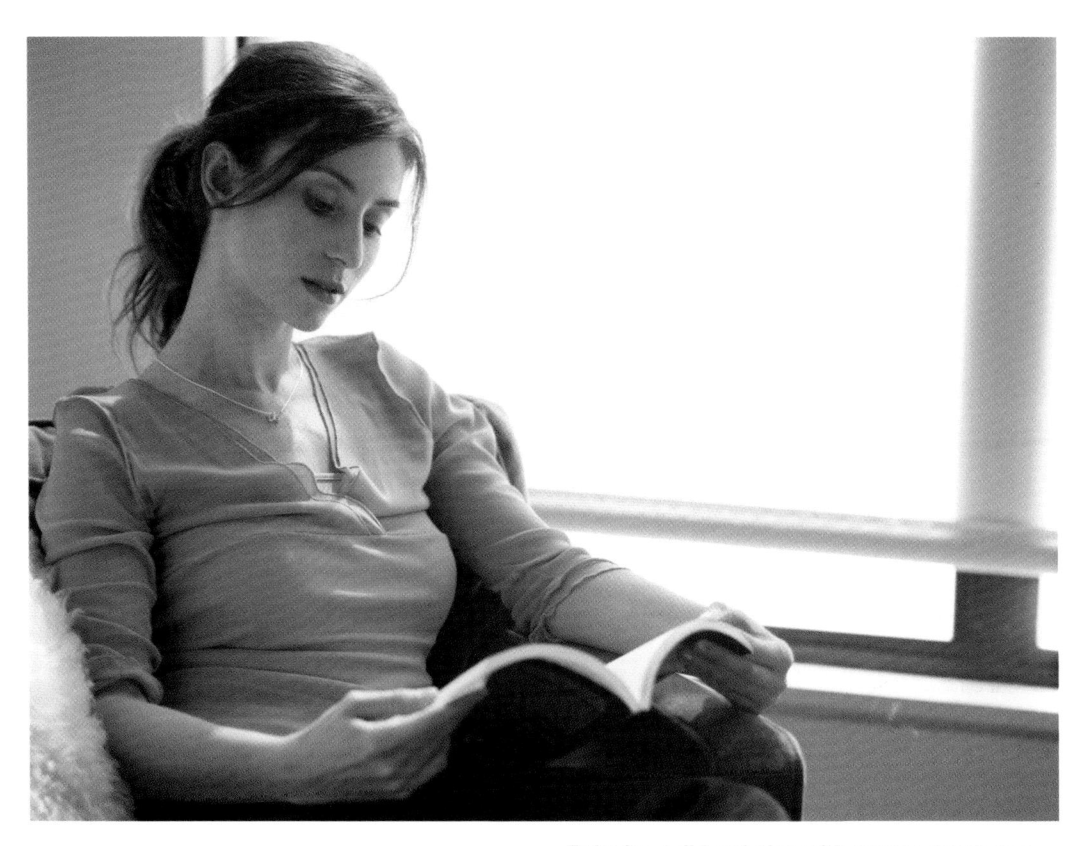

Balm is a mild sedative with many advantages over the chemical drugs: among them, that it does not create addiction, anad that it does not decreases the attention needed to manage vehicles.

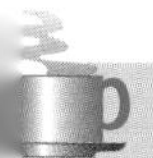

Preparation and Use

INTERNAL USE

❶ **Infusion.** 20-30 g of plant per liter of water. Drink three or four cups daily.

❷ **Dry extract.** It is usually administered in a dose of 0.5 g, three times a day.

EXTERNAL USE

❸ **Compresses.** Applied with an infusion of 30-50 g per liter of water.

❹ **Baths.** The same infusion as compresses, added to the bath water (2-3 liters per bathtub).

❺ **Frictions.** Applied with the essence dissolved in alcohol (balm alcohol).

• **Insomnia [❶,❷]**. When taken at night, it helps to overcome insomnia.

• **Menstrual pain [❶,❷]**. For centuries, it has been recommended to ease menstrual pains.

• It may be also useful for **palpitations, abdominal spasms and colics, flatulence, nausea and vomiting [❶,❷]**.

• When applied ***externally,*** it is **antiseptic, antifungal** (fights skin fungi) and **antiviral [❸,❹,❺]**, and its action has been proven helpful against the herpes virus and type 2 mixoviruses.

Passion Flower

An American anti-stress plant

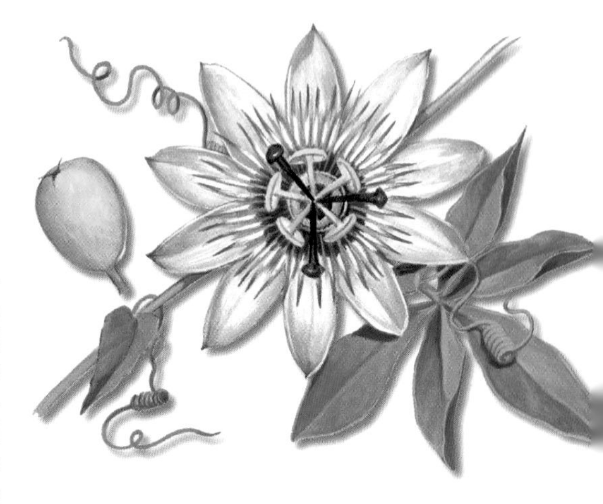

THIS PLANT attracted the attention of European travellers to the New World, who saw in the diverse organs of its beautiful flowers the representation of the instruments used in the Crucifixion: whip, nails and hammer. The plant was introduced in Europe and grown as an ornamental vine, until in the late nineteenth century it was found to have a strong sedative effect on the nervous system.

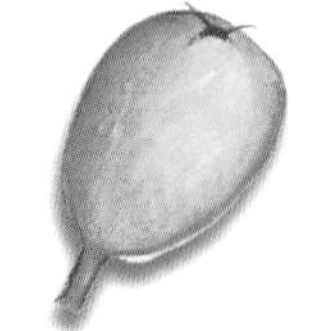

Description. *A woody-stem vine of the Passifloraceae family, with beautiful white or red flowers, divided into three lobes. The fruit is oval, fleshy, orange-colored, and its seeds are black.*

Parts used. *Flowers, leaves and fruits.*

PROPERTIES AND INDICATIONS. The ***FLOWERS*** and ***LEAVES*** of maypops (another name for this plant) contain small amounts of indole alkaloids, flavonoids, diverse steroids and pectin. It is not well known to which of these substances the plant owes its **sedative, antispasmodic and narcotic** (inductive of sleepiness) actions, though it is likely due to the combination of them all. Its main indications are:

• **Anxiety, nervousness, stress [❶]**. The passion flower acts as a mild anxiolytic, without the risk of addiction or dependence. It is the ***ideal plant*** for those people who are under nervous ***pressure.*** The *Larousse Dictionary of Healing Plants* states that: "A gift which comes from the ancient Aztec empire, the passion flower seems to be the most necessary plant in our civilization."

• **Insomnia [❶]**. The plant induces natural sleep, without drowsiness or depression on waking up. It may be administered to children, given its lack of toxicity.

• **Diverse aches and spasms [❶]**. Passion flower relaxes the hollow abdominal hollow organs whose sudden contractions provoke colics or spasms: stomach, intestines (intestinal colic), bile ducts and gall bladder (liver colics), urinary

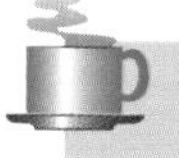

Preparation and Use

INTERNAL USE

❶ **Infusion.** The ideal way to take passion flower is with an infusion of flowers and leaves, prepared with 20-30 g per liter of water, left to rest for two or three minutes before drinking. Two or three cups daily are recommended, if desired they may be honey-sweetened. One more may be taken before bedtime in the case of insomnia.

❷ In **alcohol or drug-withdrawal treatment** the infusion is more concentrated (up to 100 g per liter), sweetened with honey. The dose depends on the patient's requirements.

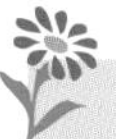

Purple Passion Flower

In Brazil and the West Indies another species of Passiflora grows, *the* Passiflora edulis *Sims.* (= Passiflora laurifolia *F. Vill.), which is a purple passion flower, with purple flowers (as its name indicates), also known as passionfruit. It is the best known species of the genus Passiflora in America.*

Purple passion flower renders a sweet, somewhat acid fruit, whose truly "tropical" flavor is present in soft drinks made with its gelatinous flesh. The oil obtained from its seeds is edible. However, ***it is not considered*** *to be* ***a true medicinal herb.***

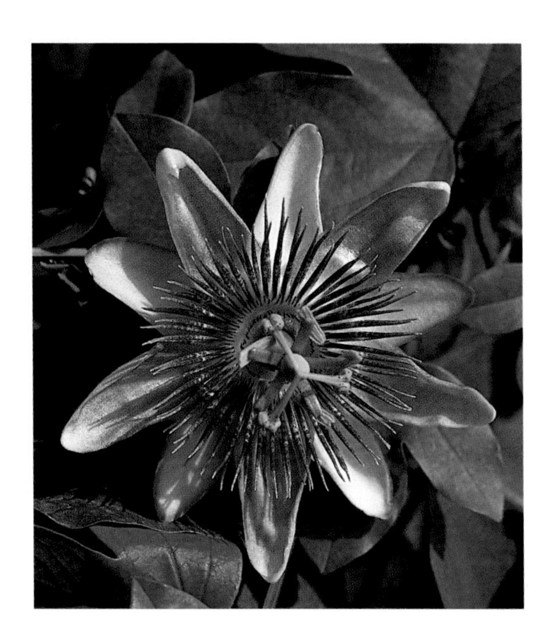

ducts (kidney colic) and uterus (dysmenorrhea). The use of the passion flower is recommended for virtually any kind of pain, even neuralgia.

- **Epilepsy** [❶]. As a ***complementary treatment,*** passion flower helps diminish the frequency and intensity of epileptic crises.
- **Alcoholism and drug-addiction** [❷]. Some interesting experiments have been conducted by administering passion flower during the first days of alcohol, heroin and other drug rehabilitation treatments. This plant makes the withdrawal symptoms (the so-called "cold turkey") more easily tolerated and with less physical consequences on the body. Its sedative action allows better endurance for drug consumption on alcoholics and drug addicts, thus overcoming the anxiety of abstinence. In these cases, the plant must be used ***under medical supervision.***

The ***FRUITS*** of the passion flower (passionfruit) are rich in provitamin A, vitamin C and organic acids. They are **refreshing and invigorating**, and are highly recommended for physical tiredness, infectious diseases, and febrile convalescence.

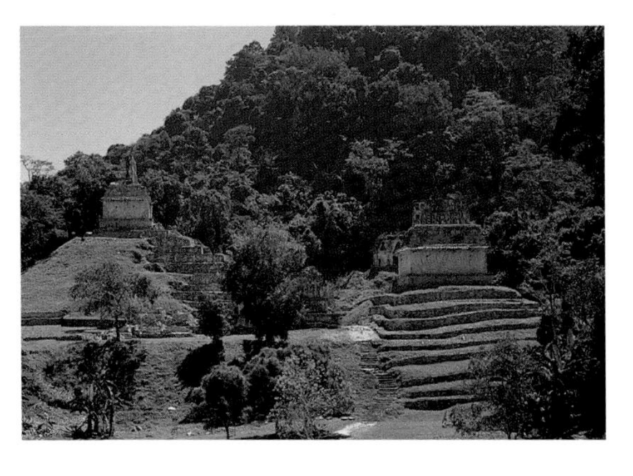

The Mayan pyramids in Palenque, in the Mexican state of Chiapas, are one of the best preserved archaeological remains of the Mayan civilization. Both Aztecs and Mayans knew and used the beautiful flowers of maypops, whose sedative effects on the nervous system were discovered in Europe in the nineteenth century.

Linden

A sedative used for nervousness, it protects the heart... and a great deal more

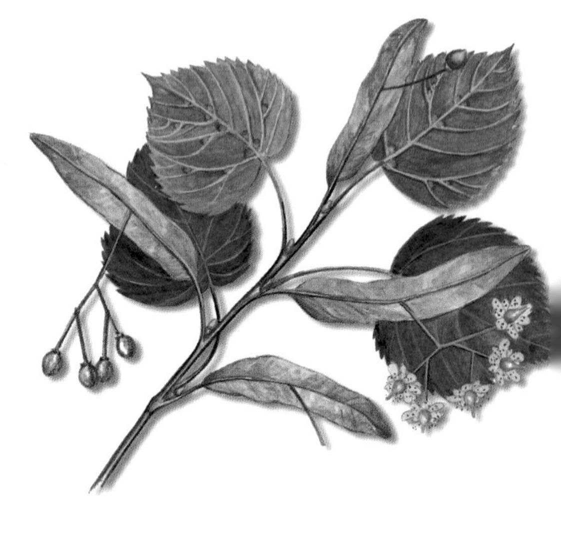

LINDEN ARE MAJESTIC trees which live for several centuries, and seem to invite us to live a peaceful and quiet life like theirs. In Central and northern European countries, the linden symbolizes the family and homelife. The use of popular lime tea (an infusion made of linden tree flowers) as sedative has its roots during the Renaissance, and is currently ***one of the most commonly used vegetal remedies***.

PROPERTIES AND INDICATIONS. Linden tree ***FLOWERS*** contain an aromatic essence rich in magnesium, with **sedative, antispasmodic, and vasodilating** properties; mucilages and small amounts of tannins, with **emollient and anti-inflammatory actions;** and flavonoid glycosides, with **diuretic and sudorific** properties.

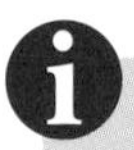

Steam Baths

*Steam baths (right picture) are recommended as **facial beauty** treatment. Boil water in a container, remove from heat and add a handful of linden flowers. The steam is directly applied to the face. Two baths daily.*

Description. *Deciduous, highly branched tree, which grows to a height of 20 m, and belongs to the Tiliaceae family. Linden leaves are serrated, heart-shaped and somewhat asymmetrical. Its flowers are milky or yellowish, with a pleasant scent.*

Parts used. *Young flowers and the bark.*

Its ***BARK*** contains polyphenols and coumarin, whose properties are **choleretic** (augment the secretion of bile), **antispasmodic** (especially active on the gall bladder), **hypotensive and vasodilator** of coronary arteries.

Its applications are diverse, however all of them are due to its sedative and relaxing effects.

- **Dysfunctions of the nervous system [❶,❷,❸]**. Due to the essence it contains, linden flowers are very useful in cases of nervous excitation, anxiety and restlessness.
- **Insomnia. [❶,❷,❸]**. Lime tea is very effective against insomnia, producing natural sleep. Unlike most synthetic narcotics and relaxant substances, lime tea does not cause drowsiness the morning after, nor does it cause addiction. However, being a gentle, non-aggressive treatment,

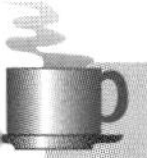

Preparation and Use

INTERNAL USE

❶ **Infusions of flowers** (lime tea). 20-40 g per liter of water. Drink three or four hot cups daily, one before bedtime. Lime tea may be sweetened with honey.

❷ **Bark decoction.** 30 g per liter of water, boil for 10 or 15 minutes. It may be mixed with lime tea in order to obtain a more complete effect.

❸ **Fluid extract.** The dose usually varies from 20 to 40 drops, three times a day, with a fourth intake at night before bedtime.

EXTERNAL USE

❹ **Linden flower baths.** Prepare them with 300-500 g of flowers infused with 1-2 liters of water, added to the water of the bathtub immediately before washing.

❺ **Compresses.** Whether for skin diseases or simply for beauty, soak compresses in an infusion of 100 g of linden flowers per liter of water, changing the compresses every five minutes. Apply daily two or three times.

lime tea acts slowly, and its effects may take several days to manifest themselves.

Warm water baths to which linden flowers are added **[❹]** have notable tranquilizing and relaxing properties, besides boosting the effects of lime tea taken orally. In the case of persistent insomnia, their results are excellent.

• **Nervous children, insomnia in children. [❶,❷,❸]**. Lime tea is also recommended by pediatricians, because it has no undesirable side effects. It is ideal for hyperactive or irritable children, but it must be administered for several days or weeks in order to render its action.

• **Respiratory dysfunctions [❶]**. The mucilaginous substances with emollient action, and the antispasmodic properties of linden flower make it recommended for bronchial catarrhs, bronchitis, asthma, influenza, and persistent cough in children. Some bark may be added for a more intense effect.

• **Heart and circulatory dysfunctions [❶,❷,❸]**. Both linden flowers and bark have vasodilating and extreme hypotensive effects. They act especially on the coronary arteries, and are recommended in the case of angina pectoris and arrhythmia, which usually effects nervous or stressed persons, who will get double results.

As discovered lately, linden flower and bark reduce viscosity of the blood, allowing it to circulate more efficiently. Hence, it favors the ***prevention*** of **heart attacks** and **thrombosis**.

• **Migraine [❷]**. Linden (especially the bark) has been shown to be useful in the treatment of migraine headaches (acute headache caused by arterial spasms), which is so difficult in chemical therapy. The action of linden is basically ***preventive,*** thus it must be taken consistently and not only when the attack comes.

• **Digestive afflictions. [❶]** Due to its choleretic and antispasmodic actions on the gall bladder, linden, and especially its flowers, is ideal for those people suffering from **gall stones** or gall bladder dysfunction (dyskinesia). It eases the expulsion of stones from the gall bladder, as well as the so-called bile mud (sand in bile), besides aiding an improved digestion in biliary dyspepsia, fat intolerance, flatulence or abdominal distension after meals.

• **Skin afflictions [❺]**. In ***external*** application, lime tea produces an observable emollient (anti-inflammatory and soothing) action on the skin. It is recommended for burns, eczema, furuncles and diverse irritations.

• **Beauty and cosmetics.** It is very useful in the fight against the effects of the wind, sun and the cold on skin (dry skin, sunburn). Its cosmetic application is to soothe and improve the appearance of skin. Steam baths with linden open up pores and cleanse the skin.

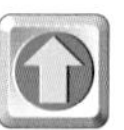

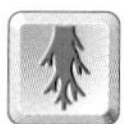

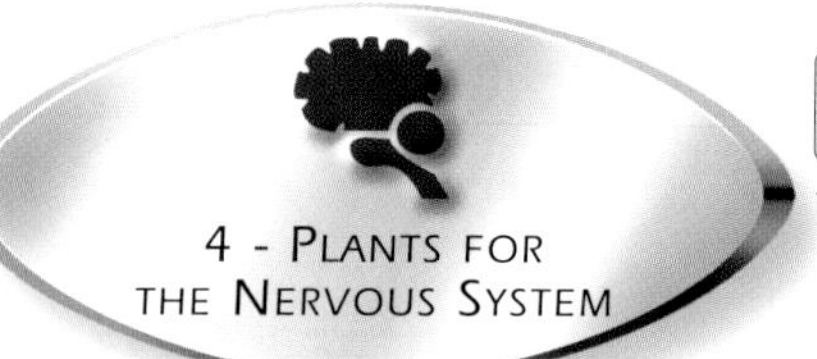

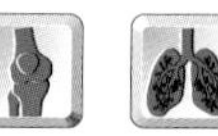

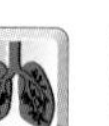

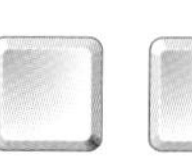

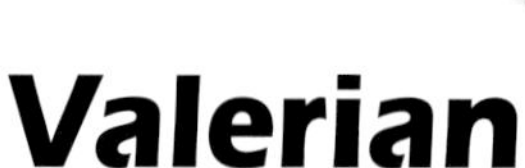

Valerian

Calms nervousness and decreases blood pressure

VALERIAN EXERTS quite different effects, depending on the living being it acts on: animals or humans. While serving as a strong stimulant for animals, it has notable sedative effects on human beings. Thus, cats become euphoric when they smell the plant, joyfully rubbing against it. The aroma of the valerian, which becomes stronger when the plant is dry, does not have any special attraction for humans, since it resembles the smell of foot sweat. It is a matter of preference!

Valerian has been employed in therapeutic science since the Renaissance, when its property to prevent epileptic attacks was discovered.

Properties and indications. The roots of Valerian have around 1% of an essential oil of antispasmodic action with many components (terpenes, borneol esters, etc.) and between 1% and 5% of valepotriats, substances which traditionally, valerian's sedative effects were attributed to. However, today it is known that the most important agent of valerian is baldrinal, which is the metabolite of the valepotriat, called valtrate.

Valerian has **tranquilizing, sedative, narcotic** (favoring sleep), **analgesic** (calms aches), **antispasmodic, and anticonvulsive** effects. It produces sedation on the whole autonomic and central nervous systems, decreasing anxiety, as well as blood pressure. Its action is quite similar to that of neuroleptic pharmaceuticals (fenotyazines and derivatives), however it lacks the latter's toxic effects. These are the indications of the valerian.

• **Autonomic Nervous System Disorders (Symptom) {❶,❷,❸}**. Anxiety, anxiety neurosis, neurasthenia and irritability, headaches, palpitations, arrhythmia, basic blood pressure hy-

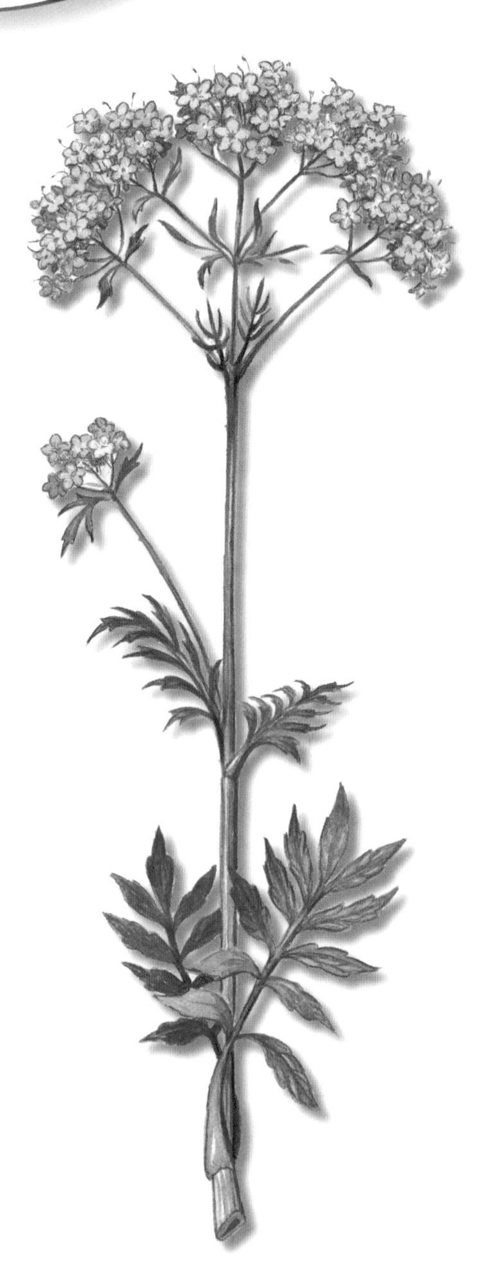

Description. *Herbaceous plant of the Valerianaceae family, with upright, hollowed, furrowed stems growing from 0.5 to 2 m high. Its little pink flowers gather in terminal clusters.*

Parts used. *Root and rhizome.*

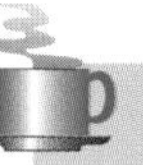

Preparation and Use

INTERNAL USE

❶ **Infusion.** 15-20 g of ground root per liter of water. Drink up to five cups daily, sweetened with honey if preferred. For insomnia, drink a cup half an hour or one hour before going to bed.

❷ **Cold extract.** 100 g of root per liter of warm water. Let it stand for approximately 12 hours. Drink three or four cups daily.

❸ **Root powder.** Three or four times a day, an intake of 1 g.

EXTERNAL USE

❹ **Compresses** of a decoction made with 50-100 g of dry root per liter of water, boiled for 10 minutes. Apply when hot to the aching areas.

❺ Warm water **baths,** with a sedative action, adding one or two liters of a decoction similar to that prepared for compresses.

pertension (with no organic cause), shivers, gastric neurosis (stomach nervousness), irritable colon, and other psychosomatic diseases.

- **Tiredness and nervous** depression [❶,❷,❸].
- **Insomnia** [❶,❷,❸]. Due to its narcotic action it renders good results when its infusion is reinforced by a bath [❺] before bedtime.
- **Epilepsy** [❶,❷,❸]. When regularly taken, it ***prevents*** epileptic attacks. However, ***it does not substitute antiepileptic treatment,*** though it may help to reduce the dose.
- **Asthma** [❶,❷,❸]. Valerian is more effective in the ***prevention*** rather than in the treatment of acute asthma attacks, as with epilepsy. Its antispasmodic and sedative actions prevents bronchial spasms, which are one of the causes of asthma, along with mucous membrane edema.
- **Pain** [❶,❷,❸]. Due to its analgesic action it is useful in the fight against sciatic and rheumatic pain. Moreover, it also acts ***externally*** [❹], applied on the affected area in order to ease pain in cases of contusions, lumbalgia, sciatica, muscular strain and rheumatic pain.

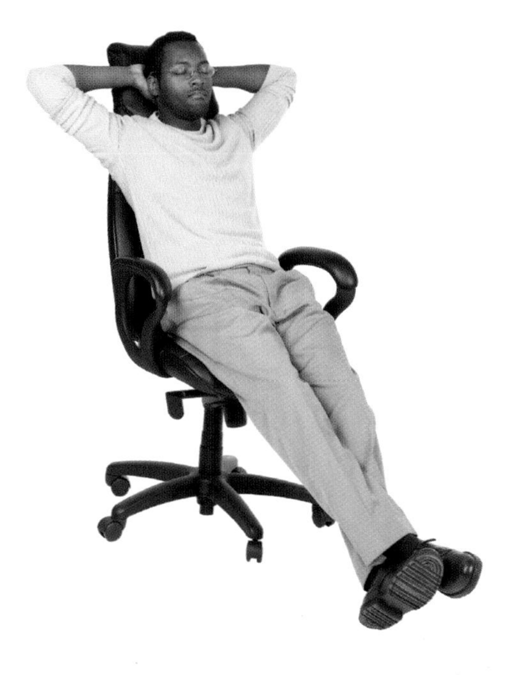

Valerian has a notable balancing effect on the autonomic nervous system, whether taken as an infusion or in medicinal baths. It is quite useful for psychosomatic diseases, nervousness, and stress.

Vervain

Alleviates migraine headaches and neuralgia

THE TEMPLE of Zeus on Mount Olympus was purified with vervain water, since this plant was regarded as a panacea, able to deliver from all evils. During the Middle Ages it was used by sorcerers and fortune tellers as a magic herb. In ancient times it was recommended as an aphrodisiac ("lights the candles"), and it is likely to be so. At present, we have come to know its true properties and applications.

PROPERTIES AND INDICATIONS. The plant contains verbenaline, a glycoside which acts on the autonomic nervous system, especially on the parasympathetic system, producing **sedative, antispasmodic, analgesic, digestive and anti-inflammatory** actions. Besides, it contains tannin and mucilage, which make it an astringent and an emollient. Thus its applications are:

- **Migraines [❶,❷]** Due to its antispasmodic action on the arterial system, it prevents migraine crises, or at least diminishes their intensity. The treatment of this ailment is quite difficult, and

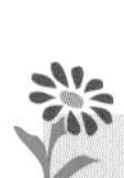

Blue Vervain

In America there is a species similar to the European vervain, known as the blue or American vervain (Verbena hastata *L.) The* ***composition and properties*** *of both species are* ***similar.*** *The blue vervain is usually employed as a* ***sedative against influenza and catarrhs,*** *especially when there are respiratory problems.*

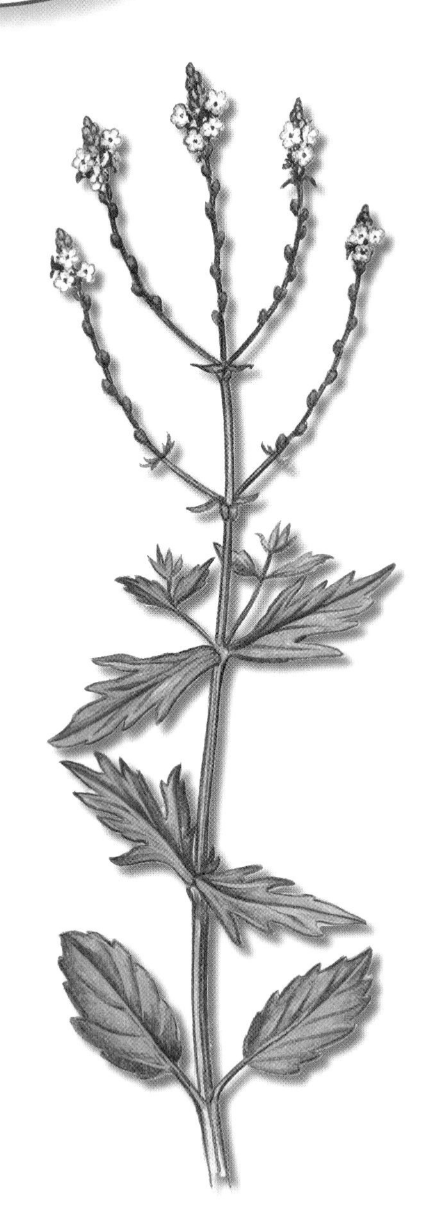

Description. *Vivacious plant of the Verbenaceae family, growing up to one meter high, with a stiff, quadrangular stem and small, mauve flowers which bloom in terminal spikes. Sour taste.*

Parts used. *The plant when blooming, the fresher, the better.*

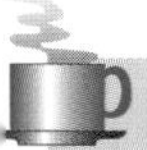

Preparation and Use

Since verbenaline degrades with drying, **fresh** plants should be used whenever possible.

INTERNAL USE

❶ **Infusion.** 15-20 g per liter of water. Drink three or four cups daily.

❷ **Decoction.** 20 g per liter, for 10 minutes. Same dose as for infusion.

EXTERNAL USE

❸ **Gargling.** The infusion or decoction recommended for internal use, though slightly more concentrated (40-50 g per liter).

❹ **Inhalations.** Breathing directly over hot decoction steam.

❺ **Hot or warm compresses.** They are made with concentrated infusion or decoction, then applied on the aching areas.

❻ **Poultices.** With a stewed plant, wrapped in a cotton fabric.

better results are obtained when vervain is ***combined*** with other plants. Unlike ergotamine-derived medicines, which are usually employed to treat migraine crises and have important side effects, vervain does not.

- **Rheumatic pain, neuralgia, sciatica.** It is applied both internally (infusion [❶] or decoction [❷]) and externally (compresses [❺] or poultices [❻]).
- **Digestive dysfunctions.** Its eupeptic action promotes digestion. The plant may be used for diarrhea and intestinal colics, given its astringent properties.
- **Relief of liver congestion [❶,❷].** Since it promotes bile secretion (**choleretic** action) it is recommended for liver dysfunctions. Its antispasmodic action also renders good results for liver **stones.**
- **Diuretic [❶,❷]** Being mildly diuretic, it is administered for **kidney stones** in order to ease pain and help eliminate stones. The same applies in the treatment of **obesity** and **cellulitis.**
- **Throat afflictions [❸].** It is highly recommended for various throat ailments such as pharyngitis, laryngitis and tonsillitis, and generally for sore throat, being applied in poultices [❻] and taken in infusion [❶].
- **Sinusitis.** Vervain is used to treat this distressful condition because of its anti-inflammatory and astringent properties. It is taken orally [❶], inhaled [❹] and applied in warm compresses [❺] on the face.

Inhalations with hot vervain decoction steam are quite useful for treating sinusitis.

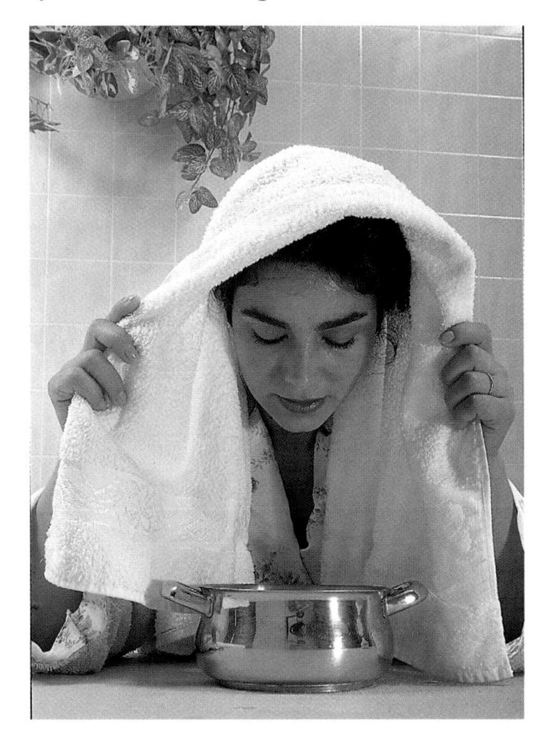

5

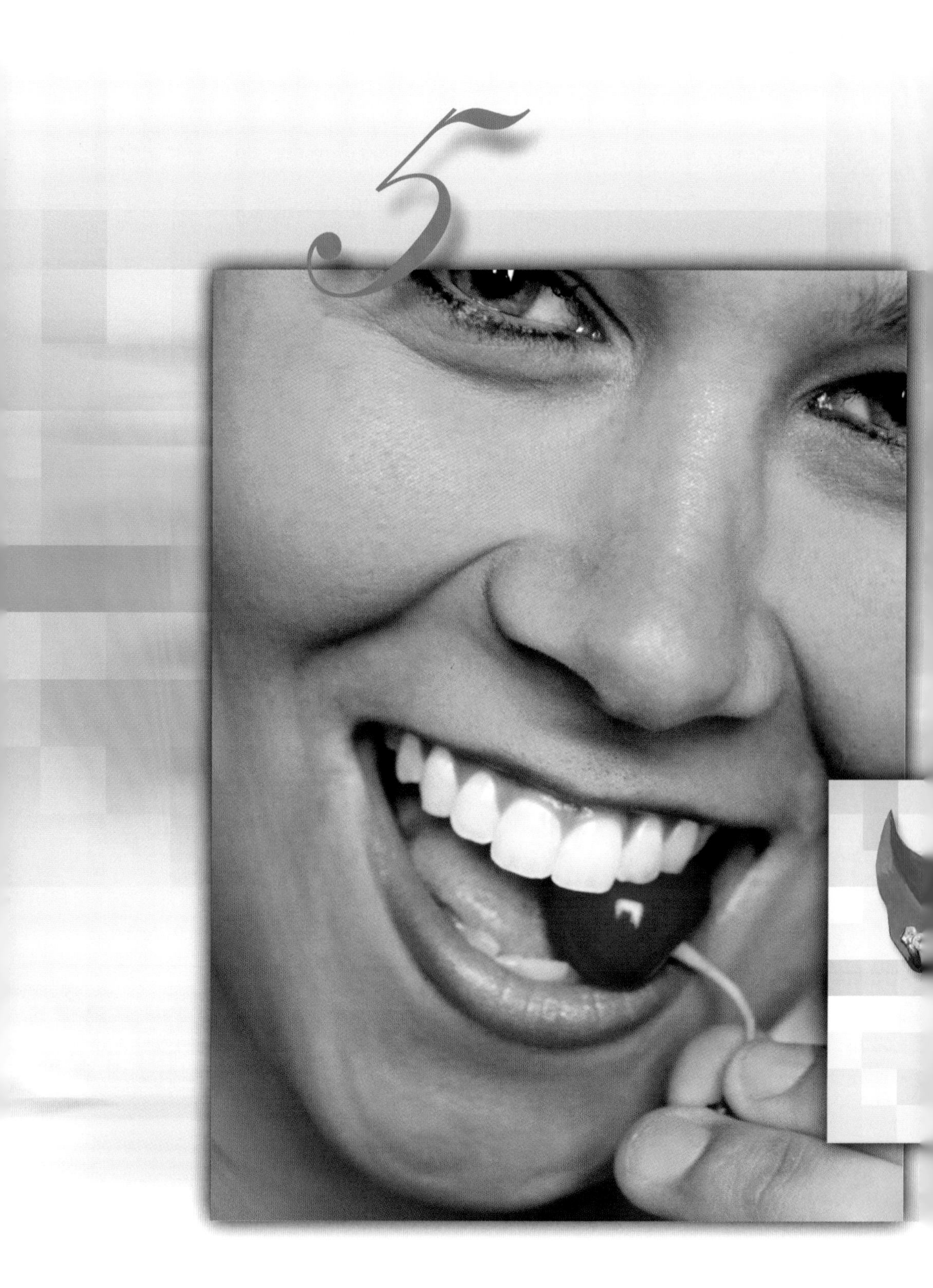

Plants for the Mouth, Nose and Throat

DISEASES	PAGES
Aphonia	92
Gingivitis	89
Hoarseness, see Aphonia	92
Laryngitis	91
Lip sores	88
Mouth ulcers	88
Mouth, bad taste in	89
Nose, bleeding	92
Nose, inflammation, see Rhinitis	91
Parodontosis	89
Pharyngitis	90
Pyorrhea, gingivitis, and parodontosis	89
Rhinitis	91
Sinusitis	91
Sore throat, see Tonsillitis and pharyngitis	90
Sores, lips	88
Teething	89
Throat, irritation	90
Toothache	89

PLANTS	PAGES
Althea	94
Bistort	93
Clove tree	96
Goldenseal	100
Hedge mustard	101
Mastic tree	98
New Jersey tea	95
Oak tree	102
Rhatany	97
Sticklewort	99

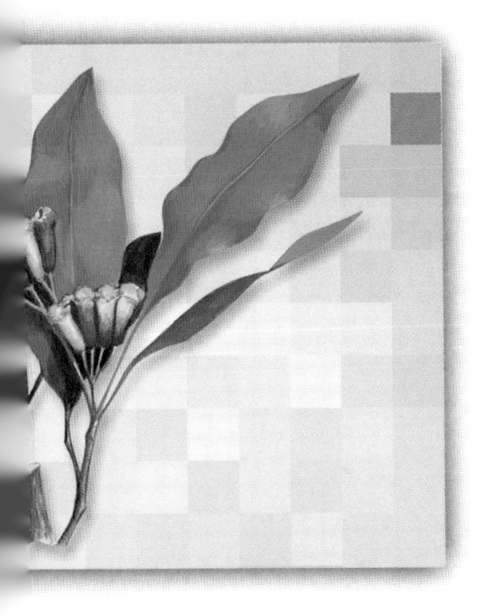

THE IMPORTANCE of oral health lies in two fundamental facts related to its anatomy and physiology:

1. In the mouth **mastication,** the first phase of the digestive process takes place. The correct function of the teeth is fundamental for good mastication and digestion.

2. The mouth contains **a wide range and amount of germs,** being one of the parts of the body where most microbes exist. These micro-organisms may cause severe infections and toxic states that influence the whole body.

The mouth, as well as the whole digestive system, is covered throughout its interior by a layer of cells called the **mucous membrane.** Inflammation of the mouth, and especially that of the mucous membrane covering it, is called **stomatitis.** Etymologically this term comes from the Greek *stoma,* which means "mouth" (and not "stomach"). It manifests itself by the reddening of the oral mucous membrane, sometimes, along with, ulcers or wounds (apthous). It mainly affects the gums, the tip of the tongue, and the internal side of the cheeks.

The most frequent causes of stomatitis are chemical irritants such as tobacco and alcoholic beverages, eating meals that are too hot, certain medicines (especially antibiotics), unsuitable dental prosthesis, and deficient oral hygiene.

Mouth rinses with medicinal herbs can significantly contribute to the ***treatment,*** and generally to the ***prevention*** of **stomatitis, gingivitis, pyorrhea,** and other oral ailments.

The ears, the nose, and the throat make up an anatomic and physiological unit, because all these organs are interconnected, and the mucous layer that covers their interior spreads to each part with no transitional joint. Each ear communicates with the pharynx through a fine duct called the Eustachian tube.

Under the term **throat** we include both the pharynx, the tonsils, and the larynx, in whose interior the voice is produced.

Paranasal sinuses form a functional unit with the nostrils. These sinuses are cavities in the facial bones, and their inflammation is called sinusitis.

The tonsils and the paranasal sinuses are especially susceptible to noxious germs, which stay in the sinuses to become infections from which toxins flow into the blood and to other organs. Often chronic or repetitive bronchitis is caused by the presence of a permanent infectious colony in the paranasal sinuses or in the tonsils.

Medicinal herbs, either locally applied in gargles, nose irrigations, or inhalations, or taken orally, provide a soothing, anti-inflammatory, and antibiotic action, as well as promoting the expulsion of the mucous, which contributes decisively to the healing, and generally, to the prevention of ailments of this important anatomic region.

MOUTH ULCERS

Definition

These are small, very painful ulcers, which tend to heal spontaneously after some days. Their causes vary widely, though they are not easy to ascertain: Viral infections, alimentary allergies, lack of B vitamins or iron, among other reasons, may cause mouth ulcers.

Treatment

Mouth rinses with ***astringent*** (which dry mucous membrane), ***antiseptic, and cicatrizant*** plants can be useful.

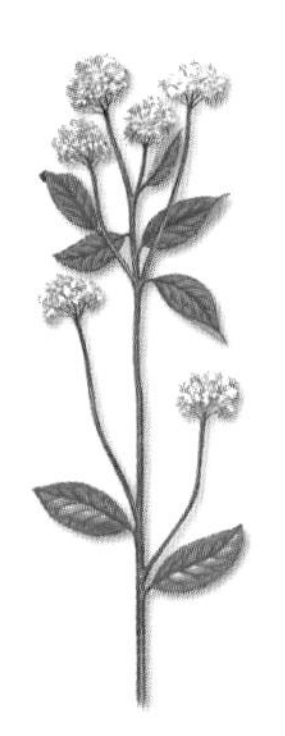

New Jersey tea

NEW JERSEY TEA	Soothes mouth mucosa
STICKLEWORT	Astringent and anti-inflammatory
MOTHER OF THYME	Antiseptic (disinfectant)
BRAMBLE	Astringent and hemostatic
SAGE	Astringent and antiseptic
ANNATTO TREE	Healing and soothing
THYME	Antiseptic

LIP SORES

Causes

Cold sores are usually caused by dryness or cold, and are painful when opening or moving the mouth. When they appear on **lip sides** they are related to the lack of certain minerals, especially of iron.

Treatment

Local treatment with compresses or poultices of ***emollient*** (soothing) and ***cicatrizant*** plants can accelerate the healing of this disease.

FENUGREEK	Anti-inflammatory and cicatrizant
PELLITORY OF THE WALL	Anti-inflammatory and emollient

BAD TASTE IN MOUTH

Causes

It may or may not be related to bad breath **(halitosis).** It is usually related to the bad functioning of the gall bladder or intestinal fermentations.

Phytotherapy

Cholagogue and digestive plants are recommended, especially the four mentioned here.

FUMITORY	Fights autointoxication caused by intestinal putrefaction
BOLDO	Favors the digestion and the emptying of the gall bladder
MILFOIL	Digestive, decreases intestinal fermentation

TEETHING

Phytotherapy

When teeth grow in milk-fed children, the gums undergo a mild inflammatory process whose discomforts may be eliminated with these plants.

ALTHEA	Softens gums and promotes tooth eruption
SAFFRON	Alleviates teething pain

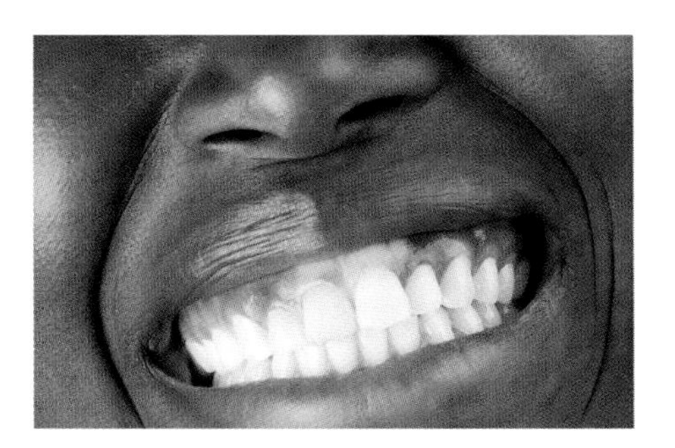

Medicinal herbs may contribute in a very positive way to oral hygiene.

TOOTHACHE

Phytotherapy

Medicinal herbs can produce a ***local analgesic*** effect when applied in mouth rinses. Thus, the undesirable side effects of internally used analgesics (injected, taken orally, etc.) are avoided.

Treatment

The ***real treatment*** of tooth inflammation that causes toothache must never be put off.

CLOVE TREE	Oral antiseptic and analgesic

PYORRHEA, GINGIVITIS AND PARODONTOSIS

Definition

From an etymological standpoint, **pyorrhea** means "pus flow," though it is only used to name the discharge of pus from the gums. Gums are separated from the teeth, and the teeth loosen and fall out.

Gingivitis is the inflammation of the gums, usually caused by pyorrhea.

Parodontosis is a wider term that includes all conditions able to alter the adherence of teeth to the jaw bone, the most frequent of which is pyorrhea.

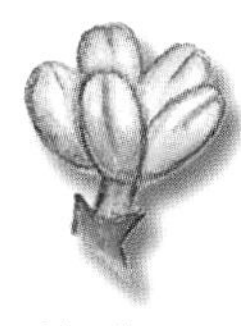

Mastic tree flower

Treatment

These conditions demand ***periodontal specialized treatment.*** Mouth rinses with these plants serve as hygienic ***complement*** of such treatment.

RHATANY	Astringent (dries mucosa) and anti-inflammatory
MASTIC TREE	Antiseptic and anti-inflammatory. Freshens breath
OAK TREE	Astringent, anti-inflammatory. Cleanses the gums
BEECH TREE	Powerful absorbent (retains dissolved particles), cleanses the gums
CINCHONA	Cicatrizant and antiseptic

TONSILLITIS AND PHARYNGITIS

Definition

Tonsillitis, or **sore throat,** is the inflammation of tonsils, usually caused by an infection, either bacterial or viral. When this inflammation extends to the entire pharyngeal mucus membrane (throat), and not only to the tonsils, it is called **pharyngitis.**

Phytotherapy

The phytotherapeutical treatment of both conditions is based on local applications, mainly gargles, with the plants mentioned here.

Repetitive pharyngeal infections in children demand the administration of plants with **antibiotic and defense-stimulating** action, such as thyme, nasturtium, and echinacea.

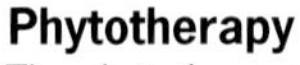

Sticklewort

VERVAIN	Anti-inflammatory and emollient
STICKLEWORT	Alleviates the inflammation and irritation of the throat
GOLDENSEAL	Antiseptic, regenerates the cells of mucosa
OAK TREE	Antiseptic and cicatrizant, alleviates itching and rashes
WALNUT	Antiseptic, cicatrizant, astringent
ANNATTO TREE	Astringent and cicatrizant
ECHINACEA	Increases defenses against infections
THYME	Antiseptic, stimulates defenses
NASTURTIUM	Natural antibiotic, cleanses the mucosa

THROAT, IRRITATION

Causes

This may be due to several causes, among them, infections (chronic pharyngitis), irritation (tobacco smoke, inhalation of chemical substances), atrophic (weakness of the mucous cells that cover the throat), and even tumors. It appears through an itching and stinging throat, dry cough, difficulty when swallowing, and mucus.

Phytotherapy

All these plants have **bechic action,** that is to say, they ease coughs caused by itching or throat irritation. They are employed both internally and locally in gargles.

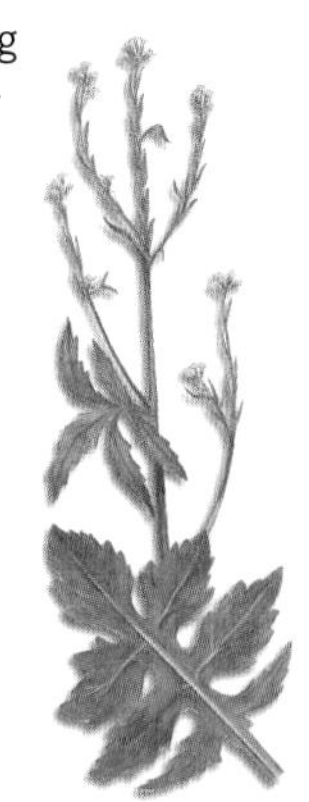

Hedge mustard

STICKLEWORT	Soothes the throat and clears the voice
OAK TREE	Antiseptic and cicatrizant, alleviates throat itching
HEDGE MUSTARD	Eases cough and throat irritation
COMMON PLANTAIN	Soothes and dries, alleviates throat irritation
LUNGWORT	Astringent, expectorant, anti-inflammatory
GARDEN VIOLET	Soothes the throat and eases cough
WILD MARJORAM	Expectorant, sedative, antitussive
FALSE ACACIA	Emollient, protects the mucosa

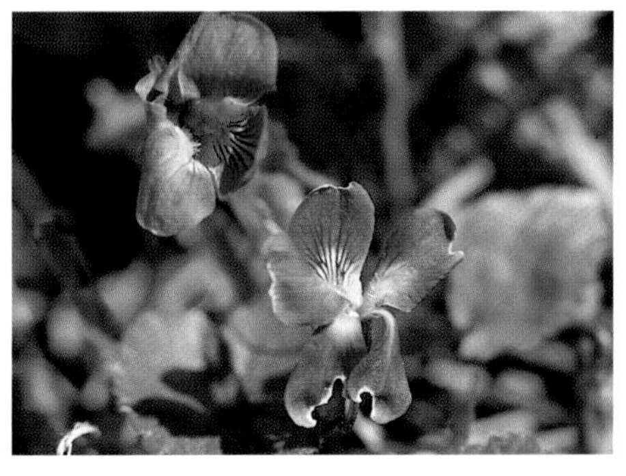

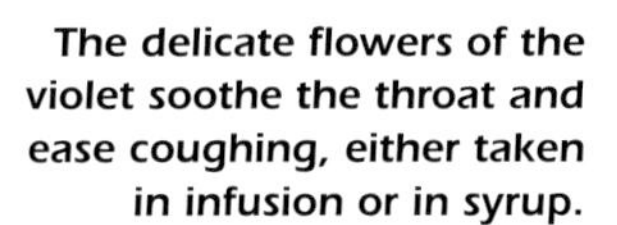

The delicate flowers of the violet soothe the throat and ease coughing, either taken in infusion or in syrup.

LARINGITIS

An inflammation of the mucous layer that covers the larynx, the organ where the voice is produced. It is accompanied by an increase in mucus production in the throat, coughing, aphonia or hoarseness, and in severe cases, breathing difficulty due to spasms of the vocal cords, which close the air passages.

VERVAIN	Anti-inflammatory and emollient
STICKLEWORT	Alleviates inflammation and irritation of the throat
HEDGE MUSTARD	Eases cough and irritation of the throat, expectorant
ICELAND MOSS	Pectoral, expectorant, antitussive
LICORICE	Promotes expectoration and reduces inflammation of the respiratory ways
COMMON PLANTAIN	Soothes and dries, alleviates throat irritation
WILD MARJORAM	Expectorant, sedative, antitussive

APHONIA

Definition

Loss of the voice. It is generally a consequence of inflammation or infection of the larynx or vocal chords (laryngitis), though it may also be caused by tumors, nervousness, and other reasons.

Hoarseness is the change in the tone of the voice, which becomes hoarse and emits less sound. It is usually caused by the same things that cause aphonia.

Phytotherapy

These plants, employed internally or in local applications, reduce the inflammation of the vocal chords and contribute to the elimination of mucus, which frequently causes aphonia or hoarseness.

HEDGE MUSTARD	Calms cough and throat irritation, expectorant
LICORICE	Promotes expectoration and reduces the inflammation of the respiratory ways
LUNGWORT	Expectorant, anti-inflammatory
GARDEN VIOLET	Soothes the throat and eases coughs
ROSE	Anti-inflammatory, antiseptic

SINUSITIS

Definition

This is the inflammation of the paranasal sinuses, small cavities in the facial bones that connect with the nostrils through small holes. The interior of these cavities or sinuses is covered by a mucous layer, whose inflammation produces headaches and other discomforts, and is slow to cure.

Phytotherapy

Besides nasal irrigations, compresses on the face are recommended, as well as inhalations of vapors or essences, and the intake of plants with ***antibiotic*** action such as radish or nasturtium.

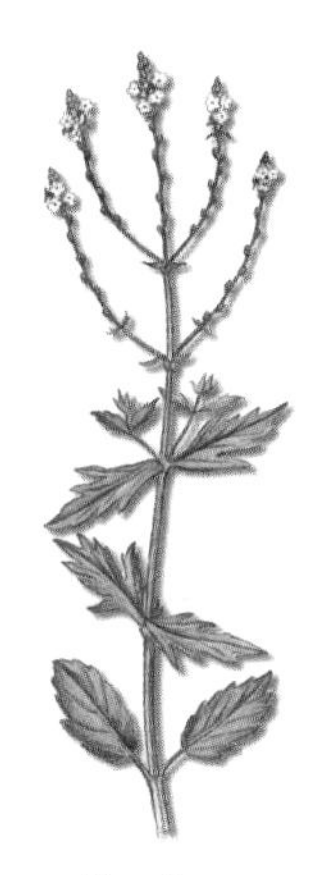

Vervain

VERVAIN	Anti-inflammatory and astringent
SILVER FIR	Balsamic and antiseptic, regenerates mucosa
PINE TREE	Balsamic and antiseptic
ROSE	Astringent, anti-inflammatory, antiseptic
ECHINACEA	Increases defenses against infection
NASTURTIUM	Natural antibiotic, cleanses mucosa

Lemon juice is a great antiseptic. When applied to the tonsils by touching them with a cotton cloth, it can destroy several types of noxious germs that are located in this part of the throat.

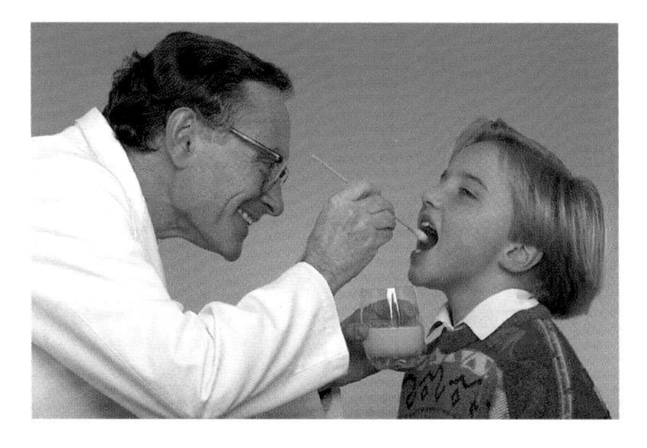

RHINITIS

This is the inflammation of the mucous membrane which covers the interior of the nose. **Astringent and antiseptic** plants are employed for nose irrigations and washings, as well as **antibiotic** herbs such as nasturtium, and **sneezing** plants such as asarum.

RED EYEBRIGHT	Antiseptic, anti-inflammatory, and astringent
GOLDENSEAL	Antiseptic, regenerates mucosa cells
PINE TREE	Balsamic and antiseptic
NASTURTIUM	Natural antibiotic, cleanses mucosa

NOSE, BLEEDING (EPISTAXIS)

Definition

This is a nasal hemorrhage. In many cases it is caused by the breaking of a tiny vein in the nostril, though it may also be related to high blood pressure.

Phytotherapy

Medicinal herbs with ***hemostatic or astringent*** action are applied in nose plugging, prepared with a gauze, or in nasal irrigations. It is better to combine this local treatment with the intake of herbal teas made with some plants with ***hemostatic or capillary protecting*** action.

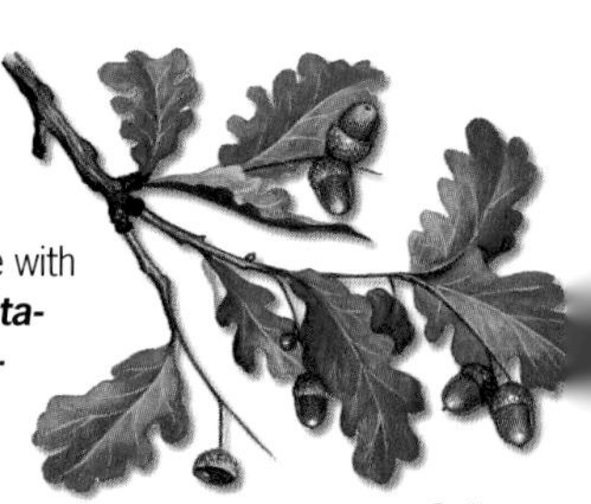

Oak tree

OAK TREE	Astringent, anti-inflammatory, and hemostatic
NETTLE	Vasoconstrictor and hemostatic
BLACKTHORN	Astringent
TORMENTIL	Astringent and hemostatic
MILFOIL	Cicatrizant, hemostatic
HORSETAIL	Hemostatic

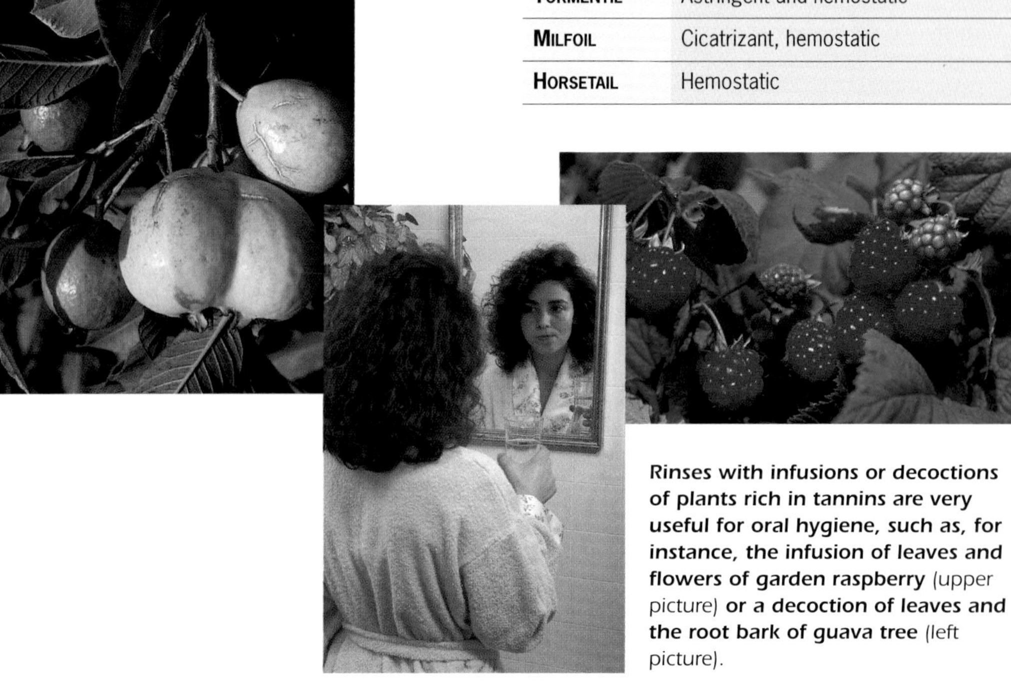

Rinses with infusions or decoctions of plants rich in tannins are very useful for oral hygiene, such as, for instance, the infusion of leaves and flowers of garden raspberry (upper picture) **or a decoction of leaves and the root bark of guava tree** (left picture).

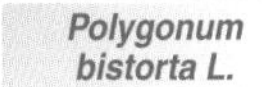

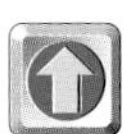
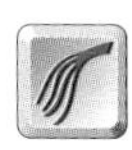
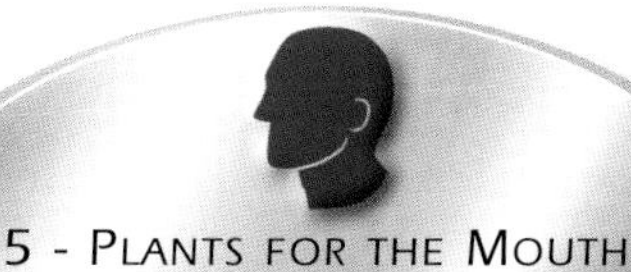

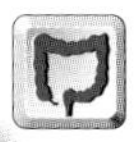
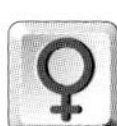
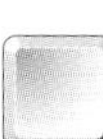
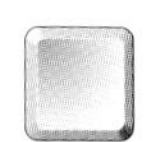

Bistort

A powerful astringent

THE RHIZOME of this plant, quite difficult to uproot, forms two angles as its name shows: bistort means twice crooked. It is reddish in color, and presents a high percentage of starch, thus being used as food in times of famine.

PROPERTIES AND INDICATIONS. The rhizome of the bistort contains plenty of galic and catechic tannins, which give the plant a strong astringent action. It is probably ***one of the most astringent plants*** known. The bistort acts ***locally*** by drying, cicatrizing and "tanning" the skin and the mucous membranes of the body. It also has **antiseptic** (fighting infections), and **hemostatic** (stopping small hemorrhages) actions. Therefore, it is recommended in the following cases:

• **Gingivitis and parodontosis [❷]** (weak and bleeding gums), applied in oral rinses with the cold extract of the rhizome.

Preparation and Use

INTERNAL USE

❶ **Decoction** with 20-30 g of ground rhizome per liter of water, drinking three or four cups daily.

EXTERNAL USE

❷ **Mouth rinses.** With the liquid of the cold extract with 60-100 g of ground rhizome per liter of water, steeping for four hours.

❸ **Vaginal irrigations.** With a decoction of 40-50 g of rhizome per liter of water.

Description. *It grows up to one meter high, this plant belongs to the Polygonaceae family. Its stem is full of joints, a usual feature of this botanical family. It has large, oval-shaped leaves, and pink flowers growing in tip spikes.*

Parts used. *The rhizome (underground stem).*

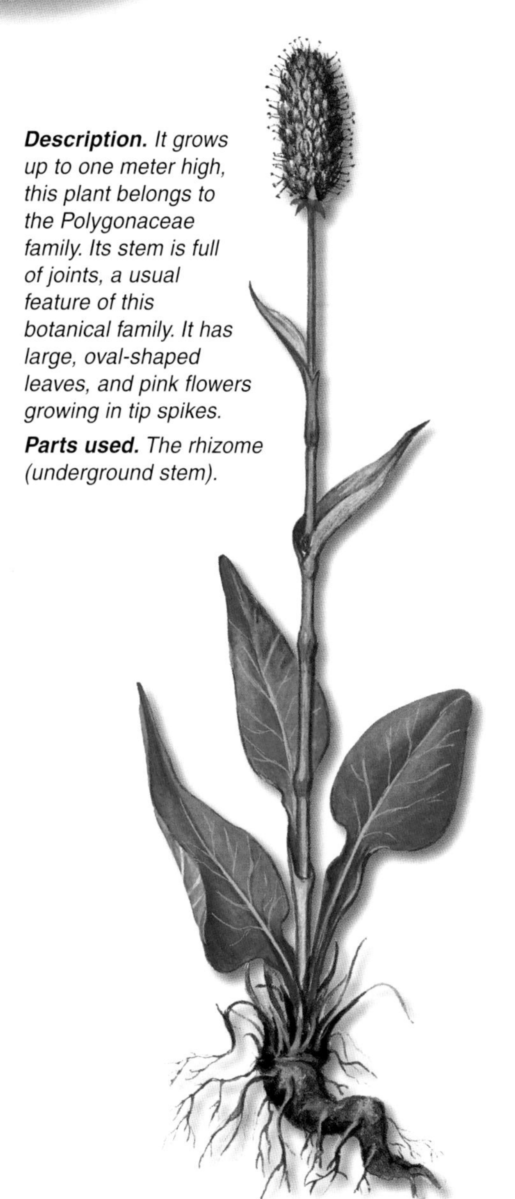

• **Stomatitis [❷]** (inflammation of the mouth mucous membrane), and **pharyngitis,** applied in mouth rinses, with the cold extract of the rhizome.

• **Diarrhea and gastro-enteritis [❶],** especially when they appear with infection and hemorrhage (dysentery, salmonellosis, cholera).

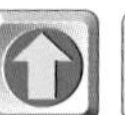
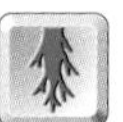
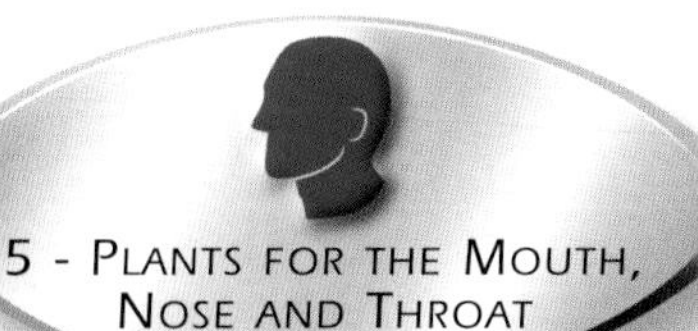

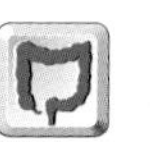
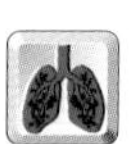
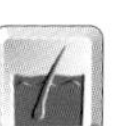

Althea

A great emollient

LIKE ITS RELATION, high mallow, althea is all sweetness and softness. Even its leaves are delicately covered with velvet-like hairs. Dioscorides already recommended this plant in the first century, and since then it has been used throughout the ages.

PROPERTIES AND INDICATIONS. All parts of the plant, and especially its root, contain mucilage, pectin, mineral salts, and vitamin C. Its properties are the same as those of the high mallow, however they are more intense due to its higher content of mucilage. It is, thus ***one of the most emollient plants*** known. Mucilage covers the **skin** and the **mucous membranes,** forming a **protective and anti-inflammatory layer.**

Its indications are very similar to those of high mallow: **laxative**, in the case of constipation, and **anti-inflammatory**, in the case of gastritis, gastroenteritis, or colitis; it also fights against respiratory afflictions, as well as against oral and other digestive mucous membrane irritations **[❶]**.

Its clean ***ROOT*** may be given to children to be chewed when teeth are erupting, because it soothes gums and eases tooth eruption.

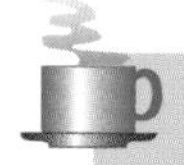

Preparation and Use

INTERNAL USE

❶ **Infusion** with 30 g of young leaves or flowers, or **decoction** with 20-30 g of root per liter of water. Drink three or four cups daily sweetened with honey.

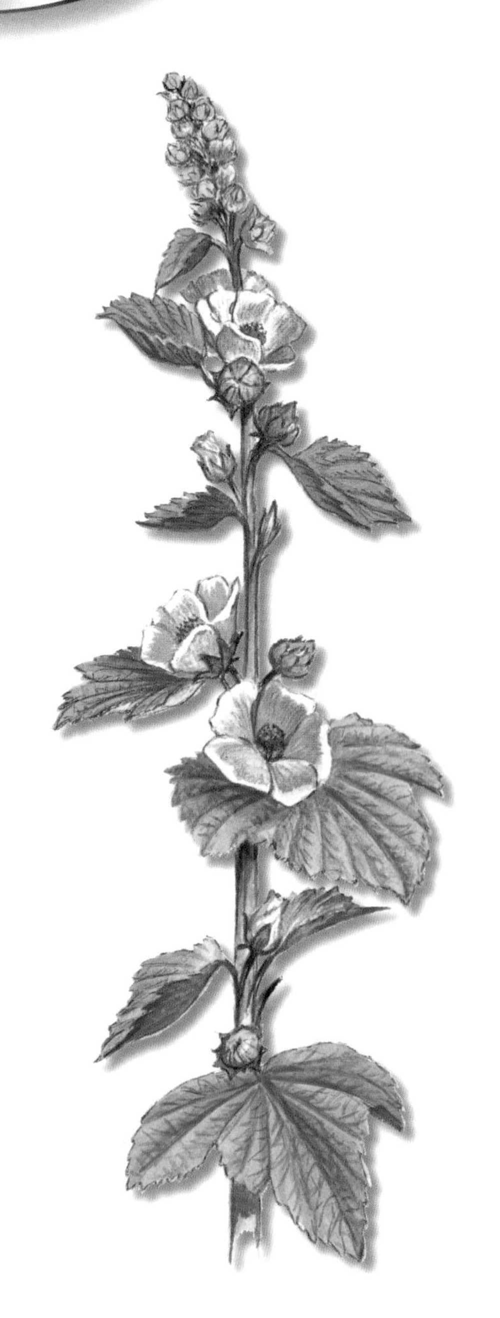

Description. *Vivacious plant of the Malvaceae family, it is hairy, and grows up to two meters high, with large, velvet-like leaves, and white flowers with five petals.*

Parts used. *The root, the leaves, and the flowers.*

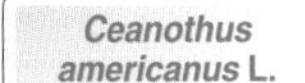

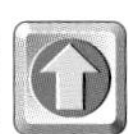
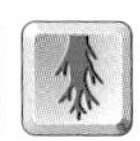
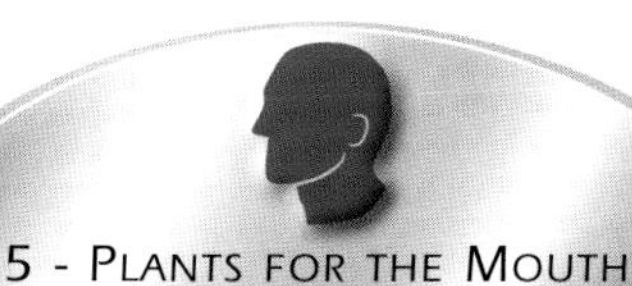

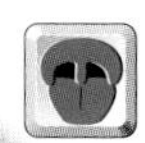
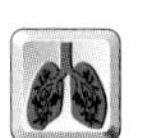
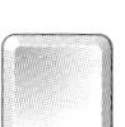
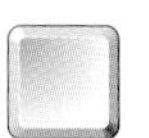

New Jersey Tea

Excellent for mouth rinses

THE SO-CALLED New Jersey tea or red root is one of the vegetal remedies used by North American natives from time immemorial. Perfectly integrated into their environment, the natives had already discovered the plant's virtues which have now been confirmed by the modern pharmaceutical industry. Its leaves were used as a substitute for tea during the United States' War of Independence.

PROPERTIES AND INDICATIONS. The bark of the root contains an alkaloid (ceanotine), tannin, resin, and traces of an essential oil. It is successfully used in the following cases:

- **Mouth and throat afflictions [❷]:** pharyngitis, sore throat, oral aphtas (sores), and other irritations, locally applied in gargles and mouth wash-offs.
- **Bronchial and lung afflictions [❶]:** bronchial catarrhs, cough, asthmatic bronchitis.

Preparation and Use

INTERNAL USE

❶ **Decoction** with a spoonful of ground bark root per cup of water. Drink two or three cups daily.

EXTERNAL USE

❷ **Rinses and gargles.** With the same decoction employed for internal use, though slightly more concentrated.

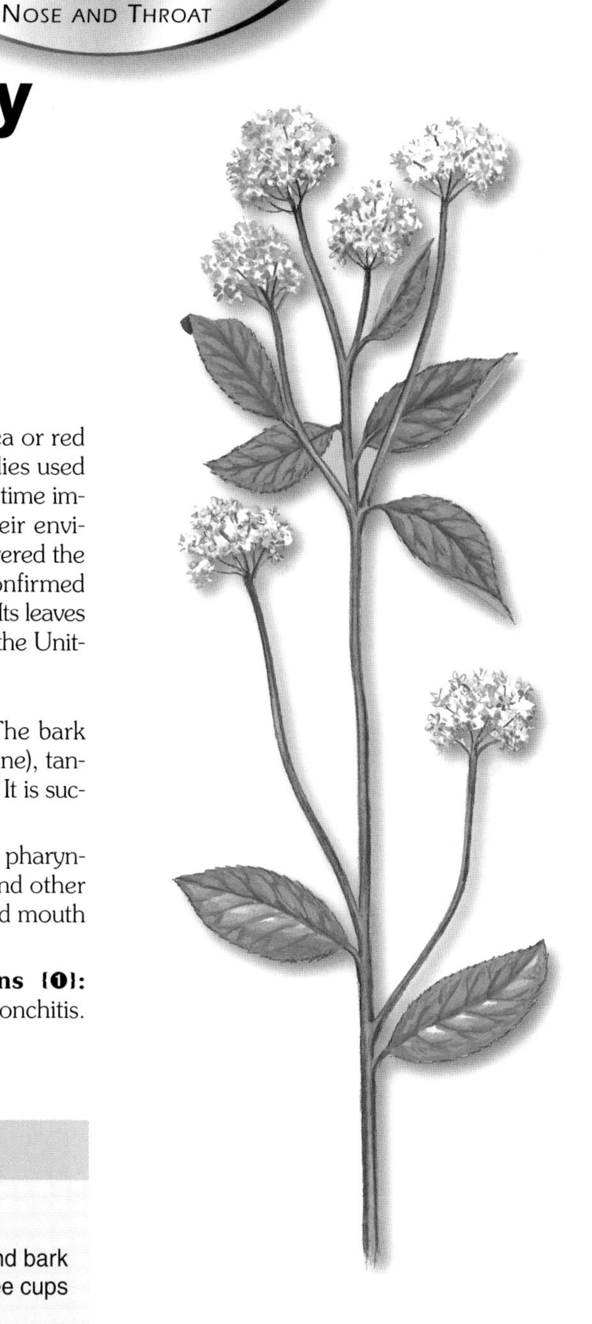

Description. *Shrub of the Ramnaceae family, growing from one to 1.5 m high. Oval, sharp-tipped, finely toothed leaves, and small, white or bluish flowers that grow from the axillary buds of the leaves.*

Parts used. *The bark of the root.*

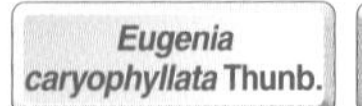

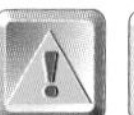
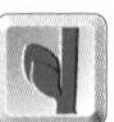
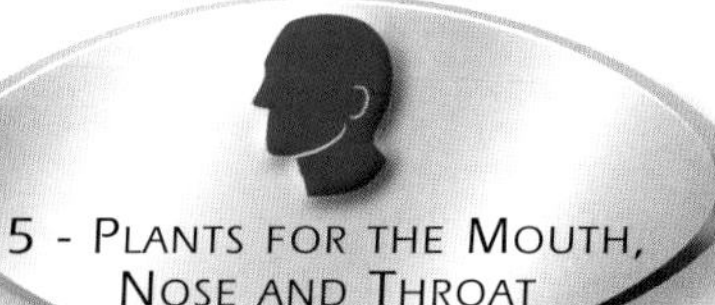

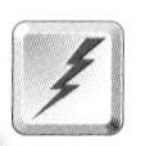
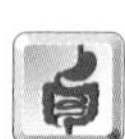
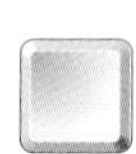
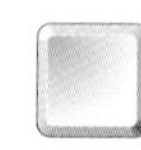

Clove Tree

Stimulant, disinfectant, and analgesic

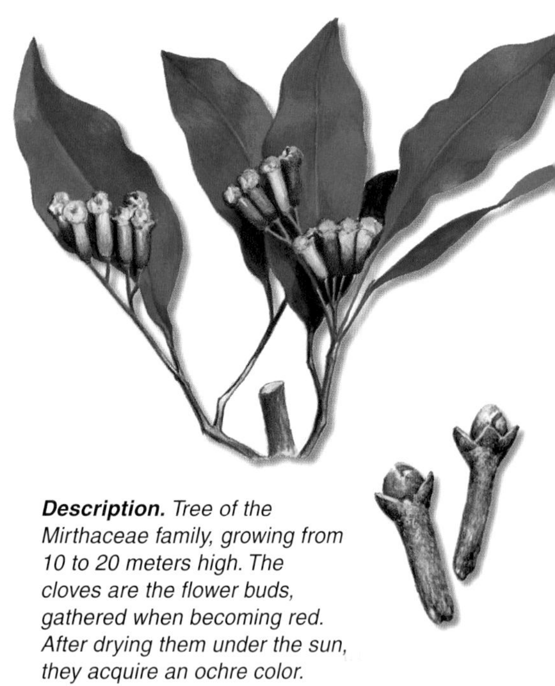

Description. *Tree of the Mirthaceae family, growing from 10 to 20 meters high. The cloves are the flower buds, gathered when becoming red. After drying them under the sun, they acquire an ochre color.*

Parts used. *Dried flower buds.*

THOSE VENERABLE Chinese physicians of the Han dynasty (206 b.c. – 220 a.d.) mention in their writings the properties of the clove tree, and especially its ability to sweeten the breath. However, until the time of great journeys in the sixteenth century, the clove tree, like many other spices, came to Europe from India in very small amounts. This fact made spices more expensive and precious.

The Portuguese seafarer Ferdinand Magellan, along with the Basque Juan Sebastian Elcano, the first to travel around the world, sailed on an expedition which in 1520 arrived at the Moluccas Islands, near China. On these islands they loaded cloves, bringing them to Spain as a precious treasure. Since then, the farming of clove trees spread to all tropical regions.

Properties and indications. Cloves contain 15 to 20% of essence, mainly formed by eugenol, along with small amounts of acetyleugenol, cariophilene, and metylamilcetone. This essence is what gives the clove its aroma, as well as its properties.

- **Oral antiseptic and analgesic.** The essence of clove, used as an oil, is included in ***toothpastes,*** orally taken ***elixirs,*** and ***perfumes.*** Its **antiseptic** power is three times superior to that of phenol. It is recommended in the case of stomatitis (inflammation of the mouth mucus membrane) or gingivitis (gum inflammation) **{❹}**. ***In local applications,*** it can temporarily ease **toothaches** caused by tooth decay **{❺}**.
- General **stimulant** **{❶,❷,❸}** of the body, though much milder than coffee.
- **Appetizer** **{❶,❷,❸}** (which stimulates the appetite), and **carminative** (eliminates intestinal gases).

Preparation and Use

Internal use

❶ **Infusion,** with two or three cloves per cup of water, drinking a cup with each meal.

❷ **Essence.** One to three drops before each meal.

❸ **Spice.** It must be sparingly used, since a single clove is enough to spice a whole meal.

External use

❹ **Mouth elixir.** Rinses with a glass of water to which some drops of clove essence have been added. It refreshes and disinfects the mouth.

❺ **Toothache.** In order to ease it, apply a **piece** of clove, or a drop of clove **essence,** on the aching tooth.

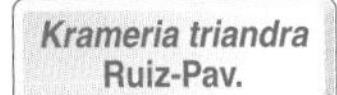

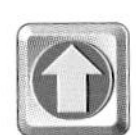
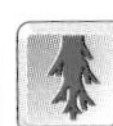
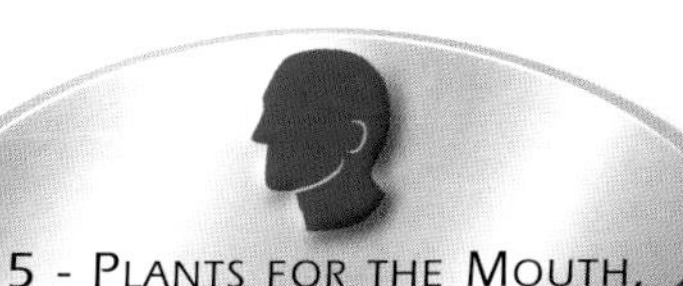

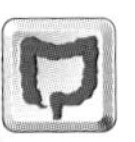
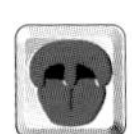
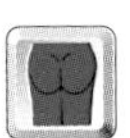
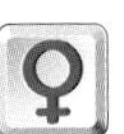
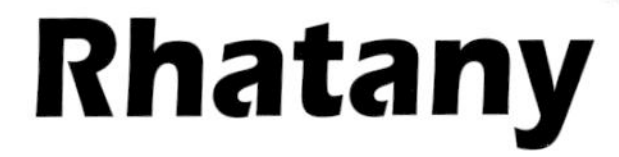

Rhatany

Powerful astringent and anti-inflammatory

THE ROOT of rhatany has been used in Peru since ancient times to clean teeth and gums. The ladies of Lima, Peru's capital city, used it in the nineteenth century to whiten their teeth for festivals and celebrations.

Properties and indications. The root contains catechic tannins, phlobaphene, krameric acid (an alkaloid), starch, mucilage, sugars, gum, and wax. Its most important active ingredient is tannin, which is not bitter, like that of the oak tree. Its strong **astringent and anti-inflammatory** action makes this plant recommended for **gastroenteritis and colitis [❶,❷,❸],** even in children.

Used ***externally***, it renders good results in the following cases:

- **Oral pharyngeal afflictions [❹]**. Stomatitis (mouth inflammation), pyorrhea, gingivitis, sore throat, pharyngitis, applied in gargles and rinses.

Preparation and Use

Internal use

❶ **Root powder.** A heaped spoonful three times a day.

❷ **Decoction** of 20 g of bark per liter of water. Drink three cups daily.

❸ **Fluid extract.** Take from ten to 20 drops, three times a day.

External use

❹ **Decoction** with 30-40 g of bark per liter of water. This decoction is used for **gargles, sitz baths, vaginal irrigations, and compresses.**

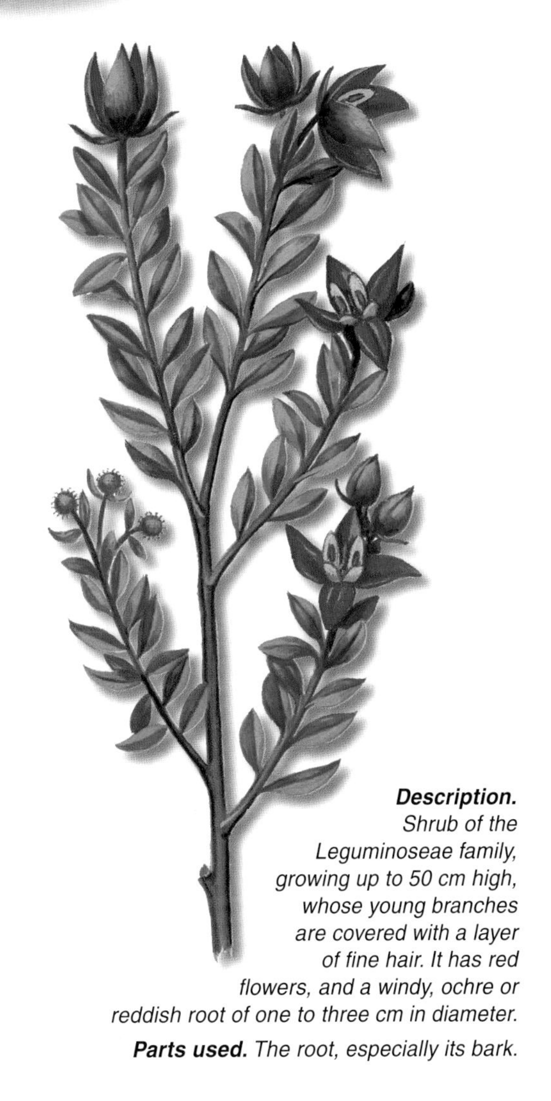

Description. *Shrub of the Leguminoseae family, growing up to 50 cm high, whose young branches are covered with a layer of fine hair. It has red flowers, and a windy, ochre or reddish root of one to three cm in diameter.*

Parts used. *The root, especially its bark.*

- **Hemorrhoids and anal fissures [❹]**, in sitz baths.
- **Leukorrhea** (vaginal flow) and **vaginitis [❹]**, in vaginal irrigations.
- **Chilblains [❹]**, in compresses soaked in a bark decoction.

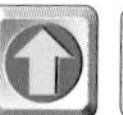
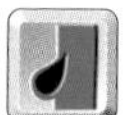
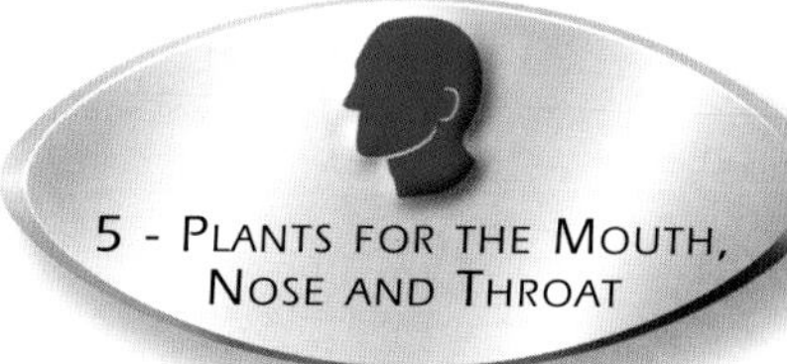

Mastic Tree

Strengthens teeth and freshens breath

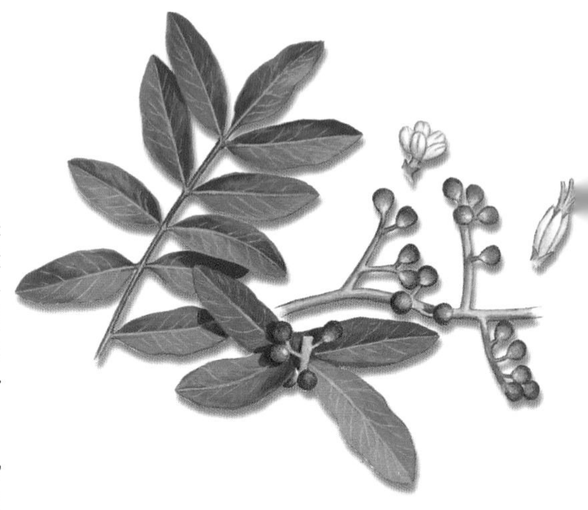

THE MASTIC is the resin that the mastic tree or lentiscus stems exude when cut on the surface. Dioscorides recommended it in the first century to "strengthen relaxed gums," and to fight bad breath. At present, it is part of many ***toothpastes and pharmaceutical preparations***.

PROPERTIES AND INDICATIONS. ***MASTIC RESIN*** contains mastitic acid, masticine, and pinene-rich essence. When chewed, it becomes a mass as soft as wax, which sticks to the teeth. Due to its **anti-inflammatory and antiseptic** action, it fights **pyorrhea** and **gingivitis** (gum inflammation) **[❶]**. It is useful in the treatment of **parodontosis** (inflammation and degeneration of the tissues that attach teeth) **[❶]**, which is the first cause of losing teeth worldwide. It also sweetens the breath, giving a fresh and clean sensation.

Its young ***LEAVES*** and ***STEMS*** contain a lower amount of active ingredients, but a higher amount of tannin. They are used in the same way as mastic resin, and in rinses with a decoction **[❷]**, in order to **reduce the inflammation of the gums and strengthen teeth**.

Description. *Shrub of the Anacardiaceae family, growing up to one meter high. Its all-year green leaves are coriaceous and hairless. The fruit is a red or black berry, the size of a pea.*

Parts used. *The mastic resin and the leaves.*

Both the mastic resin and the decoction of its leaves and stems are a good natural tooth cleanser, and are useful against pyorrhea and gum inflammation.

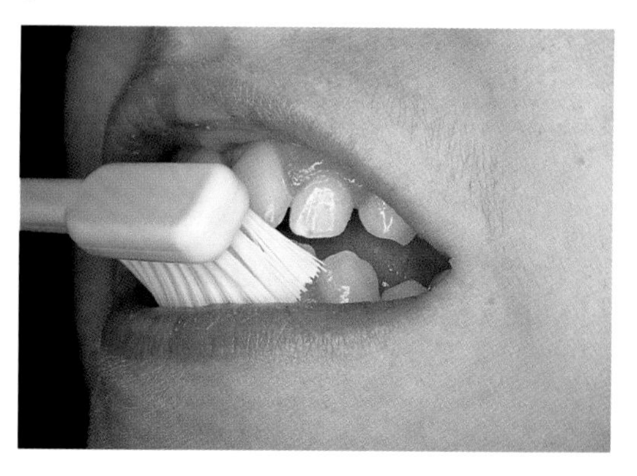

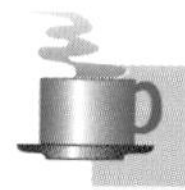

Preparation and Use

INTERNAL USE

❶ **Mastic resin,** chewed or in toothpaste.

❷ **Mouth rinses** with a decoction of young stems and leaves (100 g per liter of water), up to five times a day.

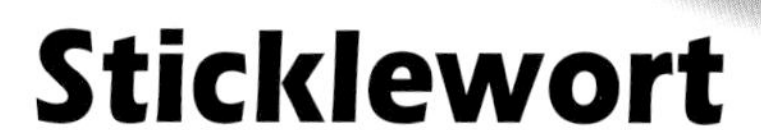

Sticklewort

Soothes and clears the throat

STICKLEWORT belongs to the *Rosaceae* family, which consists of more than 2000 species among which are some of the most beautiful plants.

PROPERTIES AND INDICATIONS. The plant contains flavonoids, essential oils, and mainly tannins, to which it owes most of its medicinal effects. Tannins act on skin and mucous membrane as **astringents,** forming a layer of coagulated proteins over them, upon which microorganisms can longer act. This fact is also the basis for skin tanning.

The infusion of sticklewort has an interesting **antidiarrheic** effect. It is also a **vermifuge** (expels intestinal worms) and is slightly **diuretic [❶].**

However, the ***greatest therapeutic use*** of this plant is when it is ***applied externally***.

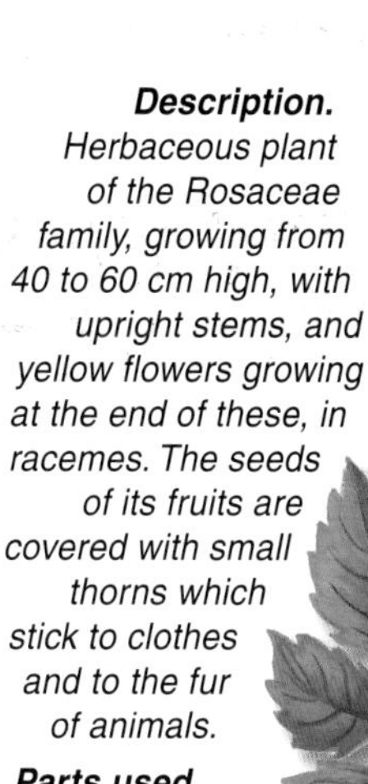
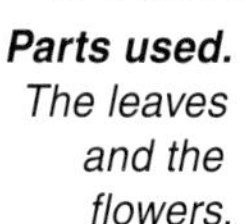
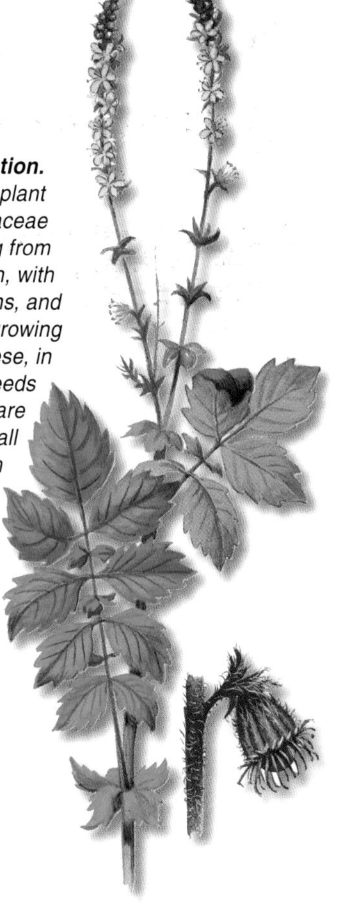

Description. *Herbaceous plant of the Rosaceae family, growing from 40 to 60 cm high, with upright stems, and yellow flowers growing at the end of these, in racemes. The seeds of its fruits are covered with small thorns which stick to clothes and to the fur of animals.*

Parts used. *The leaves and the flowers.*

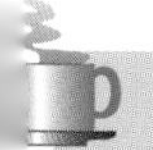

Preparation and Use

INTERNAL USE

❶ **Infusion or decoction** with 20-30 g of flowers and leaves per liter of water. Drink three or four cups a day, sweetened with honey if desired.

EXTERNAL USE

❷ **Mouth rinses and gargles,** with a concentrated decoction (100 g per liter), boiling until it reduces its volume to a third. Sage and linden may be added to this decoction. Sweeten with 50 g of honey.

❸ **Compresses** applied directly on the wounds, soaked in this concentrated decoction, without sugar.

Due to its astringent and anti-inflammatory effects on the mucous membrane, it is very useful in the following disorders:

- **Mouth sores [❷]**, applied in rinses.
- **Throat afflictions [❷]**: acute and chronic pharyngitis, tonsillitis, and laryngitis (aphonia). Gargles render good results in some cases, making the inflammation and irritation of the throat mucous membrane disappear in a few days.
- **As a cicatrizant [❸]** in torpid wounds, sores, and varicose ulcers of the legs. It is applied by putting compresses soaked in a sticklewort decoction on the affected area. The sores then dry out, and in this way cicatrization is encouraged.

Goldenseal

Effective against colds

GOLDENSEAL is a popular remedy in the United States and Canada, which is starting to be used on the rest of the American continent and Europe, due to its interesting properties.

PROPERTIES AND INDICATIONS. The rhizome of the plant contains diverse alkaloids (hydrastine and berberine, among others), essential oil, resins, and sugars, as well as vitamins A, B, and C, and mineral salts, especially phosphorus. All these substances give the plant **antiseptic, astringent, hemostatic, and anti-inflammatory** properties. It is successfully employed in the following cases:

• Nasal, pharyngeal, and bronchial **catarrhs.** Goldenseal acts effectively, by regenerating the cells of the mucous membranes, thus diminishing the production of mucus and the congestion and inflammation that accompanies catarrhs. It is applied both internally **[❶]** and externally (gargles) **[❷]**.

• **Excessive menstruation and metrorrhagia** (uterus hemorrhages) **[❶]**, because of its constricting effect on the uterus. In these cases, its use must always be under medical control.

• **Vaginitis and leukorrhea [❷]**, applied in irrigations and cleansing.

• **Pyorrhea and gingivitis** (inflammation of the gums).

• **Conjunctivitis** (eye irritations) **[❷]** in eyes baths.

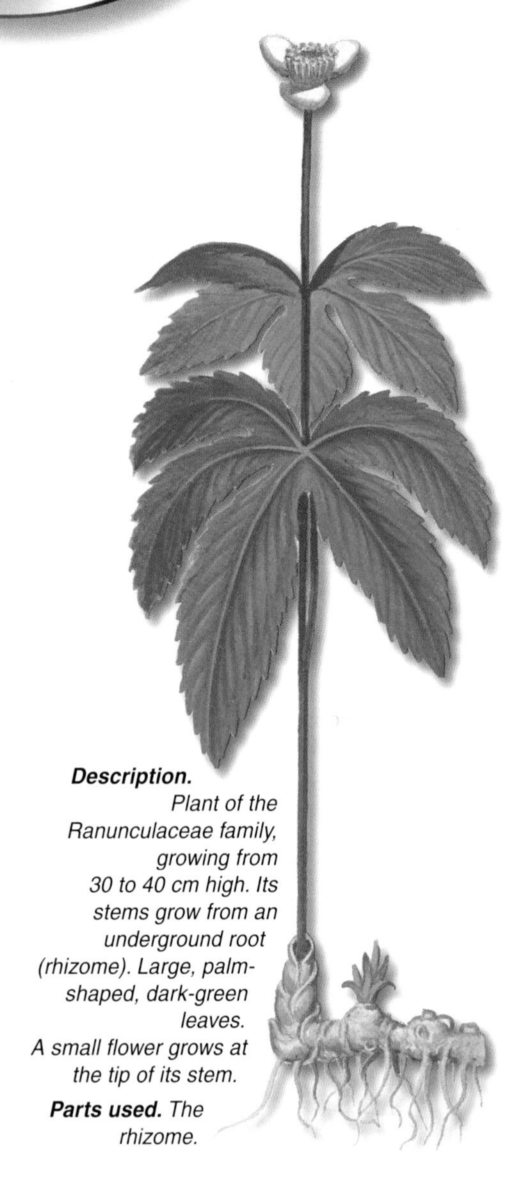

Description. *Plant of the Ranunculaceae family, growing from 30 to 40 cm high. Its stems grow from an underground root (rhizome). Large, palm-shaped, dark-green leaves. A small flower grows at the tip of its stem.*

Parts used. *The rhizome.*

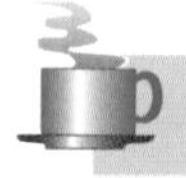

Preparation and Use

INTERNAL USE

❶ **Infusion** with a spoonful of rhizome per cup of water. Steep until cold. Drink two spoonfuls every four hours.

EXTERNAL USE

❷ The same infusion is employed in external use in the form of **gargles, rinses, irrigations, and washings.**

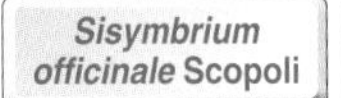
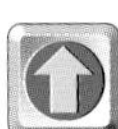
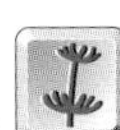
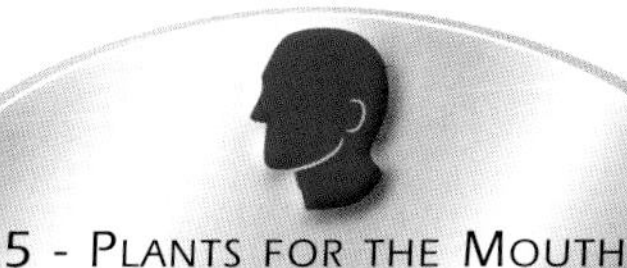
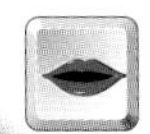
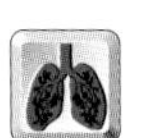

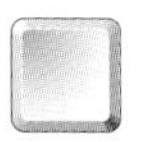

Hedge Mustard

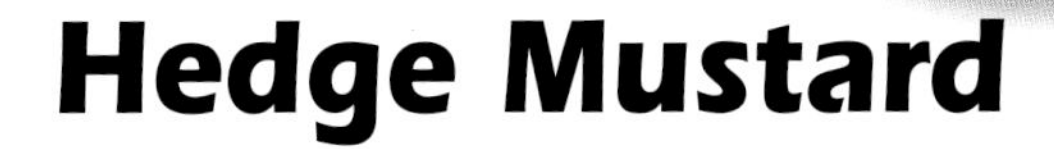

Clears the throat and reduces its inflammation

IN A TIME when microphones did not exist, singers, speakers, and actors all over Europe found in this plant the secret to keeping a clear, powerful voice.

PROPERTIES AND INDICATIONS. Hedge mustard is similar to mustard (p. 663) in appearance, flavor, and composition. It contains a sulphured essential oil that, when in contact with the mouth and pharynx mucosal membrane, provokes by means of a reflex mechanism, a greater flow of blood to the larynx and bronchi, thus promoting productive coughing.

It has **bechic** (easing cough and throat irritation), **anti-inflammatory, and expectorant** components, and it is very useful in cases of **pharyngitis, hoarseness, or aphonia** caused by laryngitis (inflammation of the vocal strings), and **bronchitis [❶,❷]**.

The best results are achieved when internal use (infusion) and external uses (mouth rinses and gargles) are combined.

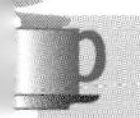

Preparation and Use

INTERNAL USE

❶ **Infusion** with 50 g of flower clusters per liter of water. Sweeten with honey and drink up to five or six hot cups a day.

EXTERNAL USE

❷ **Rinses and gargles** with the same infusion employed for internal use. Sweeten if desired. Remember not to swallow the liquid employed for rinses and gargles.

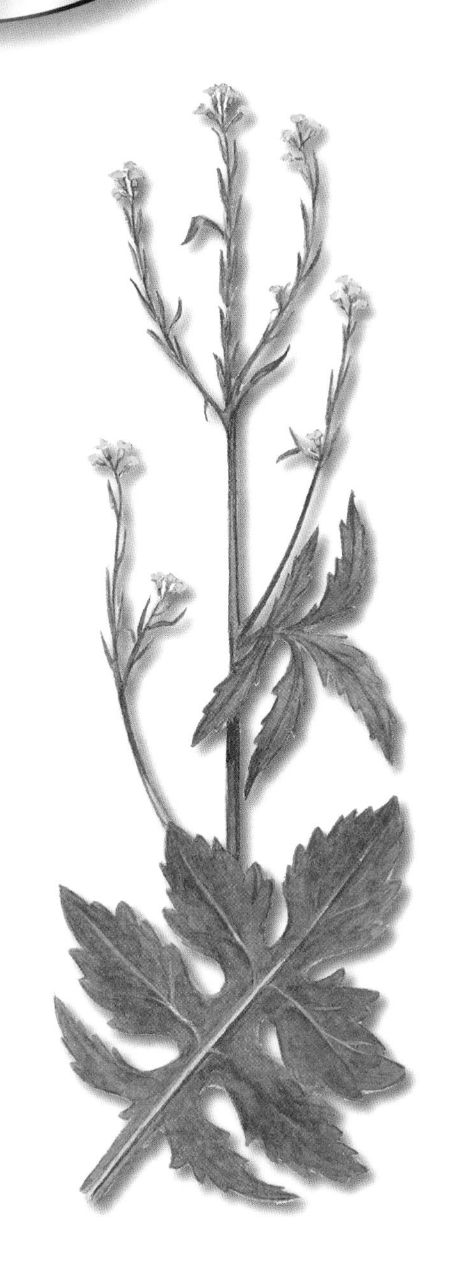

Description. *Plant of the Cruciferae family, growing from 40 to 100 cm high, with an upright, straight stem, big, deeply lobulated leaves, and small, pale yellow flowers.*

Used parts. *Flower clusters and leaves.*

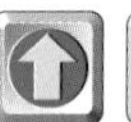
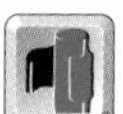
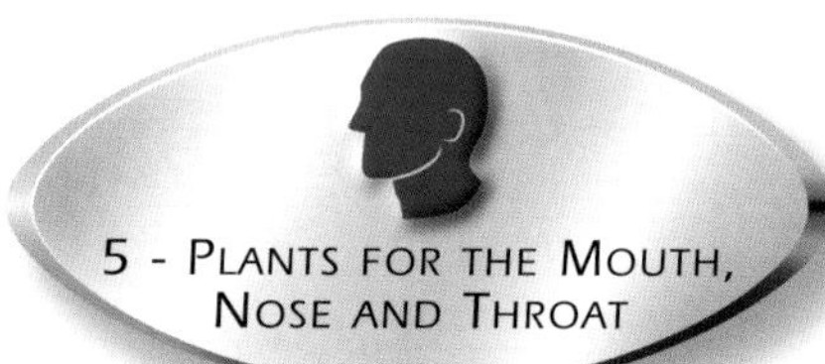

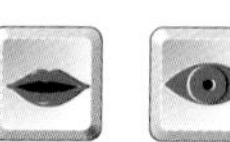
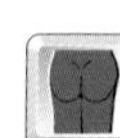
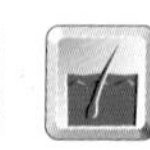

Oak Tree

Anti-inflammatory and astringent

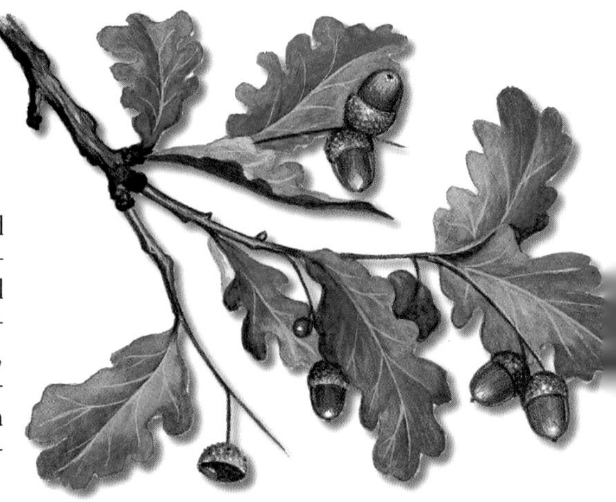

THE HUMBLE acorn is an exquisite meal for those who still have a taste, not accustomed to sophisticated and artificial modern cuisine flavors. Acorns have been a basic food for people of great physical strength, such as the Basques, for centuries. In some locations, there is a type of sweet acorn, which is even tastier than chestnuts, and may be eaten roasted like the latter.

PROPERTIES AND INDICATIONS. The ***BARK*** of all trees of the genus *Quercus* is ***very rich in tannins*** (up to 20%), among which the most outstanding is quercitanic acid. These tannins are astringent, that is to say, they dry inflamed mucous membrane and precipitate or coagulate the proteins of animal tissues. This is precisely the base for their tanning use: they dry the skin of animals, and turn it into leather.

Tannins are ***the most active astringent agents*** known. By acting on inflamed tissues, they dry and tighten them momentarily, while they are slowly substituted by healthy tissues. Tannins also have an **anti-inflammatory and analgesic** effect, and stop small surface hemorrhages (**hemostatic** action).

ACORNS also contain tannins, as well as sugars (carbohydrates) and lipids (fats) with a high biological value. They are **astringent**, and are an ideal food in the case of gastroenteritis caused by **diarrhea**, especially in children.

The ***BARK*** of oak and holm oak trees is applied in ***external use*** as a decoction **[0]** (if taken orally, though not toxic, it may provoke nausea), and has many indications due to its great healing properties.

- **Stomatitis and pharyngitis.** For oral mucous membrane and throat inflammations, it is applied in rinses or gargles several times a day, which eases the sensation of itching and stinging, besides achieving an antiseptic and cicatrizant effect.

Description. *Big tree of the Fagaceae family, with a wide crown and a thick, solid trunk, growing up to 20 m high, with lobulated, dark-green leaves with a lighter color on the underside. Acorns, its fruits, grow from large petioles hanging from its branches.*

Parts used. *The bark and the acorns.*

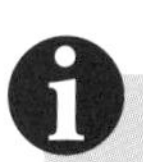

Washing the Yellow Dye

The yellow color that remains on the skin after applying oak tree remedies is caused by the action of the tannins it contains. Rubbing the skin with lemon juice will make this color disappear.

Preparation and Use

EXTERNAL USE

❶ **Decoction** with 60-80 g (around four spoonfuls) of ground oak or holm oak tree bark per liter of water, allowing it to simmer for ten minutes, then straining and applying it locally on the affected area by any of the following methods.

– **Rinses and gargles** (for mouth and throat disorders).

– **Vaginal irrigations.**

– **Sitz baths and enemas** (for anal or rectum afflictions).

– **Arm baths** (for chilblains).

– **Fomentations or hot compresses** (for aching muscles or joints).

– **Compresses,** soaking a cotton cloth or gauze and renewing it every four hours (for skin afflictions).

– **Eye baths or nose plugging.**

• **Gingivitis, parodontosis, pyorrhea**. In any kind of **gum inflammations** it helps to cleanse dirty gums. It may stabilize teeth that begin to move because of the inflammation of the gums and the tissues stabilizing teeth to the jawbone.

• **Conjunctivitis and blepharitis** (eyelid inflammation). In eye baths, or applying a compress soaked in the liquid of a decoction, every four hours. Very good results are achieved in the case of irritating or allergic conjunctivitis, as well as in styes.

• **Nose hemorrhages**. Applied in irrigations or by soaking a gauze that serves to plug the nostril. The combination with tormentil is recommended.

• **Chilblains.** Arm or foot bath, three times a day for 15 minutes, with a hot decoction of oak or holm oak tree bark. It makes reddening and skin itching disappear.

• **Hemorrhoids and anal fissures.** It reduces anal inflammation, stops the slight hemorrhage which usually accompanies these disorders, and favors the cicatrization of the painful anal fissures. It is applied in hot sitz baths, for 15 minutes, once or twice a day, as well as in enemas.

• **Skin sores and eczema.** Applied in compresses, by soaking a cotton cloth, it dries, reduces inflammation, and heals the skin.

• **Ulceration and sores** that have difficulty healing, including vascular-provoked ulcers due to bad blood circulation in the legs (varicose ulceration). Apply a compress soaked in the liquid of a decoction, renewing it every four hours.

• **Rheumatic aches.** Fomentations or hot compresses with a decoction of oak tree bark have anti-inflammatory and antirheumatic effects. They are employed to ease osteoarticular or articular aches in the neck, back, and lumbar areas, as well as in thighs and legs. People suffering from rheumatism or arthrosis will benefit from oak tree bark fomentations.

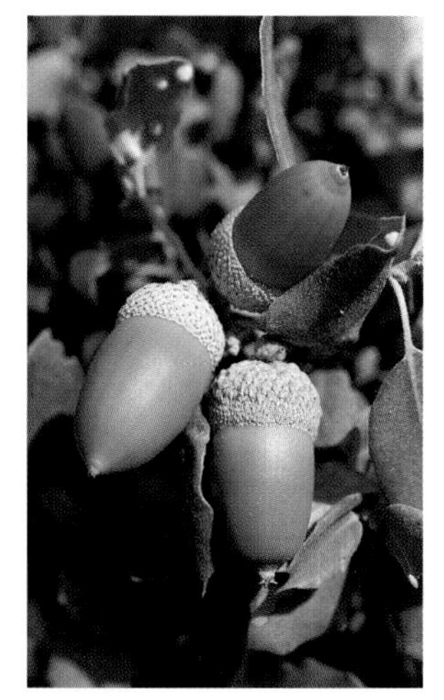

Acorns are rich in carbohydrates and fats, and have a great nutritional value. Their astringent action makes them an ideal food to combat diarrhea.

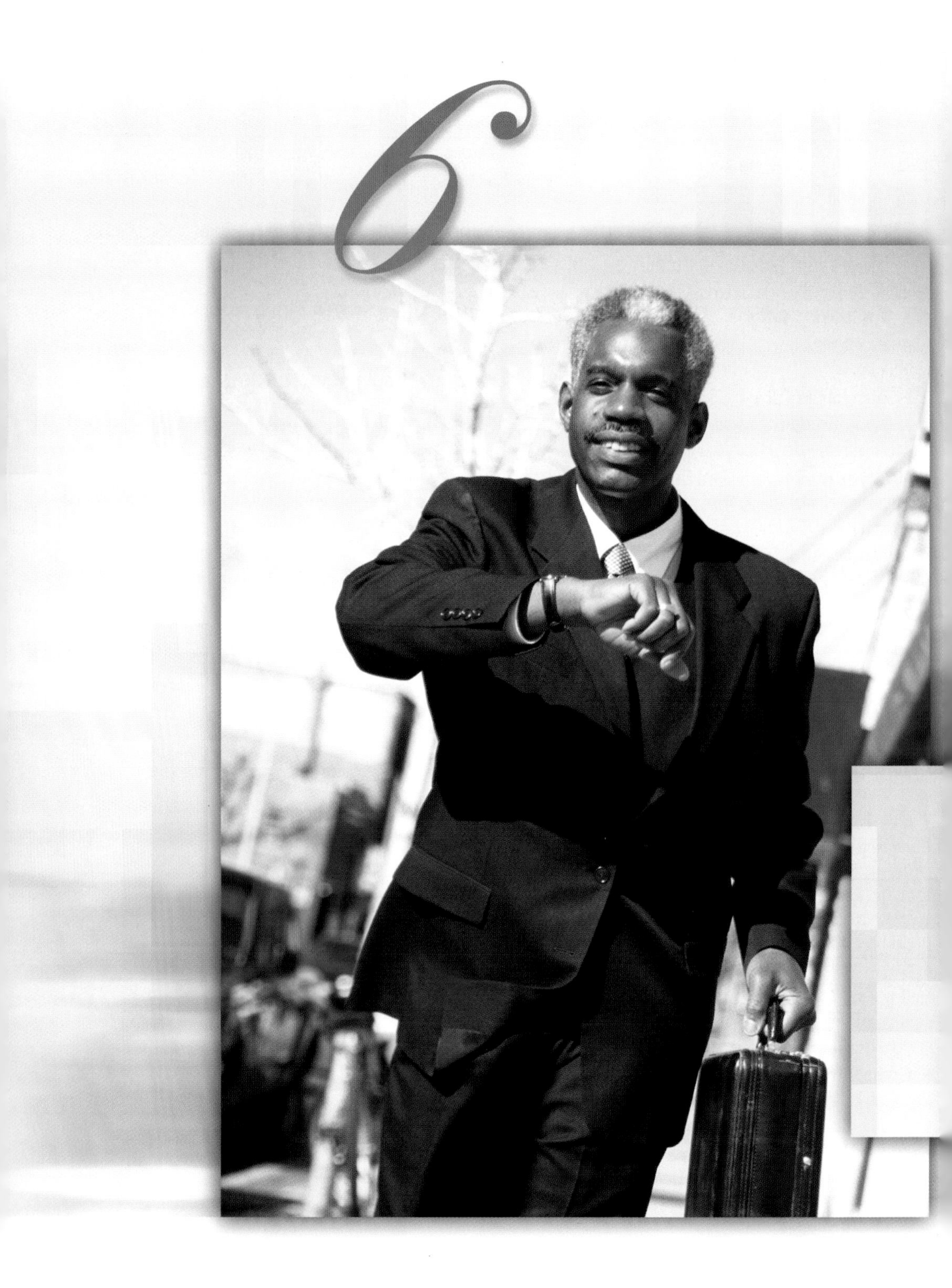

Plants for the Heart

DISEASE	PAGES
Angina pectoris	107
Arrhythmia	107
Attack, heart	107
Cardiopathy, see Heart affections	106
Coronary heart disease, see Angina pectoris	107
Heart affections	106
Heartbeat rate alteration, see Arrhythmia	107
Myocardial infarction	107
Palpitations	106
Tachycardia	106

PLANTS	PAGES
Cactus	108
Camphor tree	109
Foxglove	112
Hawthorn	110

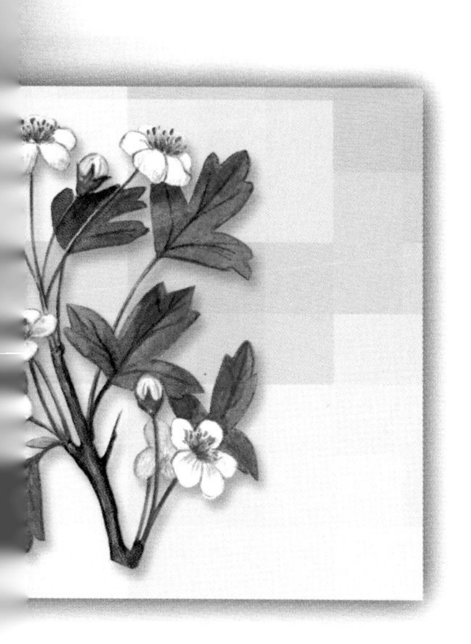

MEDICINAL HERBS exert notable actions on the heart. Those plants which augment the strength of heart contractions (called cardiotonic plants), the foxglove being the most important, are especially appreciated.

Besides strengthening the heart, medicinal herbs contribute in a decisive way to the prevention of severe heart dysfunctions, such as angina pectoris and heart attacks.

TACHYCARDIA

Definition

An increase in the heartbeat rate. When it occurs at rest, with no physical cause to explain it, it should be treated.

Phytotherapy

Usually, all cardiotonic plants, which increase heart contraction strength and thus its effectiveness, also reduce its frequency. Plants with ***sedative and balancing*** properties on the autonomic nervous system also stop tachycardia.

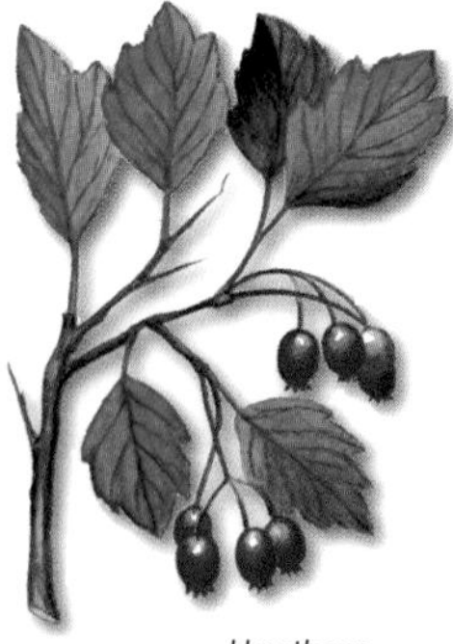

Hawthorn

HAWTHORN	Increases contraction strength of the heart and regulates its beat and rate

PALPITATIONS

Definition

This is defined as the disagreeable perception of your own heartbeat, due to a sudden change in it.

Causes

Palpitations may be caused by states of anxiety, the use of certain medicines, the consumption of toxic products such as coffee, tobacco, and alcohol, and more seldom, by certain heart dysfunctions. On an electrocardiogram they are shown as extrasystoles.

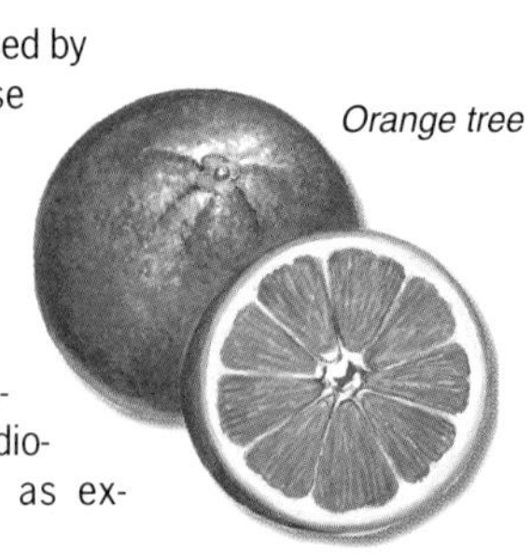

Orange tree

Phytotherapy

Besides the ***antispasmodic, sedative, and heart-invigorating*** plants we indicate, ***profound treatment*** of the underlying anxiety is required, as well as giving up the consumption of coffee, tobacco, alcohol, or other toxic substances.

ORANGE TREE	Antispasmodic, sedative
LAVENDER	Sedative balances the nervous system
BALM	Antispasmodic, sedative
VALERIAN	Antispasmodic, sedative on the central and autonomic nervous system
HAWTHORN	Increases contraction strength of the heart and regularizes beat rate

HEART AFFECTIONS

These plants are recommended for all those people suffering from any heart disease, due to their gentle ***heart-invigorating*** effect, their low sodium content (which increases blood pressure), and their diuretic effect which has no risks.

LINDEN	Vasodilator and mildly hypotensive, thins blood
HAWTHORN	Increases blood flow in coronary arteries and combats their spasms

ARRHYTHMIA

Definition

An alteration of the heartbeat rate, be it irregular, too slow (**bradycardia**), or too fast (**tachycardia**).

Causes

Arrhythmia may be a consequence of anxiety, of the use of certain medicines, of the consumption of toxic products such as coffee, tobacco, and alcohol. In these cases it is seldom severe, and disappears when the cause is corrected. However, there are other cases in which arrhythmia may be a symptom of heart dysfunctions which demand an ***accurate diagnosis*** by a professional.

LINDEN	Vasodilator, mild hypotensive
VALERIAN	Antispasmodic, sedative on the central and autonomic nervous system
HAWTHORN	Increases contraction strength of the heart and regularizes beat rate
FOXGLOVE	Cardiotonic, normalizes heartbeat rate

ANGINA PECTORIS

Definition

An affliction whose symptoms are sudden pain in the chest, occasionally passing to the left arm, with a sensation of imminent death.

Causes

This affliction is caused by a spasm or narrowing of the heart arteries, which feed the very heart muscle.

Phytotherapy

Phytotherapeutical treatment is based on ***antispasmodic*** (which alleviate the spasm of heart arteries), ***vasodilating*** (which dilate these arteries), and ***sedative*** plants.

When the arterial spasm is due to **arteriosclerosis** (thickening and narrowing) of the heart arteries, the plants recommended for this arterial affliction are also useful.

LINDEN	Vasodilator, mildly hypotensive, sedative, blood thinner
HAWTHORN	Increases blood flow in heart arteries and combats their spasms
GARLIC	Vasodilator, fluidizes blood
TINNEVELLY SENNA	Avoids dangerous defecation efforts in the case of constipation

MYOCARDIAL INFARCTION

Definition

The complete obstruction of coronary arteries, which produces death of part of the heart muscle.

Phytotherapy

Besides the recommended plants for angina pectoris, phytotherapy advises the use of plants for the ***prevention*** of heart attacks and of arteriosclerosis, an ailment which causes the obstruction of coronary arteries, as well as for the ***rehabilitation*** of people who have suffered those ailments. The ***blood-thinning*** plants also exert a preventive action.

EVENING PRIMROSE	Dilates arteries and prevents clot formation
SPIRULIN	Combats coronary arteriosclerosis because of its high content in unsaturated fatty acids

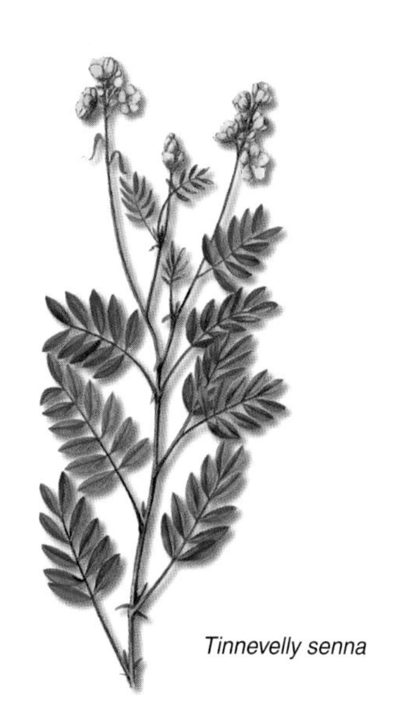

Tinnevelly senna

Cactus

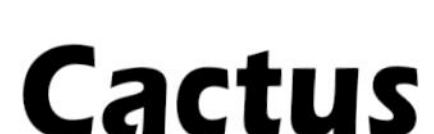

A good friend to the heart

THE BEAUTIFUL FLOWERS of this Central American cactus have very short lives. In the same night they grow, they produce their aroma, and die. However, their interesting medicinal properties remain, and these make the plant highly appreciated.

PROPERTIES AND INDICATIONS: The ***FLOWERS*** contain heart glycosides, flavonoids, and captine, an alkaloid which is very active on the heart. They have **cardiotonic, anti-arrhythmia** (regulating heartbeat), and **vasodilating** properties on the coronary arteries **[❶]**. They may complement and even substitute foxglove (p. 221). Their indications are: for coronary insufficiency, valve dysfunctions (alterations of the heart valves), heartbeat disorders (palpitations), and angina pectoris (making the sensation of oppression on the chest disappear).

The ***FLESH*** of the fruits contains mucilage with a mild **laxative** action **[❷]**, and the seeds, a **purgative** oil **[❸]**.

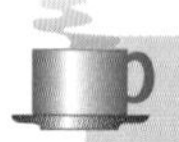

Preparation and Use

❶ **Flowers.** The safest method is to take them as **pharmaceutical preparations.**

❷ **Flesh of the fruits.** From two to ten fruits daily may be eaten.

❸ **Oil of the seeds.** From half to one spoonful is enough to obtain its purgative effect.

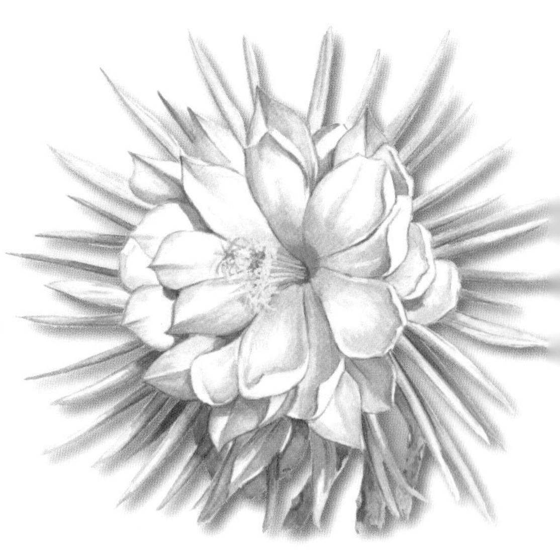

Description. *Climbing plant of the Cactaceae family, with fleshy, spiky stems from which aerial roots grow and secure the plant onto rocks and trees. Big (up to 30 cm), whitish, aromatic flowers, and ovoid berries some 8 cm large.*

Parts used. *Flowers and fruits (berries).*

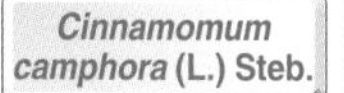

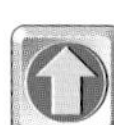
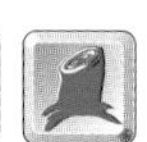
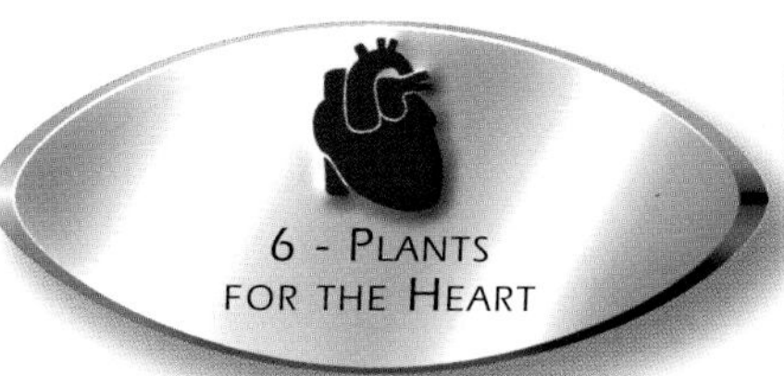

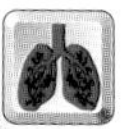
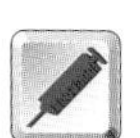
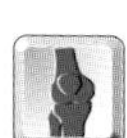
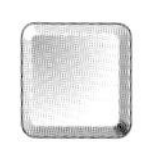

Camphor Tree

Heart and breath invigorating

THE CAMPHOR TREE is a thousand-year-old tree which begins to produce camphor when it reaches 30 years of age. In China there are camphor trees which are up to two thousand years old.

PROPERTIES AND INDICATIONS: ***CAMPHOR*** is a white, crystalline substance obtained after condensation of the essential oil, distilled from the camphor wood. These are its properties:

- **Cardiac and respiratory stimulant [❶]:** It stimulates the nervous centers of respiration and heart activity, increasing the frequency and deepness of breath, and strengthens the heart. It is used for lung congestion, fainting, hypotension, arrhythmia, and blackouts.
- **Antiseptic and febrifuge [❶]:** Very useful for influenza and colds.
- **Anaphrodisiac [❶]:** Decreases sexual excitement.
- **Antirheumatic and analgesic [❷]:** Camphor oil or alcohol is used in ***external application*** in lotions in order to alleviate rheumatic aches and neuralgia.

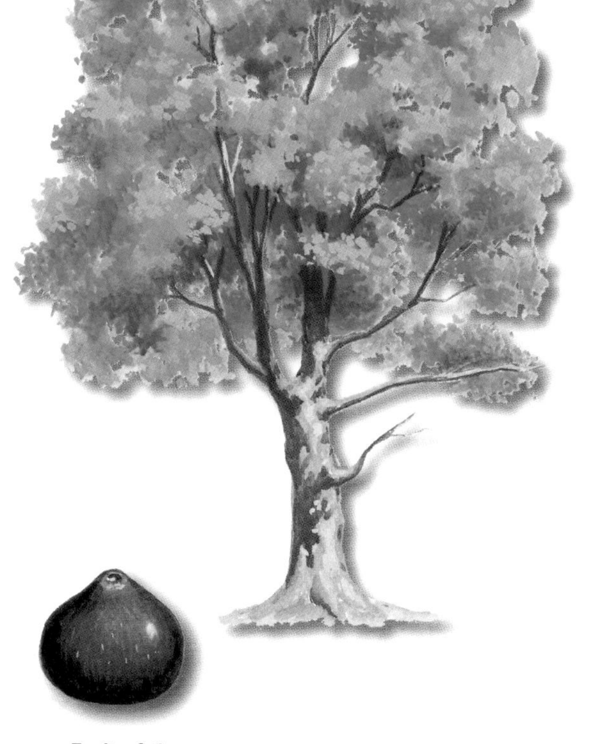

Fruit of the camphor tree.

Flower of the camphor tree.

Preparation and Use

INTERNAL USE

❶ **Camphor powder.** Up to 0.5 g a day, divided into three or four intakes.

EXTERNAL USE

❷ **Lotions and massage oils** with **camphor oil or alcohol,** which are prepared dissolving camphor in oil or in alcohol in a proportion of **10 %** alcohol.

Description. *Tree of the Lauraceae family growing up to 50 meters high. Evergreen, coriaceous leaves and small, white flowers.*

Parts used. *The essence of its wood.*

Hawthorn

Strengthens the heart and calms the nerves

"HOW DO YOU manage to breed such agile and strong goats?" a Greek peasant asked his neighbor, in the first century. "The Summer is already ending, and in the dry and rocky fields of the Mediterranean lands there does not seem to be much food for such mammals."

"I'll tell you the secret. Have you seen those spiky shrubs, with red berries? Try making your goats eat some, and in a few days you will notice the results."

Indeed, the neighbor's goats became stronger than ever before. They never seemed to tire, climbing the slopes under the heat of the Greek Summer. Perhaps this shepherd's experience was known by Dioscorides, an acute observer, brilliant botanical, and outstanding physician, who recommended this plant to give strength to the body and to heal several afflictions. Maybe its scientific name *Crataegus* arises from such an episode, since in Greek language it means "strong goats."

Hawthorn has always been highly appreciated as a remedy. However, the empirical knowledge of it, which was based upon its effects on goats, could not be scientifically proven until the

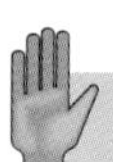

Warning

*In **high doses** (12 to 15 times more than recommended) it may produce **bradycardia** (slowing of the heartbeat rate) and **respiratory depression.** With the recommended doses there are no undesirable side effects.*

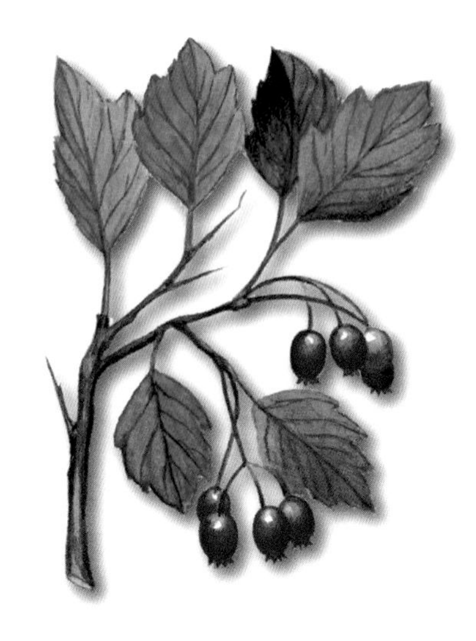

Description. *Spiky shrub of the Rosaceae family, growing from two to four meters high. Deciduous, three or five-lobulated leaves; white, aromatic flowers; red berries.*

Parts used. *The flowers and the fruits.*

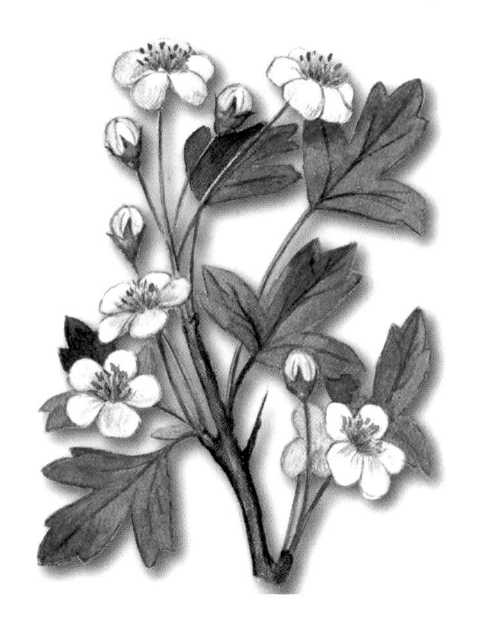

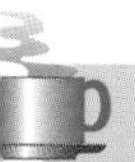

Preparation and Use

INTERNAL USE

❶ **Infusion** with 60 g of flowers (some four tablespoonfuls) per liter of water. Fresh flowers are more effective than dried ones. Drink three or four cups daily.

❷ **Fresh fruits:** Though with a lower concentration of active components, they are also effective, and a handful may be eaten three times a day.

❸ **Dry extract:** The recommended dose varies from 0.5 to 1 g, three times a day.

nineteenth century. Jennings and other American physicians of that time studied the cardiotonic properties of the hawthorn.

At present, hawthorn is well-recognized as a medicinal herb, and is part of many ***phytotherapeutical preparations***.

PROPERTIES AND INDICATIONS: Mainly its flowers, but also its fruits, contain diverse flavonic glycosides, chemically polyphenols, to which it owes its action on the heart and the circulatory system as well as triterpenic derivatives, and several biogenic amines (trimethylamine, choline, tyramine, etc.) which enhance its cardiotonic effect. The whole plant, due to the properties of the compound of these substances, is:

- **Cardiotonic [❶,❷,❸]**: A property attributed mainly to flavonoids, which inhibit (prevent) the action of ATPase (adenosyne-tri-phosphatase), an enzyme which catalyzes the splitting of ATP, the substance that serves as a source of energy for cells, including those of the heart muscle. When impeding the destruction of ATP, cells have more energy, thus there is an increase of the contractile strength of the heart, as well as a regulation of its beat rate. Hawthorn has the following indications:
  - ***Coronary insufficiency*** (heart weakness), with or without dilatation of its cavities, due to myocarditis or myocardiopathy (inflammation or degeneration of the heart muscle), valve lesions or recent myocardial infarction.
  - ***Arrhythmia*** (disorders of the heartbeat rate): extrasystole (palpitations), tachycardia, atrial fibrillation or blocking.
  - ***Angina pectoris:*** Hawthorn increases the amount of blood in the coronary arteries, and fights their spasm, which causes angina pectoris. It is a good vasodilator of coronary arteries.

The cardiotonic and antiarrhythmic effect of hawthorn is similar to that obtained with foxglove, which it can substitute with favorable results (except in acute cases). Hawthorn lacks the toxicity and the accumulative risk typical of foxglove.

- **Balancing of blood pressure [❶,❷,❸]**: Hawthorn has a balancing effect on blood pressure, since it decreases it in hypertensive people, and increases it in hypotensive people. Its balancing action on hypertension is evident and rapid, achieving more lasting effects than with other synthetic anti-hypertensives.
- **Sedative** effect on the sympathetic nervous system (sympatheticolytic effect) [❶,❷,❸]. It is useful in those persons suffering from nervousness that shows itself through a sensation of heart oppression, tachycardia, breathing difficulty, anxiety, or insomnia. It is ***one of the most effective anxiolytic*** plants (which eliminate anxiety) known.

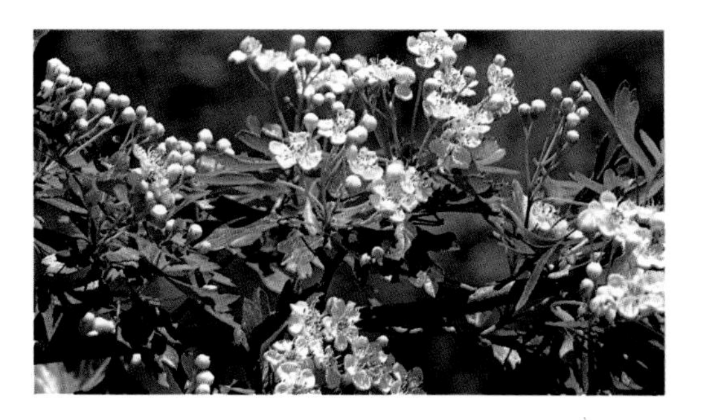

Foxglove

A powerful heart tonic that may be toxic

FOXGLOVE is a typical example of how the same plant can cure or kill. In the seventeenth century, in England, foxglove was given for the first time to an ill person who suffered from a heart-caused case of dropsy (edema in the whole body caused by heart failure). A few years later, foxglove was included in the Edinburgh *Pharmacopoeia*.

From then on, much biochemical and biological research on this plant has been carried out, whose active components have not yet been substituted by any chemical product.

At present, **foxglove glycosides** are ***widely employed*** in medicine, and ***have saved many lives*** of people with heart problems.

However, foxglove is a very toxic plant, and an infusion with a minimum part of only one leaf (10 g) may cause the death of an adult person. It is a problem of dosage. The therapeutic range is very narrow, and the toxic dose is very close to the healing one.

Because of the fact that there exist great variations in the concentration of active components depending on the place where the plants

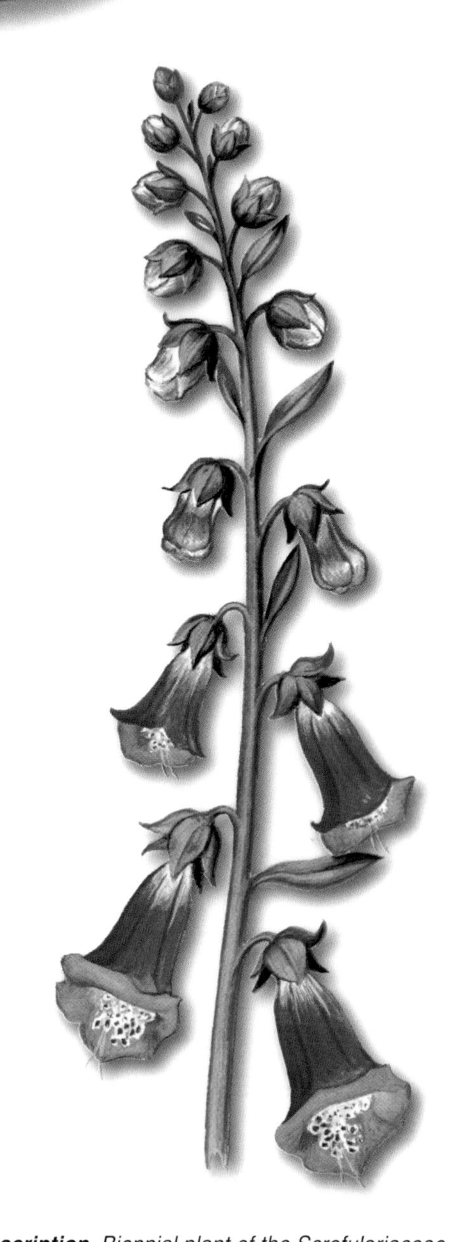

Description. *Biennial plant of the Scrofulariaceae family, growing up to one and a half meters high. Large, velvet-like, lanceolate leaves which grow from the lower part of the plant. Its flowers are finger-shaped, purple or pink colored, and grow from the top of the stem.*

Parts used. *Leaves.*

Excellent Wound Healing Agent

In external use, the leaves of this plant are an excellent wound healing agent for ***ulcers and skin wounds,*** *including* ***varicose*** *ulcers* **[❸].** *This was the main application of foxglove until its effects on the heart were discovered.*

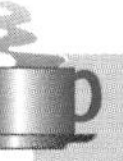

Preparation and Use

INTERNAL USE

❶ **Pharmaceutical preparations.** ***The safest and most tolerated method*** to apply foxglove is to use its extract in a pharmaceutical preparation. However, the plant when complete is more effective, though more caution is required to administer the correct dose. ***Only pharmacists and physicians*** with experience in phytotherapy can obtain the maximum advantage of this powerful plant. If correctly applied it can solve severe heart problems, and even save lives.

❷ **Infusion.** With one gram of powder obtained from ground dry leaves per 100 ml of hot water. Steep for 15 minutes. Drink during the day, by spoonfuls. ***Do not exceed this dose.*** It must never be taken continuously for more than **ten days,** because the glycosides accumulate in the body. Usually it is taken for five days, with a two-day pause.

EXTERNAL USE

❸ **Compresses.** Preparing an infusion with one or two leaves per liter of water, then soaking cotton cloths which are applied onto the affected skin area.

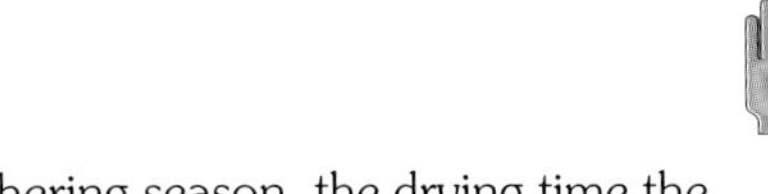

grow, the gathering season, the drying time the plant takes, etc., pharmacological industries have isolated those active principles, making them chemically pure. Thus, it is easier to dose and apply them correctly. However, their effectiveness is lower, because other substances that are usually present in the plant, and which complement the action of active components, do not appear together with chemically pure active components.

PROPERTIES AND INDICATIONS: Two kinds of substances may be distinguished in foxglove:

✓ **Non-glycosides:** Digitoflavine (yellow coloring), cyclohexanol, malic and succinic acids, tannin, and an oxidizing diastase. These substances do not have a direct effect on the heart, though they complement and improve the action of glycosides.

✓ **Glycosides:** They are responsible for the cardiotonic effects of foxglove on the heart muscle. The most important ones are digoxin and digitalin. They have the following properties:

- Increase the ***strength of heart contractions,*** improving its mechanical performance.
- Balance the ***heartbeat rate*** when it is irregular or too quick (tachycardia).

For all these reasons, the **glycosides** of foxglove are an ***indispensable remedy*** in cases of **coronary insufficiency [❶,❷]** (inability of the heart to pump the blood needed in the body), which in acute cases is clinically shown as an edema (soaking) of lungs, or as dropsy (accumulation of liquid in the cavities and tissues of the body). Moreover, they balance the heartbeat rate and have certain diuretic action, which contributes to improve the functioning of the circulatory system.

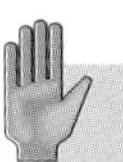

Warning

Though foxglove is a ***toxic*** *plant, accidental intoxication is rare, due to its disagreeable flavor. After chewing its leaves or flowers, it irritates the mouth, and causes nausea, vomiting, vision alterations, bradycardia, and ultimately heart failure. A few flowers may cause death in a child (and the plant is grown for decoration!).*

First aid *consists of a stomach pumping, administering purgatives, activated charcoal, and urgent transportation of the afflicted person to a hospital.*

7

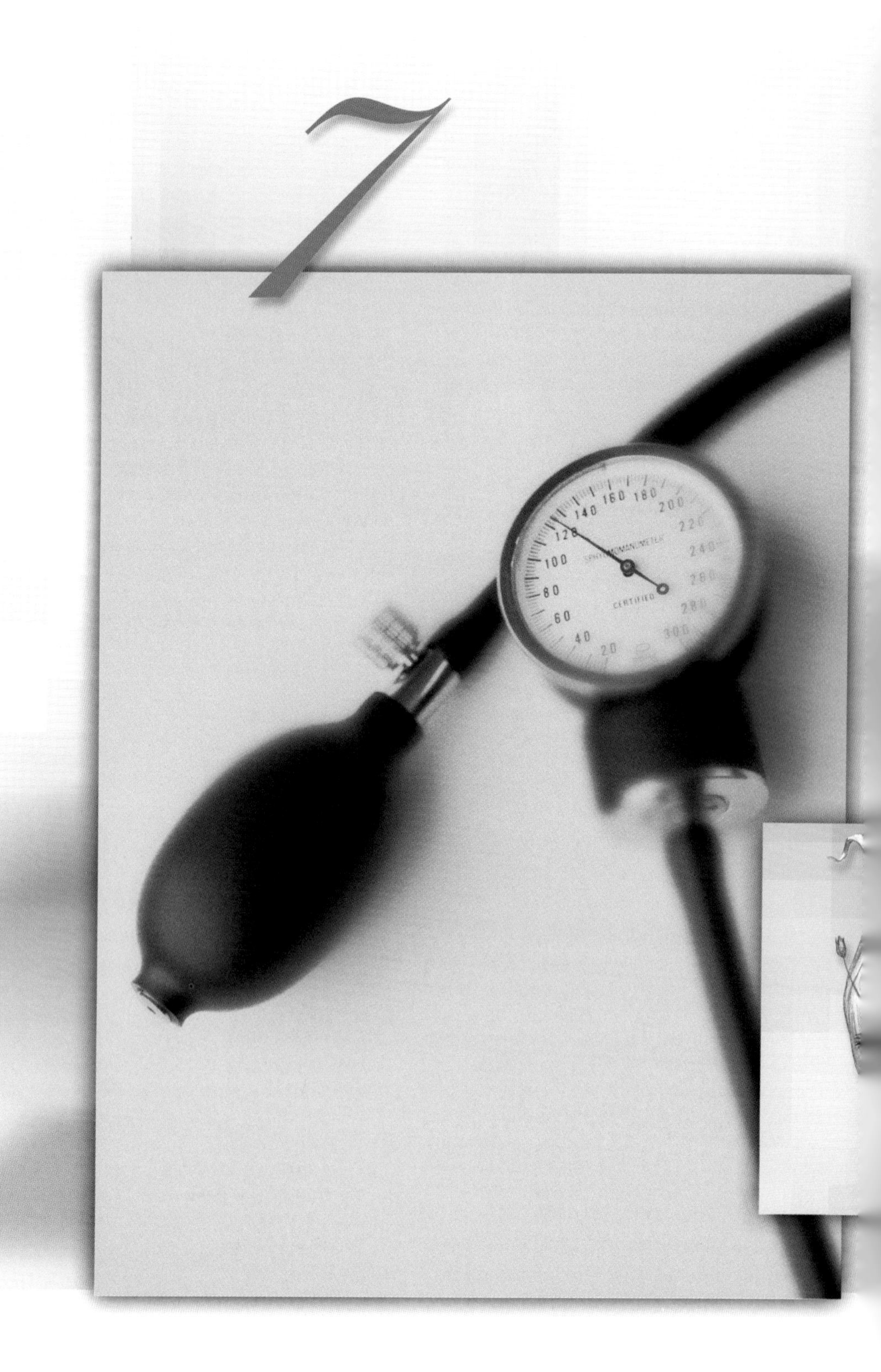

Plants for the Arteries

DISEASES	PAGES
Arteriosclerosis	117
Blood flow, lack of	117
Brain circulatory insufficiency, see Lack of blood flow	117
Chilblains	117
Cholesterol, plants against high	117
Cold, chilblains	117
Erythema pernio, see Chilblains	117
Fainting	117
High blood pressure	116
Hypertension, see High blood pressure	116
Hypotension, see Low blood pressure	116
Lack of blood flow	117
Low blood pressure	116

PLANTS	PAGES
Evening primrose	124
Garlic	118
Ginkgo	122

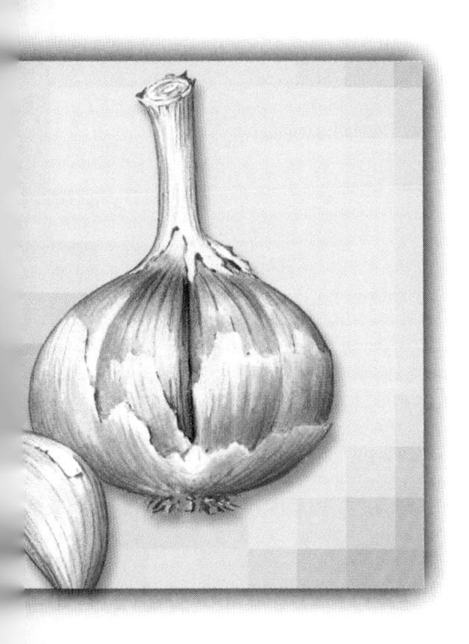

THE HEALTH of the arteries depends mainly on the quality of the blood circulating through them. Among the hundreds of substances that blood carries, cholesterol is perhaps the most harmful for the arteries.

Cholesterol is a fat which our body produces and uses for diverse biochemical functions. When there is an excess of it, it has the particular feature of covering the intima layer of arteries, provoking irritation and later a degenerative lesion. The result is the thickening of the arterial wall, and the narrowing of its diameter, known as **arteriosclerosis.** There are several factors which favor this illness, especially the following:

- The **increase of cholesterol** in the blood, usually caused by a diet rich in animal products, such as meat and its derivatives, butter, cream, cheese, and eggs.
- Arterial **hypertension.**
- **Smoking.**

Medicinal herbs also contribute to the health of arteries by decreasing **blood pressure,** and diminishing the level of **cholesterol** in the blood, by means of one of two mechanisms:

- **Decreasing the** intestinal **absorption** of cholesterol. Oat bran or apple skin retain the cholesterol in the intestine, preventing it from passing into the blood.
- **Decreasing the production** of cholesterol by the body. Vegetable oils, rich in unsaturated fatty acids such as linoleic and linolenic acids, act in this way.

LOW BLOOD PRESSURE

Definition

Low blood pressure causes tiredness, fatigue, and decreased muscular tone.

Phytotherapy

The recommended plants invigorate the nervous and circulatory systems, and are better than the habitual consumption of exciting substances such as coffee, yerba maté, or tea.

CAMPHOR TREE	Stimulates respiratory and cardiac activity nervous centers
HAWTHORN	Normalizes blood pressure
BASIL	Invigorator on the nervous and cardio-vascular systems
WINTER SAVORY	Nervous system invigorator
GINSENG	Normalizes blood pressure, both high and low
SAGE	Invigorator, stimulates suprarenal glands
ROSEMARY	General invigorator
THYME	General invigorator, helps recovery from physical exhaustion

HIGH BLOOD PRESSURE

Causes

The increase in blood pressure, wether systolic (maximum) pressure, or diastolic (minimum) pressure, can be caused by pathological reasons, such as liver dysfunctions, arteriosclerosis, or hormonal disorders. However, in many cases the cause of the disorder is unknown, hence it is called **essential hypertension.**

Phytotherapy

Phytotherapy uses ***sedative and nervous balancing plants***, ***diuretic*** plants, and ***vasodilator*** plants, with proven ***hypotensive*** efficiency, especially for essential hypertension.

LINDEN	Vasodilator, mild hypotensive, sedative, blood thinner
VALERIAN	Sedative, decreases anxiety and blood pressure
HAWTHORN	Normalizes blood pressure
GARLIC	Vasodilator, decreases both maximum and minimum blood pressure
MARJORAM	Hypotensive, decreases the tone of the sympathetic nervous system
FUMITORY	Diuretic, antispasmodic, blood thinner
GINSENG	Normalizes blood pressure, both high and low
HORSETAIL	Diuretic, remineralizer
NONI	Vasodilator, enhances arterial blood flow, antioxidant.

FAINTING

A sudden loss of consciousness, accompanied by falling over. It is usually associated with hypotension. Besides the recommended plants for hypotension, which may prevent fainting, these three may be used, which provide balance to the nervous and circulatory systems.

ORANGE TREE	Antispasmodic, sedative
LAVENDER	Sedative and nervous system balancing
BALM	Antispasmodic, sedative

LACK OF BLOOD FLOW

Also called **circulatory insufficiency,** it is characterized by an imbalance between the amount of blood needed by an organ and the amount that it actually receives through the arteries. It especially affects the brain, producing sickness, loss of memory and intellectual degeneration, among other symptoms.

GINKGO	Vasodilator, enhances blood flow

CHILBLAINS

Also called **erythema pernio,** this is a disorder of local blood flow caused by the cold, and characterized by the appearance of itching and reddening on the arms or legs. Besides these plants, applied in baths or compresses, ***capillary protecting*** plants are also recommended.

RHATANY	Astringent and anti-inflammatory
OAK TREE	Astringent, alleviates skin reddening and itching
GINKGO	Vasodilator and capillary protective
LUNGWORT	Astringent, anti-inflammatory, emollient
MILFOIL	Vulnerary, cicatrizant, antiseptic

ARTERIOSCLEROSIS AND EXCESS OF CHOLESTEROL

Definition

Thickening and narrowing of the arterial walls caused by cholesterol deposits, which produces less blood supply to the afflicted tissues.

Phytotherapy

Phytotherapy offers ***vasodilator*** plants, blood ***thinning***, and plants rich in ***trace elements*** such as silicon, which promote the regeneration of the tissues that form the arterial walls.

All plants that decrease the level of **cholesterol** prevent and avoid the manifestation of arteriosclerosis, because this fatty substance is the cause of the degeneration and narrowing of the arterial walls.

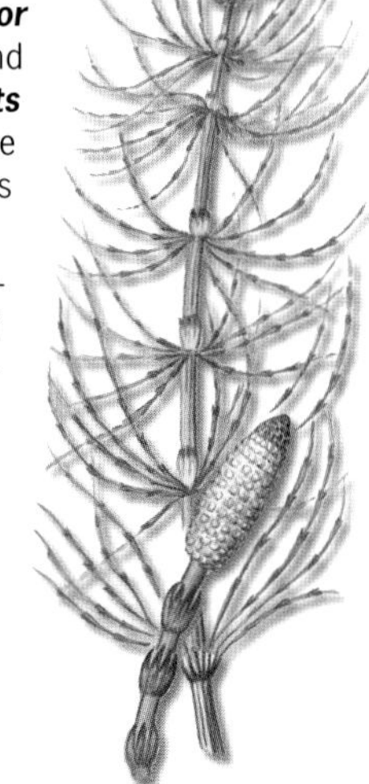
Horsetail

LINDEN	Vasodilator, mildly hypotensive, sedative, blood thinner
GARLIC	Vasodilator, blood thinner
GINKGO	Vasodilator, enhances blood flowing
DEVIL'S CLAW	Regenerates the elastic fibers of the arterial walls, decreases cholesterol level
MILFOIL	Blood thinner, enhances blood flowing
HORSETAIL	Due to its content in silicon, stimulates the regeneration of the elastic fibers of the arterial walls
NONI	Vasodilator, enhances arterial blood flow, antioxidant.

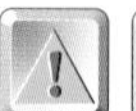

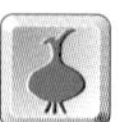

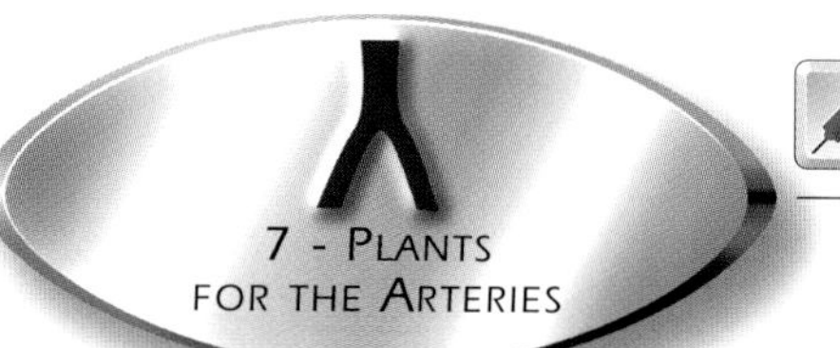

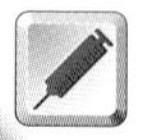

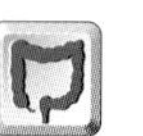

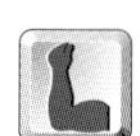

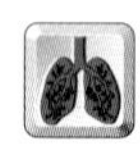

Garlic

Heals and efficiently prevents many diseases

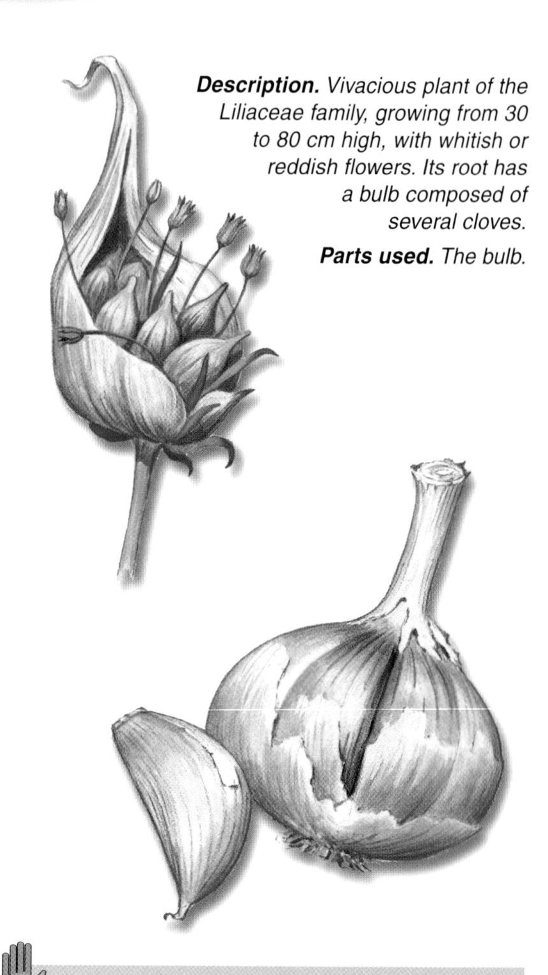

Description. *Vivacious plant of the Liliaceae family, growing from 30 to 80 cm high, with whitish or reddish flowers. Its root has a bulb composed of several cloves.*

Parts used. *The bulb.*

"IN THIS BOOK you will find all the wonderful virtues of garlic, and the ways it may be consumed in order to avoid its bad smell," said a seller to a potential client enthusiastically.

The client, after smelling the strong breath of the seller with a strong garlic aroma, asked: "Do you follow the advice of the book?"

"Of course, Sir! After eating garlic, I eat an apple and chew some parsley leaves...," the seller answered, totally unaware of the inefficiency of the method.

The truth is that those who eat garlic cannot hide it. All body secretions are impregnated with its aroma: breath, sweat, belches, winds, urine, and even the milk of breast-feeding women. Some people only eat garlic at night, then enduring in solitude its annoying smell. Other people trust in apples and parsley. And some other people accept the smell, such as the elegant French cavalry officer who, according to Mességué, had an enviable reputation among the ladies, in spite of the fact that he smelt of garlic meters away.

It is not by chance that garlic is native to central Asia, the region where people live the longest, and the incidence of cancer is the lowest known. The ancient Egyptians included garlic in the diet of the slaves who built the pyramids, according to the bas-reliefs found near the Giza sphinx.

Greeks regarded garlic as a source of physical strength, and every athlete was given a raw clove of garlic before each competition in the Olympic Games, perhaps to make them run faster. Dioscorides and Galen thought that gar-

Warning

*The use of garlic in high doses, especially when raw or in extracts, is **not recommended** in the case of **hemorrhage,** be it traumatic (wounds, accidents, etc.) or menstrual **(excessive menstruation).***

Due to its blood thinning action (see the epigraph) high doses of garlic may prolong hemorrhages and make coagulation processes more difficult to occur.

*Continuous use of **high doses** of garlic **during pregnancy is not recommended.***

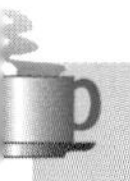

Preparation and Use

INTERNAL USE

Garlic may be eaten in many ways, including many cooking recipes. We will only mention the most recommended from a therapeutical point of view.

❶ **Raw.** Chew one to three garlic cloves preferably in the morning.

❷ **Garlic extract.** In capsules or pearls it does not cause body odor, though high doses are required to produce a therapeutic effect. The usual dose is from six to 12 capsules or pearls (600-1200 mg) daily.

❸ **Decoction of garlic cloves.** Boil a garlic bulb in a liter of water for five minutes. Drink three cups daily. This method has the disadvantage of losing part of its properties, though it avoids bad breath.

❹ **Oil and garlic sauce or emulsion.** It is perhaps the best way to administer garlic. Mash several garlic cloves in olive oil until a homogeneous paste similar to mayonnaise is obtained.

EXTERNAL USE

❺ **Enema.** Very useful against intestinal parasites. Mix two or three spoonfuls of oil and garlic sauce with one liter of warm water. Another method is introducing a clove of garlic into the anus, as if it were a suppository. This will ease anal itching in children, and provoke a strong vermifuge effect.

lic was a panacea. However, people who smelt of garlic were forbidden to enter the temples of Greek gods.

In the Middle Age, physicians used a mask impregnated with garlic when attending ill-people, especially those suffering from plagues. Later on, its fame reached America, and garlic became appreciated in Mexico, Peru, and the other territories of New Spain. Geronimo Pompa confirmed this fact in his work *Colección de Medicamentos Indígenas (Collection of Indigenous Medicines),* written in the mid-nineteenth century.

History attributes many properties to garlic, and most of them have been proven by scientific means. Perhaps garlic is ***the vegetal remedy with the most scientifically proven properties.***

PROPERTIES AND INDICATIONS. The whole plant, but especially the bulb, contains alliin (a sulphured glycoside), and enzyme (alliinase), vitamins A, B_1, B_2, C, and niacin (a vitamin of the B group). Alliin does not smell, but by the action of alliinase, which liberates and acts when garlic is mashed, it is transformed first into alliicine, and then into diallyl disulphide (the genine of the glycoside), which are the most important active principles which give garlic its typical smell.

Here is the outline of the many health properties of garlic:

- **Hypotensive [❶,❷,❸,❹].** In high doses, garlic produces a decrease in blood pressure, both maximum and minimum. It has vasodilating effects, and is thus recommended for people suffering from hypertension, arteriosclerosis, and heart dysfunctions (angina pectoris or heart attacks). Garlic is a good friend of the circulatory system.
- **Blood thinner [❶,❷,❸,❹].** Garlic helps with anticlotting of platelets (prevents an excessive tendency of platelets to group, forming clots), and fibrinolytic (disintegrates fibrin, the protein that forms blood clots). All this contributes towards thinning the blood, and makes garlic highly recommended for people who have suffered from thrombosis, embolism, or vascular accidents due to the lack of blood flow.

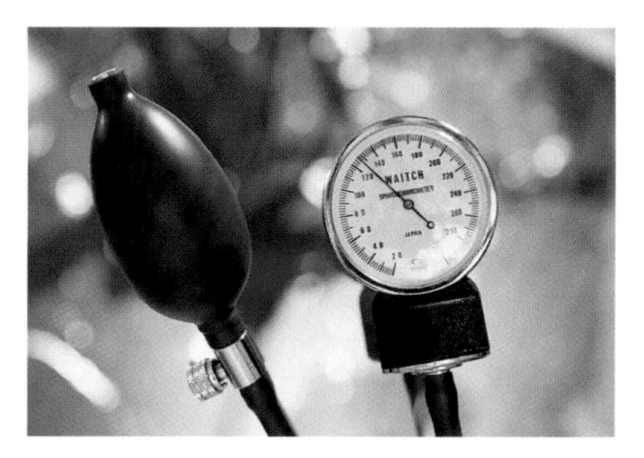

Garlic is a good friend of the circulatory system. When taken regularly it provokes a decrease in blood pressure, both of the maximum and the minimum. In order to achieve notable effects, the dose must be high (up to three cloves of garlic, or from six to 12 capsules or pearls daily).

• **Hypolidemic [❶,❷,❸,❹].** It decreases the level of LDL cholesterol (noxious cholesterol) in the blood, because it makes its absorption by the intestine more difficult. It has been proven that in the hours following a breakfast of toast with butter, the level of cholesterol increases 20%, however when the bread is rubbed with garlic, even if it has butter, this increase does not take place. This scientific observation has been published in the *Indian Journal of Nutrition* (vol. 13, n. 1).

• **Hypoglycemic [❶,❷,❸,❹].** Since it normalizes the level of sugar in blood, it is recommended for people suffering from diabetes (as a ***complement*** to other therapeutical measures), and obesity, as well as for those people with parents who have suffered from diabetes, as prevention.

• **General antibiotic and antiseptic [❶,❷,❸,❹].** Since the mid-twentieth century, the anti-infective properties of garlic have been researched. Its antibiotic action has been proven, both *in vivo* and *in vitro*, against the following micro-organisms:

- ***Escherichia coli,*** which causes intestinal dysbacteriosis and urinary infections.
- ***Salmonella typhi,*** which causes typhoid, and other *Salmonella* genus that cause severe intestinal afflictions.
- ***Shigella dysenteriae,*** which causes bacillus dysentery.
- ***Staphylococcus* and *streptococcus,*** which causes furuncles (infected blemishes) and other skin infections.
- Diverse types of **fungi, yeasts**, and some **viruses,** such as herpes. The active principles of garlic are supposed to interact with the nucleic acids of the virus, thus limiting its proliferation.

The bacteria-killing powers of garlic inside the intestine are selective with noxious bacteria, respecting the saprophytic normal flora, for which it is good. This makes garlic better than most known antibiotics, since it regulates intestinal flora instead of destroying it all.

Its use is recommended:

- In all kinds of **diarrhea, gastroenteritis, and colitis.**
- In **salmonellosis** (intestinal infections usually caused by spoiled food).
- In **intestinal bacterial imbalance** (alteration of the microbial balance of the intestine) often caused by the use of antibiotics.
- In **fermentative dyspepsia,** which cause flatulence in the colon.
- In **urinary infections** (cystitis and pyelonephritis), often caused by *Esterichia coli.*
- In diverse **bronchial affections** (acute and chronic bronchitis), because when the dysulphur of allyl is liberated through the breath, it acts directly on the bronchial mucous membrane. It is also an **expectorant and antiasthmatic.**

• **Defense stimulant [❶,❷, ❸,❹].** Garlic stimulates the activity of the defensive cells of the body, both lymphocytes and macrophages. These cells, which flow with the blood, protect us from microorganisms, and furthermore they are able to destroy cancerous cells, at least in the initial phases of tumor formation.

The consumption of garlic has a good effect on any infectious disease, augmenting the defensive ability of our body, besides directly destroying certain micro-organisms. Garlic is being used with relative success as complement in the treatment of AIDS.

• **Powerful vermifuge [❶,❸,❺]** against the most frequent types of intestinal parasites. It is especially active against ascarides and oxyuridae (little white worms which provoke anal itching in children).

• **General strengthening** of the organism, and **depurative [❶,❷,❸,❹]:** Garlic activates the chemical reactions of the body and promotes waste excretion processes (catabolism). Thus, it is recommended in states of weakness or tiredness, for people with a lack of appetite, and for those who suffer from an excess of acid wastes (gout, arthritis, certain rheumatic afflictions).

• **Detoxification [❶,❷,❸,❹],** especially recommended in the treatment to stop smoking. It normalizes the blood pressure of smokers, which is usually high, it promotes the elimination of mucus retained in the bronchi, and the regeneration of the bronchial mucous membrane, as well as helps to overcome the urge to smoke, perhaps due to the peculiar smell it gives to the breath.

• **Prevents malignant tumors [❶,❷,❸,❹],** especially digestive cancers. This is likely due to its regulating action on the intestinal flora, and normalizing action on the digestive function, though this may be related to its effects on the set of chemical reactions of the body (metabolism).

• **Corn remover.** Applying a piece of garlic mashed onto the callus, covering it with a plaster (Band-Aid). Within two or three days the corn will soften and its inflammation will be reduced, thus allowing easier extirpation.

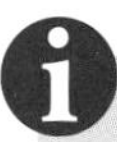

The Action of Garlic on the Cardiovascular System

LDL Cholesterol (noxious)	decrease
HDL Cholesterol (good)	slight increase
Total Cholesterol	decrease
Triglycerides	decrease
Fibrinolytic activity	increase
Platelet aggregation	reduction
Blood pressure	decrease

These results are obtained after a daily intake of 600-900 mg of deodorized garlic powder over four months. Non-aromatized garlic extracts are as active as raw garlic. Several studies show a decrease of 11-12 % in the cholesterol level and up to 17 % in the triglycerides level.

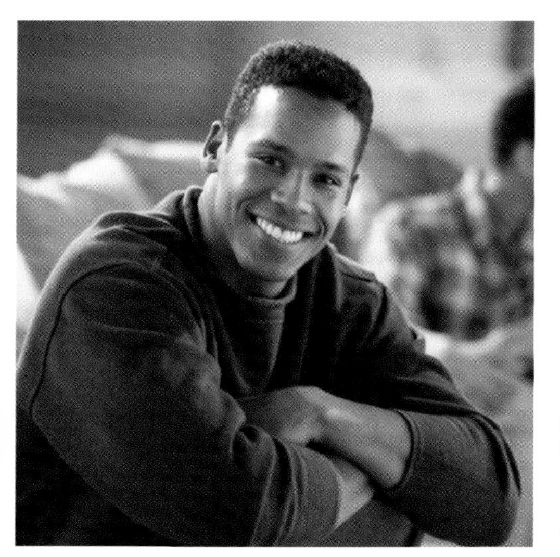

Garlic is a general invigorating plant for our body, supplying health and a sense of well-being sensation.

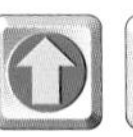
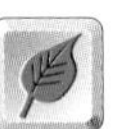
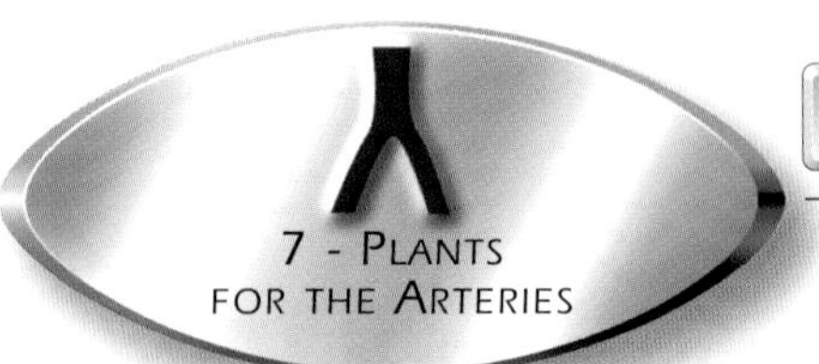

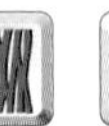
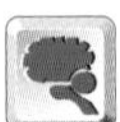
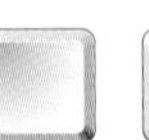
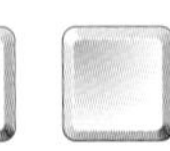

Ginkgo

Eases circulatory disorders

IT IS THE SIXTH of August, 1945. All around lie the burnt ruins of Hiroshima. The Japanese city has just been destroyed by the first atomic bomb. In what was formerly a park, a majestic ginkgo has burnt down into powder.

To the astonishment of the survivors, in the Spring of 1946, after the devastation, when the city is still in ruins, a bud grows from the carbonized trunk of the ginkgo. The old tree grew again, and became the beautiful tree we may see today in the center of the rebuilt Hiroshima.

The long-lasting life and endurance of this Asian tree seems to harmonize with its virtue of helping humans to confront the disorders of age.

For more than 4000 years, Chinese medicine has used ginkgo poultices to fight annoying chilblains. Its notable properties have been the focus of much scientific research, and at present it is contained in several ***pharmaceutical preparations.***

PROPERTIES AND INDICATIONS. The leaves contain flavonoid glycosides, chercitine, luteoline, catechines, resins, essential oil, lipids, and some substances of the terpenic group which are inherent in ginkgo: bilobalid and gingkolids A, B, and C.

As is usual in phytotherapy, the medicinal properties of the plant are brought about by the compound action of all its components, and its effects cannot be attributed to any specific component.

Ginkgo acts on the entire circulatory system, improving arterial, capillary and venous blood circulation.

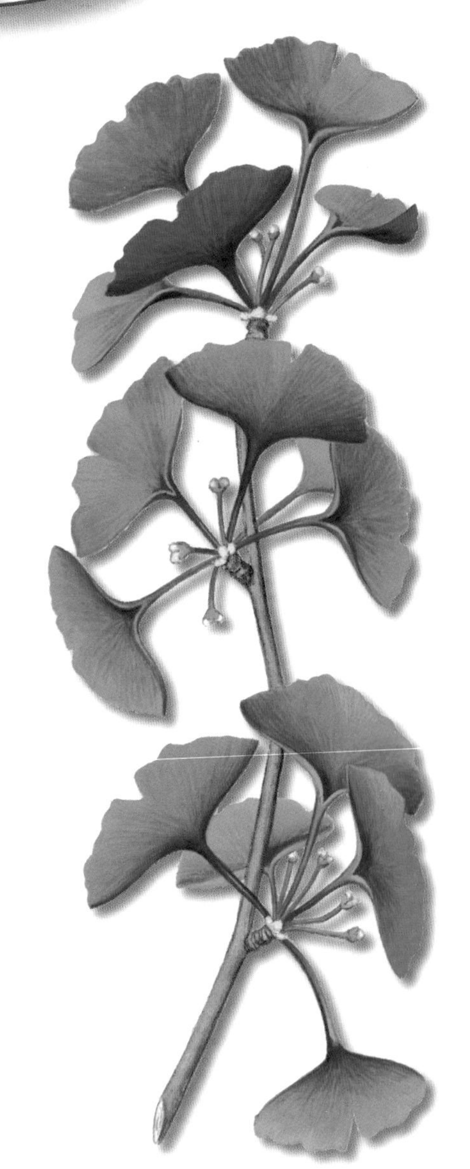

Description. *Tree of the Gingkoaceae family, growing up to 30 meters high. It is dioic (with different male and female plants), with deciduous, thick, elastic leaves that when young are divided into two lobules. Its fruit is a yellow berry, which is edible when fresh, but nauseating when too ripe.*

Parts used. *The leaves.*

Preparation and Use

INTERNAL USE

❶ **Infusion** with 40-60 g of leaves per liter of water. Drink up to three cups daily.

EXTERNAL USE

❷ **Compresses** with the same infusion, though slightly more concentrated (up to 100 g per liter), applied on the hands or feet with circulatory problems.

❸ **Poultices** of mashed leaves, applied on the affected area.

❹ **Hand and foot baths** with an infusion of up to 100 g of ginkgo leaves per liter of water. Apply warm or lukewarm, once or twice daily.

The best results are obtained combining oral intakes, with external applications.

- **Vasodilating action.** It increases perfusion (blood flow), decreasing peripheral resistance in small arteries. It also partially counteracts the disorders of arteriosclerosis.
- **Capillary protection action.** It diminishes the permeability of blood vessels, reducing edema (accumulation of liquid in the tissues).
- **Venous stimulation.** It strengthens the walls of veins, decreasing the accumulation of blood in them, and easing blood return.

These are its indications:

- **Cerebral blood insufficiency {❶}** (lack of blood flow into the brain) which manifests itself through vertigo, cephalalgia, ringing in the ears, loss of balance, memory disorders, and somnolence, among other symptoms. Those who use ginkgo say that "it clears the head."
- **Vascular brain accidents {❶}** (thrombosis, embolism, etc.). It accelerates recuperation and improves the mobility of the patients.
- **Arteriopathy in the legs** (loss of blood flow in legs) **{❶,❷,❸,❹}**: Ginkgo allows patients to walk longer distances without suffering pain.
- **Angiopathy** (blood vessel disorders) and **vaso-motor disorders {❶,❷,❸,❹}**: Reynaud's syndrome, blood vessel weakness, acroparesthesia (numbness in hand and feet), chilblains.
- **Varicose veins, phlebitis, tired legs, maleolar edema** (swollen ankles) **{❶,❷,❸,❹}**.

In the circulatory afflictions of arms and legs, it is recommended that the oral intake of ginkgo is combined with external applications in poultices, compresses, hand and foot baths.

Ginkgo is well-tolerated, and does not present undesirable side effects, nor does it raise blood pressure.

Baths with an infusion of ginkgo leaves activate blood circulation in the arms and legs. Hand baths are very effective against chilblains.

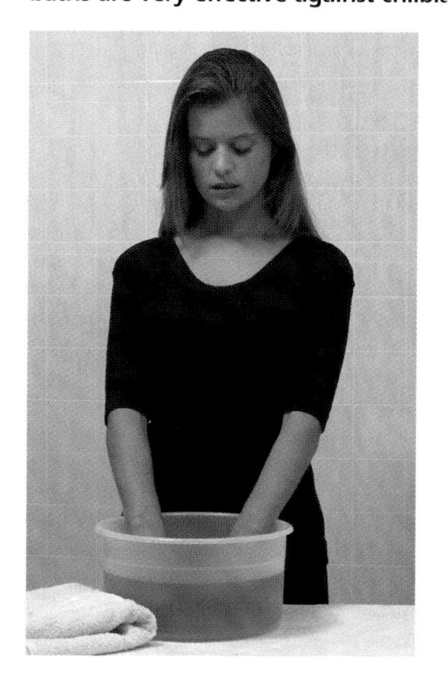

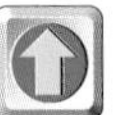
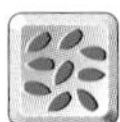
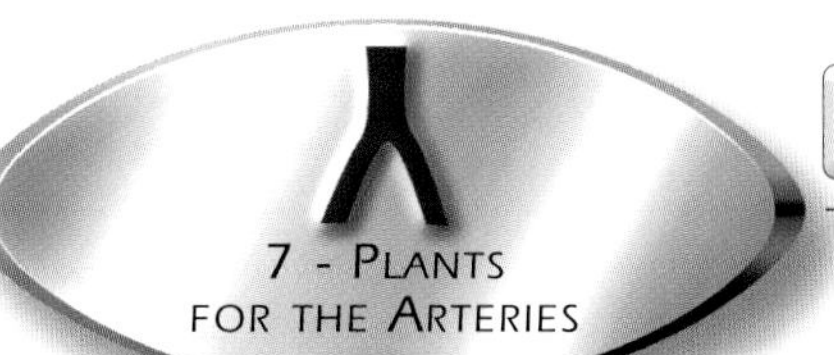

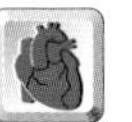
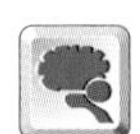
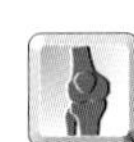
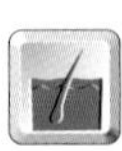

Evening Primrose

A great discovery in phytotherapy

THIS ORIGINAL plant, whose flowers open at night, was introduced in Europe in the early seventeenth century, and used as an ornamental plant. Soon, people noticed that its fleshy root was tasty, and the plant was useful not only as an ornament. In central Europe, the root of the evening primrose became a war-time food between the eighteenth and nineteenth centuries.

However, the plant was hardly appreciated until now. It is still known with pejorative names in France and Spain, related to donkeys which eat it happily.

Nonetheless, research conducted in the early eighties showed that the oil of evening primrose has interesting medicinal properties. In Germany and the United States, generally, much research has been carried out in clinics with patients suffering from circulatory, nervous, genital, and rheumatic disorders, with excellent results.

The applications of this plant, whose ***prestige and popularity*** on the phytotherapeutical world are ***growing,*** are still being investigated.

PROPERTIES AND INDICATIONS. The oil extracted from the evening primrose seeds is very rich in polyunsaturated fatty essential acids, the most outstanding of which are linoleic acid (71.5%) and linolenic acid (7-10%), whose other chemical exact names are respectively cis-linoleic acid and gamma-linolenic acid. The latter plays a very important role in the body as a chemical precursor of prostaglandins, recently discovered substances that have many metabolic functions. The evening primrose is the ***only***

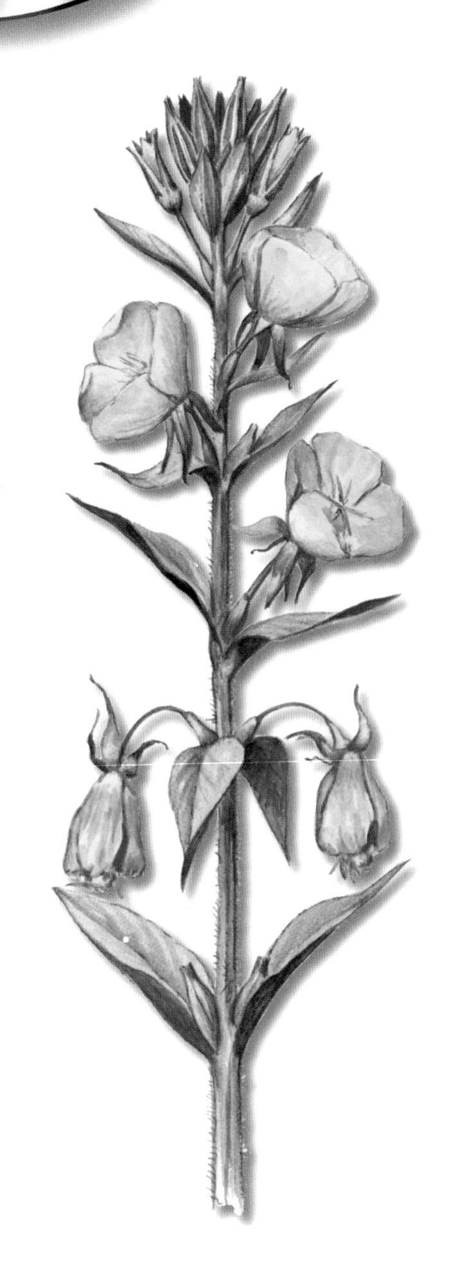

Description. *Biennial plant of the Enoteraceae family, growing up to one meter high in its second year. Upright stem, with large hairy leaves. Yellow flowers with four petals, and a sweet aroma.*

Parts used. *Seeds.*

Preparation and Use

INTERNAL USE

❶ **Capsules or pills.** The best way to take advantage of the properties of the evening primrose is by taking the oil of its seeds obtained by cold pressure, as capsules, pills or similar preparations. This is perhaps the most expensive vegetable oil known. Fortunately, the therapeutic dose is only two to four grams daily.

vegetable known with notable amounts of ***linolenic acid,*** which is also found in human milk, and is indispensable for our body (an essential fatty acid).

The linolenic acid and its immediate derivative substance, prostaglandin E1 are indispensable for the stability of the cell membranes of the whole body for the development of the nervous system, for the balance of the hormonal system, and for regulating the processes of blood coagulation, among other functions. The list of diseases in which the ***EVENING PRIMROSE OIL*** **[❶]** has been applied is thus very long:

- **High cholesterol** in the blood, and, as a general rule, in all hyperlipemia (increase in the fatty content of the blood).
- **Circulatory disorders.** Tendency toward high blood pressure and thrombosis due to the increase of platelet aggregation. It may act in prevention of cerebral vascular accidents (thrombosis, cerebral hemorrhage) and for myocardial infarction, because it dilates arteries and prevents the formation of clots and platelet aggregation.
- **Reproductive disorders.** Dysmenorrhea, irregular menstruation cycles, pre-menstrual syndrome, sterility due to ovarian insufficiency.
- **Nervous system afflictions.** Parkinson's disease, multiple sclerosis, and as a rule all afflictions caused by neuronal degeneration.
- **Behavior disorders.** Irritable children, nervousness, neurasthenia, schizophrenia.
- **Immune response disorders.** Allergies, asthma, eczema, atopic dermatitis.
- **Rheumatism.** Rheumatic arthritis and general rheumatic processes.
- **Dermatological problems.** Excess of sebaceous secretion (acne), wrinkles or skin dryness, weakness of nails and hair. We know that the Algonquin Indians of North America rubbed their skin with mashed evening primrose seeds in order to fight skin blemishes more than five centuries ago.

Due to its richness in essential fatty acids, the oil of the evening primrose decreases the level of cholesterol in the blood, improves blood circulation, and invigorates the nervous system. It is a very useful remedy for the disorders of elderly people.

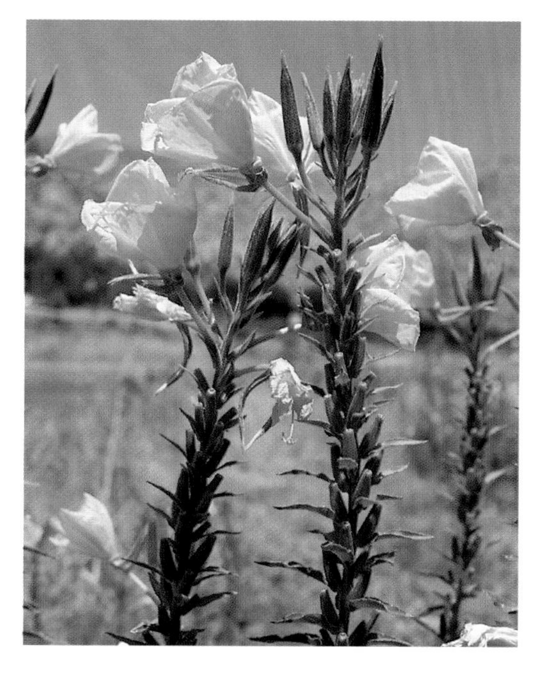

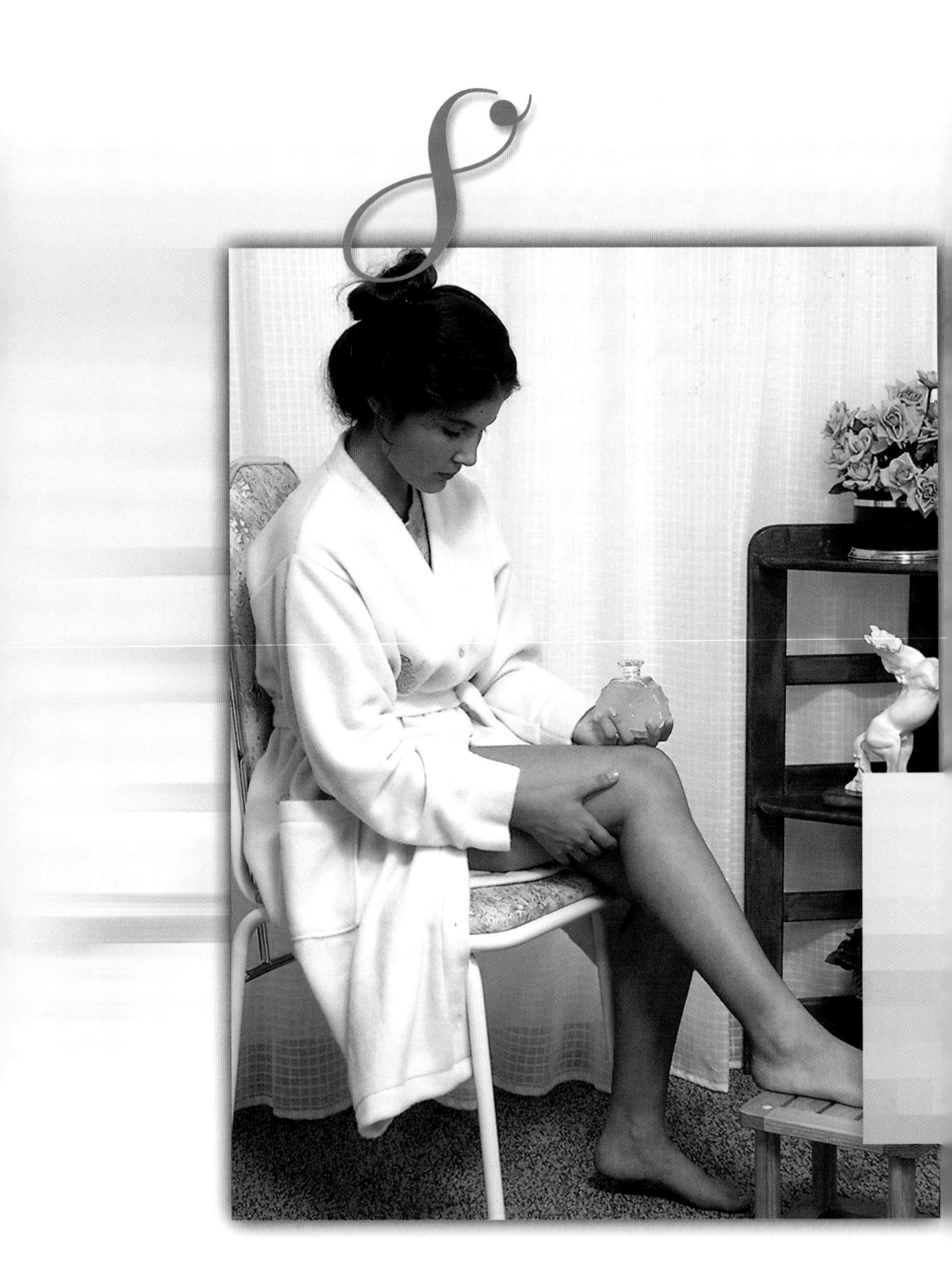

Plants for the Veins

DISEASES	PAGES
Phlebitis	128
Varicose ulceration	128
Varicose veins	128
Veins, inflammation, see Phlebitis	128

PLANTS	PAGES
Cypress	132
Horse chestnut	130
Witch hazel	129

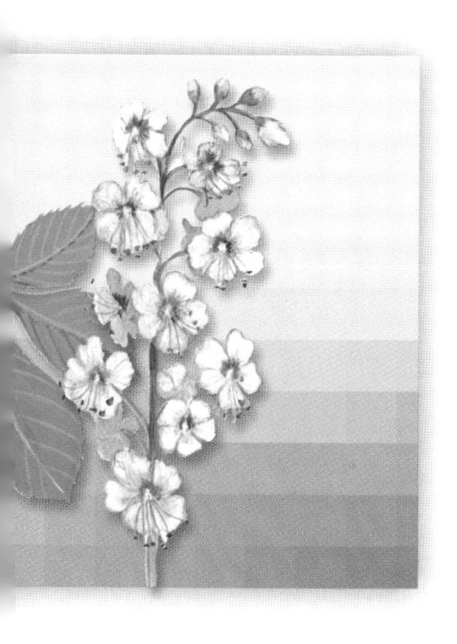

THE VEINS carry blood to the heart, after having passed through capillaries and nourished and oxygenated tissues. The blood passes through the veins with almost no pressure, thus making the return of blood from the legs especially difficult, as it has to rise against the force of gravity.

Medicinal plants contain **venotonic** substances, which promote blood flow through the veins, avoiding dilation and the formation of varicose veins. Venotonic plants are also useful for **hemorrhoids,** which are simply dilated veins in the anal area.

Compresses soaked in a decoction of certain venotonic and cicatrizant plants are an interesting addition to the treatment of **varicose ulcers** of the legs.

VARICOSE VEINS

Definition

Caused by permanent dilation of the veins. All these plants have venotonic action, that is to say, they strengthen the walls of the veins, avoiding excessive dilation. Venotonic plants also act by promoting the return of blood inside the veins.

Phytotherapy

Some of these plants also have ***capillary protecting*** properties, thus regenerating and strengthening the cells that form the tiny vessels or capillaries through which the blood flows to the tissues. This way, the edema in tissues diminishes, and blood circulation is improved.

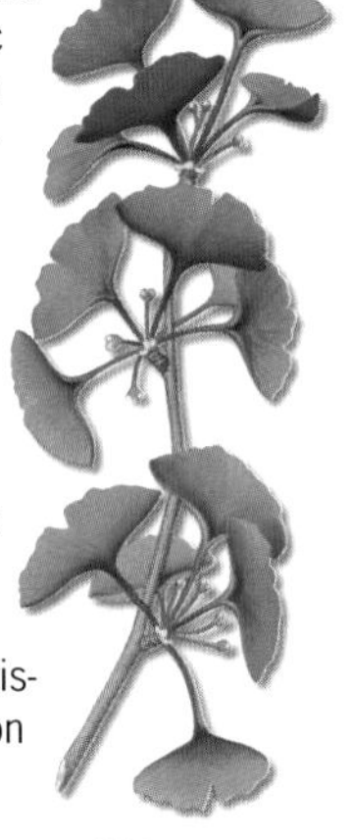

Ginkgo

ORANGE TREE	Rich in flavonoids with capillary protective action
GINKGO	Strengthens vein walls, capillary protective
HORSE CHESTNUT	Strengthens vein walls, capillary protective
CYPRESS	Venotonic
WITCH HAZEL	Enhances blood flow through the veins

VARICOSE ULCERATION

Definition

A loss of integrity of the skin, which makes it difficult to heal, and caused by an alteration in the blood circulation. It is usually related to **varicose veins and phlebitis,** and is located in the lower part of the legs, near the ankle.

Treatment

The phytotherapeutical treatment of varicose ulceration consists of the ingestion of ***venotonic*** plants, and ***capillary protecting*** plants, combined with the application of poultices and compresses on the affected area, with ***cicatrizant, antiseptic, and astringent*** plants.

STICKLEWORT	Cicatrizant (wound healer)
OAK TREE	Astringent, cicatrizant
FOXGLOVE	Cicatrizant
HORSE CHESTNUT	Venotonic, astringent, anti-inflammatory
CYPRESS	Venotonic
COMMON PLANTAIN	Emollient, astringent
PSYLLIUM	Cicatrizant, reduces the inflammation of the skin and protects it
HORSETAIL	Cicatrizant, promotes tissue regeneration
COMFREY	Cicatrizant

PHLEBITIS

Definition

An inflammation of the veins that is to say that usually occurs in varicose veins, previously dilated veins.

Phytotherapy

Besides the recommended plants for varicose veins, phytotherapeutic treatment of phlebitis requires the local application of compresses or poultices of these plants on the area affected by phlebitis.

GINKGO	Strengthens vein walls, capillary protective
HORSE CHESTNUT	Strengthens vein walls, capillary protective

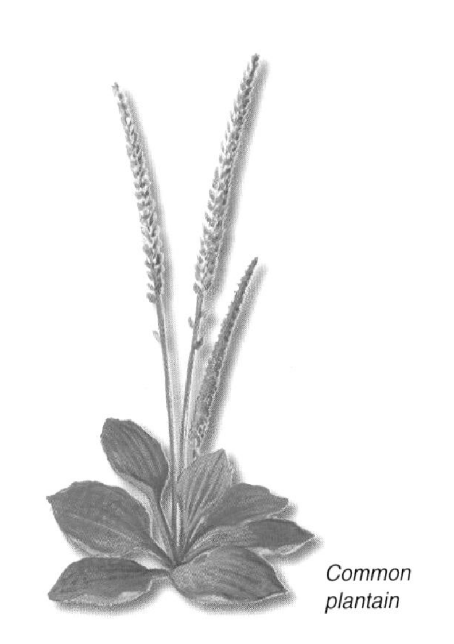

Common plantain

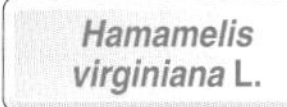

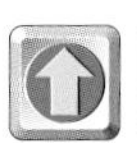

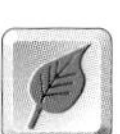

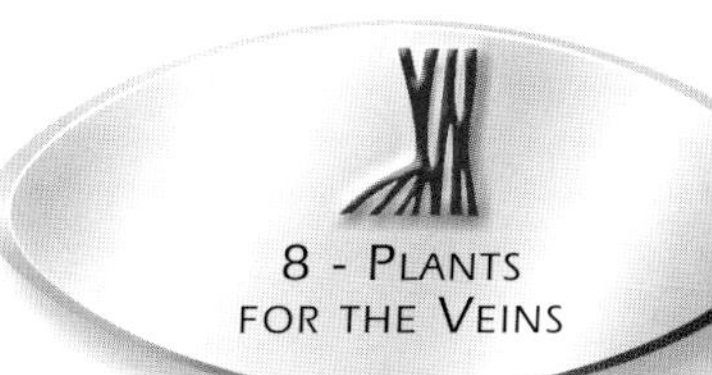

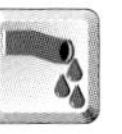

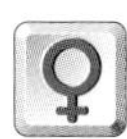

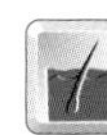

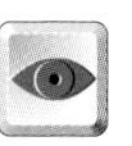

Witch Hazel

Invigorates the veins and makes the skin more beautiful

THE FRUITS of this tree are woody capsules similar to hazelnuts, and when ripe they explode noisily. Because of this, North American Indians believed that this tree was bewitched.

At present, the witch hazel is ***one of the most effective plants*** known to fight **circulatory afflictions.**

PROPERTIES AND INDICATIONS. The leaves and the bark of this tree contain several types of tannins, among which the most outstanding are hamamelitannins, as well as flavonoids and saponins. It has the following properties:

- **Venotonic.** It contracts the wall of veins, activating the blood flowing internally. Thus, it is very useful for **varicose veins, phlebitis, swollen legs, and hemorrhoids [❶,❷].**
- **Hemostatic** (stops bleeding). It strengthens the walls of veins and blood capillaries, with a similar effect to that of vitamin P (rhutine). It is employed in menopausal disorders and in **metrorrhagias** (uterine hemorrhages) **[❶,❷]**.
- **For the skin.** It activates blood flowing in the skin, and has cicatrizant and astringent effects. It is employed against dermatitis, eczema, dry skin, and wrinkles **[❹]**. It is a component of many ***beauty products.***
- **Eye sedative.** The infusion, or distilled water of witch hazel (pharmaceutical preparation) are used as eyedrops applied to wash and relax the eyes **[❸]**. They fight **conjunctivitis** caused by dust, smoke, pollution, and the irritant action of swimming pool or sea water. These eyedrops are also useful to alleviate eye **tiredness** caused by any activity demanding high visual attention, such as driving, or working with computers (because of their screens).

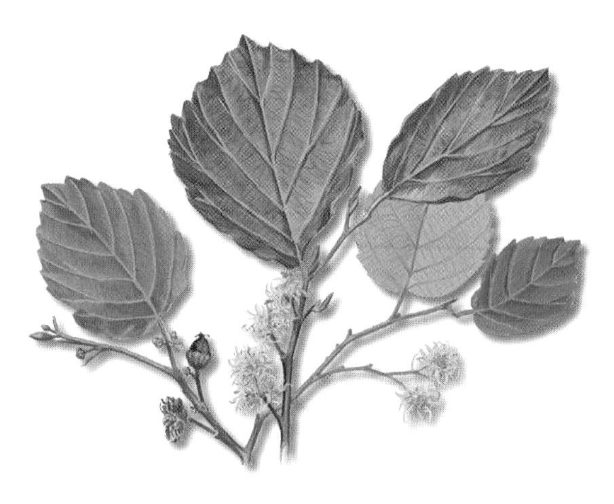

Description. *Tree of the Hamamelidaceae family, growing up to five meters high, with alternate, oval-shaped leaves, and yellow flowers of four tongue-shaped petals.*

Parts used. *The leaves and the bark.*

Preparation and Use

INTERNAL USE

❶ **Dry extract.** The normal dose is one or two grams, distributed in three daily intakes.

❷ **Infusion,** with 30-40 g of leaves and/or bark per liter of water. Drink two cups daily.

EXTERNAL USE

❸ **Eye washings,** use the same infusion as for internal use, but boil it for some minutes, and strain it well so that all dust is eliminated, or instead use distilled water of witch hazel.

❹ **Compresses,** with this infusion, applied on the afflicted skin area.

Horse Chestnut

The remedy for veins par excellence

THIS BEAUTIFUL tree was brought to Austria from Constantinople, and from there taken to other Western European countries by the gardener of the emperor Maximillian in the early seventeenth century. At that time, many new plants were coming to Europe from "the Indies" (America), and this tree was thought to be just another plant, and given its similarity with chestnuts, it was called horse chestnut. Later on, it was proven to be native to Greece and Turkey.

Its name of *hippocastannum* (the Latin term for horse chestnut) brings to mind that the Turkish people gave this plant to their old horses in order to ease coughs and asthma from which old horses frequently suffer.

The fruit of this tree has a sour taste, and people should understand from it that these fruits are not edible. Poisoning has occurred, mainly in children who have eaten great amounts.

PROPERTIES AND INDICATIONS. The bark of young branches and the seeds (chestnuts) contain several active components of great medicinal value.

✓ **Aesculin.** A coumarinic glycoside which ex-

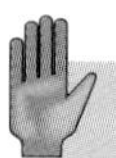

Warning

*The **seeds,** that is to say, the **chestnuts,** must not be eaten since they are **toxic.** Children must be closely watched because they may mistake these fruits for true chestnuts.*

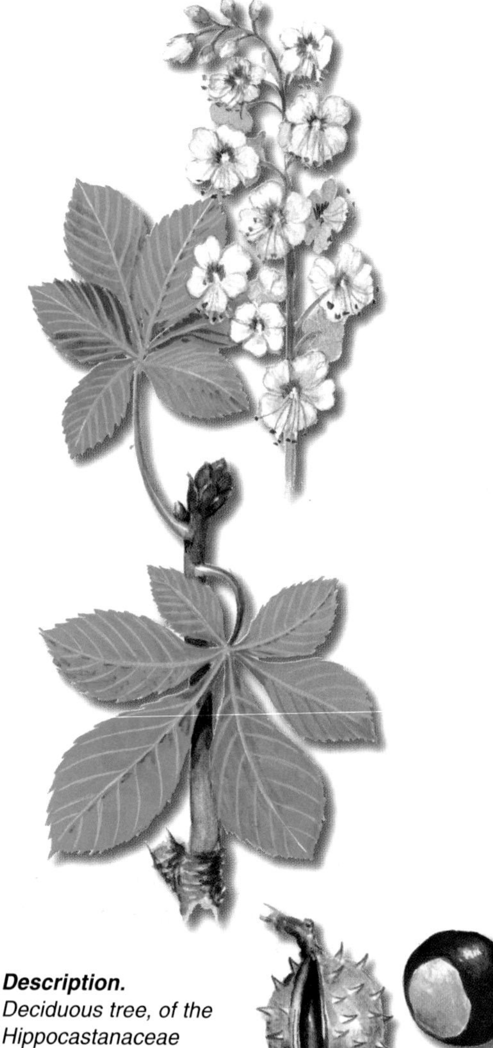

Description.
Deciduous tree, of the Hippocastanaceae family, with an attractive appearance and many leaves, growing up to 30 meters high, and living for as many years (up to 300) as the chestnut tree. Palm-shaped, large, toothed leaves growing in groups of five to nine. Its flowers are white, and gather in clusters. Its fruits are big, with a spiked coverage that contains one or two seeds resembling true chestnuts.

Parts used. *The seeds and the bark of young branches.*

Preparation and Use

INTERNAL USE

❶ **Decoction,** with 50 g of young leaves bark and/or seeds per liter of water, drinking two or three cups a day.

❷ **Dry extract.** 250 mg, three times a day.

EXTERNAL USE

❸ **Compresses** with a bark decoction, applied on the hemorrhoids or the varicose ulceration, for 5-10 minutes, three or four times a day.

❹ **Sitz baths** with this decoction, for hemorrhoids and prostate afflictions.

❺ **Bath.** Prepare a decoction with half a kilogram of ground seeds per liter of water, boil for five minutes. Then prepare a hot bath adding this decoction to the bathtub water. This will soothe and cleanse the skin better than any other soap or synthetic soap cream.

erts a powerful action on the venous system and on blood circulation in general. Aesculin is part of ***many pharmaceutical preparations,*** since no synthesized substance has superseded the effects of this vegetal product. The properties of aesculin are:

- ***Venotonic.*** It strengthens the vein wall, and as a consequence, the veins contract and blood overflow decreases, especially in the lower extremities.
- ***Capillary protection.*** It strengthens the cells that form the wall of capillary vessels, decreasing their permeability, and promoting the elimination of edema.

✓ **Triterpenic saponins** (scine) with **anti-inflammatory and anti-edema** action, which are abundant, mainly in the seeds.

✓ **Catechic** tannins, with astringent and anti-inflammatory action.

This plant is very useful for all kind of venous disorders, especially in the following cases:

- **Varicose veins** in the legs, **venous insufficiency, swollen legs [❶,❷,❸].**
- **Thrombophlebitis, varicose ulceration** in the legs [❶,❷,❸].
- **Hemorrhoids.** Eases the pain and reduces their size [❶,❷,❹].
- **Prostate.** It is very effective for congestion and hypertrophy of this gland, both taken as infusion or extract, and applied in sitz baths [❶,❷,❹]. It reduces the size of inflamed prostate, and eases the expulsion of urine.

The ***FLOUR*** of horse chestnuts is especially rich in saponins, and it is thus used in **cosmetics** and in the soap industry [❺]. It is a true vegetal soap, soothing and protecting the skin.

The horse chestnut is a beautiful tree, from whose bark and seeds a glycoside called sculine is extracted.
This natural substance forms part of many pharmaceutical preparations due to its stimulating effects on blood circulation.

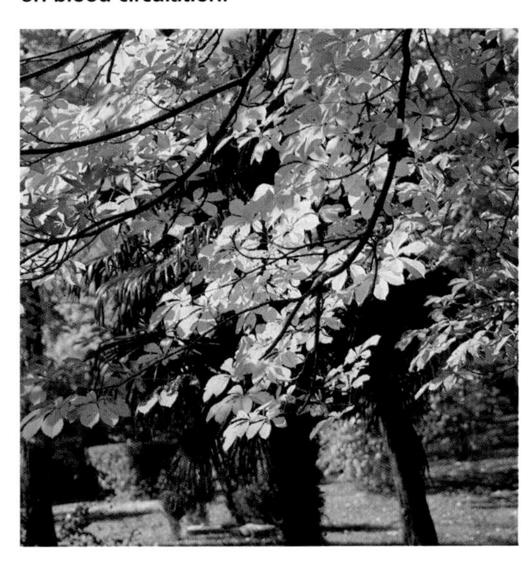

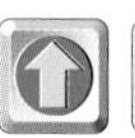

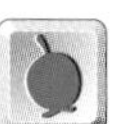

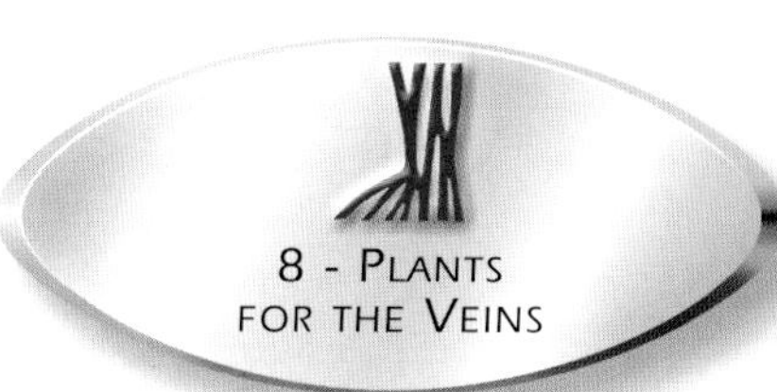

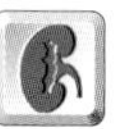

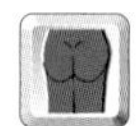

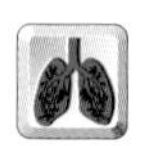

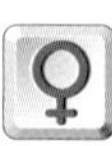

Cypress

Blood circulation and urinary bladder invigorating

THE CYPRESS is an almost a sinister tree. Firm and solemn next to graveyard gates, it points up towards the sky with its crown, and to the tombs with its elongated shadow, seeming to remind humans of the deadly destiny awaiting us. It is the tree that best symbolizes death.

However, at the same time, the cypress is a sign of life and health for many people suffering from respiratory and circulatory diseases.

In ancient Greece sick people were sent to cypress forests in order to regain health by inhaling their balsamic essences. Hippocrates and Galen recommended it as a medicinal plant. Since then, the cypress has been used successfully for over 2000 years as a healing tree.

In the Mexican state of Oaxaca there is the famous Cypress of Moctezuma or of Tule, which is 50 m high and 14 m in diameter, and belongs to a very closely related species of the common cypress. It is supposed to be 4000 or 5000 years old. The Aztecs already employed the cypress fruits (nuts) to avoid white hair and preserve its original color.

Properties and indications. In cypress wood, from its young branches, and especially from its fruits, there is from 0.2 to 1.2% of cypress essence, composed of several hydrocarbons, as well as tannin, and several aromatic substances. This tree has the following properties:

- **Powerful venotonic.** Its action is as intense as that of witch hazel, one of the most active plants known for blood circulation. The use of cypress is recommended to fight **varicose veins, varicose ulceration, and hemor-**

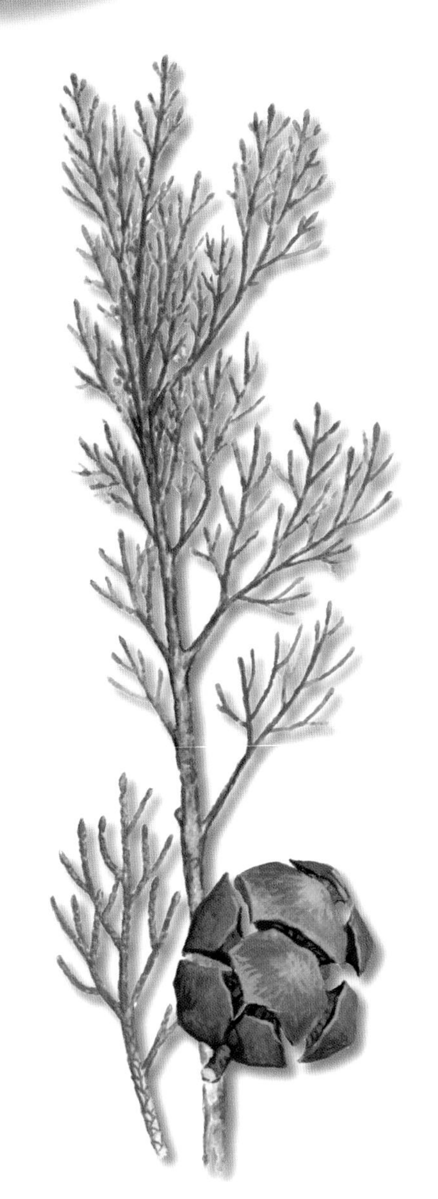

Description. *Tree of the Cupressaceae family, evergreen, growing from 20 to 25 m high. Its fruit, called the cypress nut, is polyhedral and greyish green colored.*

Parts used. *Green fruits (nuts) and wood.*

Preparation and Use

INTERNAL USE

❶ **Decoction** with 20-30 g of ground nuts (fruits), or the same amount of wood, per liter of water. Boil for ten minutes and strain. Drink one cup before each meal (three or four cups daily).

❷ **Essence.** Take from two to four drops, three times a day.

EXTERNAL USE

❸ **Sitz bath.** In order to treat hemorrhoids with a decoction similar to that employed in internal use, but with a higher concentration of nuts (some 50 g per liter). Have three baths a day, with cold water. It reduces the size of hemorrhoids and eases the pain they cause.

❹ **Inhalations.** Those people suffering from bronchial catarrh will benefit from inhalations by adding some cypress nuts or some drops of cypress essence to the water.

❺ **Compresses** on the legs, with the same decoction employed for internal use.

rhoids, and may be taken both internally [❶,❷] and in external local application [❸, ❺].

• **Vasoconstrictor** (it contracts blood vessels). It is especially recommended during the **menopause** to stop frequent metrorrhagias (uterine hemorrhages) caused by the congestion of the uterus (womb) and related to the hormonal imbalance typical at this stage of women's lives.

• **Urinary bladder strengthener.** Increases the tone of the urinary bladder, and allows better control of the autonomic nervous system on the muscles of this organ. In internal use [❶,❷] or in sitz baths [❸], it is recommended for cases of daily or night urine incontinence (enuresis), and for the prostatic syndrome (difficulty in urinating due to an increase in the size of the prostate).

• **Astringent,** due to the tannins it contains [❶]. It is used in cases of colitis or diarrhea.

• **Sudorific, diuretic, and febrifuge** (relieves fever). Very useful in bronchial catarrhs, bronchitis, colds, and influenza [❶,❹].

The **essence** of cypress also has **balsamic, antitussive, and expectorant** properties [❷].

Sitz baths with a decoction of green nuts (fruits) of the cypress alleviate prostatic syndrome, urine disorders, as well as cystitis or urine incontinence. Its effect is reinforced by drinking the decoction or cypress essence for some days.

Due to their invigorating action on the venous blood circulation, these baths are also good in the case of hemorrhoids.

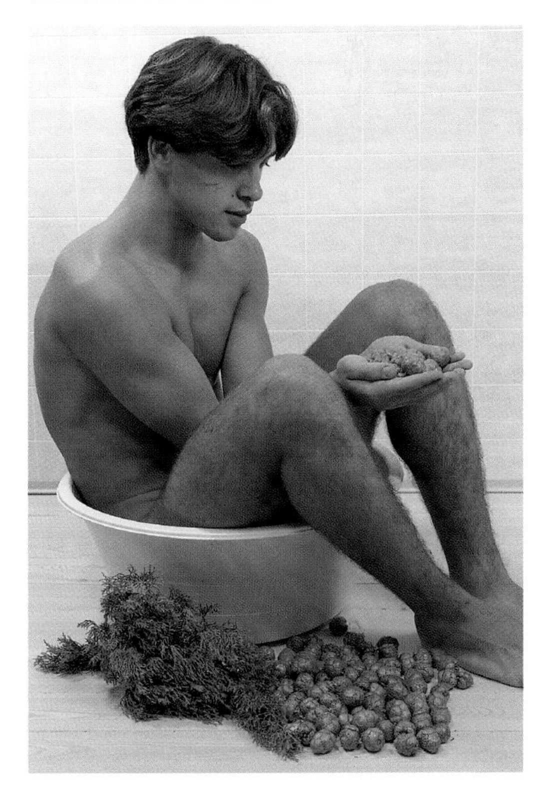

9

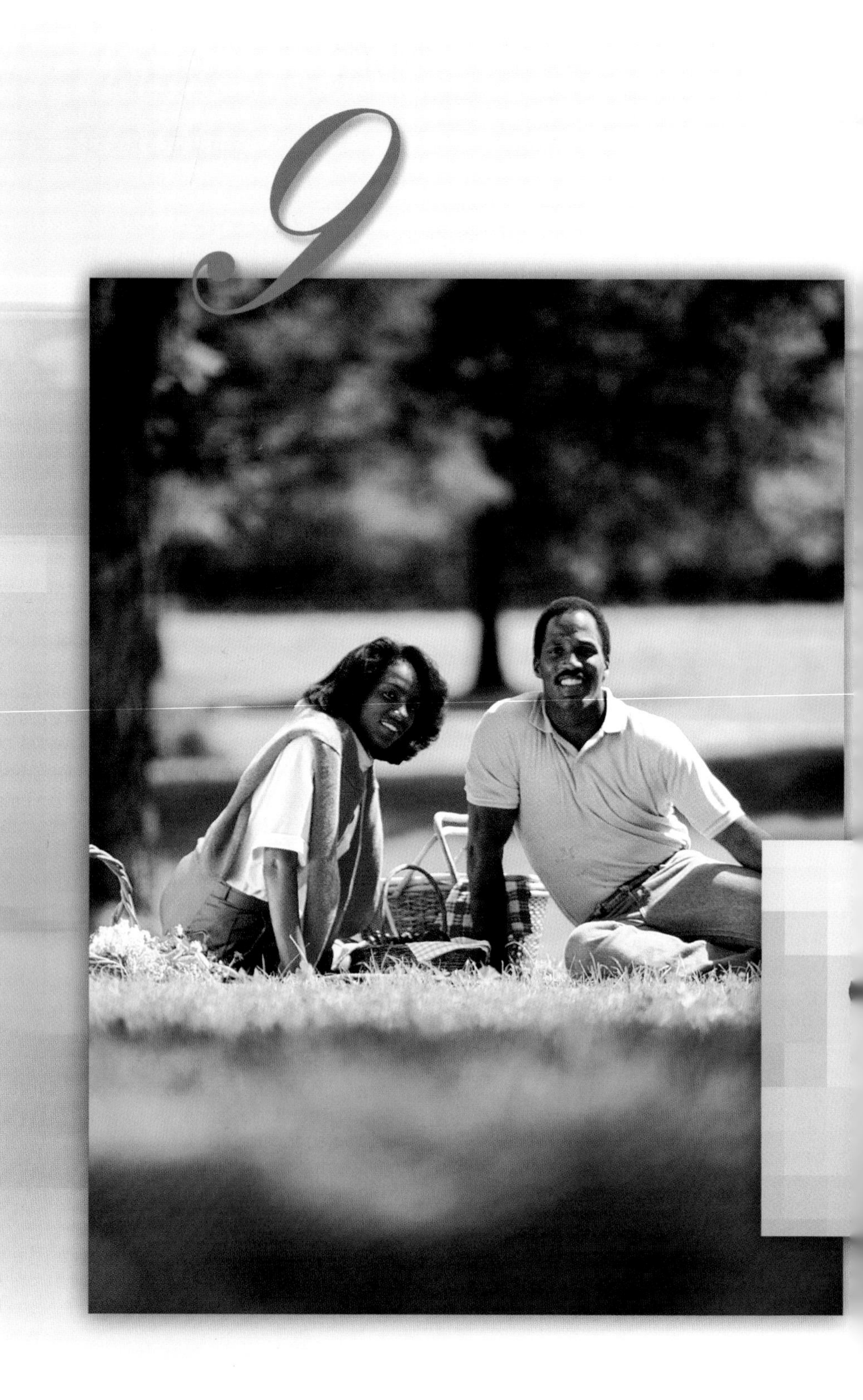

Plants for the Blood

DISEASES	PAGES
Anemia	136
Hemorrhage	136
Thrombosis	136

PLANTS	PAGES
Alfalfa	137
Nettle	142
Spirulina	140
Watercress	138

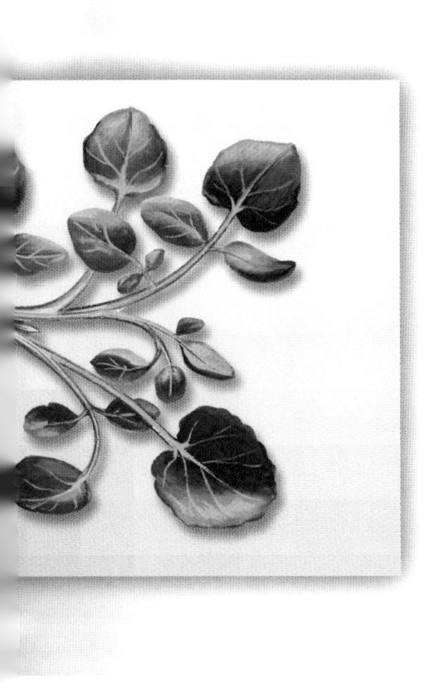

IN SOME SENSE, all medicinal herbs we consume act on the blood, since their active components are finally carried by this fluid after being absorbed in the intestine.

However, some plants act directly on the composition of the blood and on its ability to coagulate.

Certain plants are able to increase the production of erythrocytes (red blood cells), thus fighting against anemia. **Iron** in the vegetables is as useful as that of animal origin in order to form blood. The absorption of vegetal iron is slightly more difficult than that of animal iron, however it has the advantage of being usually accompanied by many vitamins and minerals. Vitamin C promotes the absorption of the iron that vegetables contain.

Hemostatic plants act by promoting the **clotting** mechanisms of the blood, by means of the vitamin K they contain, and also **clotting** tiny capillary vessels due to their astringent action.

Blood thinning plants have more therapeutic applications, and keep the blood from coagulating inside the vessels, a process known as

thrombosis. These plants make the blood more fluid, and exert an important preventive action for arterial thrombosis, especially that of the brain, heart (the origin of myocardial infarction) and femoral (that cause the lack of blood flow in legs) arteries. They act by means of one or several of the following mechanisms:

- Decreasing the excessive tendency of the blood platelets to gather and form clots: **anticlotting** action **on platelets.**
- Breaking the fibrin, a protein of the blood plasma which forms clots: **fibrinolithic** action.
- Slowing the processes of blood clotting: **anticlotting** action.

THROMBOSIS

Definition

This is the formation of a clot inside a vessel (artery or vein), which remains in the same place it is formed. When the clot moves from that place, flowing through the interior of the veins or arteries, an **embolism** is produced.

Arterial thrombosis usually occurs after an arteriosclerosis on the arterial walls.

Phytotherapy

Phytotherapy offers plants that **enhance blood circulation and make it more fluid**, thus exerting an interesting preventive action on this disorder. Plants which decrease **cholesterol** levels are also useful in the prevention of thrombosis.

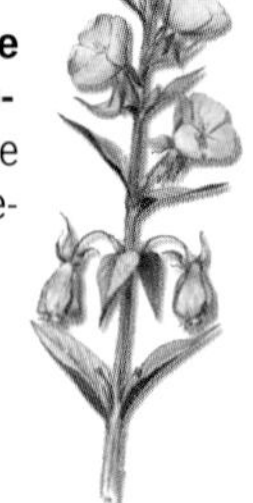

Onagra

LINDEN	Vasodilator, Hypotensive, decreases blood viscosity
GARLIC	Platelet anti-aggregant, fibrinolytic
EVENING PRIMROSE	Prevents cerebral vascular accidents, decreases platelet aggregation

ANEMIA

Definition

A decrease of the amount of blood, especially of its erythrocytes (red blood cells).

Phytotherapy

The phytotherapeutical treatment consists of using antianemic plants, rich in iron (the basic element of erythrocytes), but also with abundant amount of other minerals, vitamins (especially vitamin C), and enzymes, which activate the body. There are plants, such as ginseng, which increase the production of red blood cells.

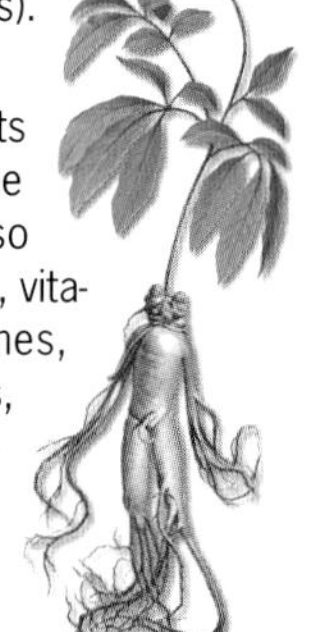

Ginseng

SPIRULINA	Contains iron, essential amino acids, and vitamin B_{12}
NETTLE	Contains iron and chlorophyll, stimulates blood red corpuscles production
GINSENG	Invigorator, stimulates blood production in the bone marrow

HEMORRHAGE

Bleeding. The plants here mentioned have ***hemostatic*** and ***vasoconstrictive*** properties. Its action is enhanced when they are taken orally and externally used.

Any abnormal **hemorrhage** should be treated by a **physician.**

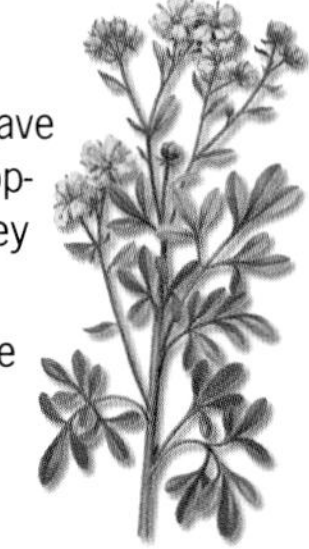

Rue

NETTLE	Contracts blood vessels, stops hemorrhages, useful in nasal and uterine bleeding
RUE	Increases resistance of capillary vessels
HORSETAIL	Hemostatic, regenerates conjunctive tissue

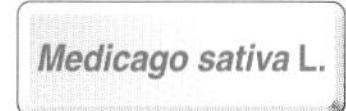
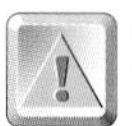
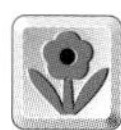
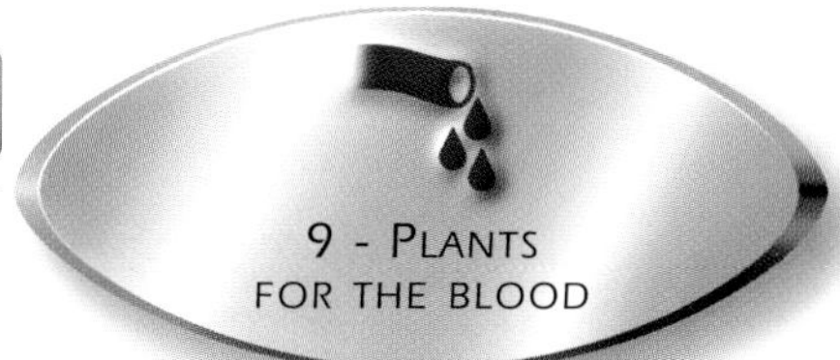

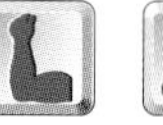
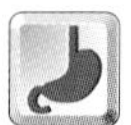
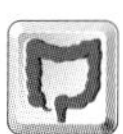
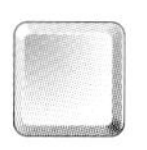

Alfalfa

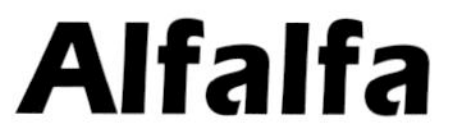

Nutritive and hemostatic

HOW LUCKY horses are, they are given alfalfa to eat! From ancient times, domestic animals have enjoyed the advantages of this nutritive plant, while their rational masters dismiss it as they regard it as an inelegant food to put on their tables.

Thanks to the modern analytical chemistry, nowadays we know the excellent properties of this humble plant, and fortunately, there are more and more people taking advantage of it.

PROPERTIES AND INDICATIONS. The ***YOUNG BUD SEEDS*** (germs) of alfalfa are rich in calcium (525 mg per 100 g, three times that of milk), phosphorus, provitamin A as betacarotene, vitamins C, B, and K, enzymes, essential trace elements, and other nutrients, besides vegetal bran.

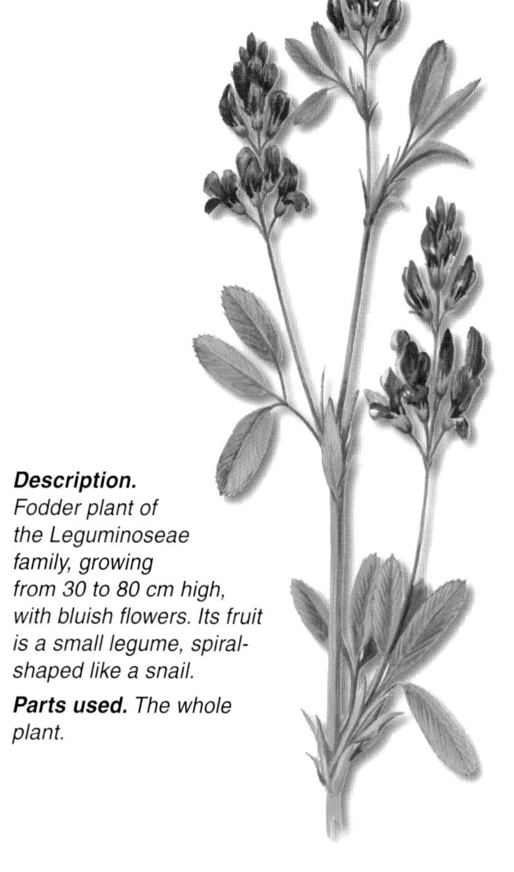

Description. *Fodder plant of the Leguminoseae family, growing from 30 to 80 cm high, with bluish flowers. Its fruit is a small legume, spiral-shaped like a snail.*

Parts used. *The whole plant.*

Preparation and Use

INTERNAL USE

❶ **Food.** The alfalfa, as many other vegetables, can be consumed raw in a salad (germs) or cooked. Its content in vitamin C withstands cooking very well.

❷ **Fresh juice.** A glass in the morning is an excellent invigorating drink.

❸ **Infusion,** with 30 g per liter of water. Drink from three to five cups a day.

❹ **Dry extract.** Half to one gram a day.

Therefore, the ***ALFALFA*** has remineralizing, invigorating, hemostatic, and infection protective properties [❶,❷,❸,❹]. It is especially recommended for:

- **Anemia** caused by lack of vitamins or minerals.
- **Malnutrition and rickets.**
- **Gastro-duodenal ulcer.**
- **Dyspepsia and intestinal fermentations,** due to its enzyme content.
- **Constipation,** because of its vegetal bran content.
- **Nose, gastric, and uterine hemorrhage.** We remind you that any ***abnormal bleeding*** must be checked out by a ***physician.***

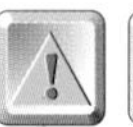
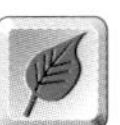
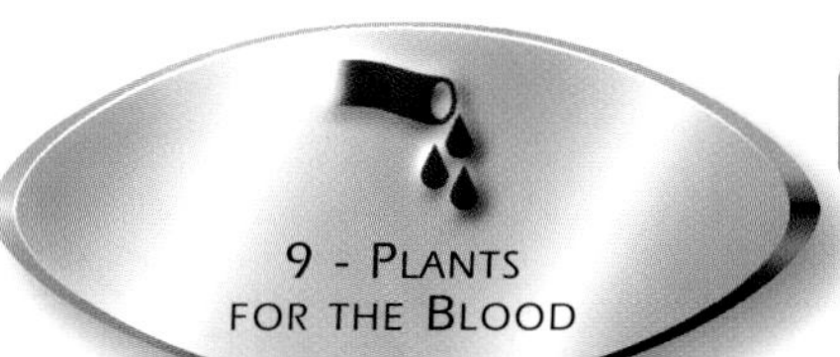

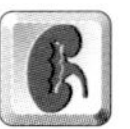
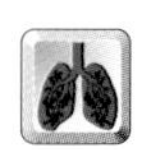
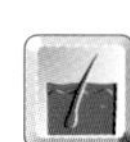
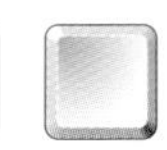

Watercress

Stimulant, depurative, and balsamic

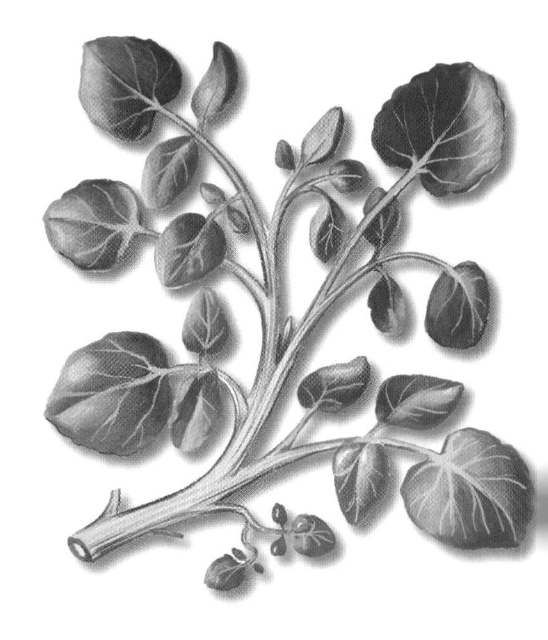

HOW HEALTHY—and cheap—those salads prepared in the countryside from wild vegetables! Watercress combines very well with dandelion, sorrel, and nettle. On a day outing, a meal like this is much more fitting than an instant soup heated on a portable stove, a tin of sardines, or a sandwich.

Anyway, take care. Enjoying nature requires knowledge, and the inhabitants of towns must acquire such knowledge. There is a Spanish saying "Those people gathering watercress, take care of monks hood." Monkshood also grows near clear waters, and is one of the most poisonous plants known. Fortunately, it is not difficult to distinguish from watercress.

The sentence, however, should have referred to other plants much more similar to watercress. The *Heloscyadium nodiflorum* is taller than watercress, with larger, light green leaves, flowers growing in umbels (flower clusters), and with

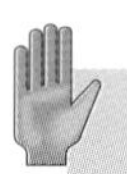

Warning

***Pregnant women** should **abstain** from watercress because of its probable abortifacient effect.*

*The consumption of **high amounts** of watercresses is not recommendable, since it can be an **irritant** for the stomach. The plants with flowers or fruits should not be used, because they are too strong.*

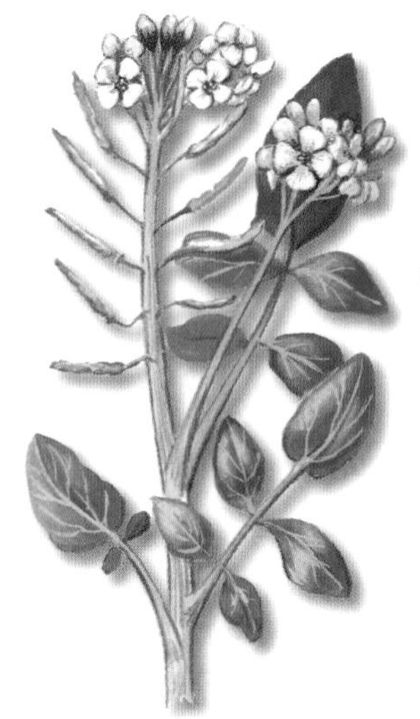

***Description.** Climbing plant of the Cruciferae family, with intense green leaves and small, white flowers. Its flavor resembles mustard, though less spicy.*

***Parts used.** The leaves and young stems.*

Preparation and Use

INTERNAL USE

❶ **Raw.** Watercress may become toxic when trying to preserve it, thus it is better to eat it young and fresh. Wash it carefully before consuming it, or keep it in salt water for half an hour, since it may house small larvae.

❷ **Juice.** Drink half a glass, sweetened with honey, with each meal.

EXTERNAL USE

❸ **Poultices,** with 100 g of fresh watercresses mashed in a mortar preferably of wood. Apply on the affected areas, wrapped in a gauze.

❹ **Lotions.** Apply the juice directly on the skin.

a flavor not so tasteful as that of watercress. Moreover, it is a ***toxic plant.***

PROPERTIES AND INDICATIONS. Watercress contains gluconasturtosid (a sulphured glycoside), iodine, and iron, as well as a bitter component, and vitamins A, C, and E. These are its properties.

- **Blood depurative and diuretic.** Recommended for gout, arthritis, obesity, and when the diet is rich in meat and fats [❶,❷].
- **invigorating.** Watercress has a soft stimulant effect on all metabolic functions [❶,❷]. It is an appetizer and activates the metabolism, since it gives important amounts of vitamins A, C, and E, besides minerals such as iodine and iron. This makes watercress very useful to help overcoming **asthenia** (weakness) states caused by **lack of vitamins or minerals.**
- **Expectorant.** Due to its content of essential sulphured oils, it promotes expectoration and relieves the congestion of the respiratory system [❶,❷]. People suffering from bronchial disorders or from emphysema can take advantage of its properties.
- **Cicatrizant.** The poultices of watercresses applied on torpid wounds or sores enhance the formation of new skin [❸]. They also **regenerate the skin** in the case of eczema, acne, and dermatosis [❸,❹]. When applied on the scalp, they **prevent hair loss** [❹].

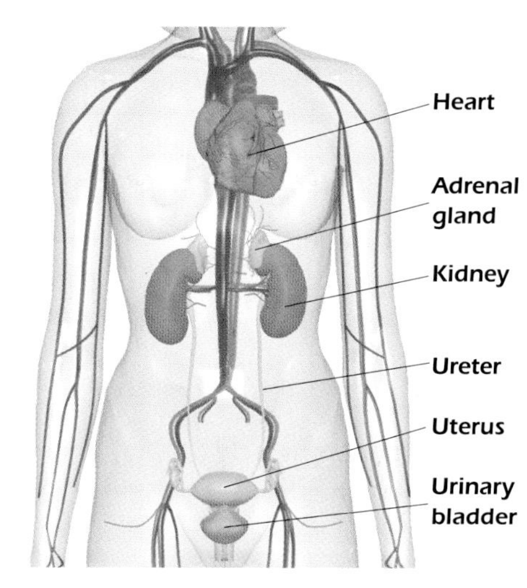

Watercress stimulate the blood cleaning function of the kidneys, enhancing the excretion of toxic wastes asuric acid.

Watercress has a notable blood depurative effect, and it is an invigorating and appetizer. One has to be sure that the water they grow in is not polluted.

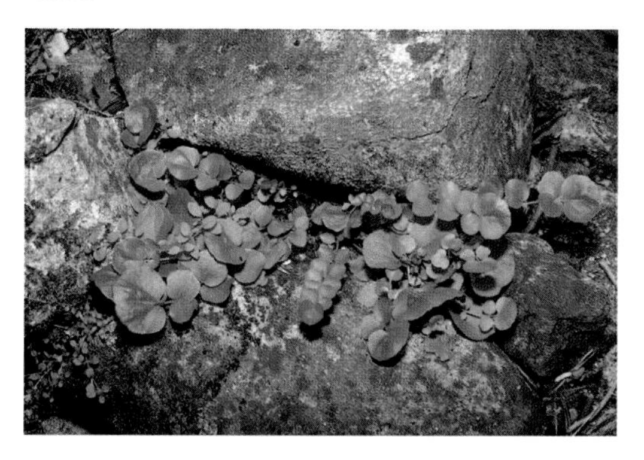

Spirulina

Small alga with great medicinal and nutritive virtues

THE MOST COMMON variety of spirulina, *Spirulina maxima,* is native to the salt lakes of the Mexican plains, such as the Totalcingo and the Texcoco lakes. In their waters are high concentrations of sodium bicarbonate and other potassium and magnesium salts, as well as minerals such as selenium, which avoid the pollution of the water.

An extensive net of water channels have been recently discovered around these Mexican lakes, intended for growing spirulina, and built by the Aztecs more than 500 years ago. These people, the Aztecs, following popular wisdom, used spirulina long before it could be watched and identified through the microscope, and modern chemistry found out its exceptional composition.

PROPERTIES AND INDICATIONS. The composition of this water vegetable, due to its nutritive richness, has been the focus of some outstanding research projects for the last few years. Besides chlorophyll, like all algae, spirulina contains:

✓ **Protein.** It is one of the richest natural sources of protein (up to 70% of its weight, while soya has 35%, and meat 20%). The protein of spirulina is complete, and has great biological value, since it contains all eight **essential amino acids** (those that our bodies cannot synthesize) in an optimum proportion, besides the other non-essential amino-acids.

✓ **Lipids** (fats: 8% of its weight), mainly unsaturated fatty acids such as linoleic, linolenic, and especially gamma-linolenic acids. Spirulina is one of the richest vegetables regarding these important substances of great value for the treatment of **arteriosclerosis.**

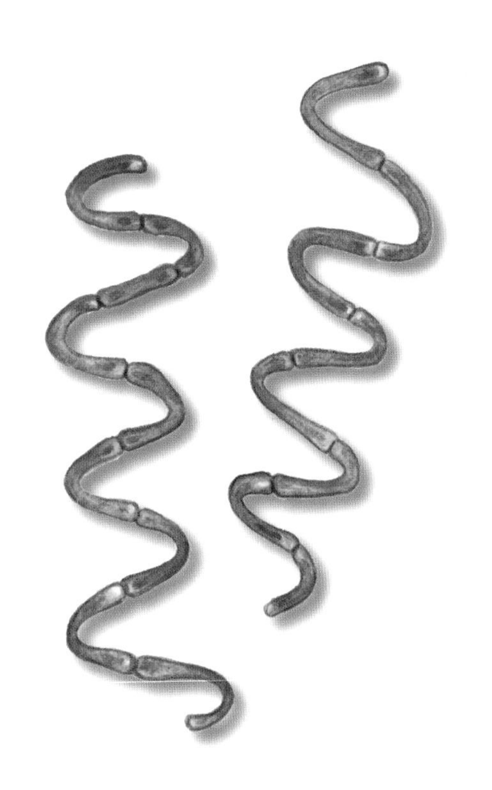

Description. *Monocellular microscopic alga of the Cyanophycea family (blue-green algae), spiral-shaped. Its size varies from 0.1 to 0.3 mm.*

Parts used. *The whole alga.*

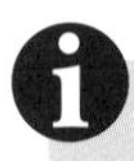

Obtaining Spirulina

When straining the water of the lakes where this alga grows, and after pulverizing and desiccating it at a 158°F (70°C) temperature, the most usually consumed form is obtained, from which the capsules and other preparations are made.

Aztecs and other peoples living close to the lakes where spirulina grows obtained it traditionally by means of sun desiccation.

Preparation and Use

INTERNAL USE

➊ **Capsules** of 400 mg to one gram of spirulina powder. This is the usual presentation. Take from three to 12 capsules a day, distributed among three intakes. In **diets for losing weight,** it is recommended to take these capsules half an hour before meals.

✓ **Sugars or carbohydrates** (18%), among them, a rare natural sugar: rhamnose, which promotes the metabolism of glucose, and has a favorable effect on **diabetes.**

✓ **Vitamins** A, B group, E, and H (biotin). Its content of vitamin B_{12} is outstanding, and exceeds even that of the mammals liver, a fact that makes spirulina a most appreciated food for people following a strict vegetarian diet, that is to say, lacking even eggs, milk, and dairy products. Actually, vitamin B_{12} is not contained in the true algae, but in a type of bacteria that usually accompany it.

✓ **Several minerals and trace elements.** Spirulina is especially rich in iron: 5.3 mg per 100 g of edible product (meat contains from two to three mg per 100 g, and liver 11 mg).

Due to its great nutritive value, spirulina has very favorable effects in many afflictions and illnesses **(➊)**:

- **Diets for losing weight.** Due to its relatively small amount of calories (360 calories per 100 g) compared with its great protein and vitamin aportion, spirulina is an optimal complement for weight loss programs. Its use helps keep a nutritive balance in hypocaloric diets, not provoking weakness or tiredness caused by nutritional deficiencies. Besides, its contents of phenylalanine, an essential amino acid that is present in relatively high amounts in spirulina, helps, according to some researchers, to reduce the sensation of hunger.
- Diseases that require a strict diet, such as **diabetes, hepatitis, or pancreatitis,** in which there exists the risk of nutritional deficiencies.
- **Anemia.** Due to its high amount of iron and essential amino-acids, it promotes the synthesis of hemoglobin, the essential part of red blood cells. It is recommended during pregnancy.
- **Malnutrition, convalescence, and physical weakness.** It acts in revitalizing and general invigorating of the body.
- **Arteriosclerosis and its disorders:** Angina pectoris, myocardial infarction, arterial ischemia (lack of blood flow), which mainly affects the legs. The favorable action of spirulina is due to its content of unsaturated fatty acids, such as the linoleic and gamma-linolenic acids.

Spirulina is a good nutritive complement for elderly people, as well as for those suffering from malnutrition, anemia, or exhaustion, due to the high amount of proteins, vitamins, and minerals it contains.

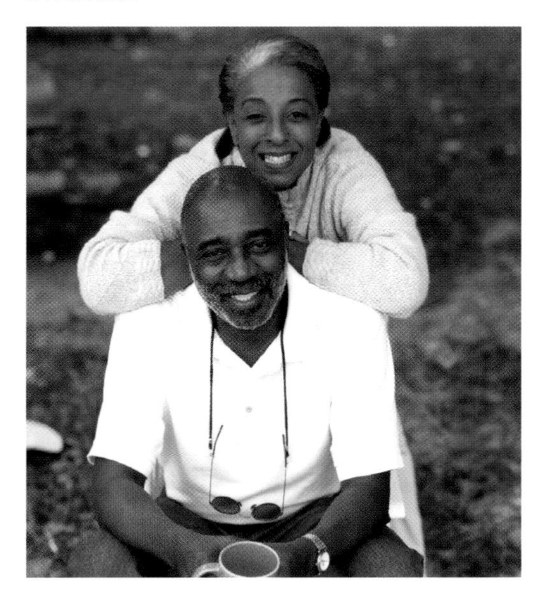

Nettle

A plant that defends itself... and defends us

IT IS A PITY that nettles are avoided by so many people, and are even regarded as a weed. If only they knew how many virtues this allegedly aggressive plant keeps!

The nettle is one of the prima donnas of phytotherapy. Its peculiar hairs make it known, even by blind people, thus one of its common names is born: herb of the blind.

PROPERTIES AND INDICATIONS. The hairs of the nettle contain histamine (1%) and acetylcholine (0.2-1%), both substances also produced by our body, and which take active part on the circulatory and digestive systems as transmitters of the nervous pulses of the autonomic nervous system. Some ten milligrams of these substances are enough to provoke a skin reaction.

The leaves contain plenty of chlorophyll, the green coloring of the vegetal world, whose chemical composition is very similar to that of hemoglobin, red-coloring our blood. They are rich in mineral salts, especially those of iron, phospho-

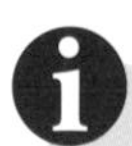

Urtications

*With a freshly gathered bunch of nettles, gently hit the skin of the joint affected by the **inflammatory or rheumatic** disorder (knee, shoulder, etc.). Then a **revulsive effect** takes place, which attracts the blood to the skin, decongesting the internal tissues.*

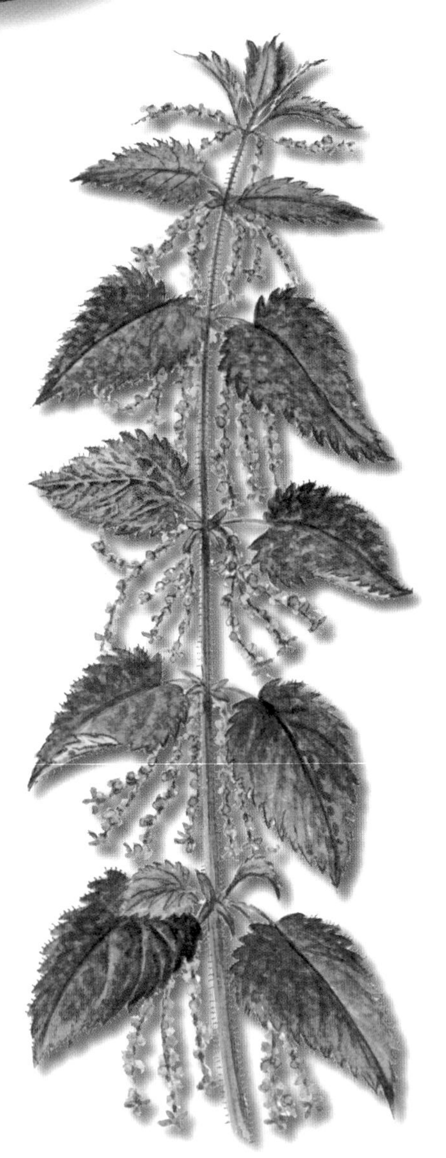

***Description.** Vivacious plant of the Urticaceae family, growing from 0.5 to 1.5 meters high. Both the stems, square-shaped, and the leaves are covered by stinging hairs. Its green-colored flowers are very small.*

***Parts used.** The whole plant, especially its leaves.*

Preparation and Use

In order to calm those people who are afraid of this plant, it may be said that after 12 hours of being gathered, its stinging effect disappears, and the plant acquires a velvet-like touch.

INTERNAL USE

❶ **Fresh juice.** The best way to take advantage of its medicinal properties, especially of its depurative effect. It is obtained by pressing its leaves or putting it in a blender. Drink half to one glass in the morning, and another one at noon.

❷ **Infusion** with 50 g per liter of water, steeping for 15 minutes. Drink three or four cups daily.

EXTERNAL USE

❸ **Lotion,** applying the juice onto the affected skin area.

❹ **Compresses,** soaked in the juice and applied onto the affected area. Change them three or four times a day.

❺ **Nose plugging.** Soak a gauze in the nettle juice, then plug it into the nostrils.

rus, magnesium, calcium, and silicon, which make them diuretic and depurative. They also contain vitamins A, C, and K, formic acid, tannin, and other substances that have not been already studied. The compound of these substances make the nettle **one of the plants with most medicinal applications.**

• **Depurative, diuretic, and alkalinizant.** Recommended for rheumatic afflictions, gout, arthritis, kidney stones, urinary sand, and as a rule whenever a depurative and diuretic action is required [❶,❷]. The nettle has a notable ability to **alkalinize** the blood, easing the expulsion of metabolic acid waste related to all these afflictions. The internal use of the plant can be combined with urtications on the affected joint.

• **Antianemic.** It is used in anemia caused by lack of iron or by loss of blood [❶,❷]. The iron and the chlorophyll that the nettle contains stimulate the production of red blood cells. The nettle also suits **convalescence, malnutrition, and exhaustion** cases, due to its invigorating and recovering effects.

• **Vasoconstrictor** (contracts blood vessels) and **hemostatic** (stops hemorrhage), especially recommended for uterine [❶,❷] and nasal **hemorrhage** [❺]. It is very useful for women with excessive menstruation. We have to insist that ***any abnormal hemorrhage*** must be checked out by a physician.

• **Digestive.** It renders good results in digestive disorders caused by atony or insufficiency of digestive organs [❶,❷]. Nettles contain small amounts of secretin, a hormone that is produced by certain glands of our intestine, and which stimulates the secretion of pancreatic juices and the motility of both the stomach and the gall bladder. This explains the fact that nettle eases the digestion and improves the assimilation of food.

• **Astringent.** It has been successfully used to calm the strong diarrhea caused by cholera [❷]. nettles are useful in all types of diarrhea, colitis, or dysentery.

• **Hypoglycemic.** Nettle leaves decrease the level of sugar in the blood, a fact which has been checked out in many patients [❶,❷]. Though it cannot substitute insulin, it allows a decrease in the antidiabetic medicine dosage.

• **Galactogene.** It increases the milk secretion of breast-feeding women [❶,❷,❹], thus being recommended while *breast-feeding.*

• **Emollient.** Due to its soothing effect, it is recommended in **chronic afflictions of the skin, e**specially eczema, eruptions, and acne [❸,❹]. It is also used for **hair loss** [❸]. Nettles clean, regenerate, and makes skin more beautiful [❸,❹]. Better results are achieved if besides using it in local applications is also employed in orally [❷].

10

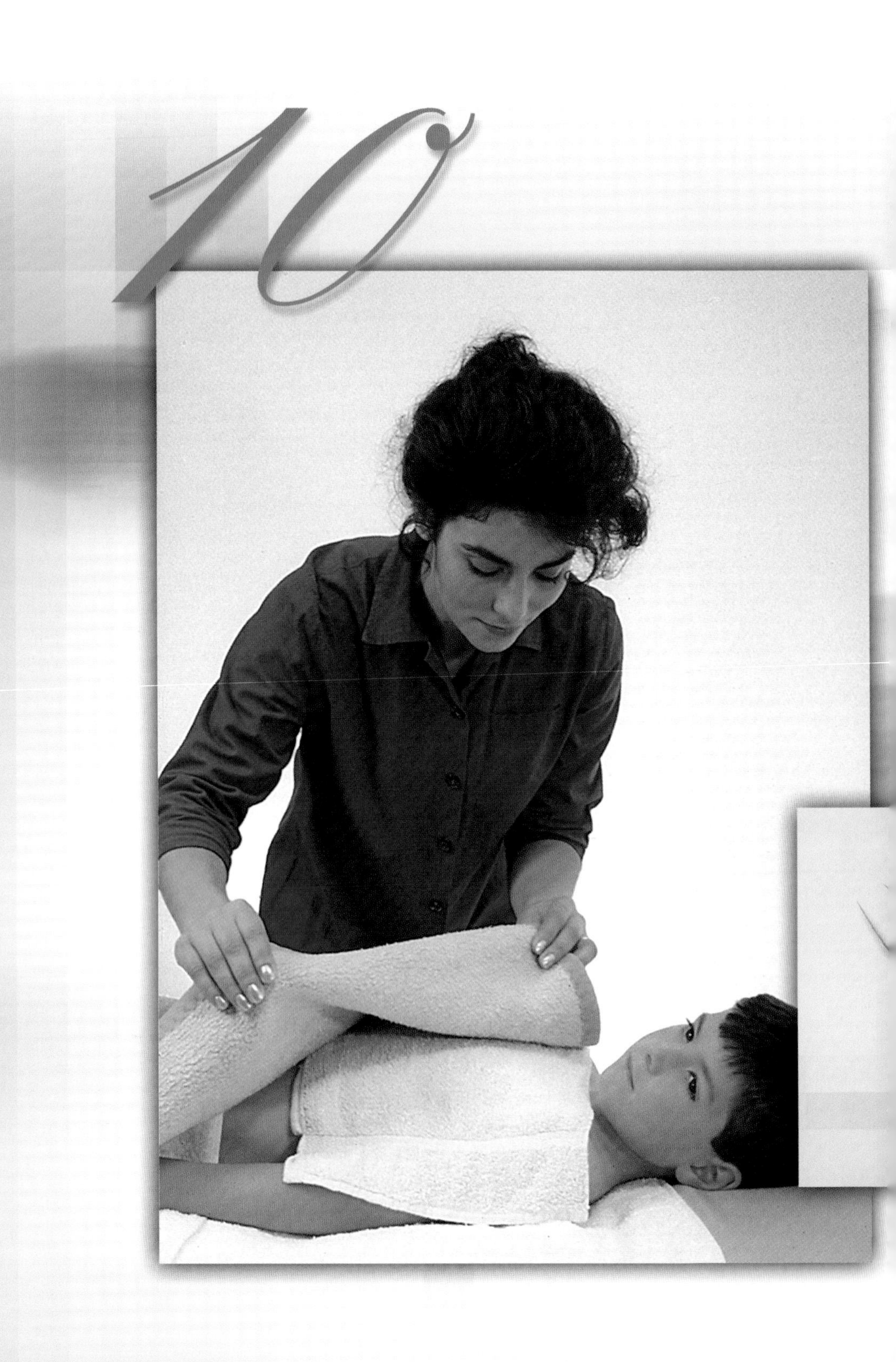

Plants for the Respiratory System

DISEASES	PAGES
Asthma	148
Bronchitis	147
Cough	148
Lung emphysema	149
Pneumonia	147

PLANTS	PAGES
Caimito	154
Canadian fir tree	151
Common plantain	162
Desert tea	155
Eucalyptus	156
Garden Violet	168
Iceland moss	152
Irish moss	153
Licorice	158
Lungwort	164
Mother of thyme	166
Pine tree	160
Silver fir	150
Sugar cane	165

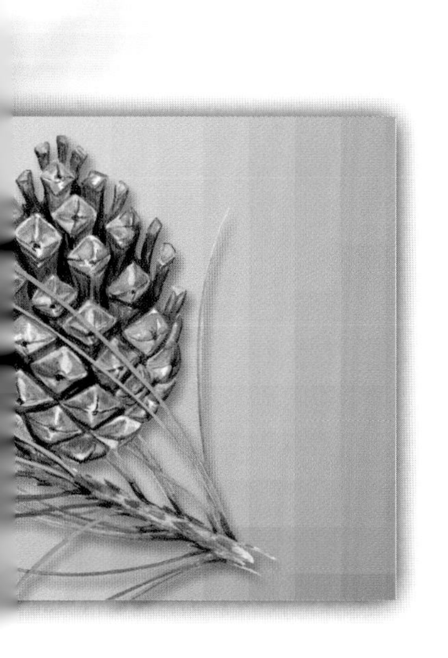

THE RESPIRATORY system is likely to be one of the systems most sensitive to the action of medicinal herbs. Many forms of phytotherapeutic treatments exert a beneficial action on the respiratory organs, for instance, the following:

- **Hot infusions or decoctions** of pectoral plants, which first act locally when passing close to the larynx and the upper areas of the high airways, and then their active components pass to the digestive tract, from there to the blood, and reach the lung and bronchial cells.
- **Syrups**. This method of preparation is traditionally employed for respiratory afflictions. Sugars usually have a balsamic action for the bronchi,

especially notable in the case of honey. Syrups should be thus prepared with honey whenever possible. They are especially recommended for children, since the flavor masks the likely bad taste of the plants they are made of.

- **Inhalation of essences**. **Aromatherapy,** that is, the use of essences or essential oils is one of the great rediscoveries of modern phytotherapy. The simple inhalation of an essence exerts medicinal actions on the respiratory system: antiseptic, bronchidilator, and mucolytic (thinning of the bronchial mucous). By breathing the aroma of eucalyptus or that of a raw sliced onion, a cough is calmed and bronchi cleared.
- **Vapor inhalations**. Water vapor is one of the most effective mucolytic substances known. The inhalation of water vapor, adding to the water some drops of an essence to achieve a better effectiveness, combines the therapeutic effects of the water with those of the employed plant.
- **Baths**, **poultices** and **fomentations** with medicinal herbs. These are other effective methods of use for treating the afflictions of the respiratory system.

All respiratory organs gain great benefits from the use of medicinal herbs. Their action is not limited to neutralizing the symptoms of any disease, but they exert a true cleansing action for excessive mucus in the interior of the airways. Besides, some plants such as nasturtium or thyme also contain antibiotic substances which prevent bacteria growth in the remanding mucus.

Every day we breathe about one thousand liters of air into our lungs. In towns, this air contains smoke, germs, and small polluting particles. Our bronchi have an effective **cleansing mechanism,** their interior being covered by a mucous layer that catches and expels the polluting particles and germs, which the air we breathe contains. Under normal conditions, this mechanism is enough to keep the bronchi clean.

However, due to the action of tobacco smoke, other smokes or irritant substances, certain noxious germs, or bad respiratory habits, the bronchi cleaning mechanism stops working effectively, and then we suffer from **bronchitis.** Medicinal herbs can then act by restoring the effective working of the bronchial mucous membrane. Obviously, the main condition to restore it is for **the cause of the dysfunction to disappear.** It would be almost useless to apply the best phytotherapeutical—or other kind of—treatments if the patient kept on smoking or breathing polluted air.

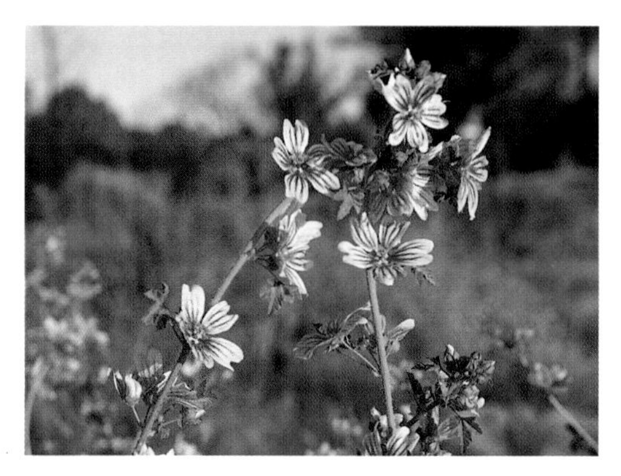

The leaves and flowers of high mallow contain a high amount of mucilage with emollient (soothing) action, as well as expectorant, antitussive, and laxative. High mallow is highly recommended for colds, influenza, and bronchitis, both for adults and children.

BRONQUITIS

Definition

It is inflammation of the mucous membrane that covers the interior of the bronchi. It is usually provoked by infectious causes, to which the inhalation of irritant smoke, such as tobacco smoke, can help it to become more severe. The symptoms are fever, cough, pain when coughing, and occasionally, breathing difficulties. When this disease appears with certain frequency, it is called **chronic bronchitis.**

Phytotherapy

The phytotherapeutic treatment consists of the ingestion and inhalation, by means of essences or vapor, of ***balsamic*** (soothing the respiratory mucous membrane), ***mucolytic*** (which break mucus and ease its elimination), ***expectorant and antibiotic*** plants. See more plants with these actions in the corresponding tables. The ones we mention here exert an interesting preventive action of new crises or relapses.

LINDEN	Emollient, antispasmodic, sedative
GOLDENSEAL	Regenerates cells of the mucosa
GARLIC	Antibiotic, expectorant
ICELAND MOSS	Pectoral, expectorant, antibiotic
EUCALYPTUS	Antiseptic, balsamic, regenerates the bronchial mucosa
LICORICE	Promotes expectoration, eases coughs, reduces inflammation of the respiratory ways
COMMON PLANTAIN	Thins secretions, reduces the inflammation of the respiratory mucosa
GARDEN VIOLET	Reduces congestion of the bronchi, eases cough, soothes respiratory mucosa
ANISE	Promotes the elimination of the bronchial mucus, helps overcoming tobacco damages
HIGH MALLOW	Expectorant, antitussive
JUNIPER	Expectorant, bronchial antiseptic
BLACK MUSTARD	Revulsive, reduces the congestion of inner organs
ANNATTO TREE	Expectorant
NASTURTIUM	Makes mucus more fluid, reduces congestion of the bronchi, eases cough

PNEUMONIA

This is an inflammation of the lung tissues usually due to infectious causes. The phytotherapeutic treatment is based in infusions and decoctions of ***pectoral and antibiotic action,*** inhalation of essences, vapors, and poultices of mustard flour, as a ***complement*** to the anti-infectious specific treatment.

Fir tree

CAMPHOR TREE	Stimulates respiratory nerve center, increasing frequency and depth of breathing
SILVER FIR	Balsamic, antiseptic, expectorant
COMMON PLANTAIN	Makes secretions more fluid, reduces the inflammation of the bronchial mucosa
GARDEN VIOLET	Reduces congestion of bronchi, eases cough, soothes respiratory mucosa
BLACK MUSTARD	Revulsive, reduces congestion on internal organs

People who perform outdoor physical exercise, such as cyclists, need to have both bronchi and lungs in optimum condition.

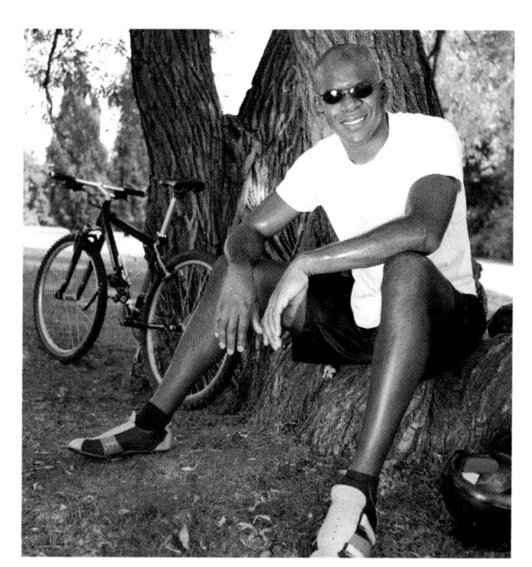

ASTHMA

Definition

A disease whose characteristics include attacks of breathing difficulty (with wheezing breath, cough, and sensation of constriction due to bronchial spasms). It is usually caused by infectious or allergic reasons.

Phytotherapy

The phytotherapeutic treatment is based on plants with ***antispasmodic*** (in order to relax the bronchial spasm), ***bronchodilator, and expectorant*** actions, such as these indicated in the table (see also the specific tables for each one of these actions). Medicinal herbs have, generally, a ***preventive action*** against new relapses.

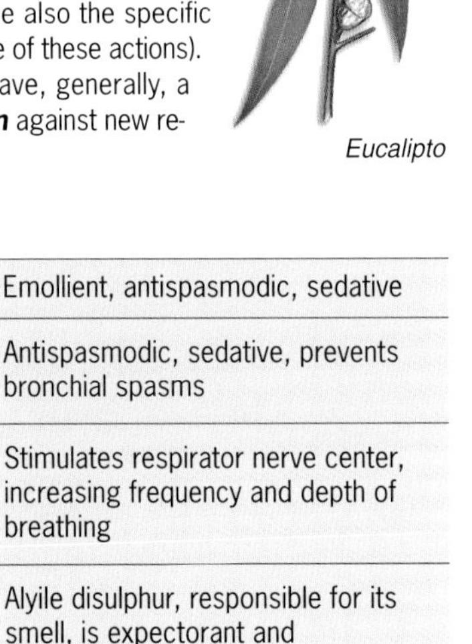

Eucalipto

LINDEN	Emollient, antispasmodic, sedative
VALERIAN	Antispasmodic, sedative, prevents bronchial spasms
CAMPHOR TREE	Stimulates respirator nerve center, increasing frequency and depth of breathing
GARLIC	Alyile disulphur, responsible for its smell, is expectorant and antiasthmatic
DESERT TEA	Relaxes bronchial muscles
SPEEDWELL	Prevents asthma crisis, antitussive
HIGH MALLOW	Expectorant, antitussive

COUGH

Causes

Coughing is, in many cases a defense mechanism of our body to expel mucus or foreign bodies located in the interior of the trachea or the bronchi. In these cases, coughing is **productive,** and expels mucus. In other cases, coughing is **dry, non productive,** and caused by an irritating focus of infectious, or more rarely tumoral, origin.

Phytotherapy

These ***antitussive*** medicinal herbs can ease coughing by means of several mechanisms: by relaxing the bronchial muscles spasm ***(antispasmodic*** action), by making mucus more liquid, which eases its expulsion ***(mucolytic*** action), or by producing nerve sedation.

PRICKLY LETTUCE	Sedative, eases irritative cough, useful for whooping cough
LINDEN	Soothing and antispasmodic on the bronchi
ICELAND MOSS	Emollient, antibiotic
EUCALYPTUS	Antiseptic and balsamic, regenerates damaged mucosal cells
MOTHER OF THYME	Eases cough, especially children
WILD MARJORAM	Expectorant, antitussive
SPEEDWELL	Antitussive, soothes the throat
HIGH MALLOW	Expectorant, antitussive
THYME	Antiseptic, antitussive, expectorant

Violet syrup is especially recommended for children with bronchial catarrh or influenza. It eases coughing, makes the bronchial secretions more fluid, and promotes perspiration.

As well as the syrup, adults can also take the garden violet in the form of a leaf and/or flower infusion.

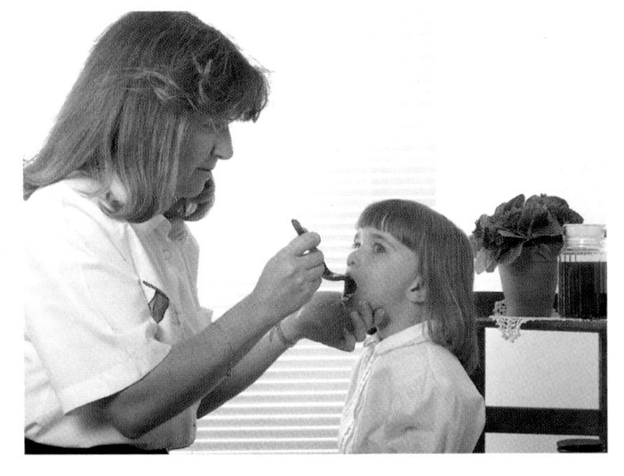

LUNG EMPHYSEMA

Definition

The exaggerated and permanent dilation of lung alveoli. It usually appears as a consequence of repeated bronchitis.

Phytotherapy

Medicinal herbs are one more element in the treatment of this affliction, with a mainly ***preventive*** action. All ***pectoral*** plants are also recommended.

WATERCRESS	Its sulphur essences promote expectoration and reduce the congestion of the respiratory system

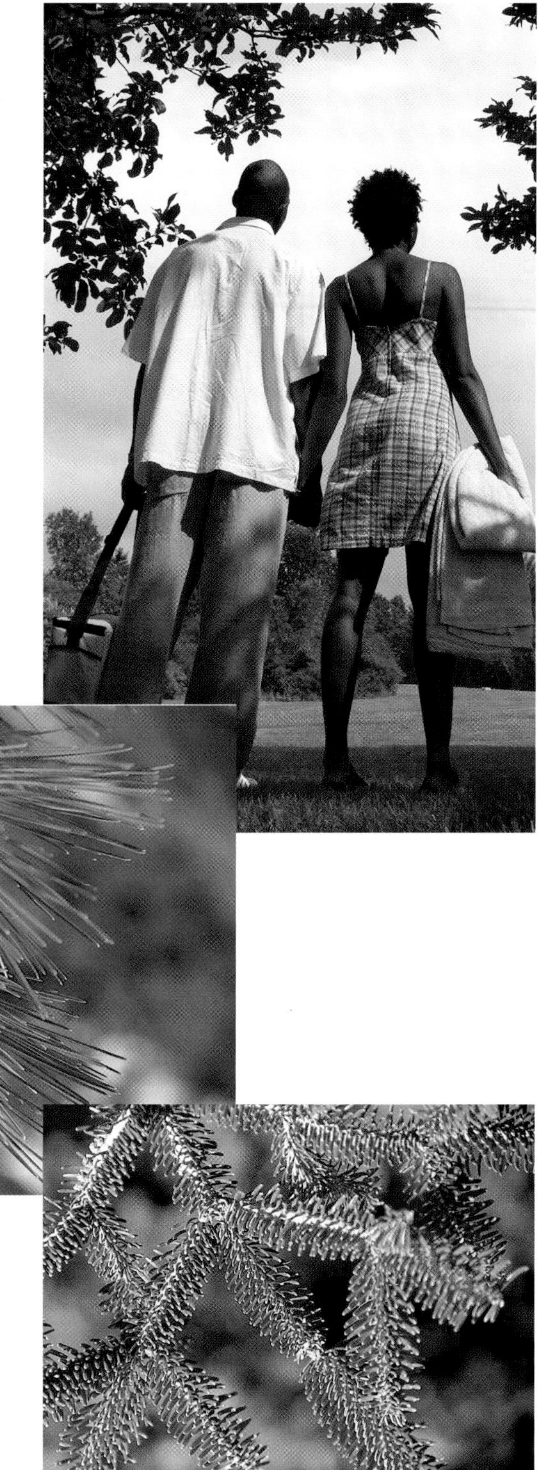

Forests in general, and especially those of conifers, are ideal places for physical exercise, since the air is full of the balsamic essence the trees exhale. The fir tree, and the pine tree, two of the more frequent Coniferae species, produce a very medicinal essence: turpentine.

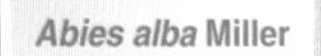
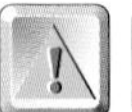
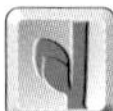
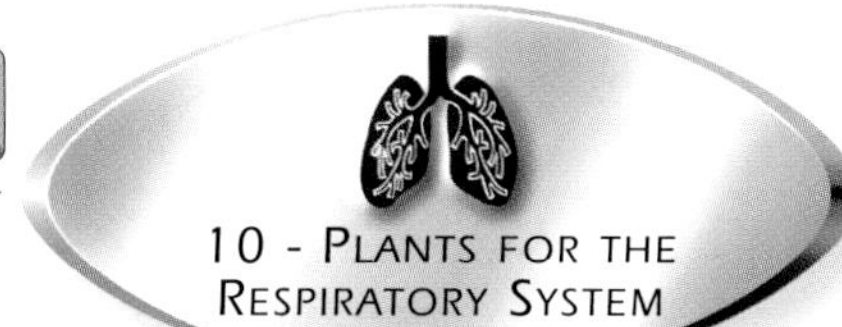

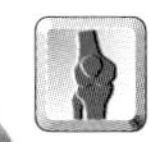
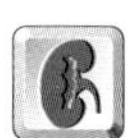
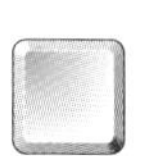
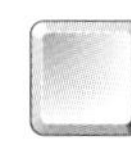

Silver Fir

Excellent for bronchitis and rheumatism

THIS MAGNIFICENT tree could perfectly be called "Doyen of the forests." Not only does it deserve attention for its great, geometrical appearance, but also for its extraordinary lifetime, living up to 800 years. During all this time, the fir tree fills the forest air with its fresh turpentine aroma, so beneficial for people suffering from bronchitis and asthma, and pleasing while strolling around the forests.

At present, fir tree turpentine is being substituted by that of the pine tree, since this is easier to harvest. Though its properties are very similar, fir tree turpentine is usually more aromatic than that of the pine tree.

The resin of the fir tree, or turpentine, accumulates in Spring under the bark and the buds. When the bark is cut, then the resin flows, a liquid as fluid as oil, whose aroma resembles that of lemon, but sour-flavored. This resin can be distilled, thus obtaining turpentine essence or turps.

PROPERTIES AND INDICATIONS. The whole plant contains tannin, essential oil, turpentine, and provitamin A. ***TURPENTINE*** is an oleo-

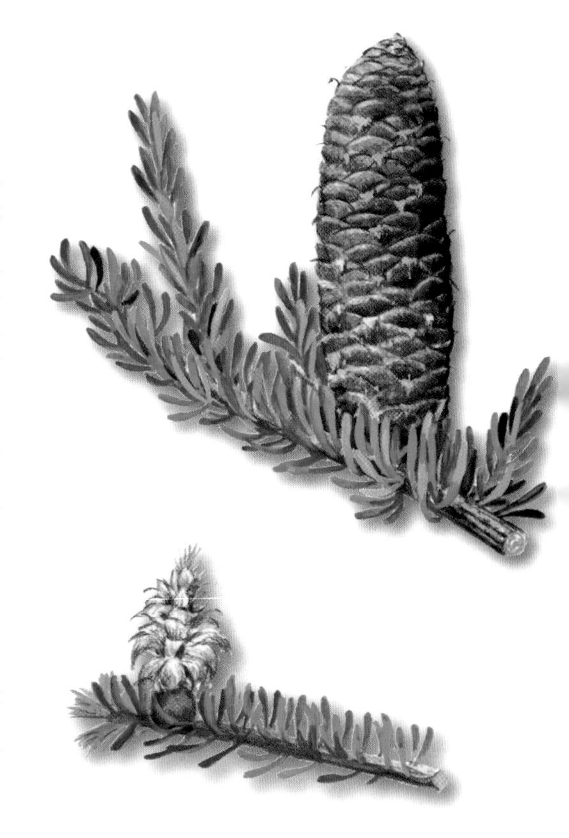

Description. *Tree of the Pinnaceae family, growing up to 50 meters high, with straight trunk, smooth, greyish bark, male and female flowers on the same tree, pine cones of around five centimeters, which, when ripe, let the scales and the seeds fall. Its aroma resembles that of lemon, and its taste is sour.*

Parts used. *The buds and the resin (turpentine).*

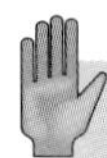

Warning

The inhalation or ingestion of ***excessive doses of turpentine*** *or its essence can produce irritation of the central nervous system, especially in children.*

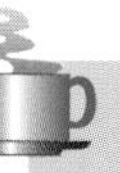

Preparation and Use

INTERNAL USE

❶ **Infusion** with 30-40 g of **buds** per liter of water, drinking three or four cups daily. The buds of the silver fir tree are sticky due to their large turpentine content, especially during Spring.

❷ **Turpentine or its essence:** three to five drops, three times a day.

EXTERNAL USE

❸ **Turpentine or its essence,** applied in **baths** (alleviating those people suffering from rheumatism or asthma), **frictions, inhalations and vapor inhalations.**

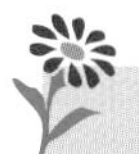

Canadian Fir Tree

In North America the Canadian fir tree (*Abies balsamea* Miller = *Abies canadiensis* L.) grows from whose resin the so-called **Canadian balm** is obtained. This balm has **the same properties** as silver fir **turpentine,** thus their medicinal applications are the same.

Besides, the Canadian balm is used in microscopic laboratory examinations, due to its special optical characteristics.

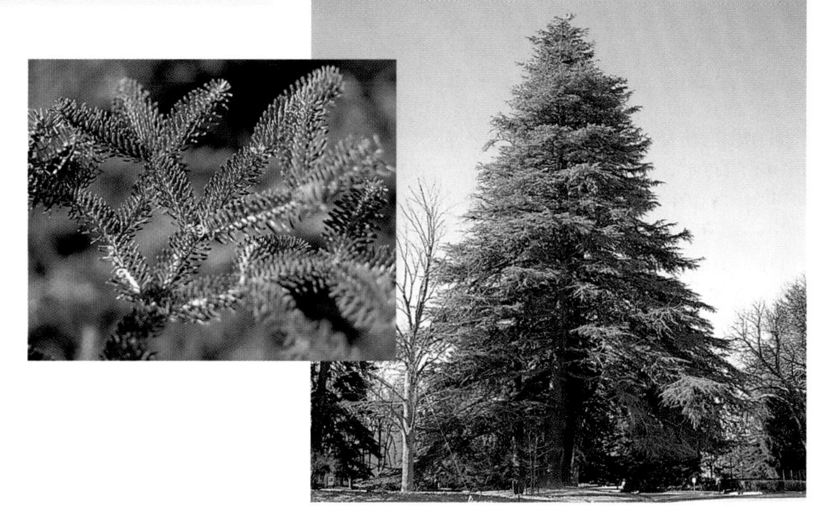

The simple fact of walking through a fir tree or pine tree forest and smelling the turpentine aroma has a beneficial effect on the respiratory system.

Besides being inhaled, the turpentine may be also applied in lotions and be taken orally.

resin, which in ***external use*** has the following properties:

• **Balsamic, antiseptic, and expectorant.** It is recommended for the afflictions of the respiratory airways: sinusitis, tracheitis, bronchitis, pneumonia, and asthma. It eases the expulsion of the mucus and regenerates the mucus membrane covering the respiratory airways [❸].

• **Revulsive** (attracts the blood to the skin, decongesting the internal organs and tissues), **antirheumatic, and vulnerary** (heals wounds and bruises). It eases rheumatic aches, sciatica, lumbago, and torticollis. Reduces the inflammation of the sprained joints, as well as bruises and muscular aches in general. It also cleans infected **wounds** and skin **sores** [❸].

• When taken ***orally,*** [❶,❷], fir tree turpentine or its essence acts in an equally good way on the **respiratory organs.** Besides, it has **diuretic and urinary antiseptic** properties, being also used as a **prevention** against the formation of **calculi and sands** in the urinary tract.

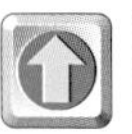

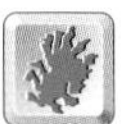

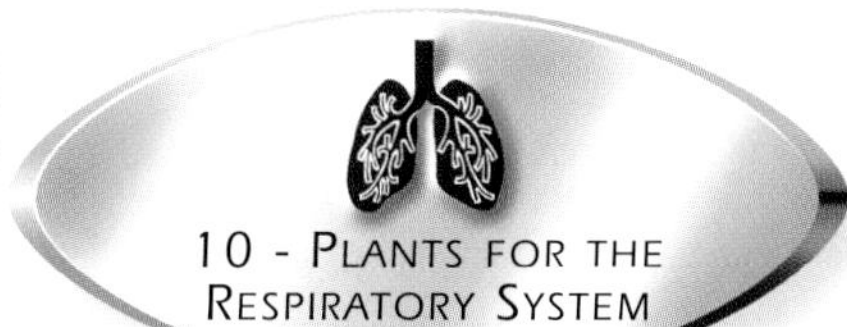

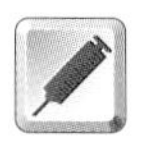

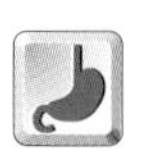

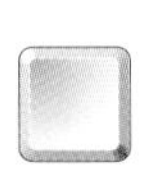

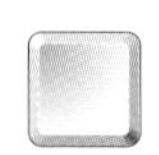

Iceland Moss

A northern remedy against colds

LICHENS, which do not have leaves or roots, are a true example of a surviving species. They adapt to cold and to dry climates, and are able to stay more than one year in a latent state.

Northern Scandinavian Laplanders have used this moss from ancient times. The great Swedish botanist Linnaeus recommended it in the eighteenth century as a medicinal herb.

Properties and indications. The plant contains cetraric acid, which gives it aperitif and invigorating properties; as well as a high amount of mucilage to which it owes its emollient (soothing) properties, and other substances such as usnic acid, which, being active in-vitro against mycobacteria that cause tuberculosis, explain the ***antibiotic*** properties of the plant.

The indications and properties of Iceland moss are the following **{❶}**:

- **Expectorant, antitussive, and pectoral.** In the case of bronchitis, catarrh, asthma, tracheitis, and laryngitis, the plant gives excellent results.
- **Antitubercular.** Iceland moss is recommended as a ***complementary*** remedy to treat pulmonary tuberculosis.
- **Antiemetic.** It helps stop persistent vomiting during pregnancy.

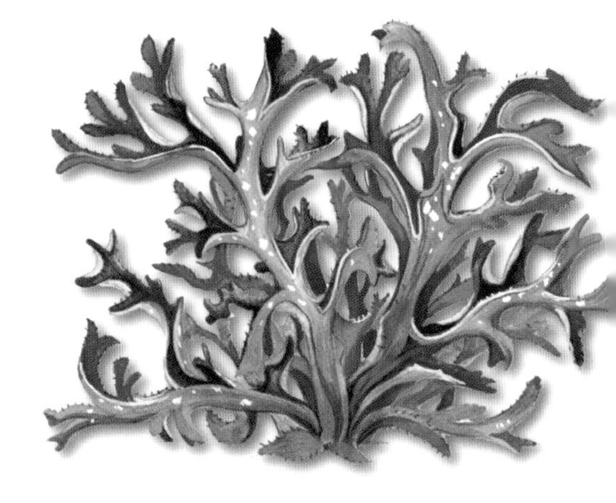

Description. *Lichen or moss five to ten cm long, of the Cetrariaceae family, with light brown stem deeply divided into unequal lobules.*

Parts used. *The dried thallus (the body of the lichen).*

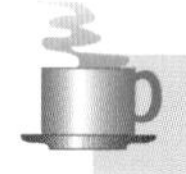

Preparation and Use

Internal use

❶ Decoction with 10-20 g per liter of water, boiling for two minutes. Change the water then in order to eliminate its sour flavor, then boil again in one and a half liters of water until it reduces to one liter. Drink three or four cups a day, hot, sweetened with honey.

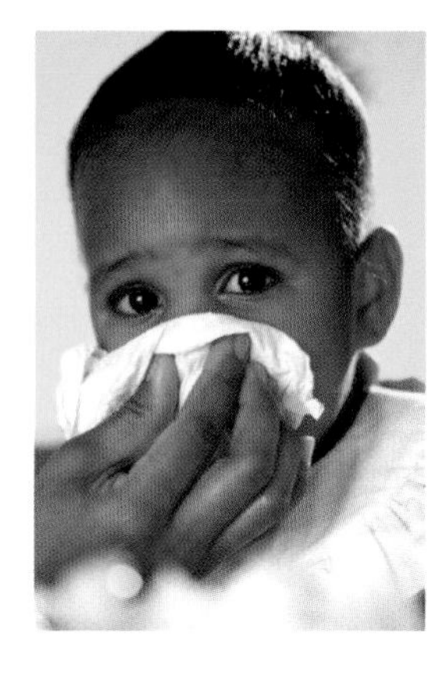

A decoction of Iceland moss is rich in mucilage, with expectorant properties.

Irish Moss

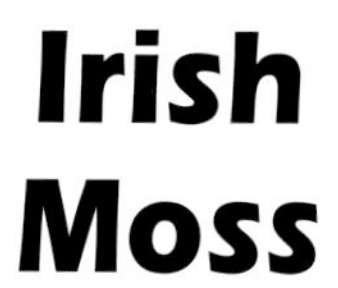

Powerful emollient

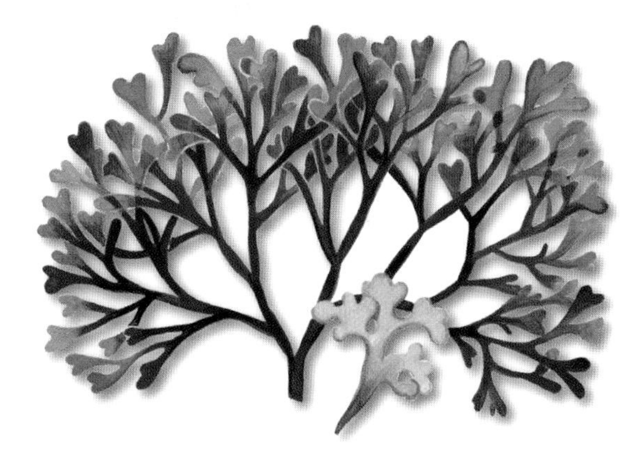

THIS FORM OF ALGAE was first used in Ireland in the mid-nineteenth century. Since then, its medicinal applications have increased more and more. The thallus of the alga has cartilaginous consistency (Latin *chondrus* = cartilage) due to the high amount of mucilage it contains.

PROPERTIES AND INDICATIONS. Besides containing 80% mucilage, the thallus is rich in iodine, provitamin D, and mineral salts. Its most important active component is the mucilage, to which Irish moss owes its **emollient, expectorant, and laxative** properties.

The use of this alga is recommended for bronchitis and catarrhs, since it promotes expectoration, eases coughs, and reduces the inflammation of the **airways.** It is also good for **gastritis** and **intestinal inflammation** caused by colitis or chronic constipation [❶]. Irish moss is widely used in ***food industry*** because of its ***jellifying*** effects.

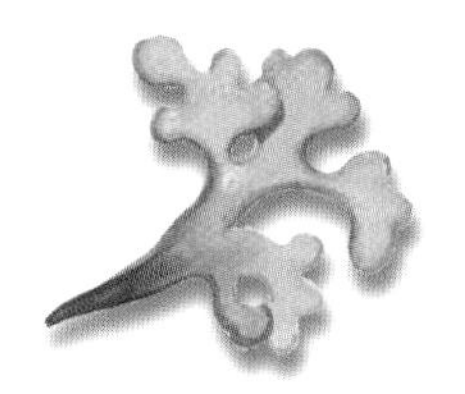

Description. *In spite of its name of moss, it is a red alga (rodophyte) of the Gigartinaceae family, whose thallus is from five to 15 cm long. Its color varies from red to ochre, when fresh, and whitish, when dry.*

Parts used. *The thallus (the whole alga).*

Preparation and Use

INTERNAL USE

❶ **Decoction** with 10 g of alga per liter of water, boiling for five minutes. Drink two or three cups daily.

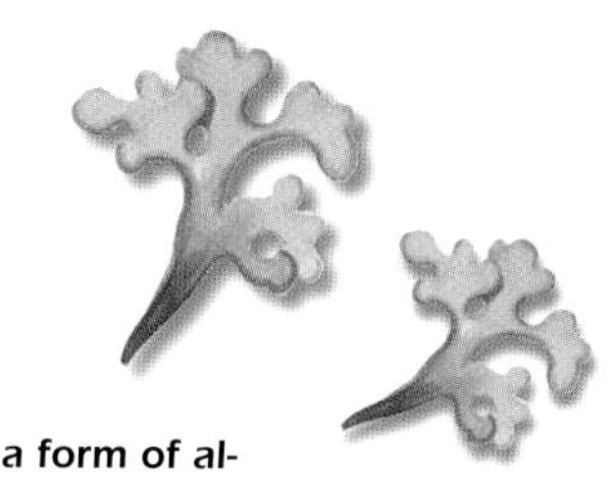

Irish moss is a form of algae with a strong soothing action on the respiratory mucous membrane.

Caimito

A tasteful and medicinal fruit

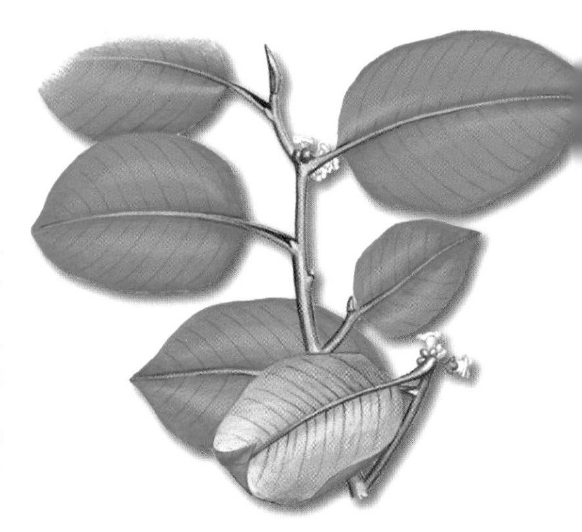

CAIMITO is one of the most flaunting trees of tropical America, with a tasteful and thirst-quenching fruit.

In is not hard to understand, because of its attractiveness and good taste, why people expect to find medicinal properties in caimito. In fact, this fruit has such properties, although they have not been scientifically proven up to now. Popular wisdom speaks in these cases.

PROPERTIES AND INDICATIONS. The flesh of its ***FRUITS*** contains 15 g of sugars (carbohydrates) per 100 g of edible part, 2 g of lipids (fats), and 1 g of proteins, as well as mineral salts, and small amounts of vitamins A, B, and C. The fruit has **astringent** properties, and is recommended for those tourists or travellers who suffer from diarrhea, a frequent disorder in tropical areas [❶].

According to tradition, its ***LEAVES,*** when their underside is applied on sores, cause them to suppurate and then to **cure;** and when their upperside is applied on wounds, stop **hemorrhage.**

The ***BARK*** of the tree and its ***LEAVES,*** and the ***FRUIT*** too, have **febrifuge and balsamic** properties (soothe respiratory mucous membrane), thus being used for bronchitis and colds [❷].

__Description.__ Tree of the Sapotaceae family, growing up to 15 m high, frequently grown as ornamental because of its fine appearance. Its leaves have silky, glowing hairs, golden on their underside. The fruit is round, of 10 cm in diameter.

__Parts used.__ The fruit, the leaves, and the bark.

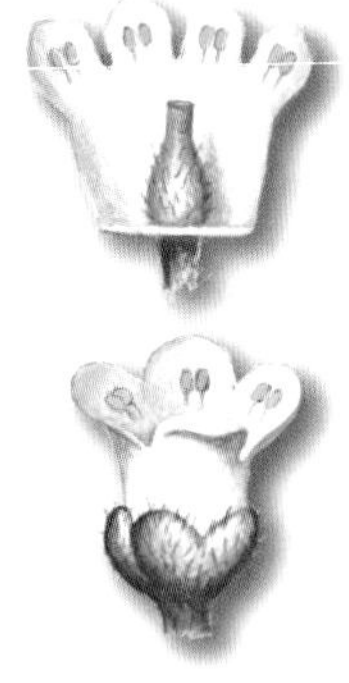

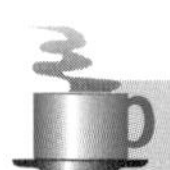

Preparation and Use

INTERNAL USE

❶ **Fruits.** These can be consumed in moderation.

❷ **Decoction** of bark and leaves, with 30-50 g per liter of water. Drink from three to five hot cups daily.

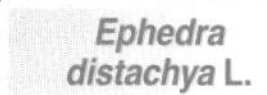

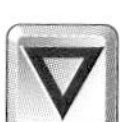
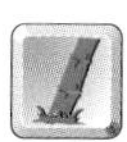
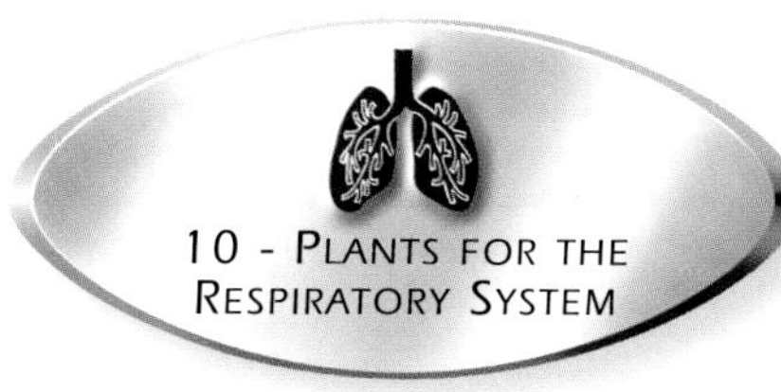

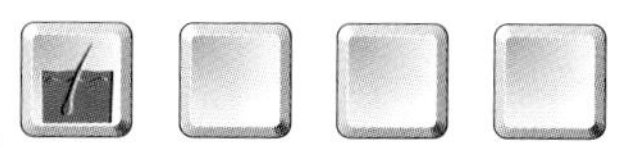

Desert Tea

Antiasthmatic and antiallergic

DESERT TEA may be the ***medicinal herb which has been used for the longest.*** It was early known in China, where it was called *mahuang* and it had been used by the Chinese for several thousand years.

Western medicine did not discover this plant until the nineteenth century. In 1926, its active principle, ephedrine, was first synthesized by Merck Laboratories, in Germany. Since then, it has become part of ***several medicines.***

PROPERTIES AND INDICATIONS. The whole plant contains ephedrine, a very active alkaloid which acts on the nervous autonomic system, as well as tannin, saponin, flavons, and an essential oil. ***Ephedrine*** acts in a way similar to adrenaline, **stimulating the sympathetic nervous system** (sympathomimetic action). It increases blood pressure, produces tachycardia, relaxes the bronchial muscles, increases perspiration and gastric and salivary secretions, and provokes mydriasis (dilation of pupils).

Its most important medical use is for **bronchial asthma,** due to its bronchidilator effect, as well as in allergic reactions (nettlerash, hay fever, etc.) since it neutralizes the **symptoms of allergy [❶]**.

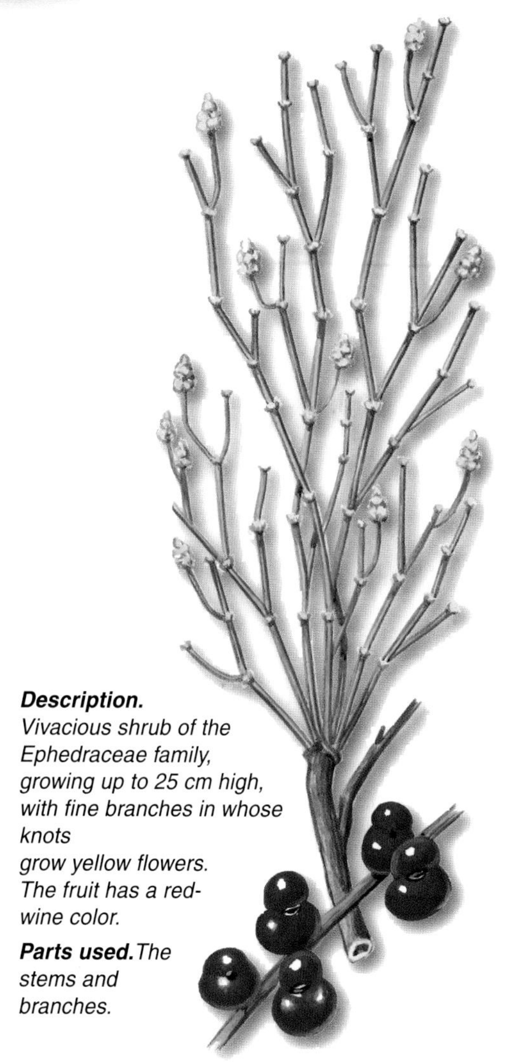

Description. *Vivacious shrub of the Ephedraceae family, growing up to 25 cm high, with fine branches in whose knots grow yellow flowers. The fruit has a red-wine color.*

Parts used. *The stems and branches.*

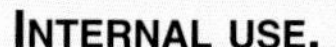

Preparation and Use

INTERNAL USE.

❶ Pharmaceutical preparations: drops, pills, suppositories.

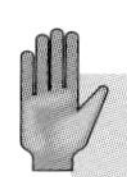

Warning

Only medical professionals *are able to correctly prescribe this plant, due to its complex actions on the human body.*

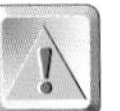

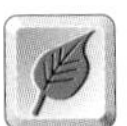

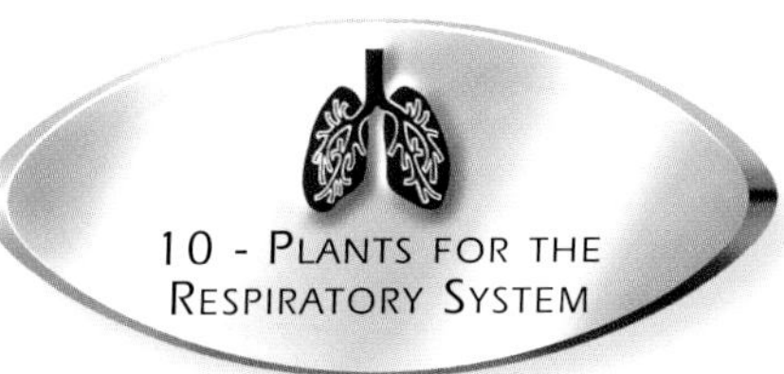

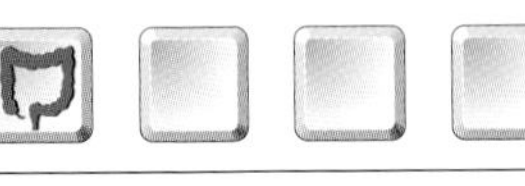

Eucalyptus

Excellent against bronchial afflictions

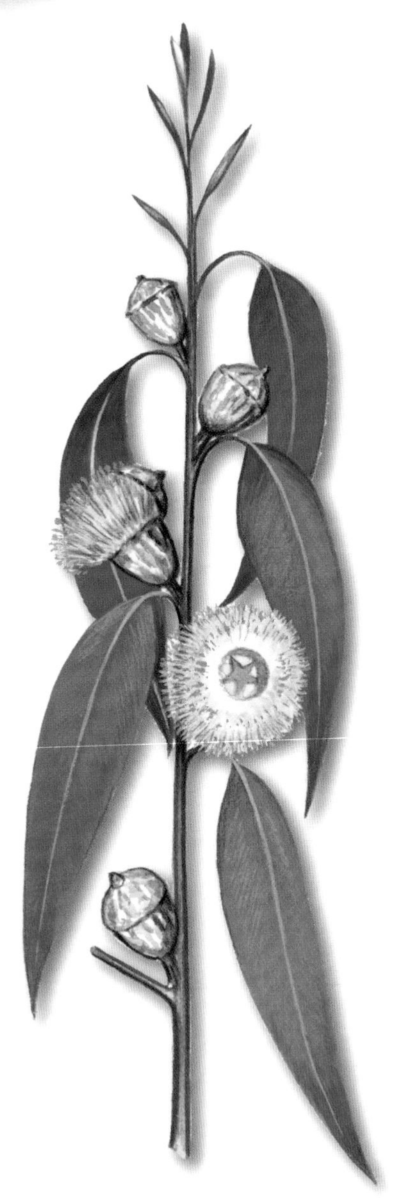

IN THE MID-NINETEENTH century, the eucalyptus was brought to Europe and America from Australia and Tasmania, where it grows up to 100 m high. It is one of the tallest trees known, with some examples reaching 180 m high.

The eucalyptus grows quickly, and absorbs a huge amount of water from the soil, thus being used to drain marshy lands and preventing anopheles (which transmits malaria) from reproducing.

However, this beautiful tree takes its toll on the soils where it is planted. It acidifies the soil and does not allow other plants to grow around it.

PROPERTIES AND INDICATIONS. Its ***LEAVES*** contain tannin, resin, fatty acids, and mainly essences in which its active components concentrate. This essence contains cyneol or eucalyptol, terpene hydrocarbons, pynene, and alymphatic and sesquiterpene alcohols. The **expectorant, balsamic, antiseptic, bronchidilator, and mild febrifuge and su-**

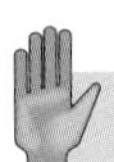

Warning

__Never__ exceed the __doses recommended__ for __internal__ use (both infusion and essence), since high doses may produce gastroenteritis and hematuria (blood in the urine). However, recommended doses will not produce any side effects.

Description. *Tall tree, growing up to 100 m high in Australia, though only to 30 m high in Europe. It belongs to the Myrtaceae family, with smooth, light colored trunk, and evergreen spear-shaped leaves.*

Parts used. *The leaves and the charcoal made from its wood.*

dorific properties of the eucalyptus are caused by this essence.

The eucalyptus is recommended in the case of all respiratory system disorders, especially in bronchial catarrh, asthma, and acute and chronic bronchitis **[❶,❷,❸]**.

Due to its antiseptic and balsamic actions on the bronchial mucous membrane, the eucalyptus helps in regenerating damaged cells, easing the expulsion of mucus, and alleviating coughs. This is ***one of the most effective plants*** known for **bronchial and pulmonary afflictions.**

The ***CHARCOAL*** of eucalyptus is a valuable remedy for these two cases:

- Accidental **poisoning** caused by toxic substances, meals in bad condition, poisonous mushrooms, etc. It acts as a universal antidote.
- **Colitis, diarrhea, intestinal flora dysfunction, or intestinal fermentation.** It adsorbs the toxin which pathological micro-organisms produce. Its effects are fantastic.

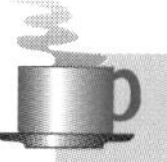

Preparation and Use

INTERNAL USE

❶ **Infusion** with two large leaves per cup of water (20-30 g per liter). Steep for ten minutes in a covered jar. Drink three cups a day, sweetened with honey.

❷ **Essence.** Administer from four to ten drops daily.

EXTERNAL USE

❸ **Vapor baths** on the chest and the head.

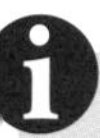

Several Effective Applications of the Eucalyptus

Vapor Baths

*These are **the best method** to take advantage of all properties of the eucalyptus. In a bowl with boiling water, place a handful of **eucalyptus leaves,** or from four to six drops of its **essence** per liter of water. The person must sit down, with a bare torso and the head over the bowl so that the vapor reaches the chest and head. The bath should last from five to ten minutes, three or four times a day.*

This vapor, as well as the evaporated eucalyptus essence, acts in two ways.

- *Directly **on the chest skin,** favoring the elimination of toxins through the skin and alleviating lung congestion.*
- ***Inhaled** into the bronchi. To the **antiseptic, balsamic, and expectorant** properties of the essence, the **mucous effects** of the water vapor are added, then breaking down the bronchi mucus and easing its elimination.*

Essence Against Coughs

Dissolve two spoonfuls of honey in half a glass of water, then add two or three drops of eucalyptus essence. Drink in the case of coughs caused by pharyngitis or laryngitis (throat infections), tracheitis, bronchitis, or bronchial catarrh.

Up to five cups daily can be taken, however the recommended dose for children should not exceed two or three cups a day.

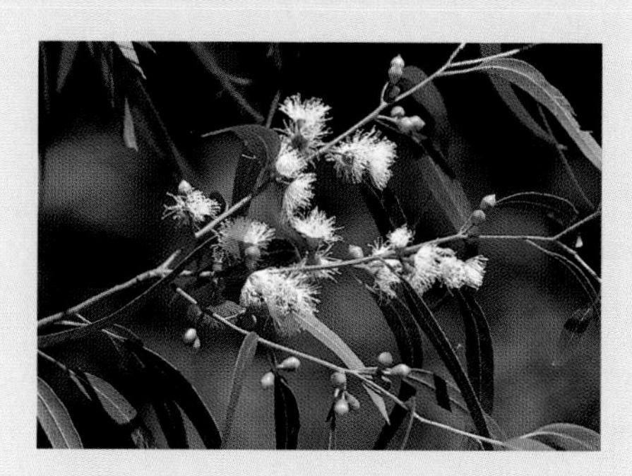

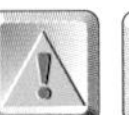
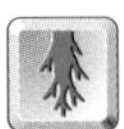
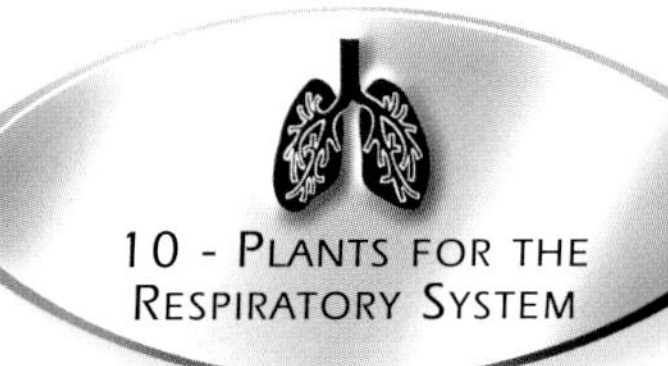

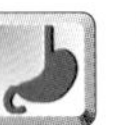
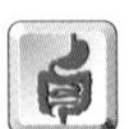
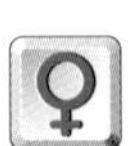
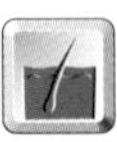

Licorice

Pectoral and digestive par excellence

"I AM GOING to 'smoke' a licorice cigar," a child says to his mate when leaving school.

"Look! There is a man selling them on the corner!" his friend replies.

Then, putting that yellow cigar between his fingers, he feels somehow older and more mature, as he enjoys the special flavor of the sweet wood (Glycyrrhiza comes from the Greek *glykys,* sweet, and *riza,* root.)

This scene can be frequently seen in many schools of southern Europe. Sucking licorice is a better habit than smoking. May this child never change those licorice cigars for true cigarettes or Havana cigars. Perhaps after starting smoking he wants to give it up. Then, someone knowing the virtues of this plant will say: "Do you remember those licorice cigars we enjoyed when leaving school? Start with them again. They will help you give up smoking, as well as restoring your body from the tobacco damage."

In fact, licorice is a good antidote for tobacco, partly due to its great digestive and pectoral properties.

PROPERTIES AND INDICATIONS. Licorice contains several groups of active substances:

✓ Triterpene **saponins,** mainly glycerin, which, unlike many saponins, does not have hemolytic properties. These saponins give the plant expectorant, antitussive, anti-inflammatory, and emollient properties.

✓ **Flavonoid substances,** especially lichirhitine and small amounts of atropine, to which it owes its antispasmodic, antibiotic, digestive, and healing properties.

✓ **Vitamins** of the B group, sugars, and resins.

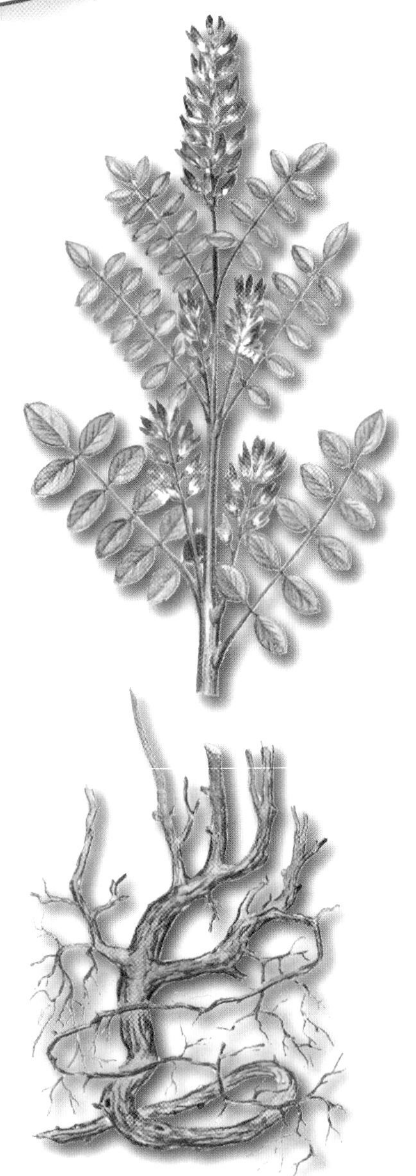

Description. *Vivacious herb of the Leguminoseae family (Papillonaceae subfamily), growing up to 1.5 m high. Its leaves are formed by small oval folioles (from seven to 17). It has blue-violet flowers, and legume-like fruits about two cm sized. From its main root grow many large rhizomes as thick as a finger.*

Parts used. *The root and the rhizome.*

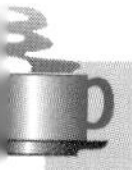

Preparation and Use

INTERNAL USE

❶ **Infusion** with 50 g of dry root per liter of water. The water must not boil, just hot water is enough, since when it boils, the infusion acquires too strong a flavor. Drink three or four cups a day.

❷ **Cold extract.** Steep for one night 40 or 50 g of ground root in one liter of cold water. Strain in the morning, and drink from three to six cups daily.

❸ **Extract.** Licorice extract is black, and is sucked in small pieces similar to pills. We do not recommend the regular use of licorice extract when sweetened with sugar. Licorice cigars (with no sugar) are better, and may be mixed with extracts of other plants such as peppermint or anise.

EXTERNAL USE

The same infusion employed for internal use can be externally applied:

❹ In **compresses** on the skin.

❺ In **eye baths.**

❻ In **mouth rinsings.**

The most important applications of licorice are the following:

- **Respiratory afflictions:** bronchitis, cough, bronchi catarrhs, pharyngitis, laryngitis, hoarseness, and tracheitis [❶,❷]. It promotes **expectoration,** easing **coughs,** and **reducing the inflammation** of the airways. It also has **antibiotic properties** against the most common pathogen bacteria of the bronchi. It is also used for tuberculosis, as a complementary treatment.

- **Digestive afflictions [❶,❷,❸].** Licorice has a notable action on the stomach, calming the acidity and quickly resolving the sensation of a heavy or upset stomach. It is successfully used in all kinds of dyspepsia, belching and gas, stomach aches, intestine and liver colics, and gastritis.

- **Gastric and duodenal ulcer.** In 1950 this sweet root was scientifically proven to be able to heal stomach and duodenal ulcers. Many people who have healed from these ulcers bear witness to this fact [❶,❷,❸]. Licorice has been proven to form a protective film over the stomach mucous membrane, then preventing the corrosive action of gastric juices to act on this mucous membrane, and allowing a quick healing. At present, licorice extract is an ***indispensable part*** of several ***anti-ulcer medicines.***

- **Tobacco addiction.** In cures of toxicity from tobacco, licorice renders good results besides contributing to the regeneration of the digestive and respiratory mucous membrane, its attractive flavor helping defeat the urge to smoke.

- **Gynecologic afflictions.** Because of its antispasmodic action this plant is used to ease menstrual aches [❶, ❷,❸].

- **Skin, eye, and mouth afflictions.** In ***external applications,*** it is used for eczema, psoriasis, impetigo, and other dermatitis [❹]; as well as in eye baths for conjunctivitis [❺], and mouth rinsings to treat stomatitis [❻].

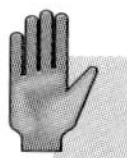

Warning

*Licorice contains small amounts of a steroid substance which stimulates the suprarenal glands. So, when consumed in **high doses** or for **long periods of time** (more than three months), it can produce symptoms of **hyperaldosteronism,** fluid retention (edema) in the joints (especially the ankles) or in the face, nausea and headache, muscle cramps, and high blood pressure.*

***Prolonged consumption** of licorice is **not recommended** in the case of arterial **hypertension, pregnancy,** or when **corticoid**-based treatments are followed.*

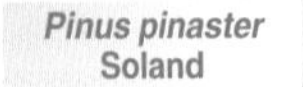

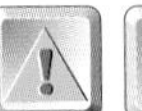
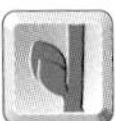
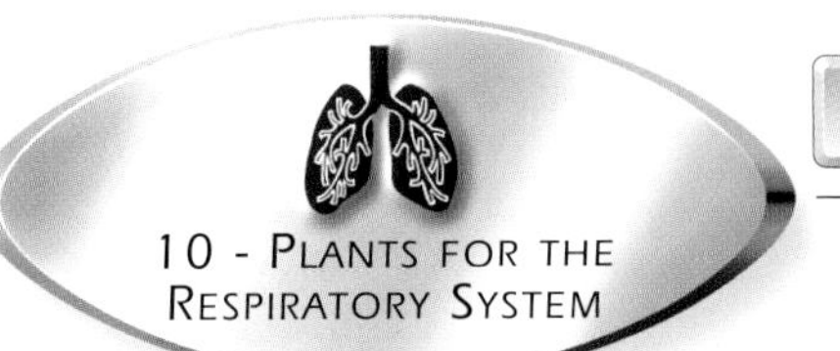

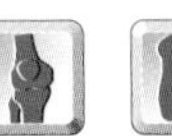
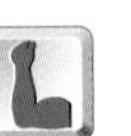
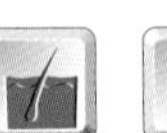
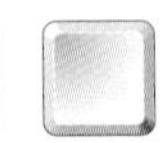

Pine Tree

Alleviates bronchitis and rheumatism

AMONG THE MANY species of pine tree known, only two have notable medicinal properties: the maritime pine tree (*Pinus pinaster* Soland), also known as cluster pine tree, and the wild pine tree (*Pinus silvestris* L.), also known as white pine tree.

The maritime pine tree has larger needles (leaves) and larger pine cones than the wild pine tree. Both species produce turpentine; however the maritime pine tree produces a larger amount.

PROPERTIES AND INDICATIONS. ***TURPENTINE*** is a fatty resin contained in the buds and the outer layers of the pine tree bark, from which it flows either naturally or due to cuts. It is formed by two main components:

✓ An **essence** (20-30%) also called ***turpentine*** (and popularly called **turps),** rich in pinene, a hydrocarbon, which is obtained after distillation, and

✓ A **resin** (70-80%), called **colophony** or Greek tar.

The ***RESIN*** is the solid residue after the essence vaporizes. The resin (colophony) is used in dressings, liniments, and ointments with **rubefacient and antirrheumatic** properties. The most widely known from ancient times is the so-called ***Royal Ointment or basilic,*** which, according to Font Quer, is made with one part of colophony, one of turpentine, one of wax, one of fat, and three of olive oil.

The ***TURPENTINE*** and its essence have **balsamic, antirrheumatic, antiseptic, diuretic, and depurative** properties, and prevent the formation of kidney and urinary **stones** [❶,❷]. The principal applications of these substances are as follows:

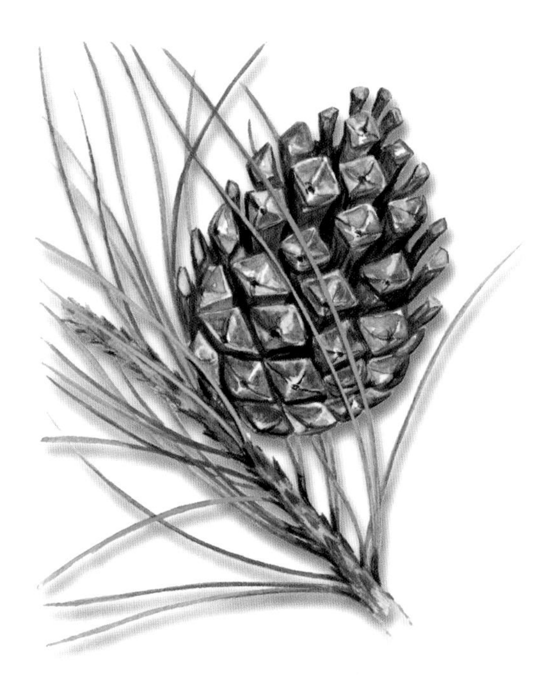

Description. *Tree of the Pinaceae family, growing from 15 to 40 m high, with evergreen, needle-shaped leaves. Male flowers (yellow stamens) and female flowers (pine cones) grow on the same tree.*

Parts used. *The buds and the resin.*

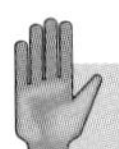

Warning

*Inhalation or ingestion of **excessive doses of turpentine** or its **essence** can produce an **irritation** of the central nervous system, especially for **children.***

Preparation and Use

INTERNAL USE

❶ **Infusion,** prepared with 20-40 g of pine buds per liter of water, drinking three or four cups daily.

❷ **Turpentine essence.** Take from three to five drops, three or four times daily.

EXTERNAL USE

❸ **Baths.** Prepare a **decoction** of 500 g of pine **buds** in four liters of water, boiling for half an hour. Strain and add the liquid to the bath-tub water (hot). A medicinal bath can be also prepared by adding 40-50 drops of **turpentine essence** to the bath water.

❹ **Massage.** With a cotton cloth soaked in turpentine (or its essence) rub the chest of people suffering from bronchitis until the skin becomes a healthy red-color. It is also applied on the joints and muscles if inflamed and aching.

❺ **Vapor inhalations.** Add a handful of pine **buds** (30-50 g) or some drops of **turpentine essence** to a bowl with one or two liters of water. Heat on an electric heater (in order to avoid combustion gases), and breathe the steam in deeply.

- **Respiratory afflictions.** Inhaled {❺}, in massage {❹}, or orally taken {❶,❷}, they are very useful in all kind of respiratory afflictions (bronchitis, asthma, etc.) as well as in the case of colds, rhinitis, and sinusitis. Hot baths {❸} with pine buds or turpentine essence give notable ease for asthma.
- **Anti-inflammatory** (revulsive). In ***external*** applications, baths, and massage {❹,❺}, both the turpentine and its resin (colophony) redden the skin, reducing any inflammation of the deeper tissues (revulsive properties). They render excellent results in the case of ***rheumatic aches,*** be they articular or muscular (lumbago, torticollis, neck aches, etc.), as well as in those produced by **throbbing or spasms.**
- **Invigorating.** The turpentine has been recently proven to have the property of stimulating the suprarenal glands, producing thus a invigorating and revitalizing effect in the whole body {❶,❷}.

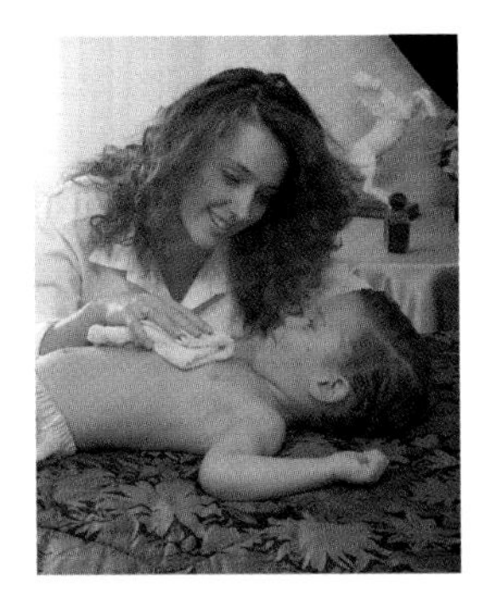

Massage with turpentine or its essence will improve the evolution of bronchial catarrhs, as well as bronchitis, both in children and adults.

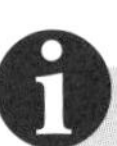

Pine Tar: A Powerful Emollient

*Pine **tar** is obtained by means of dry distillation of the trunk and the roots of the wild pine tree. This substance has a very complex chemical composition, whose principal components are phenolic substances with balsamic, expectorant, antiseptic, and mainly emollient **(skin soothing)** properties.*

*Pine tar can be taken up to one gram per day in the form of capsules or jelly pills. However, its most important application is the **external** use for **skin ailments:** dermatosis (chronic inflammation or degeneration of the skin such as eczema and psoriasis), mycosis (infection caused by fungi), and parasitosis (afflictions caused by parasites such as scabies.*

*For external use, pine tar is applied in the form of **soap, shampoo, or cream.***

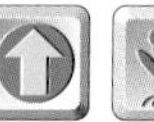

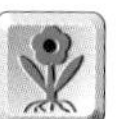

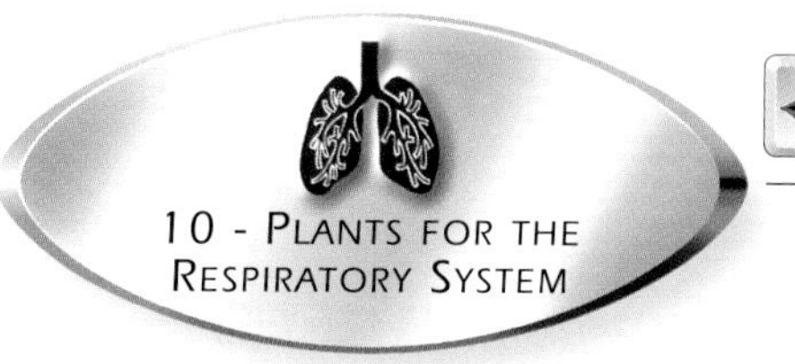

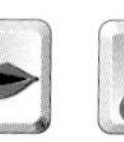

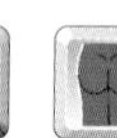

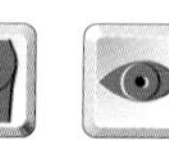

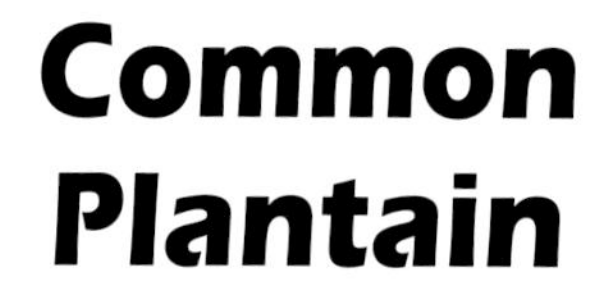

Common Plantain

Pectoral and cicatrizant

THE BOTANICAL genus ***Plantago*** comprises about 200 species, among which the most outstanding in regard to their phytotherapeutical applications are psyllium and all three species of plantain (lance-leaf plantain, common plantain, and hoary plantain), which have been used as medicinal herbs since the times of the ancient Greeks. The name *Plantago* refers to the footprint-like shape of their leaves.

PROPERTIES AND INDICATIONS. All three species of plantain contain a huge amount of mucilage, which gives them **emollient, expectorant, antitussive, and bechic** properties; tannin, to which they owe their **astringent, hemostatic, and cicatrizant** (healing) properties; pectin; and chromogenic glycosides (aucubine and catalpol), with **anti-inflammatory and antiseptic** properties.

The ***COMMON PLANTAIN*** contains as well phenolic acids, flavonoids, choline, and noscapine, an alkaloid with **antispasmodic and antitussive** properties.

Plantain soothes and dries at the same time due to the combined action of mucilage (emollient, soothing) and tannin (astringent, which produce desiccation and constriction). This fact gives plantain a wide anti-inflammatory effect, which is very useful in order to heal many respiratory and digestive mucous membrane afflictions. These are their principal applications:

• **Respiratory afflictions.** Acute or chronic bronchitis, bronchial catarrh, asthma **[❶]**. The plantain thins secretions, easing their elimination, as well as reducing the inflammation of the bronchial mucous membrane and ease coughs. The plantain has been used against pulmonary tuberculosis and pneumonia as a complement

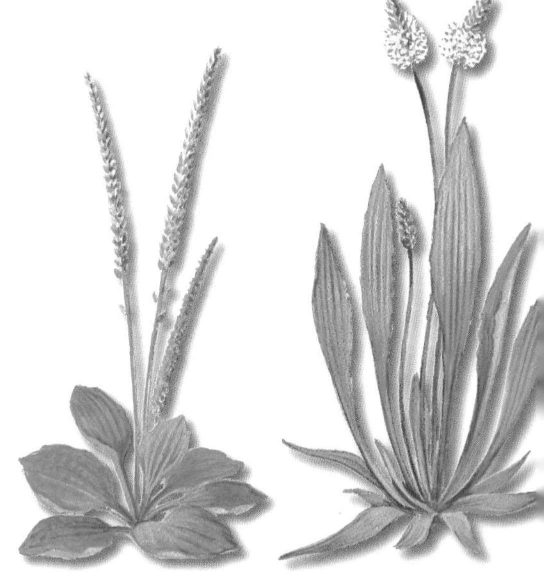

Hoary Plantain

Lance-leaf Plantain

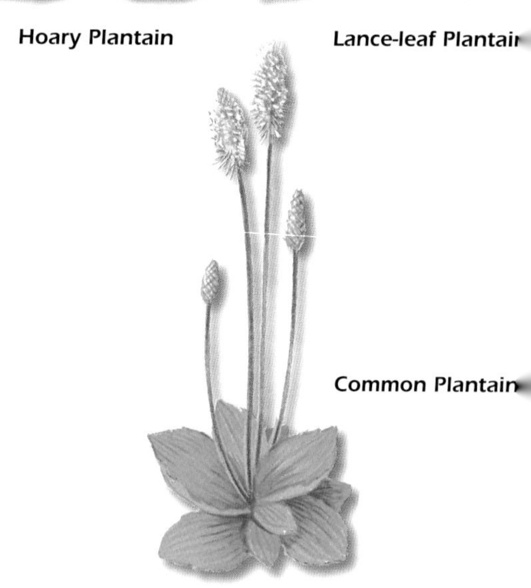

Common Plantain

Description. *Plant of the Plantaginaceae family, growing from 10 to 60 cm high. All three species have root-growing leaves with parallel nerves which join in the tip of the leaf. The length and size of the leaves are different for each species, as well as the flower spikes.*

Parts used. *The whole plant (leaves, flower spike, and root).*

Preparation and Use

INTERNAL USE

❶ **Decoction** with 20-30 g of leaves and/or root per liter of water, boiling for three to five minutes. Drink from three to five cups daily.

EXTERNAL USE

❷ The same decoction, however more concentrated (50-100 g per liter) is used in **gargles, eye irrigations, compresses on the skin, sitz baths, or enemas.**

❸ **Leaf dressings.** Previously wash the leaves, and blanch them in boiling water for one minute in order to sterilize them. Then, put them on the wounds and ulcers with the help of a pair of sterilized forceps. Fix them with a bandage and change two or three times daily.

❹ **Poultices** of boiled and mashed leaves.

to their specific treatment. Among these plants, the common plantain is the one with stronger antitussive properties.

- **Mouth and throat afflictions,** applied in gargles and mouth rinses. The plantain is recommended in the case of stomatitis (inflammation of the oral mucous membrane), gingivitis (inflammation of the gums), pharyngitis, tonsillitis, and laryngitis [❷]. The active components of the plant reduce the inflammation, heal itching and throat irritation, and alleviate coughing from whooping cough (bechic action).

- **Digestive afflictions:** colitis, aerocolia (gas in the colon), abdominal distension caused by an excess of gas or by bad digestion, intestinal putrefaction, diarrhea, dysentery, chronic constipation with inflammation of the large intestine [❶].

- **Hemorrhoids.** Sitz baths and enemas with a plantain decoction are very effective in reducing the inflammation of hemorrhoids [❷].

- **Eye ailments.** In the form of irrigation, a decoction of plantain alleviates eye diseases such as conjunctivitis and blepharitis (inflammation of the eyelids) [❷].

- **Varicose ulcers,** bleeding or suppurating **wounds, burns.** In these cases you can apply compresses with a plantain decoction [❷], or plantain leaves directly, previously blanched in boiling water [❸].

- **Insects and reptile bites.** Dr. Leclerc states that weasels rub themselves on the plantain plants before fighting snakes in order to become protected against reptile poison. In the case of bites of insects, spiders, bees, or scorpions, vigorously rub the affected area with plantain leaves, then apply a dressing [❸] or poultice made with plantain leaves [❹].

In the case of snake bites, the usual emergency treatment is required (cut the area, tourniquet, antipoisonous serum), then a lotion and a dressing or poultice with plantain leaves.

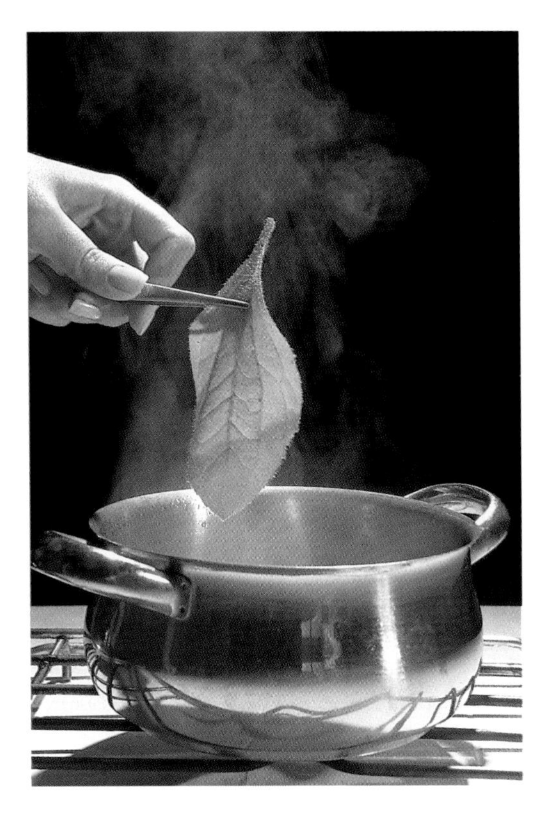

Lungwort

Pectoral and anti-inflammatory

MANY NINETEENTH and early twentieth century people suffering from tuberculosis were treated with the lungwort. At present it still is a useful plant for respiratory afflictions.

PROPERTIES AND INDICATIONS. The whole plant contains mucilage and alantoine, both substances with **emollient** properties; tannin, with astringent properties; a certain amount of saponins, which give the plant expectorant properties; salicylic acid, and potassium and calcium salts, which have **anti-inflammatory, diuretic, and sudorific** properties.

• ***Internally used*** the plant is recommended for several **respiratory ailments:** bronchial catarrh, sore throat, irritating cough, hoarseness and aphonia (taken orally and in gargles) [❶,❷]. It is very useful to combat the negative effects of tobacco on the respiratory airways [❶]. For pulmonary tuberculosis, it can be used to ***complement*** specific treatment, always ***under medical supervision.***

• In ***external*** applications, the lungwort is used to heal **wounds, bruises, skin marks, and chilblains [❸].**

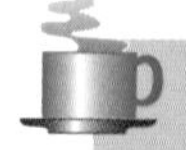

Preparation and Use

INTERNAL USE

❶ **Decoction** with 30-50 g of plant per liter of water, boiled for 15 minutes. Drink three or four cups daily, sweetened with honey.

EXTERNAL USE

❷ **Gargles** with the same infusion as for internal use.

❸ **Washing** and **compresses** with the aforementioned decoction, applied on the affected skin area.

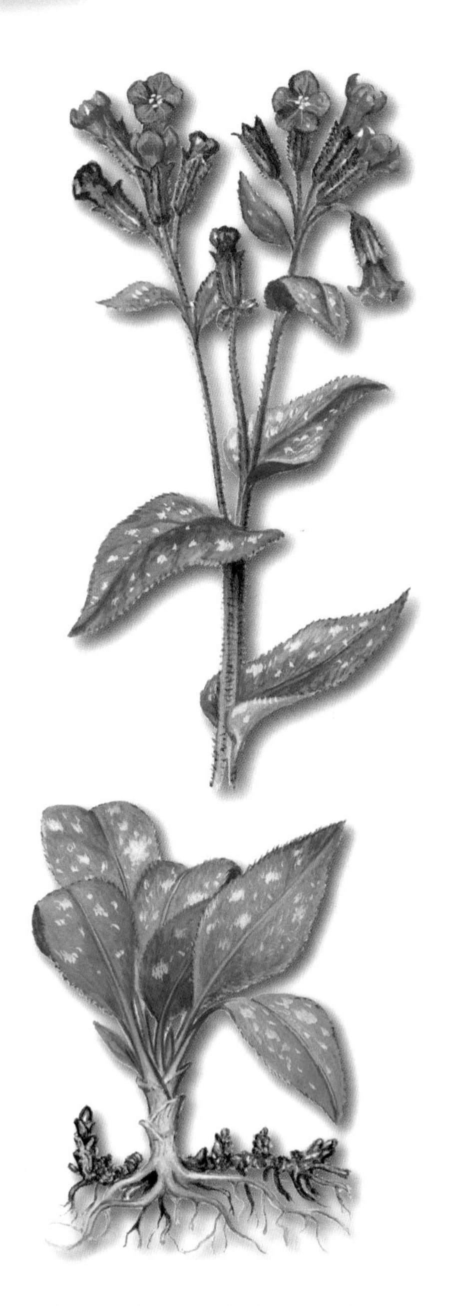

Description. *Vivacious, herbaceous plant of the Boraginaceae family, with hairy stem which grows up to 30 cm high. A pink and violet flower bouquet grows on the tip of its stem.*

Parts used. *The whole plant with flowers.*

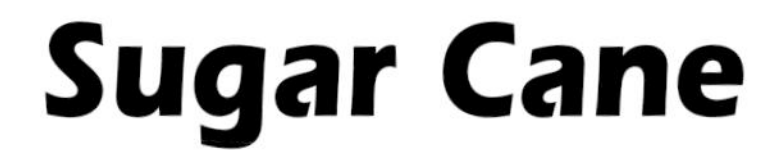

Sugar Cane

A natural candy

SUGAR cane is native to southeast Asia. The Arabs spread its cultivation throughout the Mediterranean countries, then the Spanish and Portuguese carried it to America in the sixteenth century. Cane sugar is obtained from this plant, as well as molasses, also called cane honey, which is the syrup residue after separating the sugar crystals from the cane juice.

PROPERTIES AND INDICATIONS. The sugar cane juice contains 16--20% saccharose, a disaccharide sugar, whose chemical formula is $C_{12}H_{22}O_{11}$. It also contains a high amount of mineral salts and vitamins, most of which remain in the molasses. Brown sugar (non-refined sugar) contains some molasses which gives it its color, hence it has some mineral salts and vitamins. However, refined sugar (white sugar) is pure saccharose, lacking any other nourishing substances.

Sugar cane juice [❶] and the decoction of its flesh [❷] have **pectoral** as well as **invigorating and refreshing** properties. Its use is recommended for people suffering from **bronchial catarrh, chronic bronchitis, or asthma.**

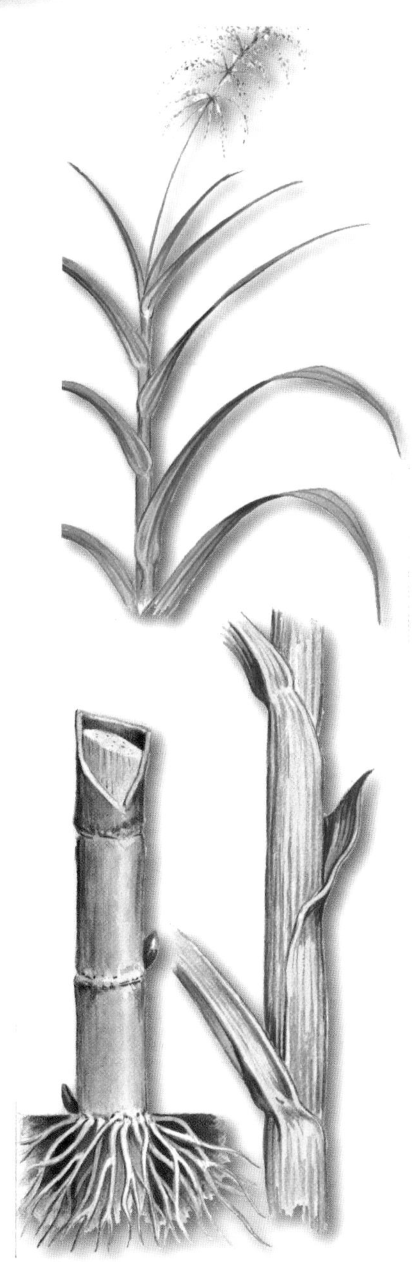

Description. *Plant of the Gramineae family, similar to the common cane, with aerial stems (canes) which grow up to 4 m high. Its flesh is sweet and juicy.*

Parts used. *The stem (cane).*

Preparation and Use

INTERNAL USE

❶ **Fresh juice,** prepared by grinding sugar canes.

❷ **Decoction,** with 250 g of peeled sugar cane per liter of water.

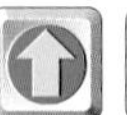
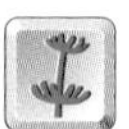
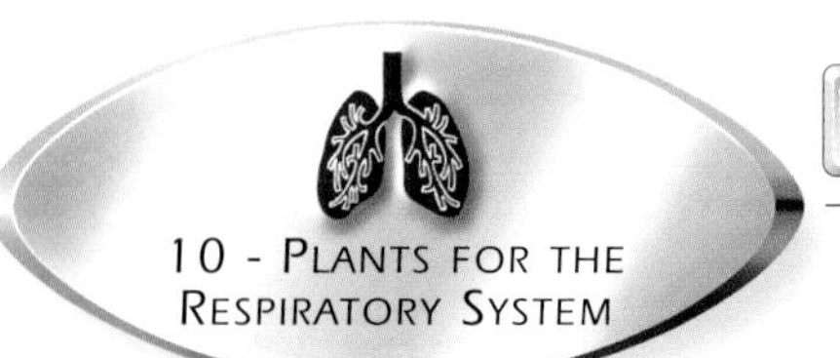

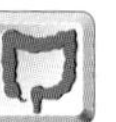
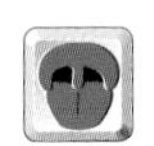
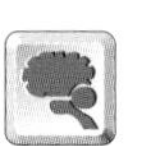
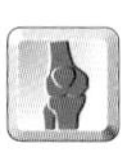

Mother of Thyme

Eases coughs and pains

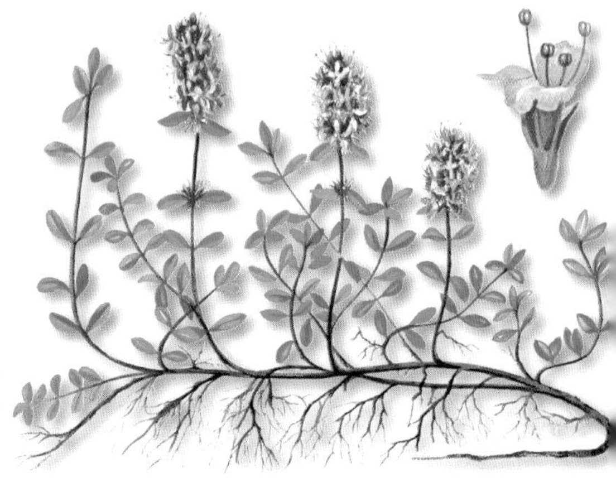

Description. *Vivacious plant of the Labiatae family, which grows up to 40 cm high, with ground stems, small, plain leaves, and pink or purple flowers growing in clusters.*

Parts used. *The flower clusters.*

LIKE OTHER PLANTS of the *Labiatae* family, such as wild marjoram, thyme, peppermint, or the European pennyroyal, mother of thyme has a pleasant smell. It is not easy to tell the difference between this plant and thyme (*Thymus vulgaris* L), particularly as there are some intermediate species. However, mother of thyme has three special features:

✓ The **upper lip** of its **calyx** is divided into three deep teeth.

✓ The **leaves** are plain, green on both sides (thyme has whitish lowersided leaves, with borders turned down).

✓ Its **aroma** resembles that of the lemon tree or balm.

PROPERTIES AND INDICATIONS. The leaves and flowers of mother of thyme contain an essence which composition varies depending on the subspecies, but always formed by cymol, thymol and carvacrol. It also contains small amounts of phenolic acids, flavonoids, and tannin. This essence gives the plant **digestive, antispasmodic, expectorant, and antiseptic** properties.

The applications of mother of thyme are similar to those of other plants of the *Labiatae* family, with several particularities:

• **Respiratory afflictions.** Mother of thyme gives good results with coughs, especially **convulsive coughing** in **children** [❶,❷]. It is also used for whooping cough and all kinds of bronchial catarrh.

• **Digestive afflictions.** Mother of thyme is used to combat stomach atony, heavy digestion, flatulence, and dyspepsia in general [❶,❷].

• **Oral and anal afflictions.** Due to its antiseptic properties, this plant is highly recommended for washings and rinsings of wounds and inflammations of the mucous membrane of the digestive system, whether in the mouth (sores or aphtas), or in the anus (anal fissure) [❹]. In gargles, it renders good results for **tonsillitis** (sore throat) or **pharyngitis.**

• **Rheumatism and neuralgia.** In ***local*** applications, mother of thyme essence eases sciatica, facial neuralgia, and in general all rheumatic pains [❺].

Preparation and Use

INTERNAL USE

❶ **Infusion** with 20-40 g of plant per liter of water. Drink from three to five cups daily, sweetened with honey if preferred. As an antitussive, take one or two spoonfuls each hour, until the cough is calmed.

❷ **Essence.** Take from three to five drops, three times a day.

EXTERNAL USE

❸ **Baths.** Add to the water of a bathtub two or three liters of a decoction made with 50-100 g of plant, boiled for five minutes.

❹ **Bathing, mouth rinsings, and gargles.** With the same infusion used internally, but more concentrated.

❺ **Compresses and friction** with the essence.

• **Depression, asthenia, and exhaustion.** Hot baths with mother of thyme, which have invigorating and revitalizing properties, render good results in this case [❸]. They are recommended both for weak children and for adults who need a natural stimulus.

A good invigorating bath is prepared by adding two or three liters of a decoction made with 50-100 g of flower clusters per liter of water, to the hot bathtub water. It gives good results with depression, asthenia, and exhaustion, both in children and in adults.

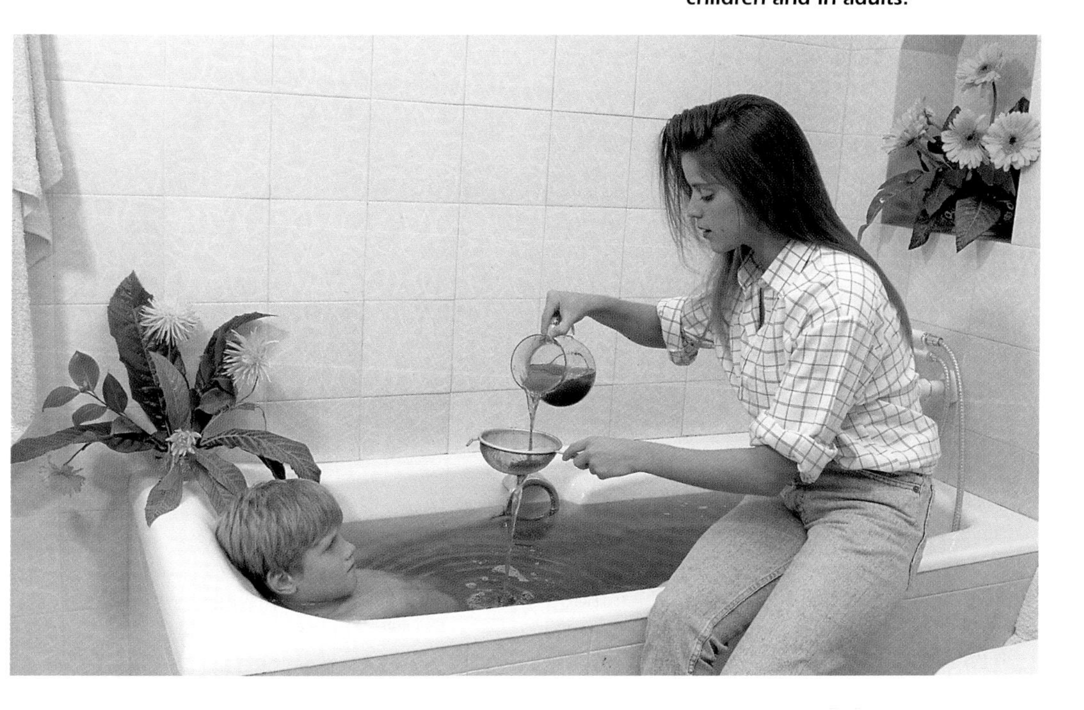

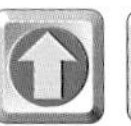
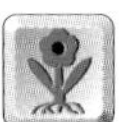
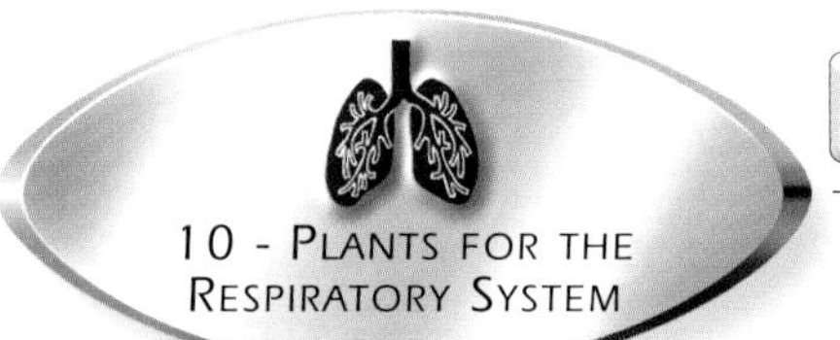

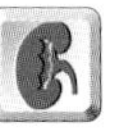
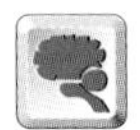
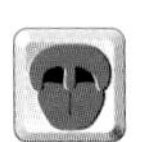
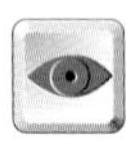

Garden Violet

Pectoral and aromatic

THE GARDEN VIOLET belongs to the same botanical family as the pansy. Both flowers are beautiful and delicate. The difference between them is that the violet has two petals growing up, and three down, while the pansy has four petals up and one down.

In the fifth century B.C., Hippocrates recommended the garden violet for the treatment of migraines. In the early twentieth century, they were supposed to heal cancer, a fact that has not been proven. The garden violet is ***one of the most appreciated pectoral plants*** in phytotherapy.

PROPERTIES AND INDICATIONS. The whole plant contains saponins (especially its root), with **expectorant and diuretic** properties; mucilage, with **emollient, bechic** (antitussive) **and laxative** properties; salicylic acid, with **anti-inflammatory and sudorific** properties; coloring substances (anthocyanins), and glycosides, to which it owes its **mild diuretic** properties, as well as essence in the flowers, which gives the plant its pleasant aroma.

The ***FLOWERS*** have the following applications:

• **Respiratory afflictions.** Due to their content in saponins, garden violet flowers make the bronchial secretions more liquid, reduce the congestion of the bronchi, and ease coughing **[❶,❷]**. The mucilage exerts a soothing and anti-inflammatory action on all mucous membranes. The mucilage of the garden violet acts specifically on the respiratory mucous membranes. The garden violet is, thus, a very useful plant in the treatment of **bronchial catarrh, bronchitis, tracheitis, and bronchial pneumonia.** They also have **sudorific** properties, thus being especially recommended when the respiratory af-

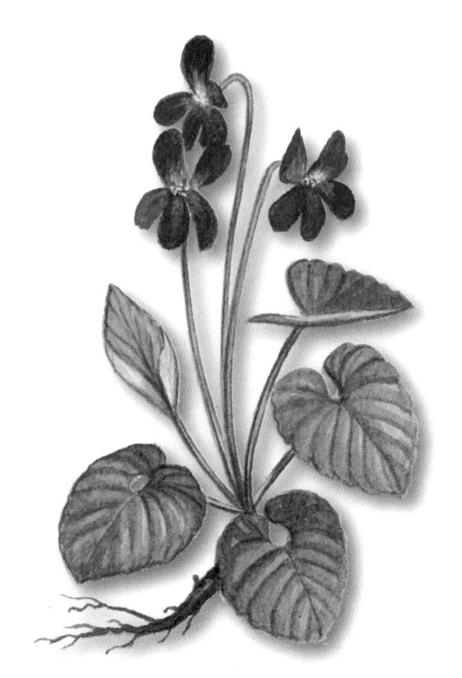

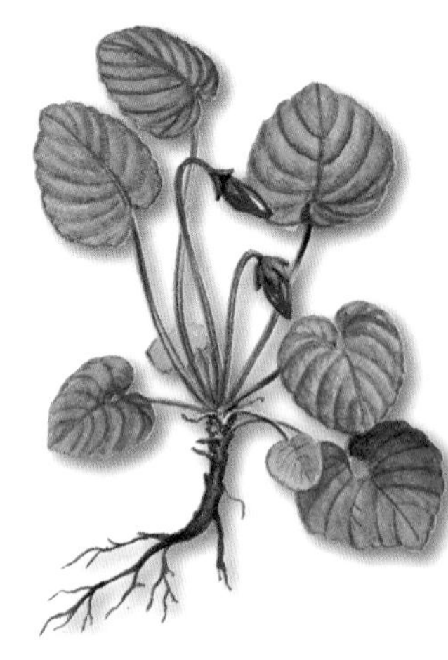

Description. *Vivacious plant of the Violaceae family, which grows from 5 to 15 cm high. It does not have aerial stems, hence its leaves and flowers grow from a central root in large peduncles. Characteristic violet flowers, (more rarely white or pink) with five petals and a strong aroma.*

Parts used. *Flowers, leaves, and roots.*

Preparation and Use

INTERNAL USE

❶ **Infusion** with 30-40 g of leaves per liter of water. Drink three or four cups daily. It has a good flavor.

❷ **Violet syrup.** The syrup can substitute the infusion, especially when given to children. It is made with 50 g of flowers in cold extract in half a liter of water for 12 hours. After straining, add 200 g of honey, and boil for five minutes. Give from one to three spoonfuls every two hours.

❸ **Vomitive decoction,** with 10-20 g of ground root and a quarter liter of water. Boil until it reduces to a half. Take one spoonful every five minutes until vomiting occurs.

❹ **Root powder,** 1-4 g dissolved in half a glass of water. The vomitive effect is more intense.

EXTERNAL USE

❺ The **same infusion** used internally is applied in **mouth rinses, gargles, eyelid cleansing, or compresses and fomentations** on the forehead.

flictions are accompanied by **fever,** as in the case of influenza. Their mild diuretic and laxative properties are good for people suffering from fever.

• **Cystitis.** The garden violet is recommended in this case due to the anti-inflammatory action exerted by the mucilage on the urinary system [❶,❷].

• **Migraines and headaches.** It has been successfully used since ancient times, though it is not known which of its active principles is responsible for this action. Garden violet flowers are traditionally applied, both orally (infusion) [❶] and in compresses or fomentations on the forehead [❺].

• **Mouth and throat afflictions.** In ***external*** applications, the violet infusion is used to make rinses or gargles in the case of stomatitis (inflammation of the mucous membrane of the mouth), gingivitis, pharyngitis, tonsillitis, laryngitis, and aphonia [❺].

• It is also applied in eye irrigations [❺] for blepharitis (inflammation of the eyelids) and conjunctivitis.

The ***LEAVES*** of the garden violet have similar properties to those of the flowers, though with a stronger **sudorific, diuretic, and laxative** effects. They are usually employed mixed with the flowers.

The ***ROOTS*** are rich in saponins, having thus emetic (vomitive) properties [❸,❹]. They are administered to induce **vomiting** for food poisoning or upset stomach.

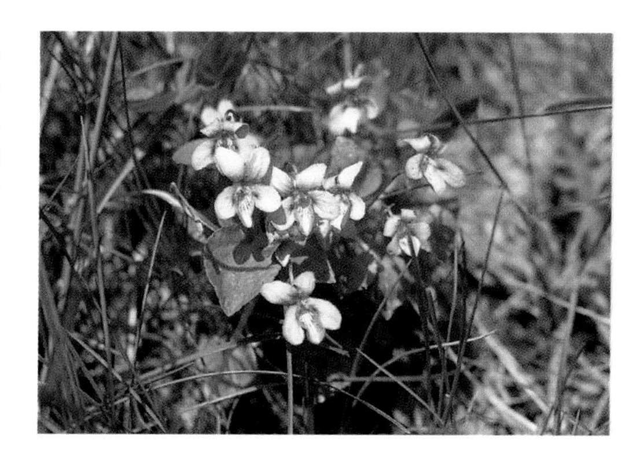

11

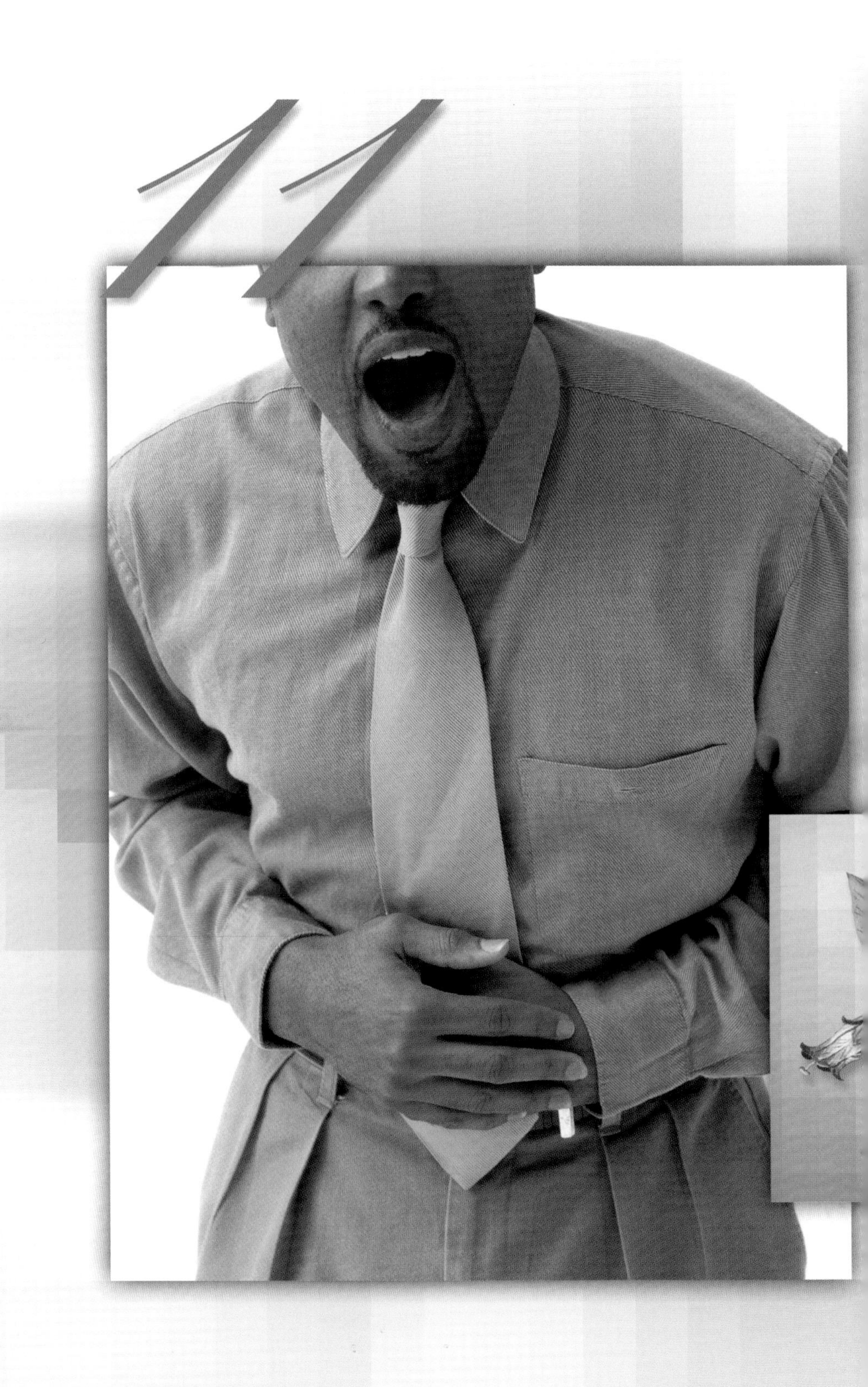

Plants for the Digestive System

DISEASES	PAGES
Anorexia, see Appetite, lack of	172
Appetite, lack of	172
Bad breath	172
Halitosis, see Bad breath	172
Lack of appetite, see Appetite, lack of	172

PLANTS	PAGES
Abelmosk	176
Basil	182
Blackthorn	184
Caraway	174
Catnip	181
Dill	173
Fennel	175
German camomile	178
Ginger	189
Guinea sorrel	177
Marjoram	183
Peppermint	180
Summer savory	187
Tiny savory	187
Vanilla	188
White savory	187
Winter savory	186

ALMOST ALL medicinal herbs produce effects on the digestive system. Those we describe in this chapter act on all digestive organs, including the stomach, the intestine, the liver and the pancreas. These plants promote digestion through two basic actions:

- **By activating the peristaltic movements,** or contractions, of the digestive tract, which cause the passage of the intestines contents. When these contractions are not intense enough, or not effective, the bolus does not pass adequately, thus digestion is slow and the intestine becomes bloated.
- **By increasing the production of digestive juices** in the stomach, the intestine, and the pancreas. A lack of juices makes digestion slower.

A correct, natural, healthy diet is required for these plants to be really effective. There is no medicinal herb or medicine which is able to compensate negative effects caused by an unhealthy diet.

BAD BREATH

Abnormal smell of the exhaled air, usually caused by mouth (pyorrhea), gastric (retention of food in the stomach), or intestinal (fermentation) disorders. Besides these plants, all those used in the case of ***pyorrhea***, ***dyspepsia***, and ***intestinal fermentation*** can be administered.

MASTIC TREE	Freshens breath, fights pyorrhea
EUCALYPTUS	Fights intestinal fermentation, eliminates intestinal toxins causing bad breath
EUROPEAN PENNYROYAL	Fights intestinal fermentation

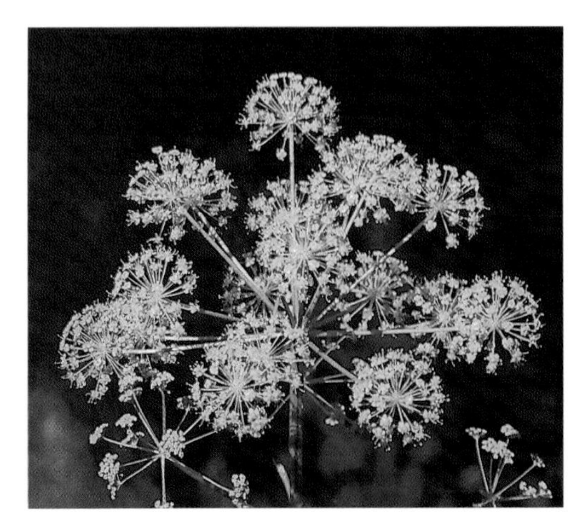

APPETITE, LACK OF

Causes

Any of the disorders affecting the digestive system, from the esophagus to the intestine, can produce lack of appetite. This can also be caused by psychological disorders (anorexia nervosa).

Treatment

Before trying any treatment, a professional should ***diagnose the causes*** of the lack of appetite.

BLACKTHORN	Stimulates digestive processes, appetizer, invigorator
WINTER SAVORY	Increases appetite, promotes digestion, eliminates gas
GENTIAN	Contains bitters which stimulate secretions of all digestive glands
LAUREL	Promotes digestion, increases appetite
MUGWORT	Increases appetite, stimulates stomach emptying
MILFOIL	Invigorates digestive organs
CINCHONA	Appetizer, invigorator, fights intestinal fermentation

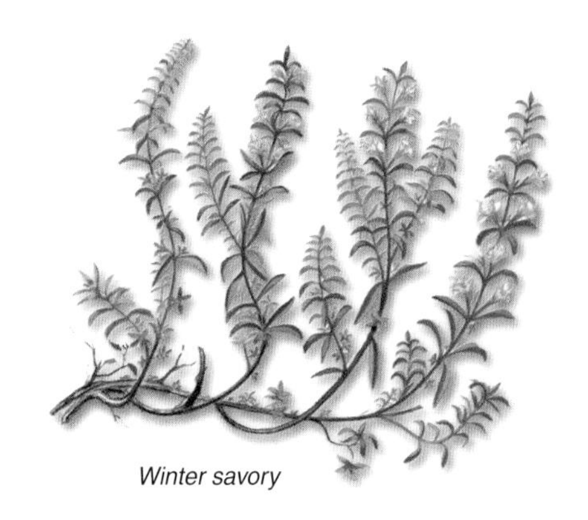

Winter savory

Fennel belongs to the "Umbelliferae" botanical family, as well as anise, cumin, and coriander, among other plants. All these plants contain essences with digestive and carminative (against intestinal gas) properties.

Dill

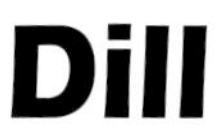

Appetizer and antiflatulent

DILL IS ONE of the oldest medicinal herbs. The Egyptians, the Greeks, and the Romans knew and appreciated it, using the plant as a remedy and seasoning herb.

Dill looks quite similar to fennel. The sixteenth century Spanish physician Andrés de Laguna said, "If would be easy to mistake dill for fennel by sight alone, but they are easily distinguished by taste."

Actually, dill has a harder, more spicy taste than fennel, though the properties of both plants are similar.

PROPERTIES AND INDICATIONS. Dill seeds contain an essence (3-4%), whose most important component is carvone. This essence has a ***powerful*** **carminative** (eliminates intestinal flatulence and gas), **appetizer, diuretic, galactogenic** (increases milk production), and mild sedative properties. It also has **emmenagogue** (stimulant of the menstruation) properties.

Its most important use is for **hiccups and belching** in children, as well as excessive **gas** in the stomach (aerophagia), and intestinal **flatulence** in **adults [❶]**.

It is also used as **sedative** for vomiting, and as a milk-production **stimulating** substance for **breast-feeding women.**

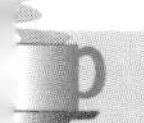

Preparation and Use

INTERNAL USE

❶ **Infusion** with a tablespoonful (about 15 g) of seeds per half a liter of water. Drink two or three cups a day after meals.

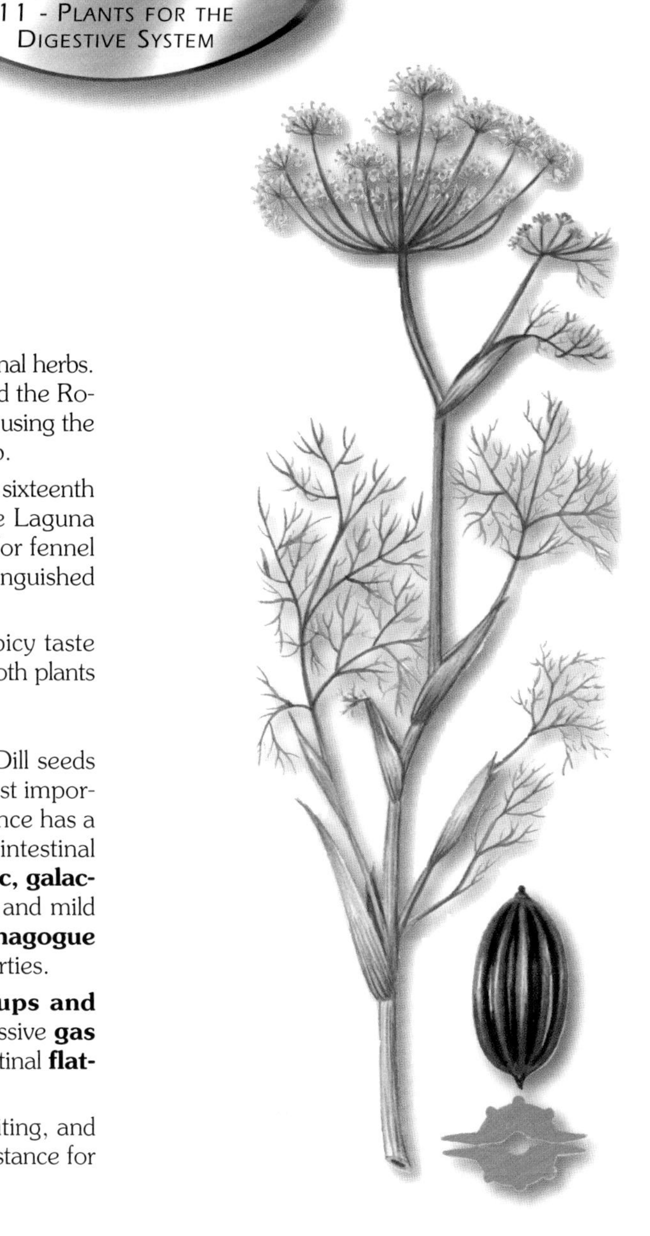

Description. *Herbaceous plant of the Umbelliferae family, which grows from 30 to 50 cm high, with hollow stem and yellow flowers growing in umbels with unequal radii.*

Parts used. *The seeds.*

Caraway

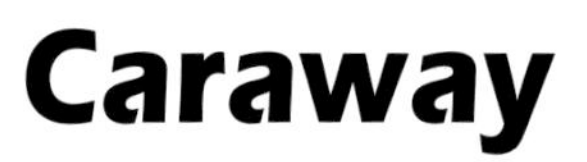

Fights against digestive gas

NATIVE to Mediterranean countries, caraway has been used for centuries as a seasoning plant. Bread, vegetables, pies, cheese, and many other meals and sauces take advantage of the aroma of this plant.

PROPERTIES AND INDICATIONS. As happens with other plants of the Umbelliferae family, such as anise or fennel, caraway contains a high amount of essences, the most abundant being carvone, to which the plant's fruits owe their carminative (anti-flatulent) properties.

Caraway is one of the plants with a stronger carminative property, thus being recommended whenever there is an excess of gas.

Caraway cures flatulence, and eases intestinal spasms [❶,❷]. It is ***very useful*** for **babies with excess gases,** to whom it can be administered mixed with their milk [❸].

This plant has also **eupeptic** (promotes digestion), and **mildly diuretic** properties, and favors **milk secretion** (galactogenic) of breastfeeding women [❶,❷].

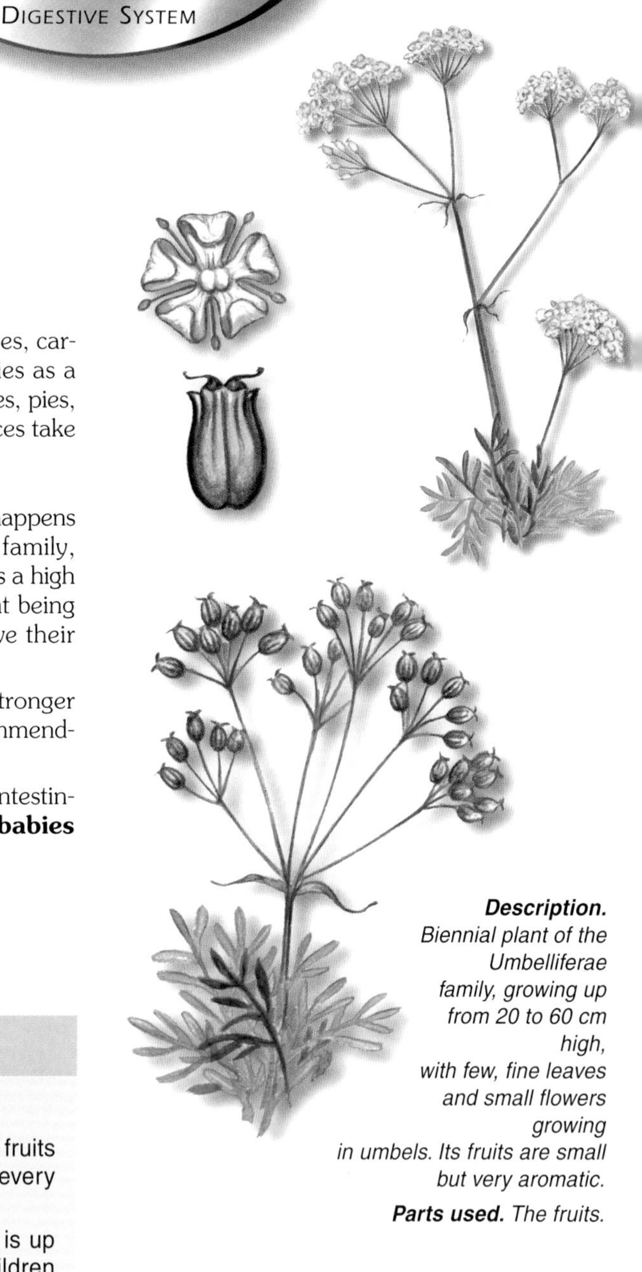

Description. *Biennial plant of the Umbelliferae family, growing up from 20 to 60 cm high, with few, fine leaves and small flowers growing in umbels. Its fruits are small but very aromatic.*

Parts used. *The fruits.*

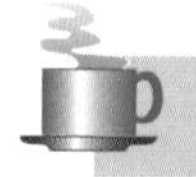

Preparation and Use

INTERNAL USE

❶ **Infusion** with half a teaspoonful of fruits per cup of water. Drink a cup after every meal.

❷ **Essence.** The recommended dose is up to three drops, three times a day. Children still on milk should be given one or two drops in some sweetened water, two or three times a day.

❸ **Mixed with milk.** Add half a teaspoonful per liter of milk, or boil it in one liter of water, with which the milk will be prepared. Strain and administer.

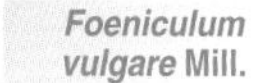

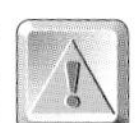
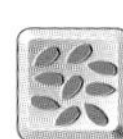
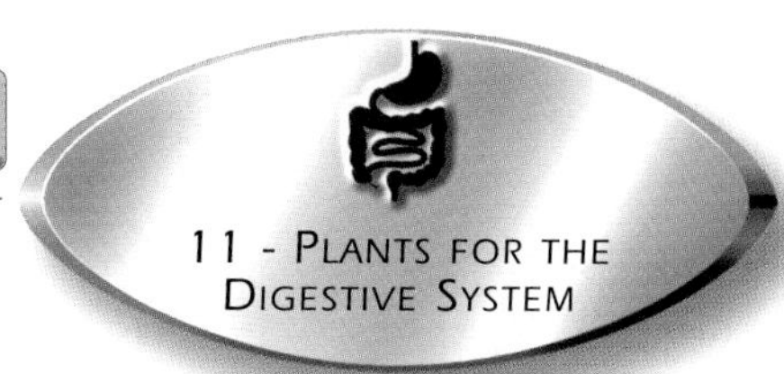

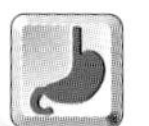
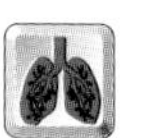
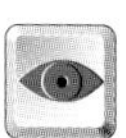
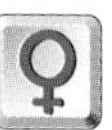

Fennel

It cleans the stomach and eyes

IN INDIA, a tradition says that this plant is "the pearl among aphrodisiacs," thus it is part of potions which allegedly arouse sexual desire. However, its main current applications are those related to the digestive and respiratory systems.

PROPERTIES AND INDICATIONS. The whole plant, and especially its seeds, contains an essence rich in anetol, estragol, and terpenic hydrocarbons. Let us see its properties and indications:

• **Carminative.** Fennel eases the expulsion of intestinal gas, and stimulates the peristaltic movements of the intestine **[❶,❷]**. It has mild laxative properties.

• **Digestive.** It promotes the emptying of the stomach, as well as digestion. The plant renders good results with bloated stomach, slow digestion, and excess of gas in the stomach, as well as in belches **[❶,❷]**.

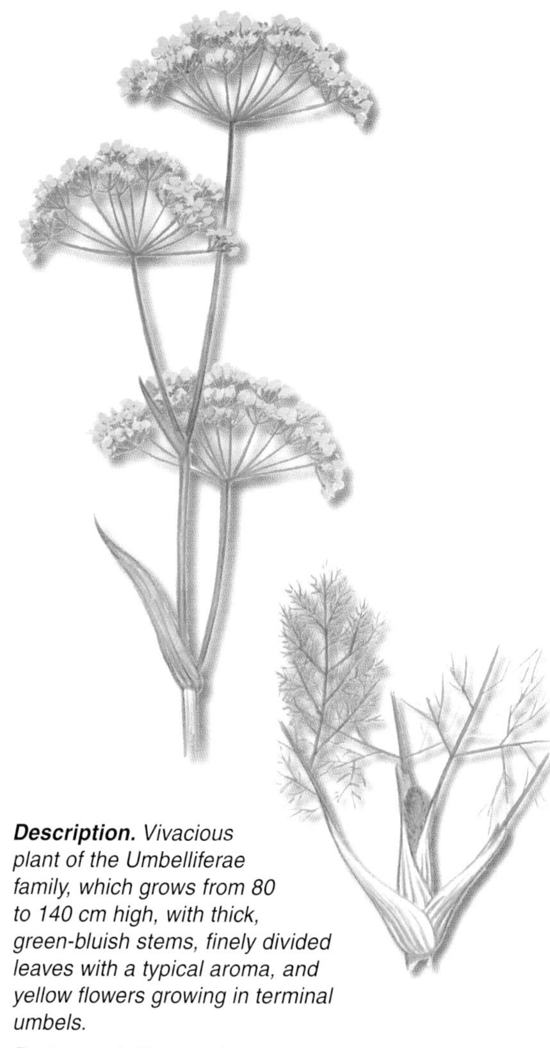

Description. *Vivacious plant of the Umbelliferae family, which grows from 80 to 140 cm high, with thick, green-bluish stems, finely divided leaves with a typical aroma, and yellow flowers growing in terminal umbels.*

Parts used. *The seeds.*

Preparation and Use

INTERNAL USE

❶ **Infusion** with one teaspoonful of seeds per cup of water. Drink three or four cups a day after meals. In the case of a cold, sweeten this infusion with honey.

❷ **Essence.** The usual dose is from one to three drops, two or three times a day.

EXTERNAL USE

❸ **Eye washing** with the same infusion used internally.

• **Expectorant.** Fennel is recommended for bronchial catarrh and colds **[❶,❷]**.

• **Galactogenic.** It increases the production of milk in breast-feeding women **[❶,❷]**.

• In ***external*** applications, the plant is used for eye irrigation or eye baths for chronic **conjunctivitis [❸].**

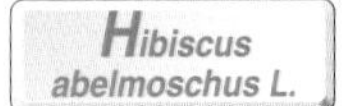

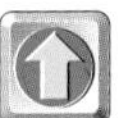
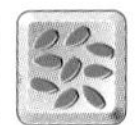
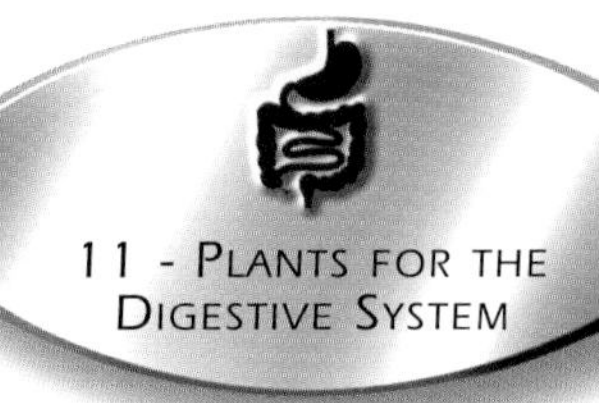

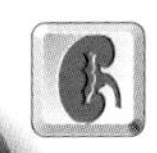
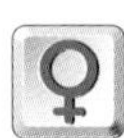
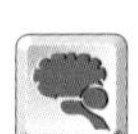

Abelmosk

A relaxing, sedative fragrance

THE SEEDS of the abelmosk are very appreciated by Indian and Arabic perfume makers, and the Arabs also use this plant as an aphrodisiac. When rubbed or heated, the abelmosk seeds give an intense aroma which resembles that of amber and musk. In some places of Central America, these seeds are added to coffee in order to give it more fragrance.

PROPERTIES AND INDICATIONS. The seeds of the abelmosk contain an essential oil with a strong **antispasmodic** effect, which is able to relax the muscles of internal cavernous organs when suffering from spasms. Therefore, they are successfully used to ease the pain for intestine, bile, or kidney **colic,** as well as in that of uterine spasms of **dysmenorrhea** (painful menstruation) **[❶].** They have also a **sedative** effect on the **nervous** system.

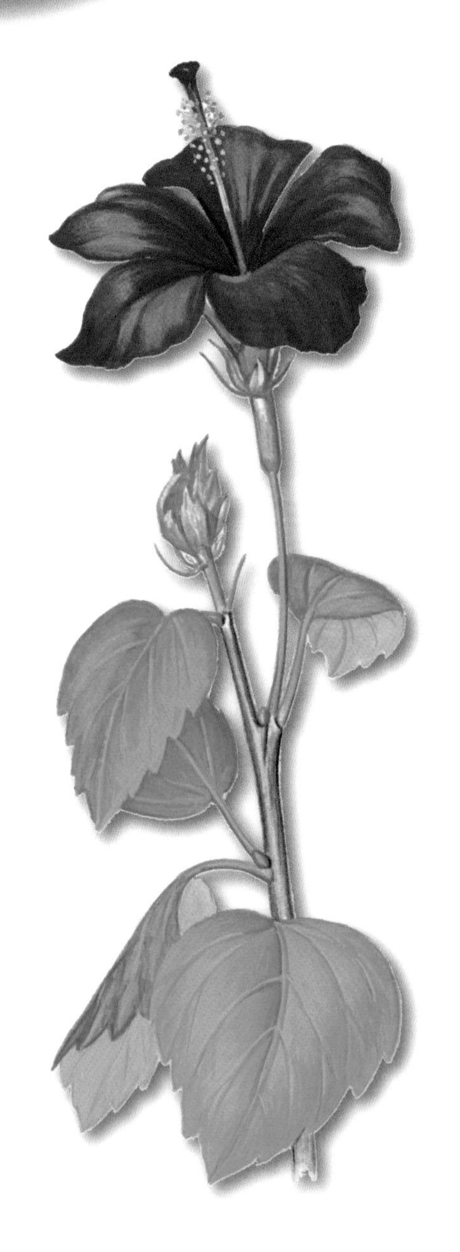

__Description.__ Shrub of the Malvaceae family, which grows up to two meters high, with unequally lobulated leaves, large, exuberant, yellow or red flowers that contain kidney-shaped seeds with greyish mark lines.

__Parts used.__ The seeds.

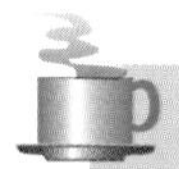

Preparation and Use

INTERNAL USE

❶ **Infusion** with 50 g of seeds per liter of water. Drink two or three cups daily.

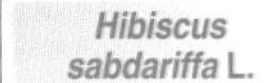

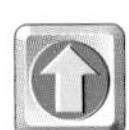
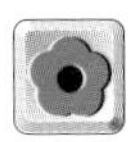
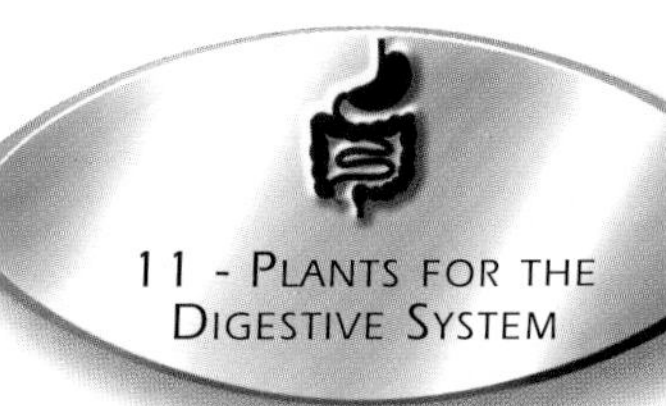

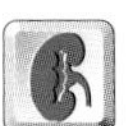
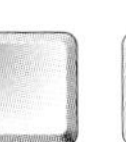
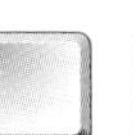
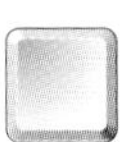

Guinea Sorrel

A beautiful flower which invigorates and refreshes

HIBISCUS is a botanical genus which consist of some 200 species, many of these being used as ornamental plants in gardens and parks because of their beautiful flowers.

PROPERTIES AND INDICATIONS. The sepals of Guinea sorrel flowers contain hibiscic acid, as well as a mixture of organic acids (malic, citric, and tartaric), and a red coloring substance, with the following properties:

- **Invigorating and digestive.** Because of their content in organic acids, Guinea sorrel infusion has a stimulant effect on the digestive function, and an invigorating effect on the whole body **[❶]**.
- **Mildly laxative.** The emollient (soothing) properties of Guinea sorrel on the digestive mucous membrane causes an easing of the intestinal evacuation **[❶]**.
- **Diuretic.** The flowers of Guinea sorrel have a mild, however effective, diuretic effect, being thus recommended for people suffering from obesity and from heart disorders **[❶]**.
- **Natural additive.** The mild acid flavor of Guinea sorrel, and the red coloring its flowers give to other substances are two reasons why these flowers are used as a ***natural additive*** in order to enhance the appearance and flavor of medicinal herbs or prepared meals **[❶]**.

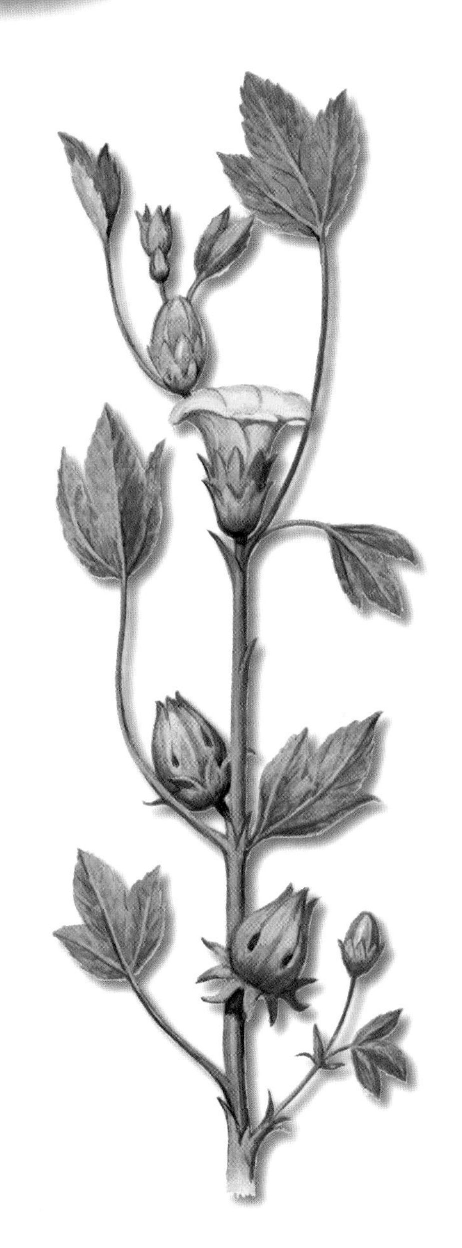

__Description.__ Shrub of the Malvaceae family, which grows up to two meters high. Its leaves have from three to five lobules, and it has yellow or reddish flowers.

__Parts used.__ The flowers with their calyx.

Preparation and Use

INTERNAL USE

❶ **Infusion** with a handful of flowers (with their calyx) per liter of water. Sweeten and take it cold as any other soft drink.

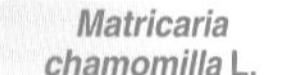

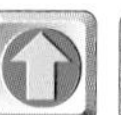

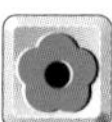

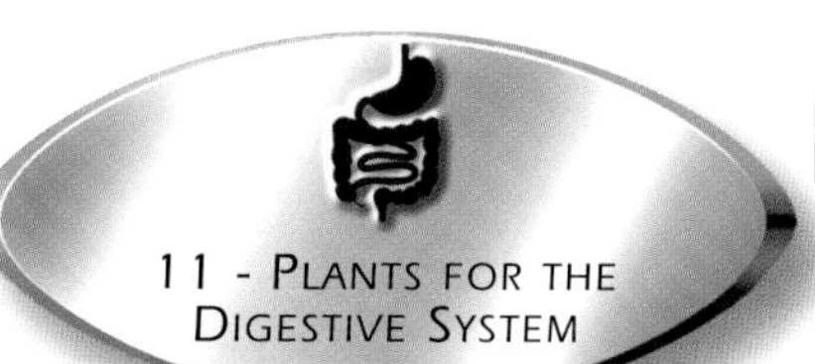

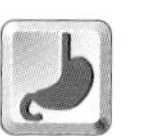

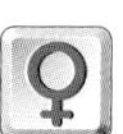

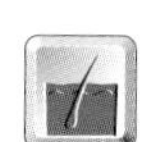

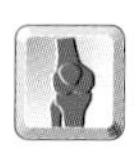

German Camomile

The digestive infusion par excellence

WHEN TALKING about herbal teas, many people immediately think about camomile. We could say that camomile makes *The Herbal Tea par excellence.*

"Bring a cup of camomile infusion to this patient before taking the saline solution away," the surgeon says to a nursing student.

Both of them are facing a teenage patient who has undergone surgery because of a perforated acute appendicitis. His digestive process has been stopped due to the peritonitis (inflammation of the peritoneum, the membrane covering the interior of the abdomen and its organs) produced by the appendicitis.

"Doctor, why do you always recommend a camomile infusion for post-operative patients?" the would-be nurse asks after the visit has finished.

"For many years I have been sticking to the rule of beginning oral diet for post-operative patients with a camomile infusion. Camomile stimulates the peristaltic movements of the intes-

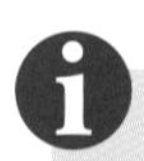

Other Uses of Camomile

- **Against insects.** *Little bags of camomile in the wardrobe make moths and other insects go away.*
- **Relaxing.** *When adding a camomile infusion to the bath water.*
- **Hair cosmetic.** *Brown or blonde hair, when washed with a camomile infusion, becomes brighter and more beautiful.*

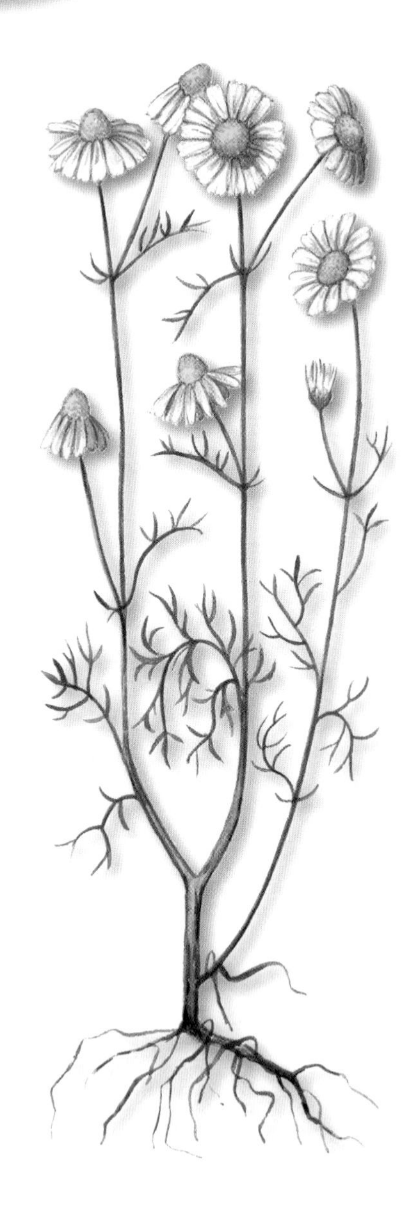

Description. *Herbaceous plant of the Compositae family, which grows from 20 to 50 cm high, with very branched stem, and daisy-like flowers which gather in flower heads of about two centimeters in diameter. It has a characteristic aroma, and sour flavor.*

Parts used. *The flower heads.*

Preparation and Use

INTERNAL USE

➊ **Infusion** with 5-10 g of flower heads per liter of water (5-6 flower heads per cup). Drink from three to six hot cups daily.

EXTERNAL USE

➋ Eye, nose, or anal **washing,** with a slightly more concentrated infusion (up to 50 g of flower heads per liter of water). Steep for 15-20 minutes, and strain well before using.

➌ **Baths.** Add to the water of a bathtub from two to four liters of concentrated infusion. These lukewarm baths have a strong relaxing and sedative effect.

➍ **Compresses** with the aforementioned concentrated infusion, applied on the affected skin area.

➎ **Friction** with **camomile oil.** Prepare the camomile oil by heating for three hours in a double boiler 100 g of flower heads in half a liter of olive oil. Strain the mixture and keep in a bottle.

tine, thus recovering the digestive functions which have been stopped by peritonitis."

PROPERTIES AND INDICATIONS. The most important active component of camomile is its essence, whose main components are camazulene (with anti-inflammatory properties), and bisabolor (with sedative properties). It also contains coumaric and flavonic substances, as well as a invigorating bitter principle. The plant has many properties which have been proven by scientific research.

• **Sedative and antispasmodic.** It is useful for stomach and intestinal spasms caused by nervousness or anxiety [➊,➌]. It is also used in any type of colic, and especially in the case of liver and kidney colic, because of its relaxing and sedative properties [➊,➌].

• **Carminative and intestinal invigorating.** Although it may seem to be a paradox, camomile also stimulates the movements of the digestive tract. It is thus recommended for post-operative patients and for those who suffer from excess of gas, which camomile helps expel because of its carminative properties [➊]. Actually, the action of camomile is that of regulating and balancing the functions of the intestine.

• **Eupeptic.** An infusion of camomile is recommended for bloated or upset stomach. It alleviates the nausea and vomiting, and softly stimulates the appetite [➊]. All sour camomile species have a stronger eupeptic action.

• **Emmenagogue.** This plant stimulates menstrual functions, normalizing its amount and regularity, as well as alleviating menstrual aches. Dioscorides called it Matricaria, from the Latin word *matrix* (womb).

• **Febrifuge and sudorific.** Given that it raises the temperature and provokes perspiration, it is recommended for people with a fever, especially children [➊].

• **Analgesic.** Camomile eases headaches and some cases of neuralgia [➊].

• **Antiallergic.** Some calming properties of camomile on allergic reactions, such as asthma, and allergic rhinitis and conjunctivitis, has been proven. It is recommended for healing acute allergic crises, as well as being an ongoing treatment in order to prevent them. The best results are obtained when combining internal applications (herbal teas) [➊] with external ones (eyedrops, nose irrigations) [➋].

• **Healing agent, emollient, and antiseptic.** In ***external*** applications, camomile renders good results for washing any wound, sore, and skin infection [➋]. The camazulene has been proven to be effective against hemolytic streptococcus, golden staphylococcus, and *Proteus*. A camomile infusion is an adequate ***eyedrop*** for eye bathing in the case of conjunctivitis or eye irritation [➋]. It is also used as an anti-inflammatory, applied in compresses on eczema, rashes, and other skin afflictions [➌]. Anal cleansing with an infusion of camomile reduces the inflammation of hemorrhoids [➋].

• **Antirrheumatic.** The oil of camomile is used for massage in lumbago, stiff neck, bruises, and rheumatic aches [➎].

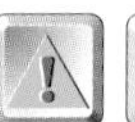
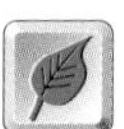
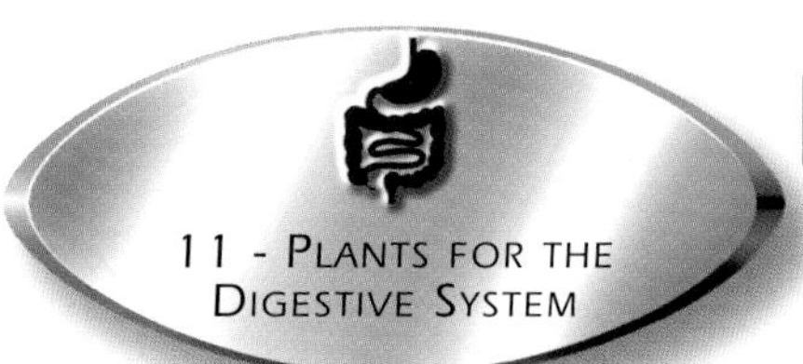

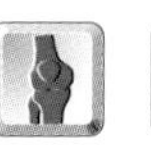
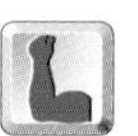
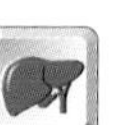
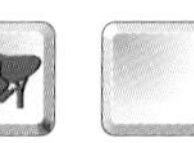

Peppermint

Invigorates and eases pains

THERE ARE MANY species and varieties of peppermint that, even cross-pollinated, preserve their medicinal properties.

PROPERTIES AND INDICATIONS. The plant contains from one to three percent of an essence with complex composition with more than 100 components, the most outstanding of which is menthol, an alcohol to which the plant owes many of its properties: **digestive, carminative** (eliminates intestinal gas and putrefaction), **choleretic, antiseptic, analgesic, invigorating, and aphrodisiac** in high doses. The essence contains polyphenolic substances with **antiviral** properties on the **A hepatitis** virus.

- ***Internally used,*** it is recommended for dyspepsia, intestinal gas, headaches and migraines, digestive colics and spasms, gastric atony, type A (viral) hepatitis, and physical exhaustion **[❶,❷]**.
- ***In external applications,*** massages with its essence in alcoholic dissolution (menthol alcohol) alleviate **rheumatic and muscular aches,** as well as **neuralgias [❸]**.

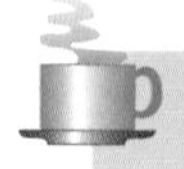

Preparation and Use

INTERNAL USE

❶ **Infusion** with 10-20 g of leaves and flower clusters per liter of water. Drink from three to five cups daily.

❷ **Essence.** The recommended dose is from one to three drops, up to three times a day.

EXTERNAL USE

❸ **Compresses and lotions,** applied with the essence or with menthol alcohol.

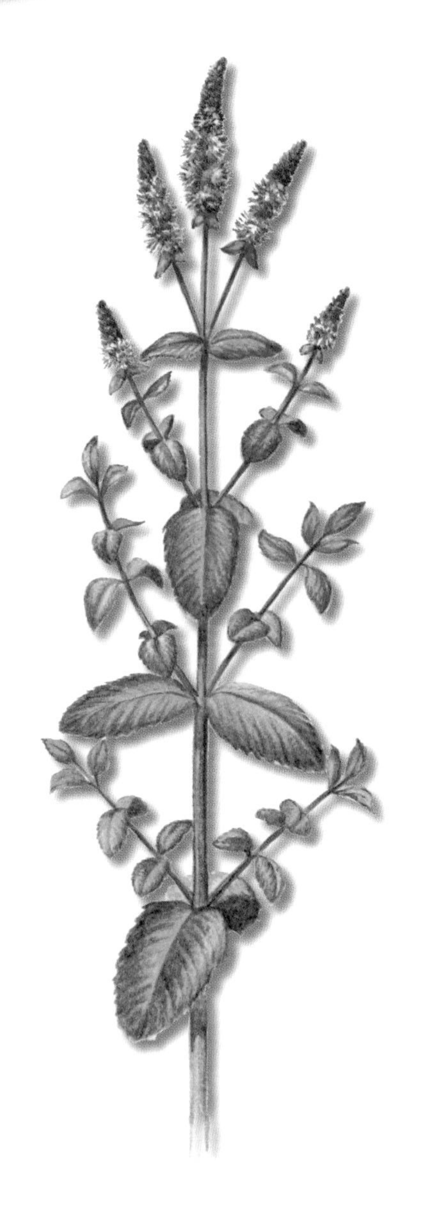

Description. *Herbaceous plant of the Labiatae family, with quadrangular, violet stem growing from 40 to 80 cm high. Its flower clusters are pink or violet, growing in terminal spikes.*

Parts used. *The leaves and the flower clusters.*

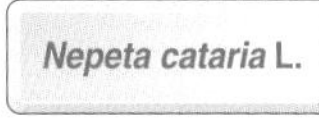

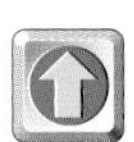
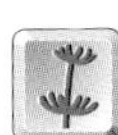
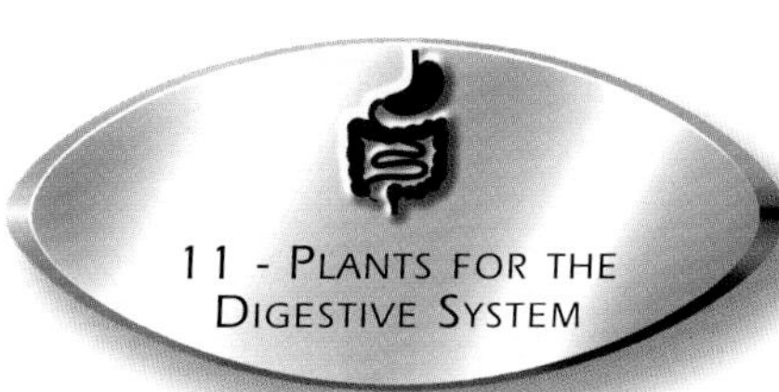

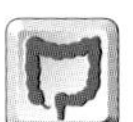
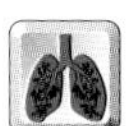

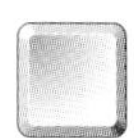

Catnip

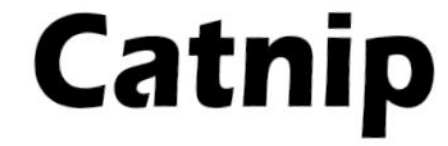

Eases colic pain

CATS ARE ESPECIALLY attracted by the aroma of this plant, and perhaps they also use catnip as a medicinal herb. Catnip teas resemble those of peppermint, although not as aromatic. Catnip has been passed over in recent times, however it has interesting properties.

PROPERTIES AND INDICATIONS. The whole plant contains an essence rich in carvacrol and thymol, as well as lactone and nepetalic acid. It has antispasmodic, antidiarrheic, carminative (eliminates intestinal gas), and pectoral properties. It is mainly used to alleviate **diarrhea** and its **colic** pain [❶]; and as **antiflatulent and pectoral,** in the case of bronchial catarrh [❶].

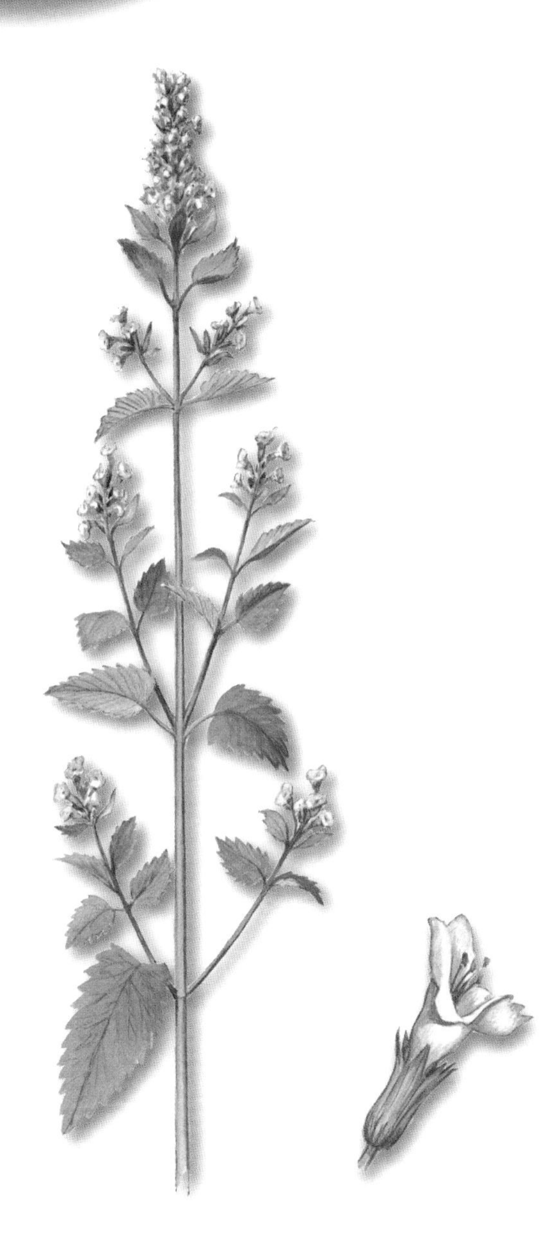

Preparation and Use

INTERNAL USE

❶ **Infusion** with 30 g of plant per liter of water. Drink one hot cup after every meal (three or four cups daily), which may be sweetened with honey if desired.

Description. *Vivacious plant of the Labiatae family, growing from 20 to 60 cm high, with pink or yellowish flowers (unlike balm). The whole plant gives off a typical peppermint scent.*

Parts used. *The leaves and the flower clusters.*

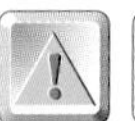

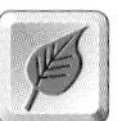

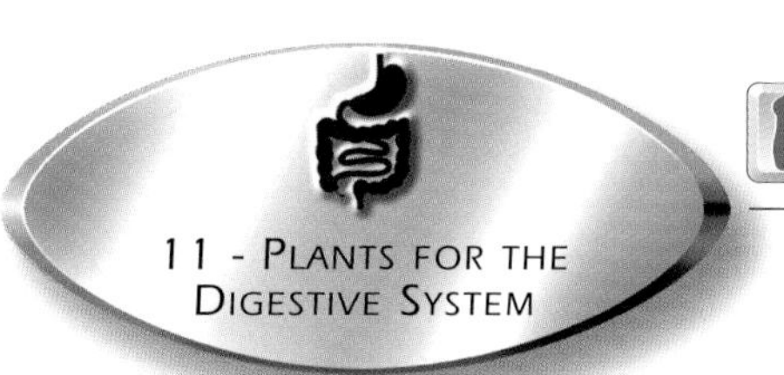

Basil

Eases digestion and invigorates

BESIDES ITS pleasant aroma, this highly appreciated seasoning plant has interesting medicinal properties.

PROPERTIES AND INDICATIONS. To this essence the plant owes the following properties:

- **Antispasmodic.** Basil calms nervous **digestive disorders,** such as digestive spasms (stomach nervousness), aerophagia (excess of gas and belches), and nervous dyspepsia (slow digestion caused by nervous tension). It also eases migraines caused by, or associated with, bad digestion **{❶,❷}**.
- Nervous and cardiovascular system **invigoration.** It is recommended for **asthenia, nervous exhaustion,** fatigue, and arterial **hypotension** (low blood pressure) **{❶,❸,❹}**.
- **Galactogenic.** Basil increases the production of milk in breast-feeding women **{❶,❷}**.
- **Emmenagogue.** The plant eases menstruation and the pain caused by uterine spasms or congestion **{❶,❷}**.

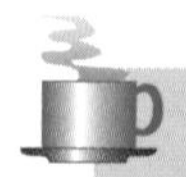

Preparation and Use

INTERNAL USE

❶ **Infusion** with 20-30 g of leaves and flowers per liter of water. Drink after every meal a hot cup, sweetened with honey to enhance its effect.

❷ **Essence.** The recommended dose is from two to five drops, three times a day.

EXTERNAL USE

❸ Invigorating **lotion** with the essence.

❹ **Baths.** Adding the essence to the bath water to take advantage of its invigorating effects.

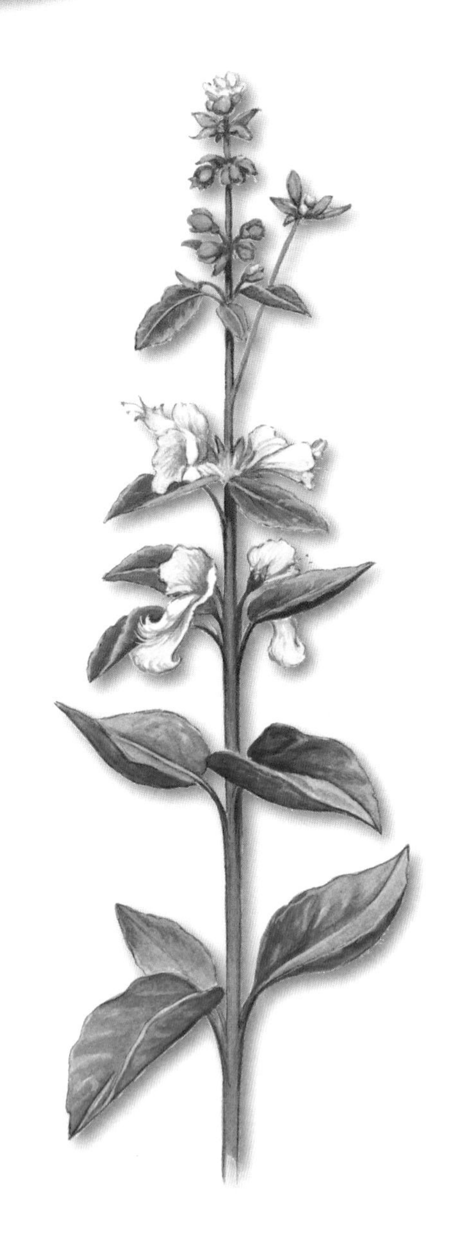

Description. *Herbaceous, vivacious plant of the Labiatae family, which grows up to 50 cm high, with lanceolated, light green leaves, and white or pink flowers growing in terminal bouquets.*

Parts used. *The leaves and flowers.*

Marjoram

Sedative and digestive

DUE TO ITS SIMILARITY with wild marjoram, a plant that, as its name says, indeed grows wild in Europe, it was called native marjoram.

PROPERTIES AND INDICATIONS. The active principles of marjoram are concentrated in its essence, which is rich in terpenic substances such as terpineol. This essence has the following properties.

- **Antispasmodic and digestive.** The plant is very useful for flatulence **(carminative** properties), nervous spasms of the stomach, and bloated stomach **[❶,❷]**.
- **Sedative.** It is recommended to combat psychological excitation, nervousness, and insomnia. It is a good remedy against anxiety **[❶,❷]**.
- **Antirrheumatic.** When ***externally*** applied, the essence eases rheumatic aches and muscle contractions. In lotions **[❸]**, or added to the bath water, it also has invigorating properties **[❹]**.

Preparation and Use

INTERNAL USE

❶ **Infusion** with 40-50 g of flower clusters per liter of water. Drink up to three cups daily.

❷ **Essence.** The recommended dose varies from four to six drops three times a day.

EXTERNAL USE

❸ **Lotions** with the essence dissolved in alcohol (10-20 drops in 100 cc. of alcohol).

❹ **Baths,** adding some drops of the essence to the bath water in order to achieve a notable antirrheumatic effect.

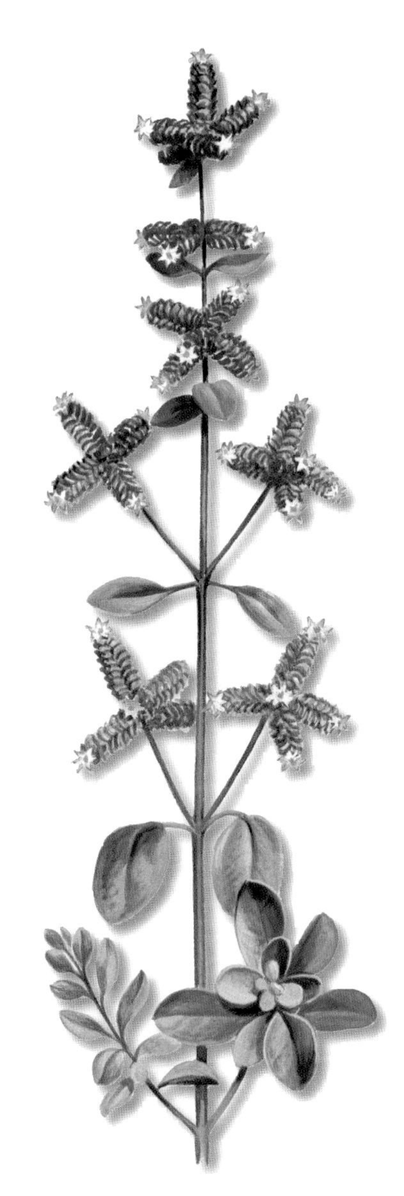

Description. *Vivacious plant of the Labiatae family, which grows from 15 to 40 cm high, with white or pink flowers growing in clusters in the tip of the stems. Its aroma could be described as being between that of peppermint and thyme.*

Parts used. *The flower clusters.*

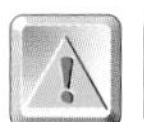
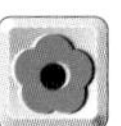
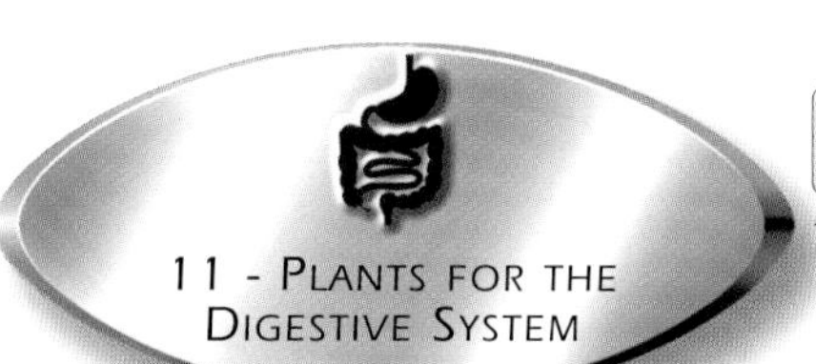

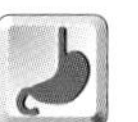
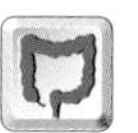
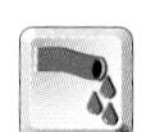
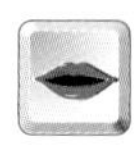

Blackthorn

Refreshing, invigorating, and appetizer

"LET US WALK in the forest, there we will gather some blackthorn berries."

These small wild prunes refresh walkers and are Fall food for doves, thrushes, and other birds. They have a slightly rough, but pleasant flavor. Their medicinal properties are not extraordinary, and their effects could be produced by the physical exercise done when gathering them.

However, it is worth to take advantage of this humble and happy wild fruit.

PROPERTIES AND INDICATIONS. Blackthorn ***FLOWERS*** contain amigdaline (a cyanogenetic glycoside), coumarine derivatives, and flavonic glycosides. They have **laxative, diuretic, and depurative** properties. The **laxative** properties are mild, and are accompanied by an **antispasmodic** (relaxing) action on the muscles covering the large intestine. They are highly recommended for the spasm-caused con-

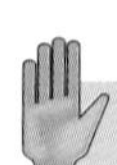

Warning

*The **almonds** of the sloes, as many other of the Rosaceae family, liberate hydrocyanic acid, which is a powerful poison. So they **must never be eaten or ground.***

*The **bark** of the branches and the root also contains hydrocyanic or prussic acid, another toxic substance. Therefore, the bark **must not be used,** although some people recommends it as an astringent substance.*

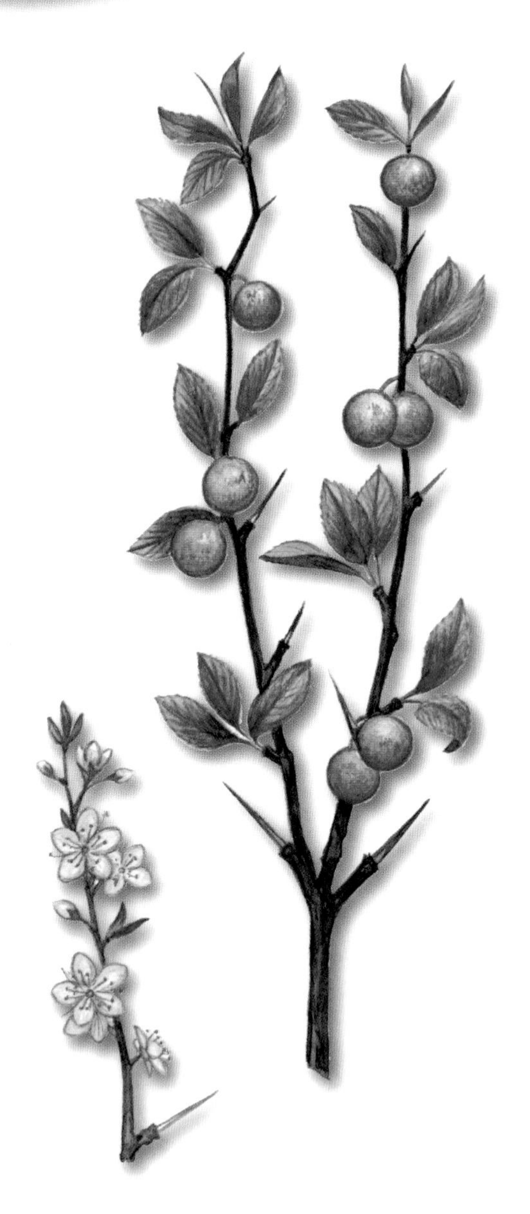

***Description.** Shrub of the Rosaceae family, which grows from one to three meters high, which dark-ochre bark and many woody thorns. Its flowers are ivory-white, small.*
The fruit is a round berry, dark-blue when ripe.

***Parts used.** The flowers and the fruits (sloes).*

Preparation and Use

INTERNAL USE

❶ **Infusion** with 60 g of flowers per liter of water. Drink a cup in the morning every day.

❷ **Fruits.** Sloes can be eaten fresh, or boiled in water (only two minutes) to eliminate their rough flavor.

❸ **Syrup,** prepared with half a kg of **fruits,** the same amount of sugar, and a glass of water. Boil the mixture for 15 minutes. The resulting red, pleasantly tasting syrup, must be strained, and taken by spoonfuls as an antidiarrheic or appetizer.

❹ **Decoction** with 100 sloes per liter of water, boiling on low heat for 10 minutes. Strain and take by the spoonful.

EXTERNAL USE

❺ **Nasal plugging** with a gauze soaked in the aforementioned decoction.

❻ **Mouth rinses and gargles,** with the decoction used in internal application.

stipation which takes place in so-called **irritable colon [❶]**.

The ***FRUIT*** (sloes) contain tannin (hence their strong flavor), flavonic substances, malic acid, saccharose, pectin, gum, and vitamin C. Unlike the flowers, they have **astringent** properties, being thus useful for mild diarrhea and intestinal upset. Moreover, they have **eupeptic** (stimulate digestive processes), **appetizer, and invigorating** properties on the whole body **[❷,❸,❹]**.

Sloes give those people eating them an increase in appetite and an invigorating and refreshing feeling. They can be eaten fresh, cooked, or used as of syrup.

The liquid obtained from the sloes decoction is used to stop **epistaxis** (nasal hemorrhages), by soaking a nasal packing in it **[❺].** It is also useful for gargles and rinses to treat **gingivitis** (inflammation of the gums) and **pharyngitis [❻]**.

Fresh, cooked, or in the form of syrup, sloes are appetizing and stimulate digestive processes.

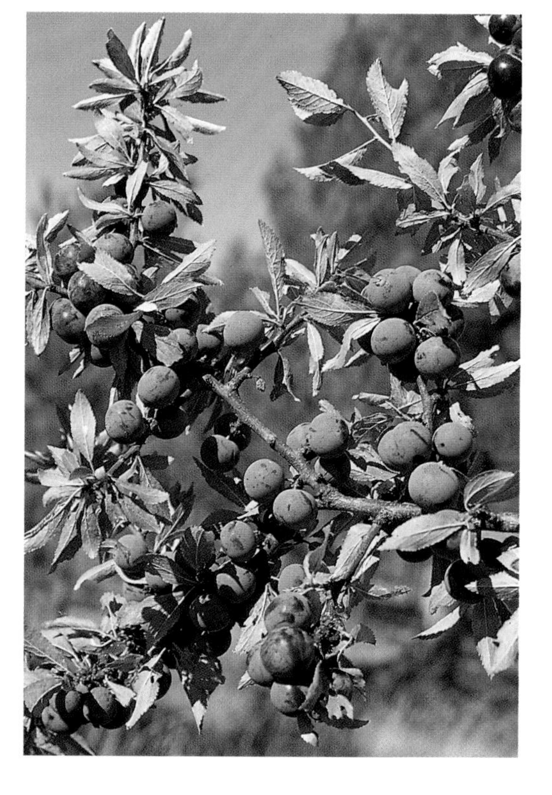

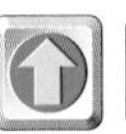
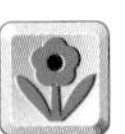
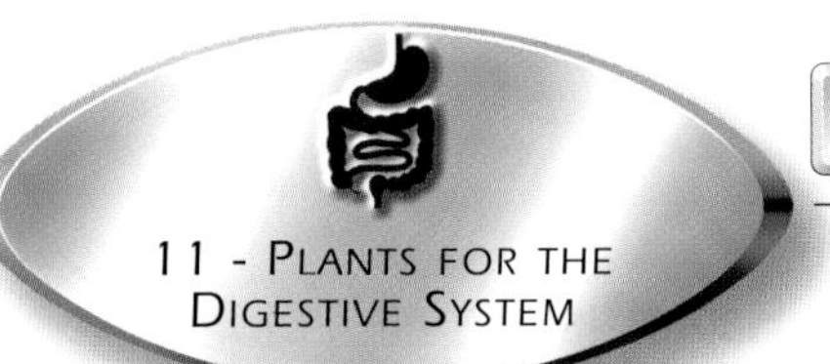
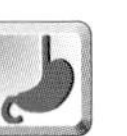
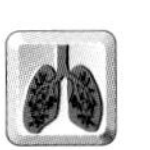
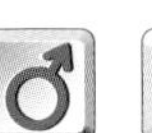
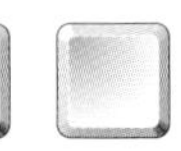

Winter Savory

Carminative, invigorating, and aphrodisiac

WINTER SAVORY is a truly sensual plant. Its strong aroma seems to prove it. It is not strange, thus, that for ages its seasoning and aphrodisiac virtues were known. It is said that ancient Greeks dedicated this plant to the god Dionysus, called Bacchus by the Romans, in whose honor many orgiastic festivals were celebrated. Winter savory encourages digestion and promotes vital functions. The Middle Age monks were not allowed to cultivate this plant in their gardens.

In Mediterranean areas, especially in Andalusia, one of the typical dishes is olives seasoned with Winter savory.

PROPERTIES AND INDICATIONS. Winter savory contains up to one percent of an essential oil rich in carvacrol and cymol, which gives the plant **stimulant, carminative, antispasmodic, vermifuge, diuretic, and pectoral** properties. The oil also contains tannin and polyphenolic substances.

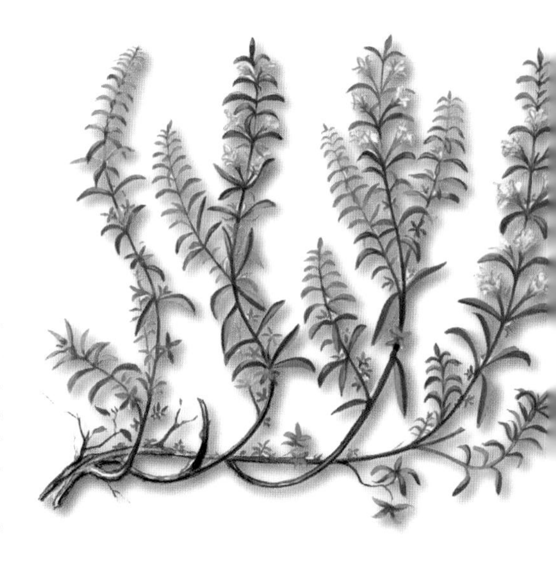

Description. *Shrub, growing up to 25-30 cm high, of the Labiatae family. Winter savory calls attention because of its aroma in any place. It has fine, small, point-tipped leaves with small holes in which the essence-producing glands are housed. The flowers are small, pink or white, and divided into two lips.*

Parts used. *Leaves, flowers, and stems.*

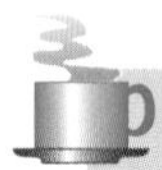

Preparation and Use

INTERNAL USE

❶ **Infusion** with 20 g of plant per liter of water. Drink up to three or four cups daily.

❷ **Essence.** The recommended dose is from three to five drops after every meal.

• The plant also features **appetizer** properties, and serves to ease digestion. Moreover, its **carminative** properties are interesting. According to Font Quer, the outstanding Spanish pharmacist and botanist, Winter savory "fights the winds of the stomach and intestine." There's nothing better than Winter savory to season dishes. Besides, it relaxes the muscles of the intestine **(antispasmodic** properties), being thus useful for abdominal spasms and diarrhea **[❶,❷]**. It is recommended for people suffering from

Cuisine Applications

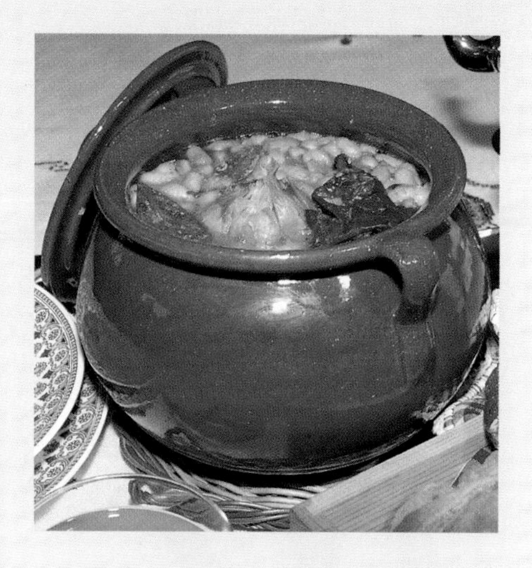

- *In **stews,** savory can be used both fresh and dry, and even ground by means of a pepper mill. Its essence is also used as seasoning.*
- *As a **seasoning for raw olives.** This recipe has a long tradition in southern Spanish villages. Olives are put in water for some days, changing water until it is clear, and the olives lose their sour flavor. Then, put the the olives in water and add savory (a handful per liter), salt, garlic, and orange rind (in the case of black olives), or lemon rind (in the case of green olives). Satisfaction is guaranteed.*

gastritis, and it also presents some vermifuge properties.

- For the **nervous system,** it offers mild **invigorating** properties, being thus recommended for chronic fatigue, weakness, low blood pressure, and asthenia {❶,❷}. Of course, the use of Winter savory must be ***accompanied*** by other natural treatments within the frame of a reinvigorating cure.
- Its **aphrodisiac** properties are not overwhelming and dramatic, but discrete and progressive {❶,❷}. When a stronger action is wanted, Winter savory should be combined with other plants (see p. 602).
- It is mildly **diuretic and depurative,** and is thus recommended for people suffering from obesity, arthritis, and gout {❶,❷}.
- It has **balsamic and expectorant** properties because of the essential oil it contains. Winter savory is thus useful for acute and chronic bronchitis, as well as asthma {❶,❷}.

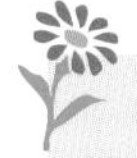

Summer Savory

There are several savory species, all of them **similar in regards to their composition and properties.** One of them is **summer savory** (*Satureja hortensis* L.), which is sometimes called oregano and marjoram.

Besides its medicinal properties, summer savory is cultivated because of its ***leaves,*** which serve as **seasoning.** The essence is also a valued seasoning.

White savory (*Satureja fruticosa* Béguinot) grows in Catalonia (Spain). In Mediterranean Spanish regions, you will find **fine** or **tiny savory** (*Satureja odorata* Lagasca).

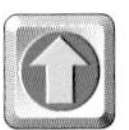
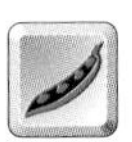
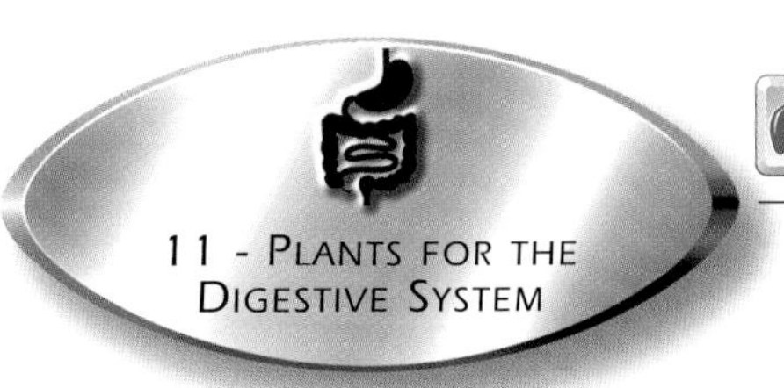

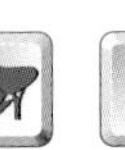
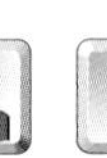
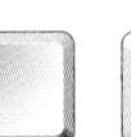
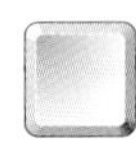

Vanilla

Fragranceand digestive

FOR MANY AGES, Mexican Aztecs used vanilla as an fragrance (flavoring) for their favorite drink, made with cocoa grains and corn flour. The Spanish carried it to Europe in the late sixteenth century, but the plant did not take roots. In 1836, a Belgian botanist found the vanilla tree could only be pollinated by an insect which lives in Mexico. Anywhere else it needed artificial pollination.

PROPERTIES AND INDICATIONS. The active principle of vanilla is vanillosid, a glycoside which, during the drying process becomes vanillin, the substance which gives vanilla its typical aroma. Vanilla has **stomachic, digestive, choleretic** (increases the bile secretion), mildly **invigorating,** and, according to some people, aphrodisiac properties **[❶,❷]**.

Although its present use is only as a **seasoning,** it is worth remembering its **invigorating** benefits to the digestive functions.

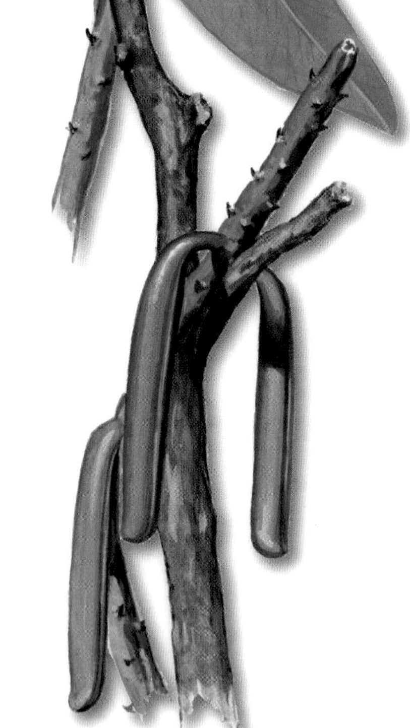

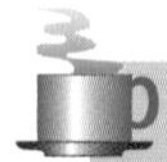

Preparation and Use

INTERNAL USE

❶ Vanilla is used as **vanilla sugar, syrup, or tincture.**

❷ However, the most usual method to obtain its authentic aroma is by **boiling its pods with** the substance you want to flavor: chocolate, infusions, desserts, etc.

Description. *Climbing plant of the Orquidaceae family, whose stems may grow up to 30 m long. It has aerial roots which it sticks to the tree that serves its as support. It has fleshy leaves, and large (15 cm) blackish-ochre pods with many seeds.*

Parts used. *The green pods.*

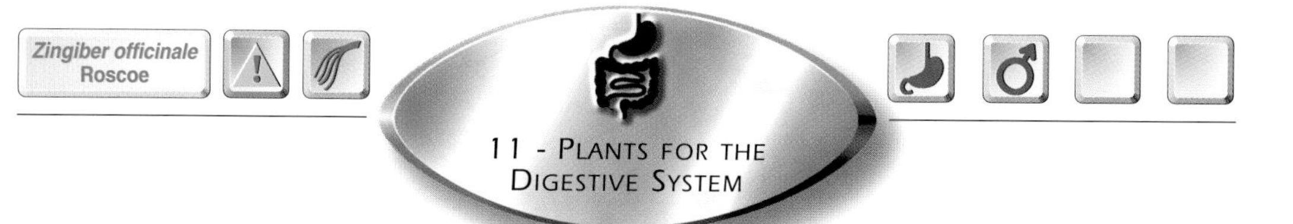

Ginger

Helps digestion

TRADERS carried ginger from Eastern Asia to the Mediterranean coast. In Rome it became the most appreciated spice, only second to pepper. Dioscorides (first century A.D.) knew it and recommended it for those with weak stomachs.

During the whole Middle Age it was exported to Europe, where it was highly appreciated, but it could never be cultivated there. In the early sixteenth century, the Spaniard Francisco de Mendoza was first to carry its seeds to the "New World," then its cultivation quickly spread along the West Indies, Mexico, and Peru.

PROPERTIES AND INDICATIONS. Ginger contains an essential oil with several terpene derivatives, which give the plant its **digestive and carminative** (prevents the formation of gas in the digestive system) properties.

It is also **sudorific,** and in India there is a belief which says it has aphrodisiac properties.

Ginger is recommended to treat **exhaustion, lack of appetite, bloated stomach, and flatulence [❶,❷]**.

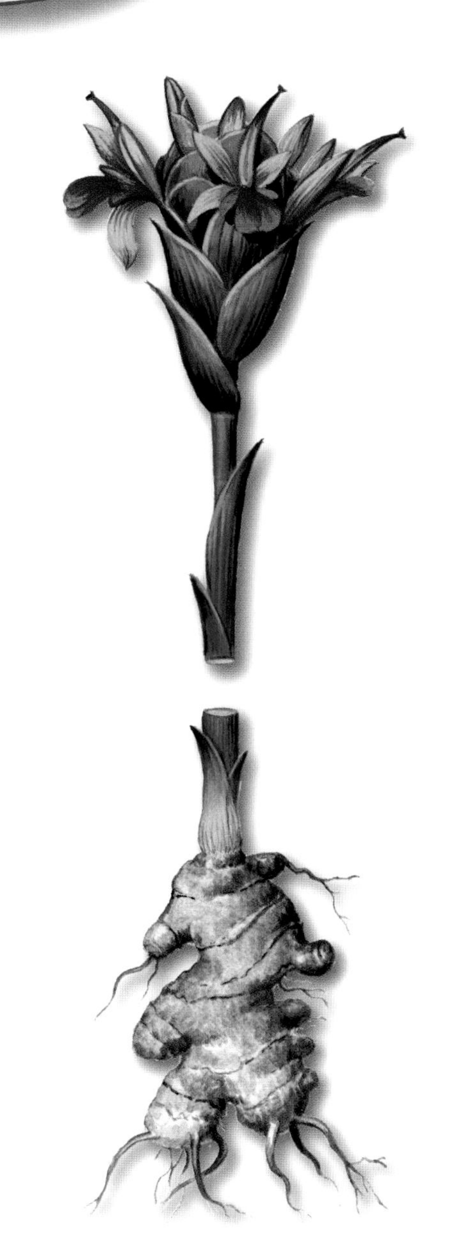

Preparation and Use

INTERNAL USE

❶ **Seasoning.** In **small amounts** for raw and cooked foods.

❷ **Infusion** with two grams of ground rhizome per half a liter of water. Drink a cup after every meal. **Never exceed** the recommended dose.

Description. *Vivacious plant of the Zingiberaceae family, growing up to 1-1.3 m high, with exuberant flowers resembling orchids. It reproduces by means of its aromatic rhizome.*

Parts used. *The rhizome (underground stem).*

12

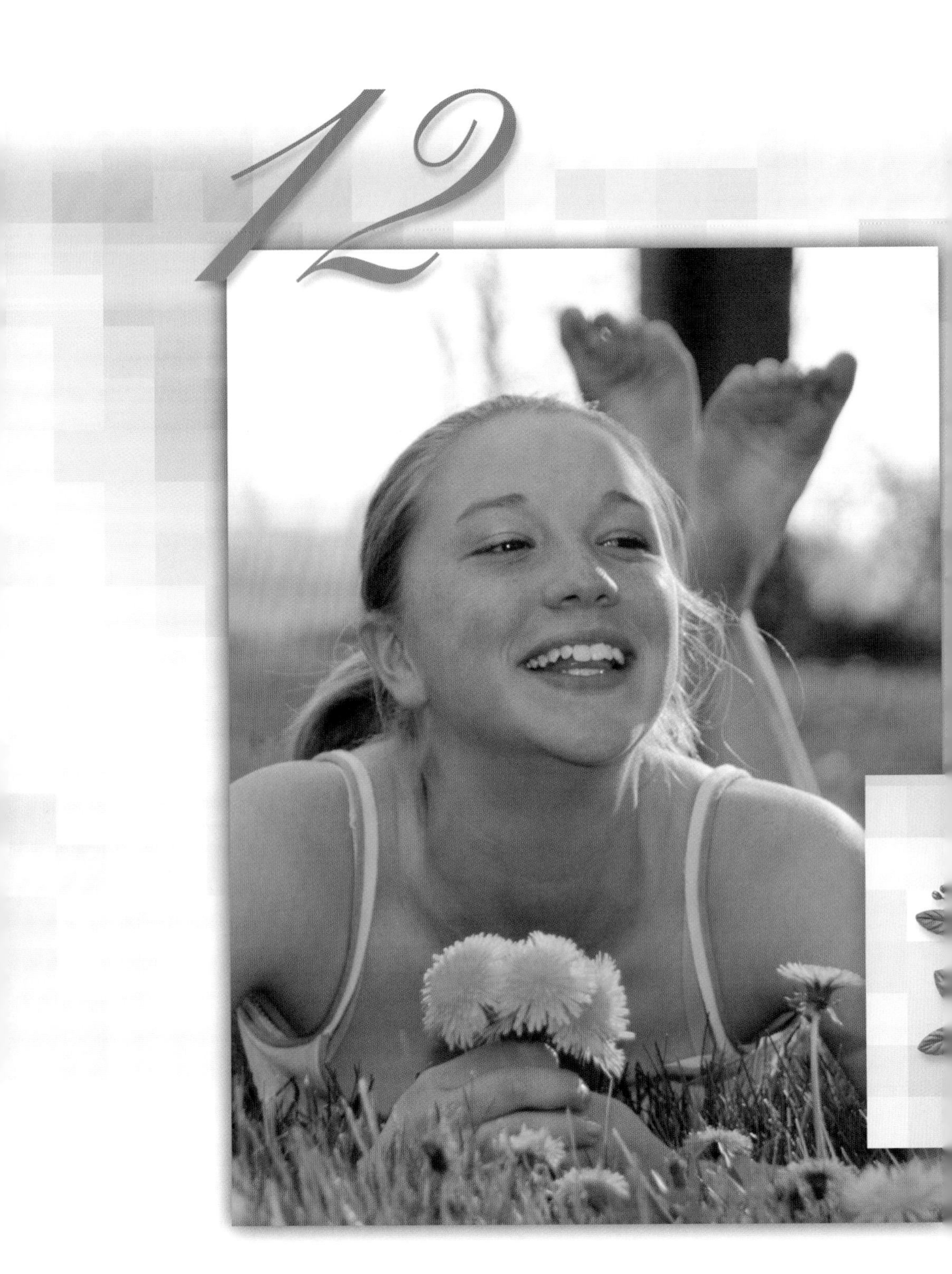

Plants for the Liver

DISEASES	PAGES
Ascitis, see Fluid in the abdomen	192
Biliary colic	193
Cholelithiasis, see Gall bladder dysfunction	193
Cirrhosis, see Hepatitis	192
Fluid in the abdomen	192
Gall bladder, dysfunction	193
Hepatic colic, see Biliary colic	193
Hepatitis	192
Liver insufficiency, see Liver, dysfunction	192
Liver stones, see Gall bladder dysfunction	193
Liver, dysfunction	192
Liver, toxicity	193
Pancreatic, insufficiency	193
Portal hypertension, see Fluid in the abdomen	192

PLANTS	PAGES
Artichoke	197
Barberry	194
Boldo	198
Dandelion	202
Fumitory	196
Milk thistle	200

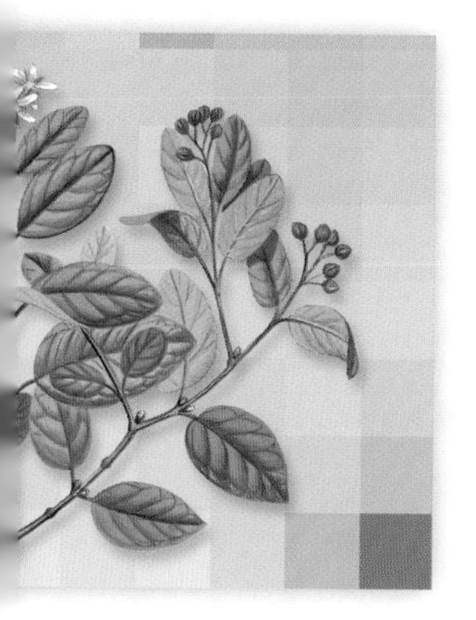

MEDICINAL HERBS exert two types of actions on the hepatobiliary system: choleretic and cholagogue. Bile production is one of the basic functions of the liver.

Plants with **choleretic** properties increase the amount of bile secreted by the liver. Bile is stored in the gall bladder, until the passing of food produces its emptying in the intestine. By increasing bile production, choleretic plants reduce the congestion of the liver and promote digestion. They are especially useful for liver disorders, such as hepatitis.

Plants with **cholagogue** properties ease the emptying of the bile stored in the gall bladder to the duodenum. Cholagogue plants stop gall bladder and Oddi sphincter spasms, alleviating pain and encouraging the correct functioning of the biliary system. They are used for biliary dyskinesia (slow gall bladder), biliary dyspepsia, and cholelithiasis (gall stones).

LIVER, DYSFUNCTION

Definition

The liver is the biggest gland in our body. Many chemical reactions take place in it. It has three main functions:

1. **Transformation** of nutrients into other nutrients
2. **Bile** production, which is needed to digest fats.
3. Blood **cleansing,** by neutralizing and eliminating many foreign and toxic substances flowing into the blood system.

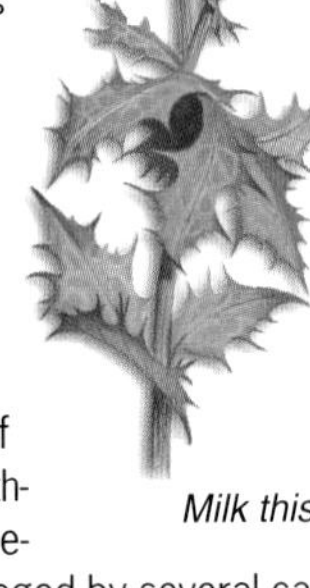

Milk thistle

Phytotherapy

Many of these plants have **choleretic** properties, that is, they favor bile secretion by hepatic cells. Hence, they reduce the congestion of the liver, and enhance its function. Other plants stimulate regeneration of hepatic cells when they have been damaged by several causes (viruses, medicines, toxic substances, etc.).

VERVAIN	Reduces liver congestion, antispasmodic
BARBERRY	Promotes evacuation of bile, digestive invigorant
FUMITORY	Reduces liver congestion, reduces toxicity
BOLDO	Powerful choleretic and cholagogue, promotes bile emptying
MILK THISTLE	Stimulates regeneration of damaged hepatic cells
DANDELION	Increases bile production and promotes its emptying
CHICORY	Promotes bile secretion, relieves liver congestion
GENTIAN	Stimulates secretion and emptying of bile
ALDER BUCKTHORN	Promotes good functioning of the liver
CALENDULA	Increases bile production

HEPATITIS

Definition

It is the inflammation of the live,r usually caused by any virus. Its main symptom is **jaundice,** a yellowish coloring of the skin due to the inability of the liver to eliminate bile, then it passes to the blood and permeates the skin and other tissues.

Phytotherapy

Medicinal herb based treatment tries to enhance liver function so that this gland recovers to its best working conditions. The same plants can be used as complementary substances in the treatment of **cirrhosis.** Besides these herbs, all those with ***choleretic*** properties are useful.

SPIRULINA	Supplies nutrients with a high biologic value
PEPPERMINT	Its essence is active against hepatitis A virus
MILK THISTLE	Stimulates regeneration of damaged hepatic cells
DANDELION	Relieves liver congestion, promotes liver detoxifying functions

FLUID IN THE ABDOMEN

Definition

The accumulation of liquids in the peritoneal cavity is called **ascitis.** Its most frequent cause is hepatic **cirrhosis.**

Phytotherapy

These plants activate blood flowing in the portal system, reduce the congestion of the liver, and promote the elimination of abdominal fluids. Hence, they improve the resolution of hepatic cirrhosis.

CHICORY	Activates portal circulation, reduces liver congestion
JAVAN TEA	Intensive diuretic, rich in potassium salts, cholagogue
BLACK ELDER	Purgative, diuretic

GALL BLADDER, DYSFUNCTION

Definition

The gall bladder must empty the bile stored at the right time so that digestion continues normally. However, the bile emptying mechanism suffers from frequent disorders, which are shown in bloated stomach, pain in the liver area, or in the omoplates, nausea, and headaches. In many cases, these disorders are caused by **cholelithiasis** (gall stones) or **biliary mud** (thick bile).

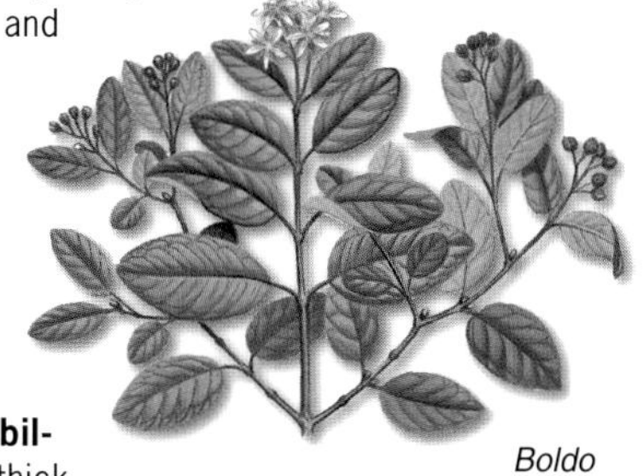

Boldo

Phytotherapy

Phytotherapy has plants able to regulate the bile emptying mechanism and make bile more liquid, thus avoiding the formation of new gall stones. All ***cholagogue*** plants are also useful.

LINDEN	Antispasmodic, improves functioning of gall bladder
BARBERRY	Cholagogue, improves heavy digestion
BOLDO	Powerful choleretic and cholagogue, normalizes bile emptying
DANDELION	Increases bile production and promotes its emptying
GENTIAN	Choleretic and cholagogue, improves biliary dyskinesia, stomachic tonic
JAVAN TEA	Corrects atony of the gall bladder
ST. JOHNSWORT	Promotes gall bladder functioning

BILIARY COLIC

Definition

Biliary colic takes place when the gall bladder tries to expel a stone or calculus formed in its interior. It is an acute disorder which may last for several days, with spasmodic contractions of the gall bladder and of the ducts by which the bile flows into the small intestine. This shows itself through pain, nausea, vomiting, and general discomfort.

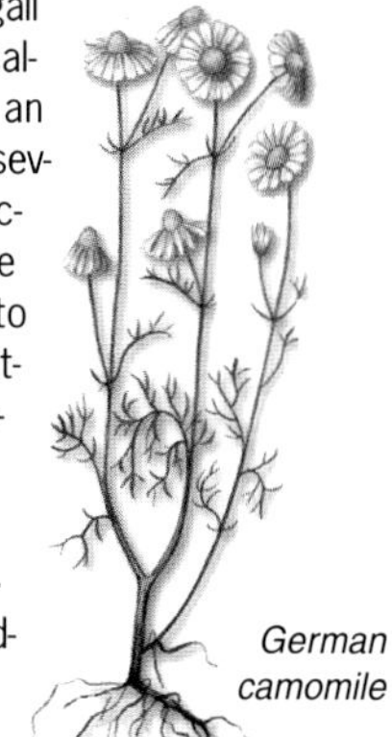

German camomile

Phytotherapy

Besides these plants, all ***antispasmodic*** plants are also recommended.

PASSION FLOWER	Relaxes hollow abdominal organs such as the gall bladder
GERMAN CAMOMILE	Antispasmodic, sedative
FLAX	Antispasmodic, sedative, anti-inflammatory
DEVIL'S CLAW	Relaxes colic spasms

PANCREATIC, INSUFFICIENCY

All three plants mentioned here promote exocrine function of the pancreas, increasing the production of pancreatic juice, which is needed for digestion.

NETTLE	Stimulates production of pancreatic juice

LIVER, TOXICITY

When liver cells have been damaged by medicines, chemical products, or poisonous mushrooms, any of these two plants can help enhancing the anti-poisonous functions of the liver and regenerating its cells.

MILK THISTLE	Stimulates regeneration of damaged hepatic cells

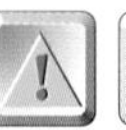

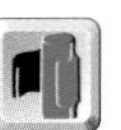

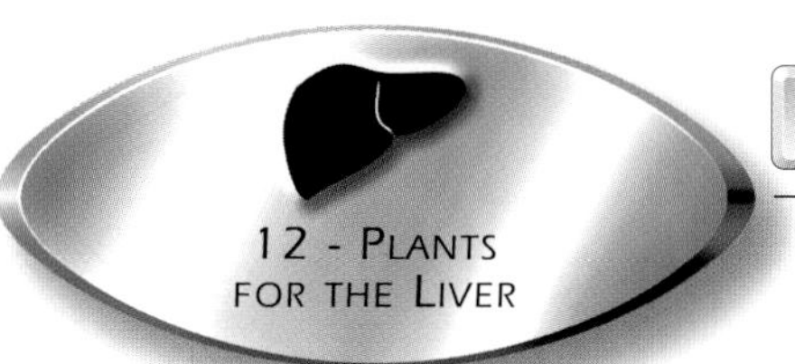

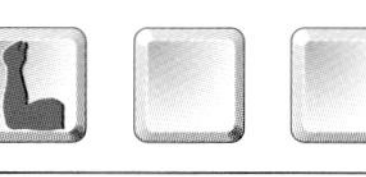

Barberry

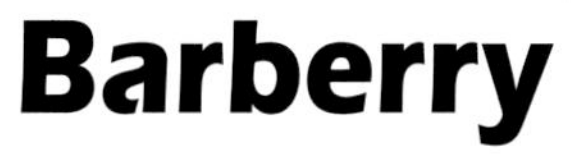

Digestive and invigorating

WHEN WALKING in mountainous, dry places, it is pleasant to meet this shrub, somewhat hostile in appearance because of its spiked thorns, however with exquisite fruit. Until mid-Fall, walkers can enjoy this refreshing, natural gift. To be so pleasant, they have a cool flavor, somewhere between sweet and sour.

PROPERTIES AND INDICATIONS. The whole plant except the berries contains very active alkaloids, which can be poisonous.

The ***ROOT'S BARK*** of the barberry is the part of the plant with a higher content in barberine. It has the following properties:

• **Cholagogue and digestive.** By promoting the emptying of bile, it reduces the congestion of the liver and the bile system, thus reducing bloated stomach [❶]. It acts as a digestive tonic, increasing appetite.

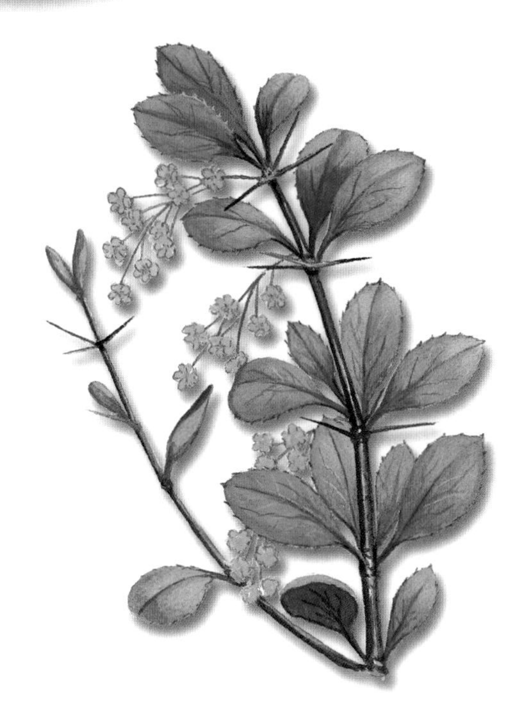

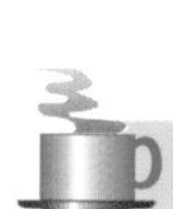

Preparation and Use

INTERNAL USE

❶ **Infusion or decoction** with 40 g of root's bark per liter of water. The maximum dose is three cups daily.

❷ **Syrup,** made with mashed fruits, then straining and adding twice its weigh of sugar in order to avoid fermentation. The syrup obtained can be used to make a quenching drink all the year around.

❸ **Jelly.** Barberries are also used to prepare delicious jellies.

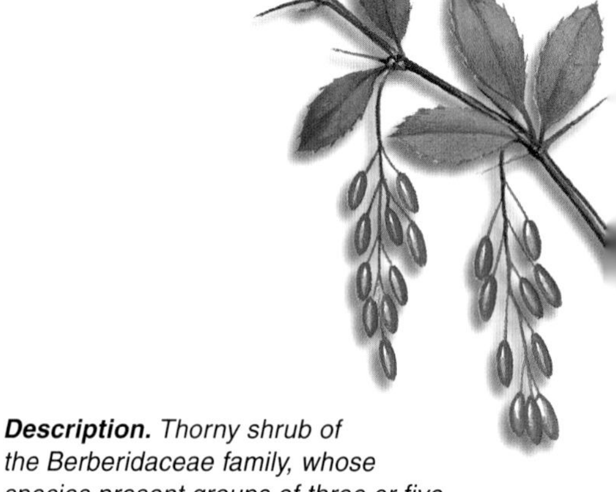

Description. *Thorny shrub of the Berberidaceae family, whose species present groups of three or five thorns on each knot. Yellow flowers, and oval, little, red or purple berries growing in clusters. The bark of the trunk and of the root is yellowish, and it has been used to dye wool and other fabrics.*

Parts used. *The bark of the root and the berries.*

Warning

*Due to its content in **barberine,** an alkaloid similar to morphine, the **root's bark** of the barberry must be carefully used, **never exceeding** the prescribed **doses.***

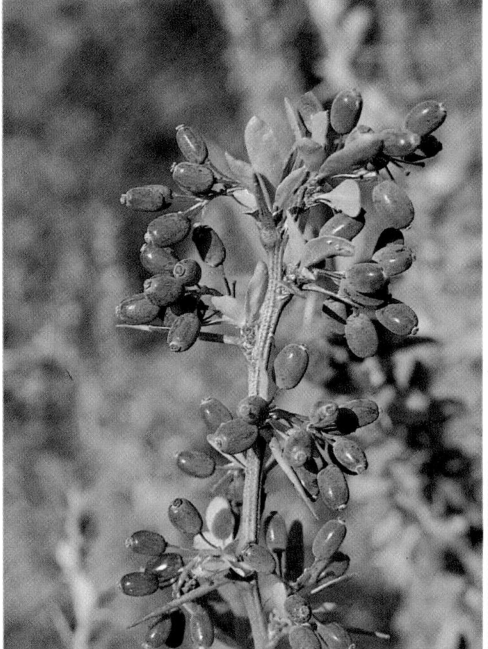

• **Laxative.** It eases constipation when the latter is caused by an insufficient bile secretion [❶].

• **Heart and circulatory invigorating.** It has been traditionally used as a stimulant substance for exhaustion or febrile diseases [❶].

• **Diuretic and febrifuge,** although with mild effects [❶].

Its ***FRUITS*** (berries) contain glucose and levulose, vitamin C, and citric and malic acids. Both fresh, in the form of juice, or in syrup, barberries are effective in refreshing and thirst quenching. They have a **mild laxative effect.** Barberry juice and syrup are ideal in quenching the thirst of **people with fever,** since it decreases their temperature, invigorates and stimulates them [❷,❸].

Barberries should be gathered in the late Summer or in Fall. They can be used freely, as they contain no alkaloids.

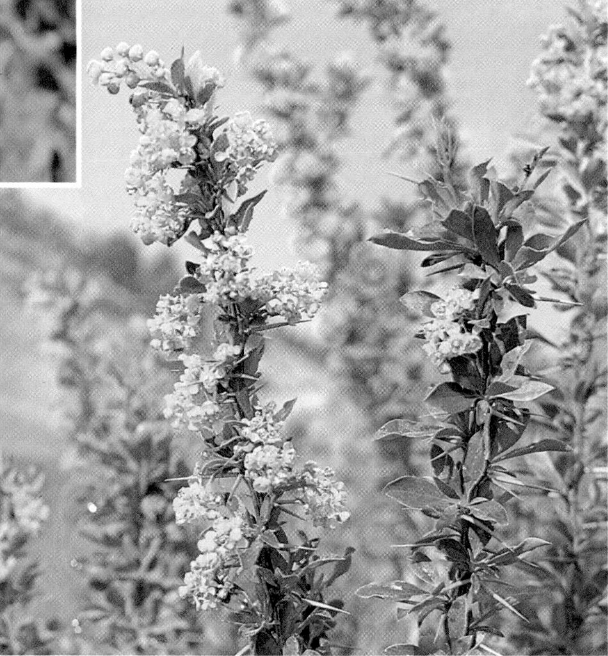

The root's bark of the barberry has positive effects on the gall bladder. By promoting the emptying of bile to the duodenum, improves bloated stomach and bile-caused dyspepsia.

The fruits of the barberry (barberries) are recommended for fever caused by influenza or by other afflictions: they decrease temperature and have invigorating properties.

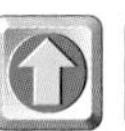
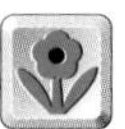
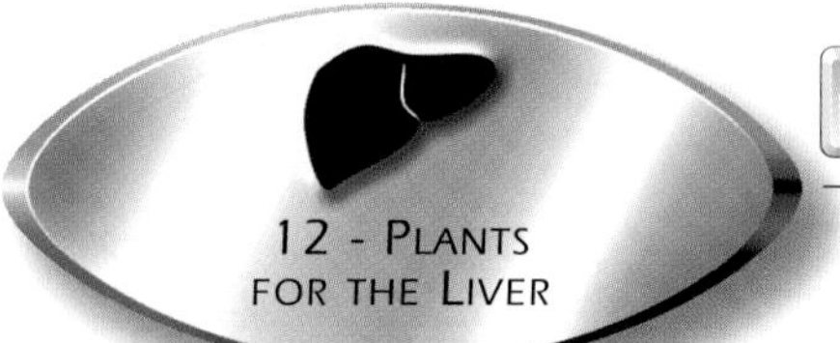

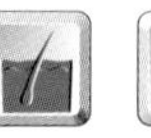
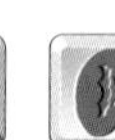
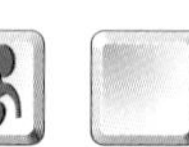

Fumitory

Relieves congestion of the liver and toxicity

THE NAME OF this plant could be derived from either of two facts. First, when the plant is cut or mashed, it makes anyone shed tears as if it was smoke. Second, its sterling-grey leaves resemble the smoke of a fire, while the flowers seem like the fire itself.

Properties and indications. The whole plant contains flavonic substances with **antispasmodic and choleretic** properties; potassium salts, to which it owes its **diuretic and depurative** properties, and several alkaloids which are derived from the isoquinoline (fumarine), which give the plant **antihistaminic** and **anti-inflammatory** properties.

It has the following indications:

- **Skin eczemas and rashes,** caused by **autointoxication** (internal toxicity) with intestinal putrefaction, kidney and liver insufficiency, or allergies [❶,❷,❸].
- **Hepatic affections:** congestion and dysfunctions of the liver or chronic hepatitis, because of its choleretic effect [❶,❷,❸].
- **Arterial hypertension,** given its diuretic, antispasmodic, depurative, and blood thinning properties [❶,❷,❸].

Preparation and Use

Internal use

❶ **Infusion** with 50 g of plant per liter of water. Drink a cup before every meal.

❷ **Juice of the fresh plant,** sweetened with honey. Half a glass before every meal.

❸ **Dry extract.** One gram before every meal.

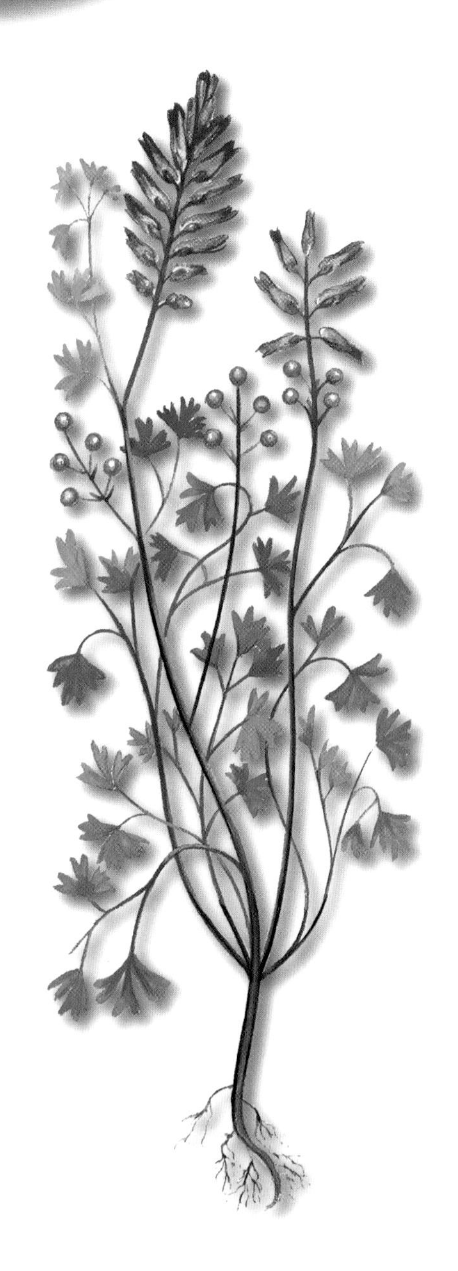

Description. *Annual plant of the Fumariaceae family, growing from 20 to 70 cm high, with greyish-green leaves and pink or red flowers. It has an acid smell and a sour taste.*

Parts used. *The whole plant, except its root.*

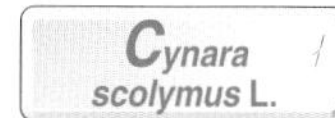

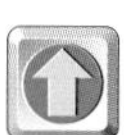
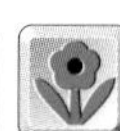
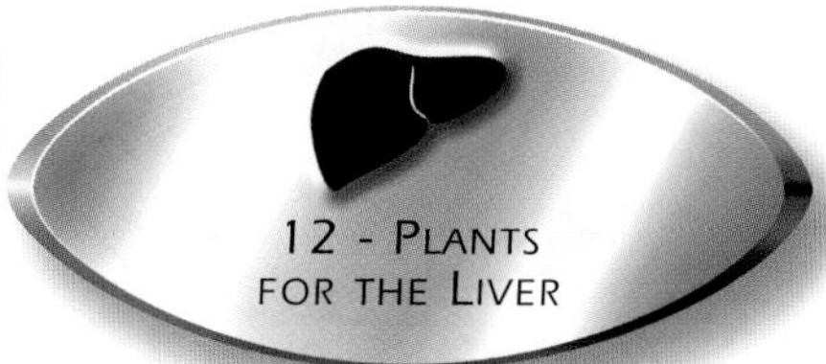

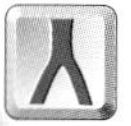
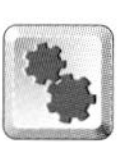
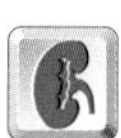
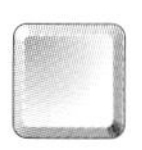

Artichoke

Regenerates the liver and decreases cholesterol

ARTICHOKE EXTRACTS are part of the composition of several ***medicines*** because of their notable medicinal actions on the liver and the body.

PROPERTIES AND INDICATIONS. The active components of artichoke, which concentrate mainly in its leaves, are cynarine (a bitter component), and flavonic derivatives of the luteine. The plant is rich in enzymes, inulin (a sugar quite well tolerated by diabetic people, see p. 80), potassium and manganese. Although the proper artichoke, that is to say, the flower head of the plant, also shares the aforementioned medicinal properties, the leaves, stem and/or roots of the plant should be used in order to achieve an important therapeutic effect. The properties of the artichoke plant are as follows.

• **Choleretic** (increases bile secretion) and **hepatoprotective** (antitoxic). It is recommended for dyspepsia or biliary colic, and hepatic insufficiency [❶,❷,❸]. In the case of **hepatitis,** artichoke is ***highly recommended.***

• **Hypolipemic.** The plant decreases the level of cholesterol in the blood, as well as other lipids, being thus ***recommended*** for **arteriosclerosis** [❶,❷,❸].

• **Hypoglycemic.** Due to its content in inuline, artichoke is an ideal food for people suffering from **diabetes** [❶,❷,❸]. It promotes the decrease of the level of sugar in the blood.

• **Diuretic, depurative, and urea eliminating.** Very appropriated for albuminuria and kidney insufficiency [❶,❷,❸].

Description. *Plant of the Compositae family, growing up to 1.5 m high, with large, segmented, greyish-green leaves, and violet flower heads surrounded by bracts (false leaves) with edible base.*

Parts used. *The leaves, stem and root of the plant, and the flower heads (artichokes).*

Preparation and Use

INTERNAL USE

❶ **Infusion** of leaves, stem and/or root: 50-100 g per liter of water. Drink three cups daily, before meals if possible.

❷ **Fresh juice,** prepared with the leaves. Drink a glass with every meal.

❸ **Dry extract.** The recommended dose is one or two grams daily, if the sour flavor of infusions or juice is not well tolerated.

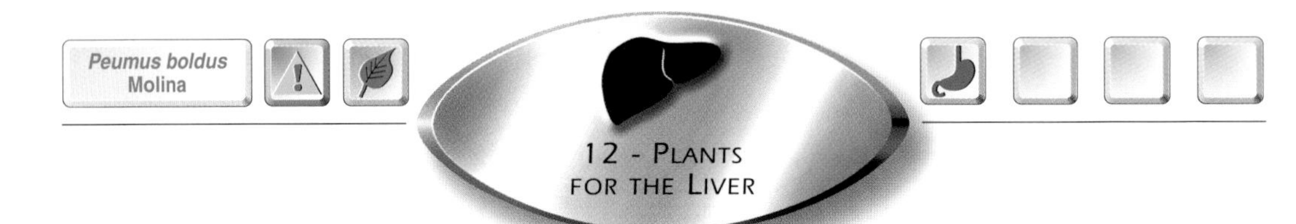

Boldo

Normalizes the function of the gall bladder

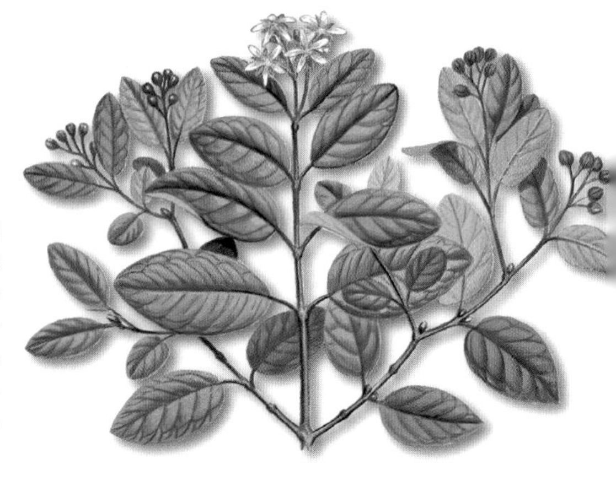

BOLDO IS ONE of the medicinal plants ***most used*** in preparing ***medicines*** for the treatment of **liver** and **gall bladder** diseases. There are several medicines, laboratory produced, in whose composition boldo is an essential part. This plant has some properties that could never be achieved by any chemically synthesized product.

It is a highly appreciated plant in Chile. Native Andean Indians used boldo because of its stomachic and digestive properties. It can be currently found in pharmacies and herb shops of Europe and America, and still with its primitive Araucanian name.

Description. *Tree or shrub of the Monimiaceae family, growing up to 5 m high, with elliptic, rough leaves, and white or yellowish flowers. The whole plant gives an aroma similar to that of peppermint.*

Parts used. *The leaves.*

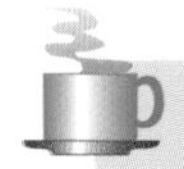

Preparation and Use

INTERNAL USE

❶ **Infusion** with 10-20 g of leaves per liter of water. Drink a cup before meals, up to four daily.

❷ **Dry extract.** One gram, three or four times a day, before meals.

PROPERTIES AND INDICATIONS. The leaves of boldo contain around 20 alkaloids which are derived from aporfine, the most important of which is boldine, making 25-30% of the whole. They also contain essential oil, which gives the plant its typical smell. In this essential oil there are eucalyptol, ascaridol, and cymol. The leaves also contain several flavonoids and glycosides (boldoglycine).

The most outstanding properties of boldo are as follow:

• **Choleretic** (increases the bile production in the liver), and **cholagogue** (promotes the emptying of the gall bladder). Hence, boldo leaves are recommended for hepatic congestion and biliary dyskinesia (disorders in gall bladder functions), and biliary colic {❶,❷}.

Boldo is also useful for **biliary lithiasis** (gall stones), as well as to alleviate digestive discomfort and the sensation of distension after meals, quite characteristic of this ailment {❶,❷}. Actually, boldo is not able to dissolve gall stones, or to provoke their expulsion. However, it has been proven that boldo produces changes in the chemical composition and the physical properties of the bile. Hence, it makes bile more fluid, and less lithogenic (which tends to form stones or calculi). Boldo, thus, prevents the bile from forming new stones, or those existing to grow.

- **Eupeptic** (eases digestion) **and appetizer.** Boldo is recommended for bloated stomach and slow digestion, lack of appetite, and bad breath (sour) {❶,❷}.
- **Mildly laxative,** probably as a consequence of the higher flow of bile in the intestine, which this plant provokes {❶,❷}.

Boldo is usually taken ***in association*** with other choleretic and cholagogue plants (artichoke, rosemary) or laxative (alder buckthorn, tinnevelly senna, etc.).

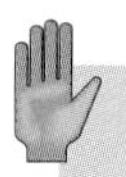

Warning

Never exceed the prescribed dose *(four cups a day) since in high doses boldo has narcotic and anesthetic properties, acting on the central nervous system. These effects only occur when taken in high doses, and never with those doses recommended here.*

Even though its effect on the fetus have not been proven, ***pregnant*** *women should* ***abstain*** *from this plant.*

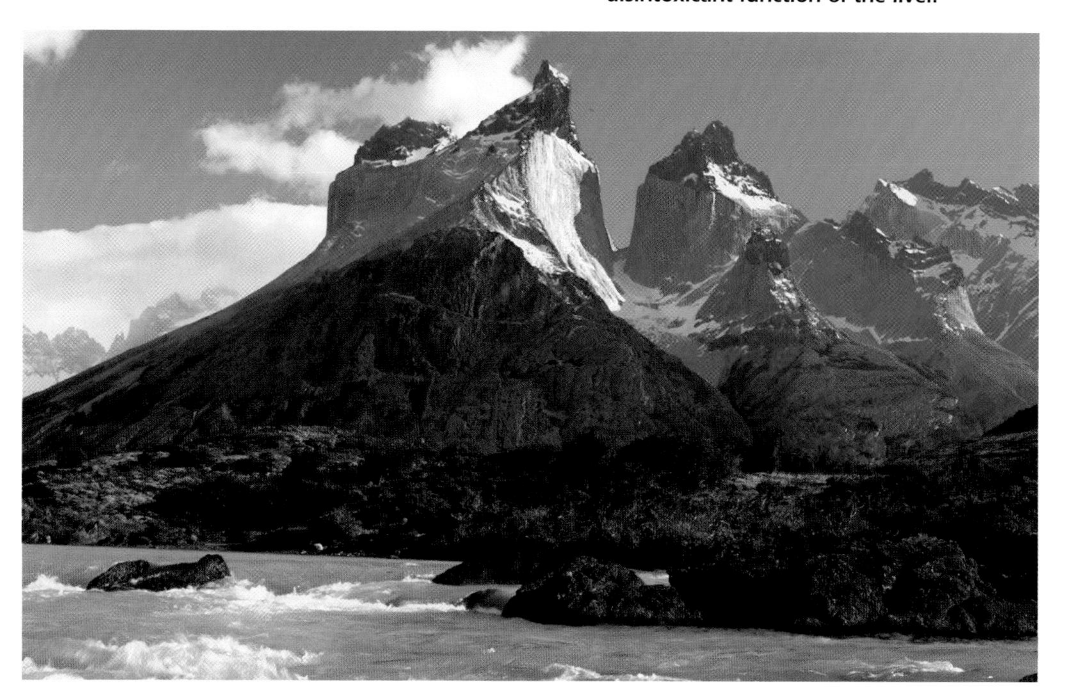

A magnificent view of the Paine Towers (Chile). Boldo is native to the mountainous Andean areas of South America, though at present it is being cultivated in Italy and North Africa. The consumption of boldo has proven to improve skin eczemas. This is likely to occur since the plant promotes the disintoxicant function of the liver.

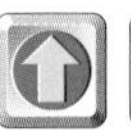
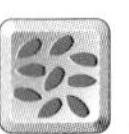
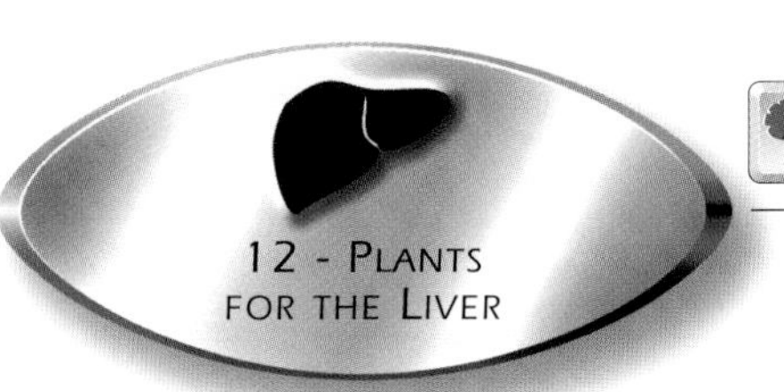

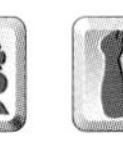
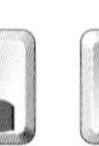
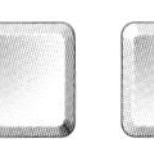
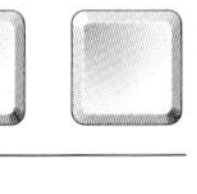

Milk Thistle

Regenerates hepatic cells

THE PRICKLES of thistles are defenses protecting a valuable medicinal treasure. Many people, however, dismiss these plants, thinking these are rough vegetables only fit for donkeys. Hence, in many Latin countries this plant is given the name of donkey thistle, in spite of its doubtless medicinal properties.

Many people would be surprised when knowing that from this thistle a powerful substance against liver disorders is extracted: **silimarine,** which makes part of several ***pharmaceutical preparations.***

Late scientific developments, which made it possible to know the chemical composition of many plants, allowed physicians to surrender many popular myths about plants. Hence, we can currently use medicinal herbs in a more effective, steady manner than before.

Properties and indications. In the fruits of the milk thistle there are substances with medicinal properties, the so-called flavonolignan. Dr. Coll (of the Pharmacognosis and Pharmacodynamics Laboratory of Barcelona's Pharmacy College) points out that these complex substances are formed by a flavonoid (taxifoline) and a phenolpropanic molecule (coniferilic alcohol). The mixture of several types (isomers) of flavonolignanes is called silimarine.

Silimarine is able to stimulate regeneration of hepatic cells damaged by toxic substances such as ethyl alcohol or carbon tetrachloride, as well as phalloidine, a substance contained in the *Amanita phalloides,* the most poisonous of all mushrooms. Silimarine stimulates protein synthesis in hepatic cells, and it has important anti-inflammatory properties on the mesenchyme (supporting fiber tissue) of the liver.

Hence, the milk thistle is highly recommended in the following cases:

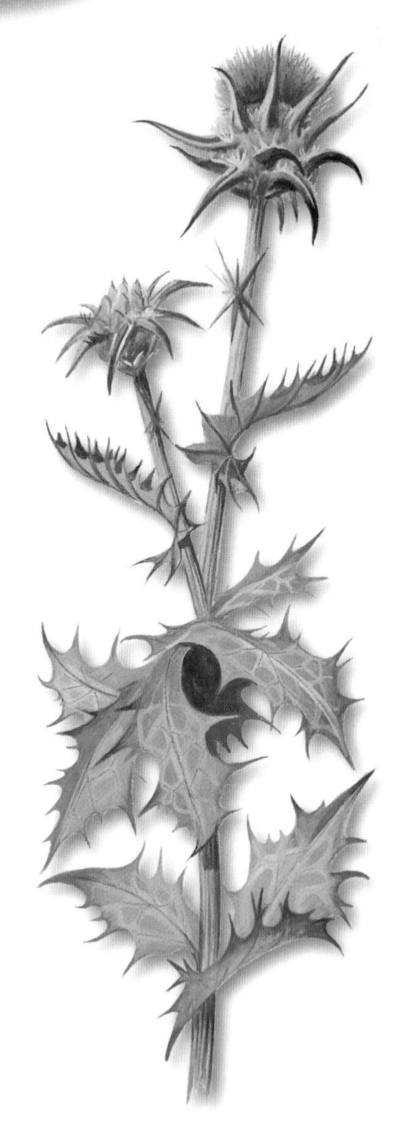

Description. *Plant of prickly appearance, growing up to two meters high, of the Compositae family, with large, prickly, white-stained leaves. Its flower heads are pink or purple, and the fruits are hard, dark colored.*

Parts used. *The fruits (seeds), the leaves and the root.*

Preparation and Use

INTERNAL USE

❶ **Salads.** Young leaves without prickles, as well as flower hearts (like artichokes) can be eaten raw, as Sahara Bedouins do. These are exquisite meals.

❷ **Infusion or decoction** with 30-50 g of mashed or ground fruits per liter of water, to which some leaves or roots can be added. Drink from three to five cups daily. The dose can be exceeded with no risk, since the milk thistle has no toxic effects.

❸ **Dry extract.** The recommended dose is 0.5-1 g, twice a day.

- **Fatty degeneration of the liver,** both caused by alcohol or by other toxic substances {❶,❸}.
- **Inflammation of the liver,** caused by medicines, such as those with anti-inflammatory, tuberculostatic, anovulatory, or psychological effects {❶,❸}.
- **Poisoning with hepatotoxic substances,** such as carbon tetrachloride, organic-phosphoric insecticides, and mushrooms of the genus *Amanita (Amanita phalloides, Amanita verna, Amanita virosa)* {❶,❸}.
- Acute viral **hepatitis,** chronic hepatitis, alcoholic hepatitis (inflammation of the liver caused by alcoholic beverage consumption) {❶,❸}.
- **Hepatic insufficiency or congestion,** with or without jaundice {❶,❸}.
- **Hepatic cirrhosis {❶,❸}.**

In all these cases, silimarine stimulates the regeneration of damaged liver cells and restores their normal functions. However, ***this plant does not completely heal cirrhosis, nor any other treatment*** does up to now, if necrosis has already occurred (death or destruction of liver cells). Nonetheless, even in the most severe cases, an improvement is expected.

The ***FRUITS*** of the milk thistle, and in less proportion, its leaves and root, contain other active substances (biogenic amines, essential oil, albuminoid substances, and tannin), which could explain its balancing action on the autonomic nervous system that controls the tone of blood vessels. Therefore, the plant is successfully used in the cases of:

- **Migraines and neuralgias {❷}.**
- **Exhaustion and asthenia** (fatigue) {❷}.
- **Kinetosis** (nausea and vomiting when travelling): drink a cup of herbal tea before departing {❷}.
- **Allergic reactions:** hay fever, asthma, nettlerash {❷}.

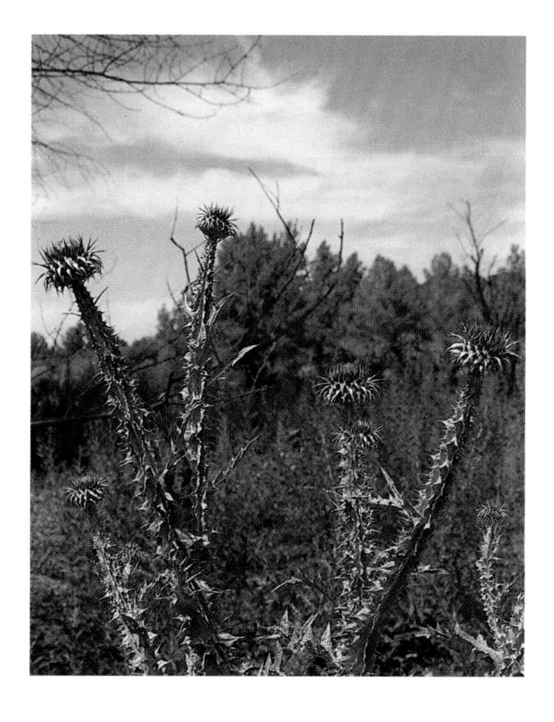

Dandelion

Good for the liver and kidneys

"DON'T PLAY WITH those yellow flowers. You will be wetting the bed tonight!" a peasant mother tells her children.

"Why, Mum?"

"Look. This plant is called lion's tooth because of its leaves' shape. But in France, where it is common, it is called *pissenlit,* which means bed-wetting."

Truly, the dandelion is a great diuretic plant, and component of many depurative cures of Spring, to which many people are fond in Saxon countries.

Who has never blown those white, hairy spheres which contain the seeds of dandelion? Their easy dispersion allowed the plant, native to northern Europe, to spread around the whole world. Many people world-wide have taken advantage of its medicinal properties.

PROPERTIES AND INDICATIONS. The leaves and root of dandelion contain a bitter component similar to that of chicory, to which the plant

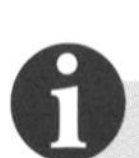

Coffee Substitute

A substitutive infusion for coffee is prepared with the ***toasted roots*** *of the dandelion. The advantage is that this infusion lacks any noxious effect of coffee.*

It has a pleasant flavor, and ***has almost all the medicinal properties*** *of the plant.*

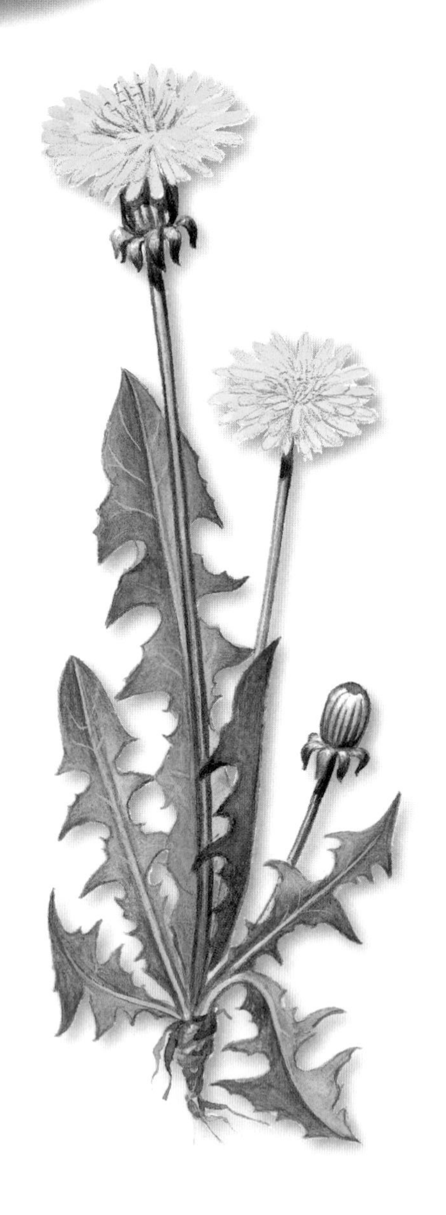

Description. *Vivacious plant of the Compositae family, growing up to 30 cm high, with deeply toothed or lobular leaves growing from the base. Flower stems also grow from this base, and in their tip there is a bright yellow flower head.*

Parts used. *Leaves and root.*

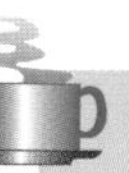

Preparation and Use

INTERNAL USE

❶ **Salads.** Its pleasant, gently sour flavor is good gently in Spring salads in which dandelion can play an important role as an ingredient. These salads will have appetizer and depurative properties. They can be dressed with lemon and oil.

❷ **Fresh juice.** Pressing or grinding its leaves and root. Take two or three spoonfuls before every meal. When a significant **depurative** effect is needed, the treatment must last for one to one and a half months, in Spring.

❸ **Infusion,** with 60 g of leaves and root per liter of water. Drink one cup before every meal.

owes its invigorating and digestive properties, as well as inuline. The leaves also contain flavonoids, coumarinic substances, and vitamins B and C. The properties of the dandelion are as follows:

• **Appetizer, digestive, and stomachic invigorator.** It increases the secretions of all digestive glands, promoting digestion and improving digestive ability [❶,❷,❸]. The dandelion increases the production of saliva and gastric, intestinal, and pancreatic juices, as well as bile. Moreover, it stimulates the muscles of the whole digestive system. Hence, it accelerates and stimulates all digestive processes, both physical and chemical.

• **Choleretic** (increases bile production) and **cholagogue** (promotes the emptying of the gall bladder). Its action on the liver and the gall bladder is similar to that on other digestive organs, though more intense. It is ***one of the plants with most active action on biliary functions,*** so it is especially recommended for people suffering from the following disorders:

- **Hepatic insufficiency, hepatitis, and cirrhosis.** It can ***increase bile*** production ***up to three*** times, relieving liver congestion and easing its disintoxicating function.
- **Biliary dyskinesia.** Gall bladder disorders.
- **Cholelithiasis** (gall stones). Though dandelion is not able to dissolve the calculi, it promotes a better function of the gall bladder while a ***definitive treatment*** is applied.

• **Diuretic and depurative.** One of its strongest effects. The dandelion increases the production of urine, and promotes the elimination of acid metabolic waste. It is recommended for people suffering from gout and arthritis [❷]. As the French saying goes, "Dandelion cleans the kidney filter, and dries the liver sponge."

• **Mild laxative,** non irritating. It is especially useful for intestinal atony. Its laxative properties, along with the **depurative** effect, make of this plant a good remedy for eczema, rashes, furuncles, and cellulitis, which are often caused by internal toxicity due to constipation [❶,❷,❸].

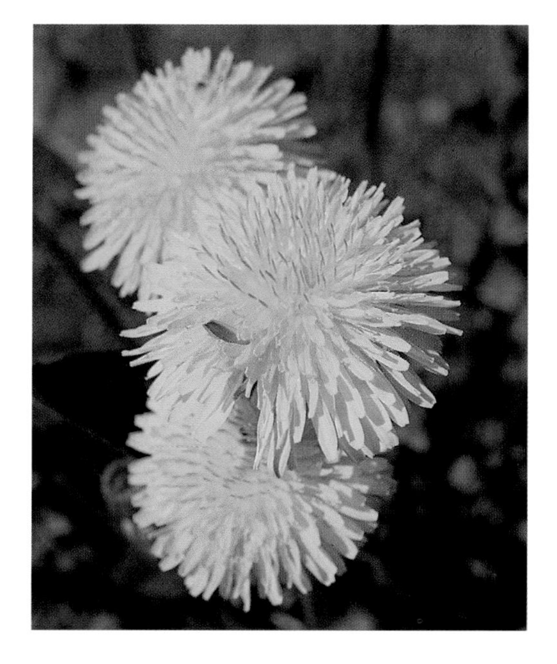

13

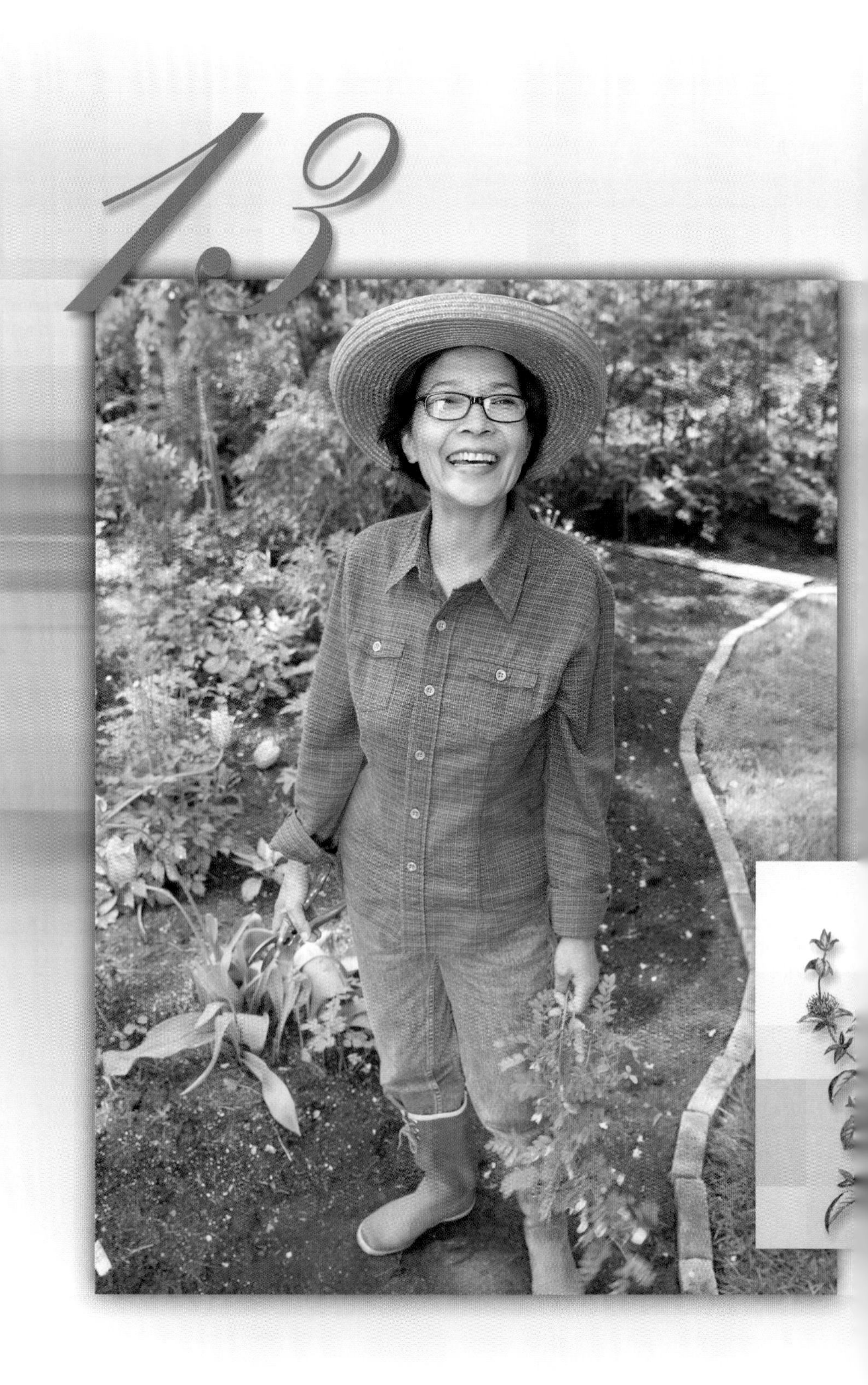

Plants for the Stomach

DISEASES	PAGES
Ache, stomach	208
Acidity, stomach	206
Belches, see Stomach gas	207
Bloated stomach	207
Chronic gastritis	208
Digestion, disorders, see Dyspepsia	207
Dyspepsia	207
Gas, stomach	207
Gastric juice, lack of	206
Gastritis	209
Gastritis, chronic	208
Hypochlorhydria, see Lack of gastric juice	206
Lack of gastric juice	206
Nervousness, stomach	208
Stomach ache	208
Stomach acidity	206
Stomach gas	207
Stomach nervousness	208
Stomach ulcer	209
Ulcer, stomach	209
Vomiting	208

PLANTS	PAGES
American pennyroyal	227
Anise	230
Chicory	212
Chinese cinnamon	215
Cinnamon tree	214
Coriander	216
Cumin	218
European pennyroyal	226
False acacia	232
Fenugreek	234
Gentian	220
Ipecac	210
Laurel	224
Lavender cotton	233
Lemon verbena	225
Quassia	229
Rock's tea	223
Saffron	217
Speedwell	235
Star anise	222
Turmeric	219
Wild marjoram	228
Wormseed	211

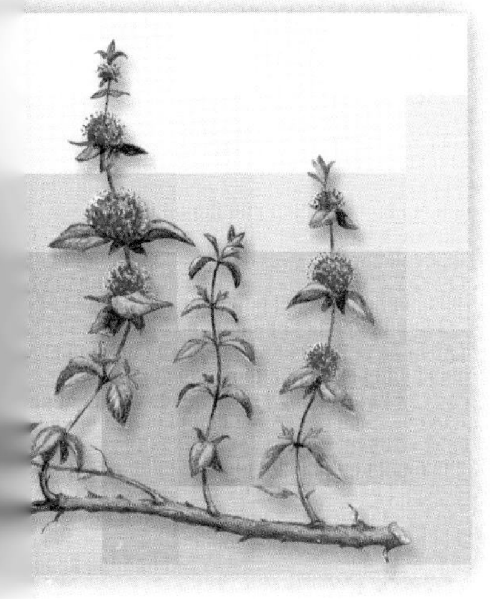

THE STOMACH is very sensitive to the action of medicinal herbs, perhaps because, when they are taken orally, they have to spend some time inside that digestive organ.

Most plants act **directly on the mucous membrane** covering the inner layer of the stomach. Some plants provide a **protective coat** of mucilage, such as the false acacia. Other plants dry and **reduce the inflammation** of the gastric mucous membrane since they have astringent properties, such as burnet or Lady's mantle. Still others balance any **excess of acidity,** such as carrot, cassava, or pumpkin.

Nonetheless, there are also some plants which

act on the stomach **through the blood;** after passing into the blood when in the intestine. The stomach walls have many blood vessels through which a high amount of blood flows. Certain vegetal active components need blood in order to exert their action, such as angelica, licorice, or milfoil. Hence, these active components do not exert their action when passing through the stomach, but after being absorbed into the blood.

Every day the stomach manufactures up to four liters of **gastric juice,** which basically consists of water, hydrochloric acid, pepsin, mucoproteins, and an antianemic factor, known as Castle's intrinsic factor. Many medicinal herbs increase the production of gastric juice, without irritating or inflaming the stomach mucous membrane, thus promoting and accelerating all digestive processes.

Medicinal herbs also exert a notable healing action toward **gastric ulcers,** the most frequent ailment of the stomach. Licorice, cabbage (almost all varieties), and calendula are outstanding because of their ability to heal ulcers; false acacia, cassava, flax, and psyllium are important plants which exert a protective action on the gastric mucous membrane. These herbs coat the inside of the stomach to prevent its walls from being in touch with the corrosive hydrochloric acid of the gastric juices.

STOMACH ACIDITY

Definition

This symptom is also known as **pyrosis,** and it appears through a sensation of burning, which is usually located in the commonly called "stomach mouth," which anatomically is the part of the digestive tract which joins the esophagus and the stomach. The stomach always has a required acidity level for digestion, however it is not perceived as acid. Acid sensation is actually perceived in the esophagus, when stomach acid flows up, leaving the stomach and reaching the lower area of the esophagus.

Phytotherapy

Phytotherapy provides us with plants able to protect the digestive mucous membrane, and to absorb or neutralize acid excess. Unlike antacid medicines, medicinal herbs do not present ***backlash effects*** (increase of acidity after the medicine effects have passed).

Psyllium

FALSE ACACIA	Emollient, protects mucosa from acid excess
PSYLLIUM	Protects digestive mucosa
FUCUS	Absorbs gastric juice and decreases acidity

LACK OF GASTRIC JUICE

Definition

Gastric juice is necessary for digestion, although most of its components are later reabsorbed in the intestine. A lack of gastric juice affects in a negative manner all digestive processes, causing **bloated** stomach, intestinal **fermentation,** and even **anemia.**

Phytotherapy

Some medicinal herbs can increase the production of gastric juice by ***stimulating the secreting glands.*** As a rule, all ***bitter*** plants, and all ***spices and seasoning or flavoring plants,*** increase the production of gastric juice.

Before administering any herb to increase gastric juice production, ***an accurate diagnosis of the cause*** of the lack of gastric juice is required, so that any malignant ailment may be adequately treated.

CINNAMON TREE	Increases production of gastric juice and stomach motility
TURMERIC	Stimulates secretion of gastric juice
GENTIAN	Its bitter principles excitate secretion of all digestive glands
EUROPEAN PENNYROYAL	Favours digestive processes
MILFOIL	Due to its bitter principle, increases juice secretion

BLOATED STOMACH

Definition

This disorder is also known as **hypotonia or gastric ptosis.** It is caused by dilatation of the stomach due to an **excess** of food or **obstacles** when emptying. However, in most cases this ailment has **physical constitution** causes. It usually happens to tall, thin people, of leptosomatic constitution, and shows itself through **gastric dyspepsia's** symptoms.

Phytotherapy

The medicinal herbs recommended here invigorate the stomach and stimulate its emptying, thus contributing to alleviation of the discomforts of gastric ptosis.

PEPPERMINT	Digestive, invigorant
GENTIAN	Powerful stomach invigorant
MUGWORT	Stimulates stomach emptying

Licorice

STOMACH GAS

Gas in the stomach is frequently produced by **nervous** causes or **diet transgressions.** These plants have ***carminative*** properties, that is to say, they eliminate any excess gastric gases or flatulence. As in any other case, the ***causative agent*** must be ***always identified.***

LICORICE	Eliminates gas and fights stomach belches
CARAWAY	Fights intestinal gas and belches
FENNEL	Promotes expulsion of digestive gas
BASIL	Calms excess of gas and belches
MARJORAM	Antiflatulent, calms nervous spasms of the stomach

DYSPEPSIA

Definition

This is a disorder which shows itself through **difficult digestion,** a bloating or painful sensation in the stomach, flatulence, and burning, usually after meals. The term dyspepsia also describes any **mild epigastric discomfort,** whether located in the stomach, the biliary channels, or the intestine.

Causes

Bad digestion or **gastric dyspepsia** may be ***caused by* alimentary, nervous, or functional reasons.** Actually, in this case there is no organic damage to the digestive system. However, it may be also caused by ***organic* reasons,** such as gastric or duodenal **ulcer,** stomach **cancer,** pyloric valve **stenosis** (a narrowing of this valve, at the base of the stomach) and other severe ailments.

Treatment

Of course, ***unhealthy diet habits*** which frequently cause dyspepsia, such as incorrect chewing; excess of food, especially fatty food; toxic substances such as tobacco, alcoholic beverages, or coffee; ***must be corrected*** in all cases.

NETTLE	Stimulates digestive juice secretion and stomach motility
LICORICE	Calms acidity and makes bloated stomach sensation disappear
FENNEL	Promotes stomach emptying and digestion
GERMAN CAMOMILE	Alleviates nausea and vomiting, increases appetite
PEPPERMINT	Invigorates digestive processes
WINTER SAVORY	Increases appetite, promotes digestion, eliminates gas
BOLDO	Promotes digestion, appetizer
ROCK'S TEA	Digestive, astringent
LEMON VERBENA	Digestive, antispasmodic, carminative
EUROPEAN PENNYROYAL	Promotes digestive processes, increases juice secretion
MILFOIL	Digestive tonic, increases production of gastric juice
ALOE	Appetizer, stomachic
CINCHONA	Appetizer, invigorator, fights intestinal fermentation

STOMACH ACHE

The most frequent causes of stomach aches are **dyspepsia**, gastro-duodenal **ulcer,** and **gastric nervous** (neuritis stomach). These plants contribute in an effective, physiological way to alleviate stomach aches, however they must ***only be administered after the causative agent*** of the aching has been ***identified.***

ORANGE TREE	Calms gastric aches with a nervous cause
LICORICE	Calms acidity and stomach ache
PSYLLIUM	Mucilage it contains creates a protective layer on the stomach and intestine

VOMITING

Besides the herbs mentioned here, all those with ***antispasmodic*** properties are useful, since they prevent stomach spasms which are usually associated with vomiting. Of course, the ***causative agent*** of vomiting ***must always be identified.***

BALM	Antispasmodic, sedative, digestive
MILK THISTLE	Calms sickness and vomiting when travelling
SAGE	Digestive, antispasmodic, calms vomiting and cholic pains

CHRONIC GASTRITIS

Definition

Diagnosis of chronic gastritis must be based on a stomach biopsy. This disease is more commonly the sign of some underlying disorder such as gastric or duodenal ulcers, iron deficiency anemia, or other diseases that involve the stomach. It can be also related to a decrease in gastric juice production.

Phytotherapy

These plants ***invigorate*** digestive functions and ***promote the regeneration*** of the atrophied gastric mucosa, which is the most important symptom of chronic gastritis.

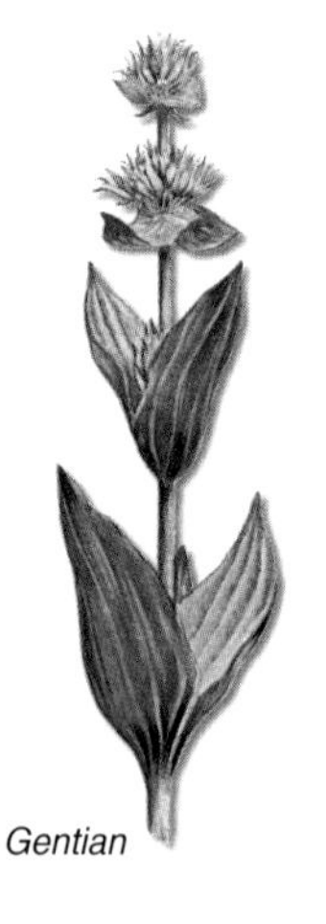
Gentian

TURMERIC	Stimulates production of gastric juice
GENTIAN	Increases secretion of all digestive glands
MILFOIL	Invigorates digestive organs, increases motility and juice secretion in the stomach

STOMACH NERVOUSNESS

Definition

Emotional states have a decisive influence on stomach functions through the autonomic nervous system. This fact was experimentally proven by Pavlov with his famous dogs. Almost half of the total amount of visits to digestive specialists have nervous causes.

Phytotherapy

These plants combat stomach **spasms** and **balance** the autonomic nervous system, thus avoiding gastric discomfort caused by an excited emotional state.

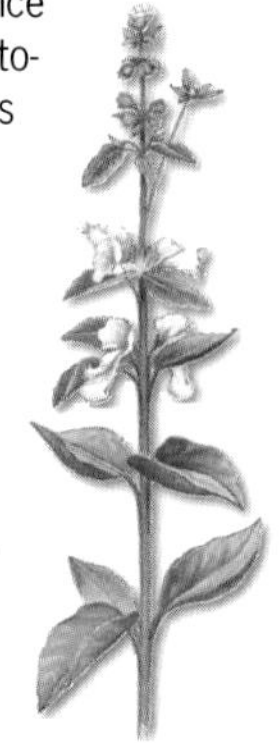
Basil

ORANGE TREE	Calms stomach spasms, sedative
VALERIAN	Sedative, calms pain, antispasmodic, decreases anxiety
BASIL	Calms gastric spasms, enhances slow digestion caused by nervous stress
MARJORAM	Calms nervous spasms of the stomach and heavy digestion
WILD MARJORAM	Sedative, antispasmodic, carminative

GASTRITIS

Definition

Gastritis is an inflammation of the stomach lining that can be **caused** by many factors, including irritation by agents such as drugs, alcohol, and chemical products and medicines (especially aspirin and other anti-inflammatory substances); food which is too hot or too cold, inadequate chewing caused by tooth problems or fast swallowing; and bacterial and viral infections, such as hepatitis and influenza.

Treatment

Besides **correcting the causes,** treatment of gastritis requires a **mild diet** (which may include raw, well chewed meals), and administration of one or several of these plants with **soothing and protective** properties.

LICORICE	Calms acidity and dyspepsia
FLAX	Anti-inflammatory and emollient, promotes regeneration of damaged digestive mucosa
PSYLLIUM	Creates a protective layer inside the digestive tract
CALENDULA	Cicatrizant and anti-inflammatory on the digestive mucosa

STOMACH ULCER

Definition

Also known as ***gastro-duodenal*** and ***gastric ulcer,*** since it commonly occurs in the stomach wall, and in the duodenum near the junction with the stomach. It is a pitting of the stomach mucous membrane, often from 0.5 to 2 cm in diameter, which may heal and open again several times during the year.

Causes

It may be ***caused*** by **exogenous** (listed in the gastritis epigraph) or **endogenous** reasons, related to organic constitution.

Hydrochloric acid of the gastric juice is one of the causative agents of ulcers. Certain micro-organisms also play a role in ulcer formation.

Phytotherapy

The plants here mentioned can decisively contribute to healing gastro-duodenal ulcers, though ***healing will never be complete as long as the causative agents are not eliminated.***

LICORICE	Eases acidity and dyspepsia, creates a protective layer on the stomach mucosa
FALSE ACACIA	Protects the stomach mucosa from an excess of acid
FLAX	Anti-inflammatory and emollient, promotes regeneration of damaged digestive mucosa
PSYLLIUM	Creates a protective layer inside the digestive tract
CALENDULA	Healing and anti-inflammatory on the digestive mucosa
ROSE	Calms stress related to the genesis of ulcers
FUCUS	Absorbs excess of acidity
NONI	Anti-inflammatory and ulcer healing

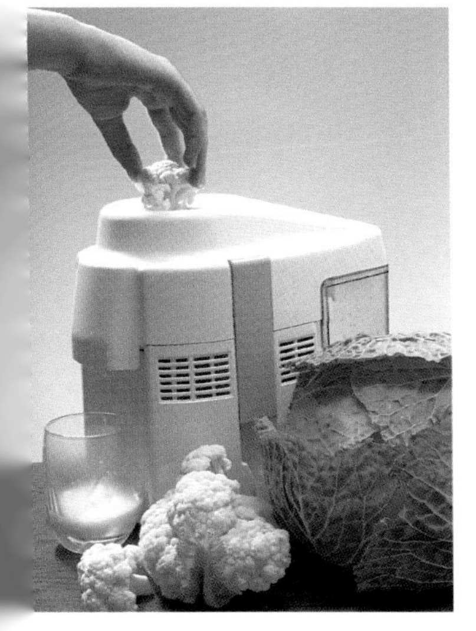

In addition to the plants mentioned in this chapter, raw cabbage juice has notable antiulcer and wound healing properties on the stomach.

It has been proven that some peptic ulcers were healed after drinking from half to one glass of cabbage juice before meals for three weeks.

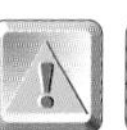
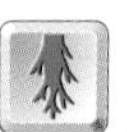
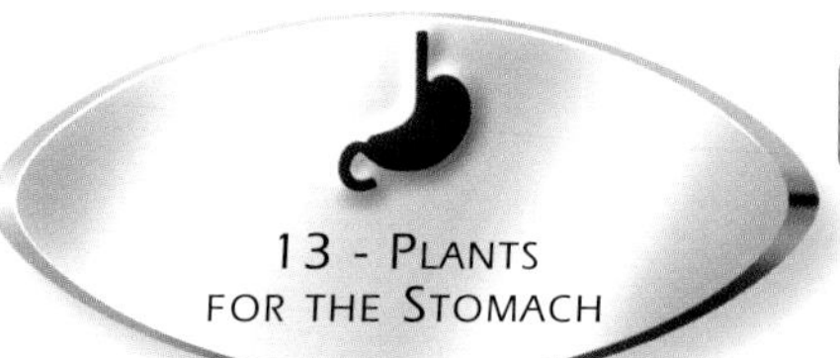

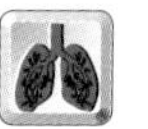
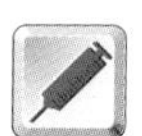

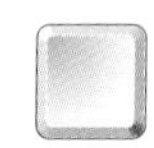

Ipecac

Vomitive, expectorant, and antidysentery

IN 1912 the active components of ipecac were discovered. Since then it has been part of ***many pharmaceutical preparations.***

PROPERTIES AND INDICATIONS. The root of ipecac contains emetine and other alkaloids, as well as ipecac acid and saponins. Its properties are as follows:

- **Emetic.** Ipecac, because of emetine, easily induces vomiting [❶,❷]. It is used to empty the stomach in the case of **poisoning,** when a stomach washing cannot be performed.
- **Expectorant.** The saponins and emetine it contains give the plant an intense expectorant action in low doses, thus being part of ***several bronchial syrups* [❸].**
- **Amoeba-killer.** Emetine destroys amoebas which cause amoebic dysentery and amoebic disorders of the liver. In these cases, the use of any of the existing ***pharmaceutical preparations*** based in emetine is recommended.

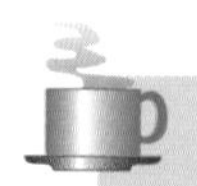

Preparation and Use

INTERNAL USE

❶ **Root powder.** Four to six grams dissolved into water. For children, the dose is 0.1 g per year of age. It is used as a **vomitive and expectorant.**

❷ **Syrup.** One or two spoonfuls will induce vomiting.

❸ **Infusion** with 8 g of ground root in 250 ml of water. As an expectorant, take only four or five spoonfuls per hour, to avoid vomiting.

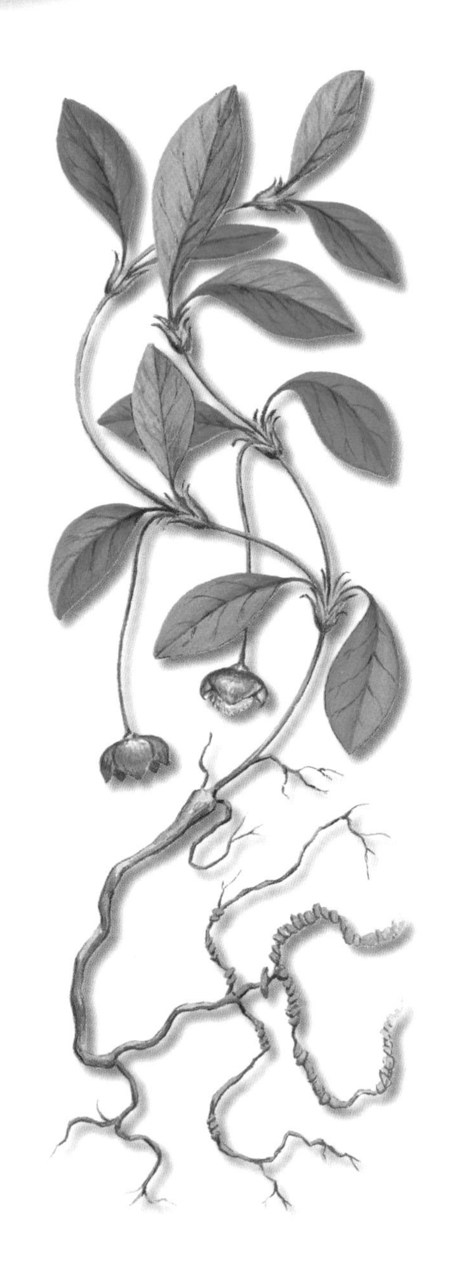

Description. *Shrub of the Rubiaceae family, growing from 30 to 50 cm high, with large, ringed roots, and small, white flowers growing in terminal heads.*

Parts used. *The root, ground into powder.*

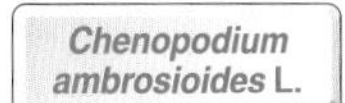
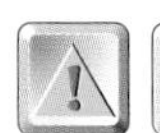
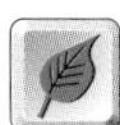
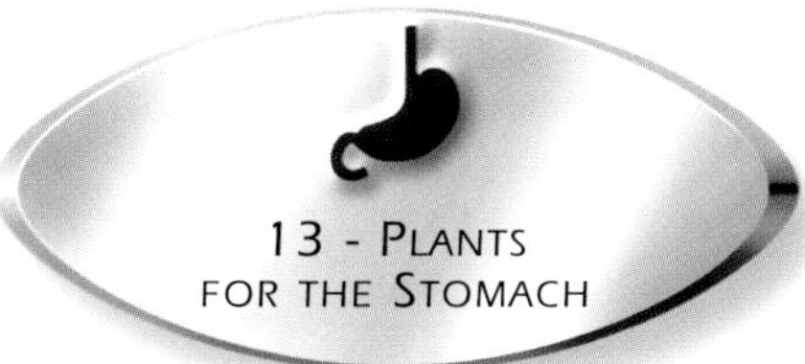

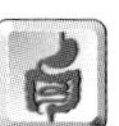
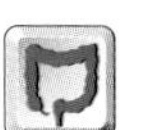
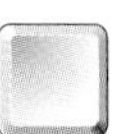
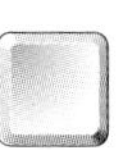

Wormseed

Digestive invigorator and vermifuge

BEFORE THE ARRIVAL of Columbus, ancient Mexican people used wormseed because of its medicinal properties. Its leaves and flowers have a strong scent due to the essential oil they contain.

PROPERTIES AND INDICATIONS. The essence of wormseed consists of terpene hydrocarbons (cymene, limonene, terpinene, etc.) and ascaridol. It has the following properties:

- **Stomachic invigorator and carminative** (expels intestinal gas). Its use renders good results for indigestion, stomach ache, flatulence, and lack of appetite **[❶]**.
- **Anthelmintic and vermifuge** (kills intestinal parasites). This is its most important application **[❶]**. It is ***very effective*** against ascaris and anchilostomae, but not so against tapeworms and oxyuridae.

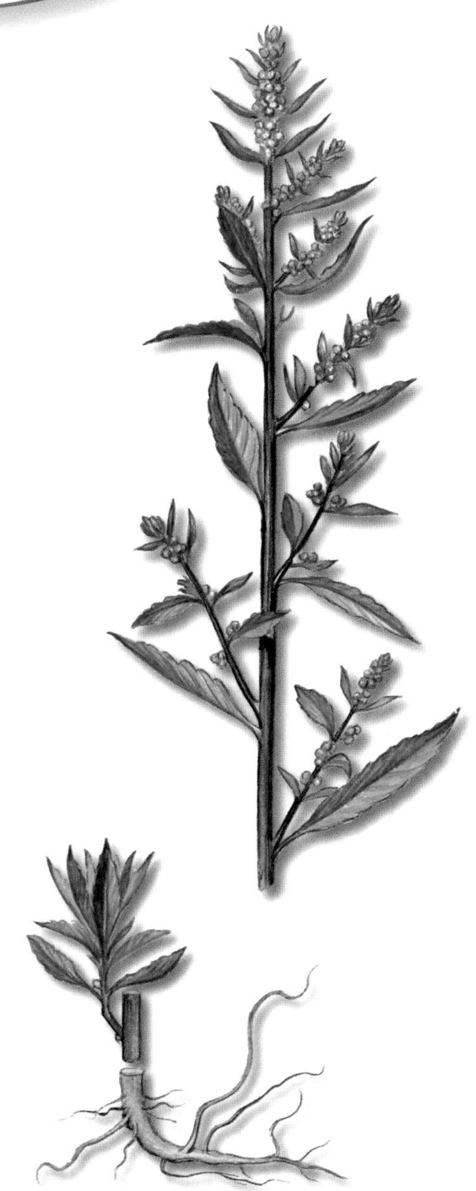

Preparation and Use

INTERNAL USE

❶ **Infusion** with 15-20 g of leaves and flowers per liter of water. As a **stomachic invigorator,** drink a cup after each meal. As a **vermifuge,** drink a cup in the morning on an empty stomach, for three days. Administer a **laxative after** every wormseed intake in order to expel parasites (for instance, castor bean, aloe, or cascara sagrada).

Description. *Herbaceous, vivacious or evergreen plant of the Chenopodiaceae family, which grows from 40 to 100 cm high, with branched stem and yellowish or greenish small flowers growing in terminal spikes.*

Parts used. *Leaves and flowers.*

Chicory

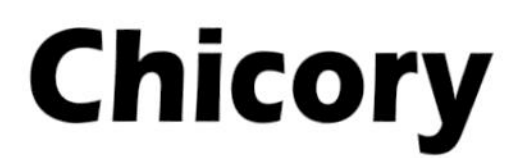

A coffee substitute which lacks undesirable effects

CHICORY is a gift for walkers. Until midsummer roadsides retain the sky blue color of chicory flowers, contrasting with the golden landscape. The plant can hardly go unnoticed, even for people who have never heard about it. It seems to suggest, "Use me! Enjoy my properties!"

Chicory is ***one of the most beneficial*** plants known, since in addition to its extraordinary medicinal properties it can pleasantly substitute coffee. In times of shortage, when expensive coffee cannot be bought, this humble plant can be used. It has not been highly appreciated, perhaps because it is abundant and cheap.

"Chicory," some people say with nostalgia. "We drank it during the war, when there was no coffee."

It is interesting to point out that, in this case, the substitute—chicory—is better than the original product—coffee.

PROPERTIES AND INDICATIONS. Already known and used by ancient Egyptians, Galen said of this plant that it was a ***"friend of the liver."*** Both its roots and its leaves contain in-

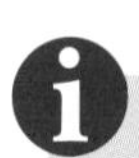

Chicory Coffee

Chicory root, gathered in Fall, is then dried, toasted, and ground in order to obtain "chicory coffee". It can be mixed with oat malt, which gives the infusion a more pleasant flavor.

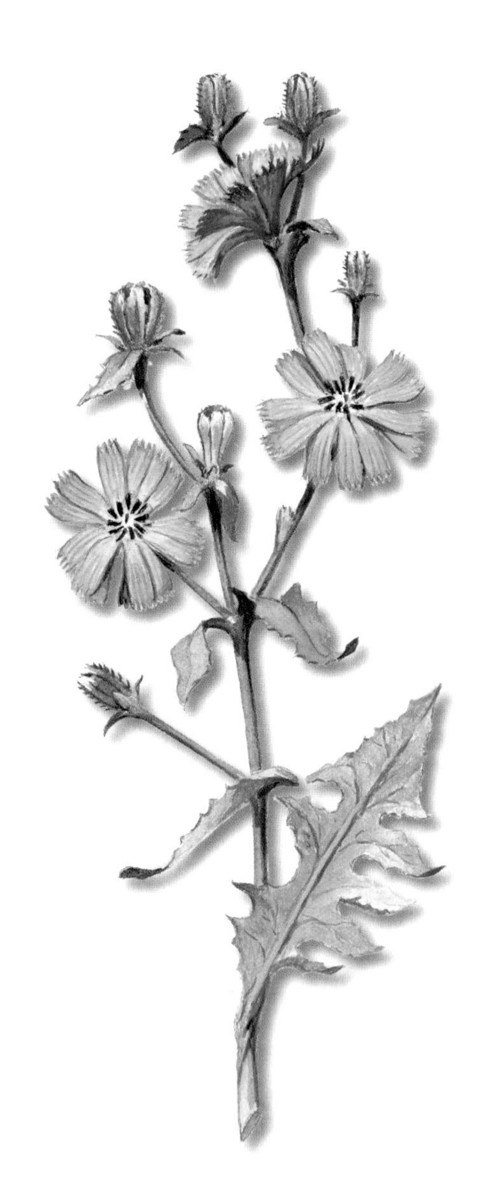

Description. *Herbaceous, vivacious plant of the Compositae family, with an upright stem which grows from 50 to 60 cm high. Its beautiful blue flowers have petals with five pointed ends, and close at night or when the weather is bad. All parts of the plant, including its latex, have a bitter flavor.*

Parts used. *Young leaves and root.*

Preparation and Use

INTERNAL USE

❶ **Salads.** Raw leaves of chicory, when cut before the plant blooms, have a pleasant, bitter flavor. Excellent wild plant salads are prepared with these leaves and with dandelion and garlic, dressing the dish with lemon juice and olive oil.

❷ **Fresh juice.** People who want more powerful effects can drink fresh juice of chicory leaves, which is obtained by pressing them on a cloth, or with an electric blender. It has a bitter flavor, but **it will encourage a strong appetite.** for lack of appetite, half a glass is recommended before each meal.

❸ **Infusion,** with 30 g of fresh leaves and root per liter of water. Drink two or three cups daily: as an **appetizer** before meals, and as a **digestive,** after meals. This infusion must not be sweetened to achieve the most benefit from its stimulating bitter flavor.

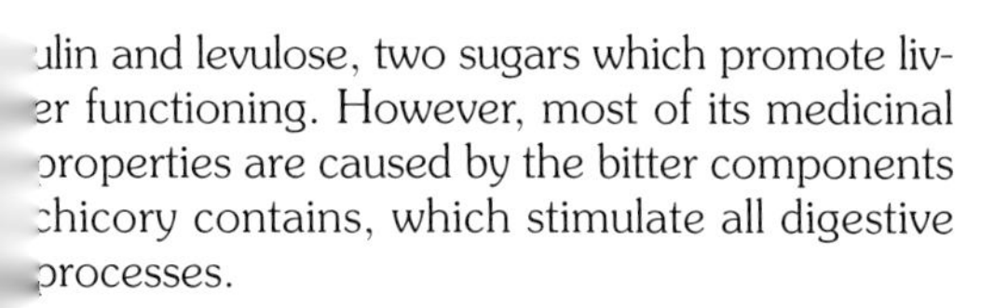

ulin and levulose, two sugars which promote liver functioning. However, most of its medicinal properties are caused by the bitter components chicory contains, which stimulate all digestive processes.

• In the stomach it has **eupeptic** properties, increasing the production of gastric juice. Hence, it is useful for **bloated stomach,** if one drinks a chicory infusion after meals instead of a teaspoonful of bicarbonate. Moreover, when taken before meals, it has **powerful appetizer** properties, **giving an appetite to children and adults.**

• In the liver it promotes bile secretion (**choleretic** action), which is needed for digestion of fat. It also **activates circulation and relieves liver congestion.**

Chicory also activates intestinal motility (**laxative** action). A cup of chicory infusion on an empty stomach in the morning helps combat intestinal laziness and constipation. It also has mild **vermifuge** properties, which help to expel intestinal parasites.

Therefore, the recommended uses of chicory are as follows: **lack of appetite, gastric atony, bloated stomach, biliary dyspepsia** caused by a deficient functioning of the gall bladder, **liver congestion, portal hypertension, constipation, and intestinal parasites [❶,❷,❸].**

Chicory also has mild **diuretic and depurative** properties, hence it is recommended for **gout and arthritis [❶,❷,❸].**

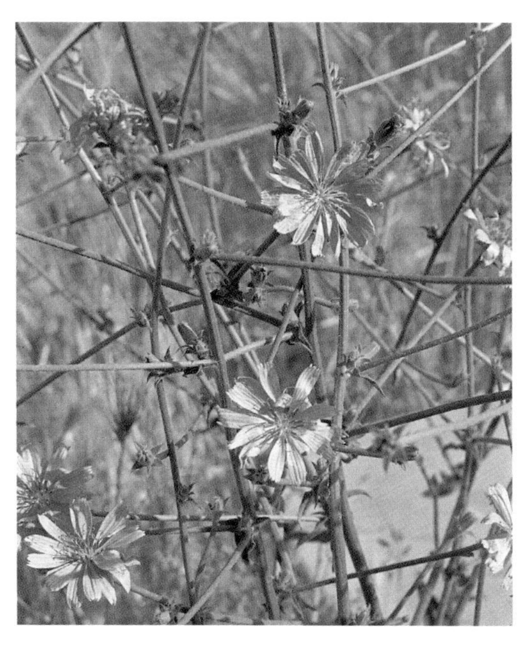

The appreciated chicory root is gathered after the plant has grown its typical, flamboyant blue flowers.

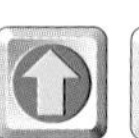

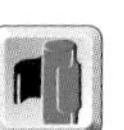

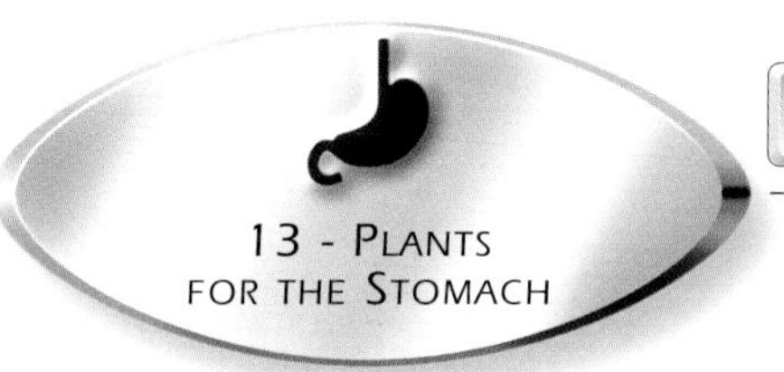

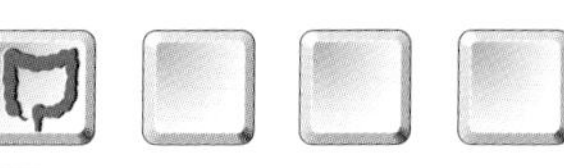

Cinnamon Tree

An exquisite seasoning which helps digestion

THE CINNAMON TREE was already known and used in China in 2500 B.C., and was as valuable as gold. Ancient Egyptians used it to embalm mummies. Cinnamon was also appreciated among Israelites, and Moses was told to use it, as well as other spices, in making the Holy Ointment which the objects of the Sanctuary and the priests were to be anointed with (Exodus, 30: 23).

Cinnamon was one of the spices which indirectly contributed to the Discovery of America, since Columbus sailed towards the West with the aim of making the journey to India shorter. It was cinnamon, and other appreciated Eastern products, that were brought from India. During the seventeenth and eighteenth centuries, cinnamon became the most profiting spice for Dutch traders.

Cinnamon, which is still highly valued in modern cuisine, has notable medicinal properties.

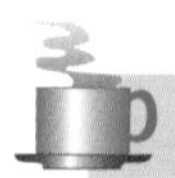

Preparation and Use

Internal use

❶ **Seasoning.** Both cinnamon sticks and ground cinnamon are used as seasoning in different cookery recipes.

❷ **Infusion.** When a more intense effect is required, prepare an infusion with one or two cinnamon sticks of about 10 cm long per cup of water. Add a couple of lemon slices, if wanted. It is more effective when not sweetened. Drink a cup after each meal.

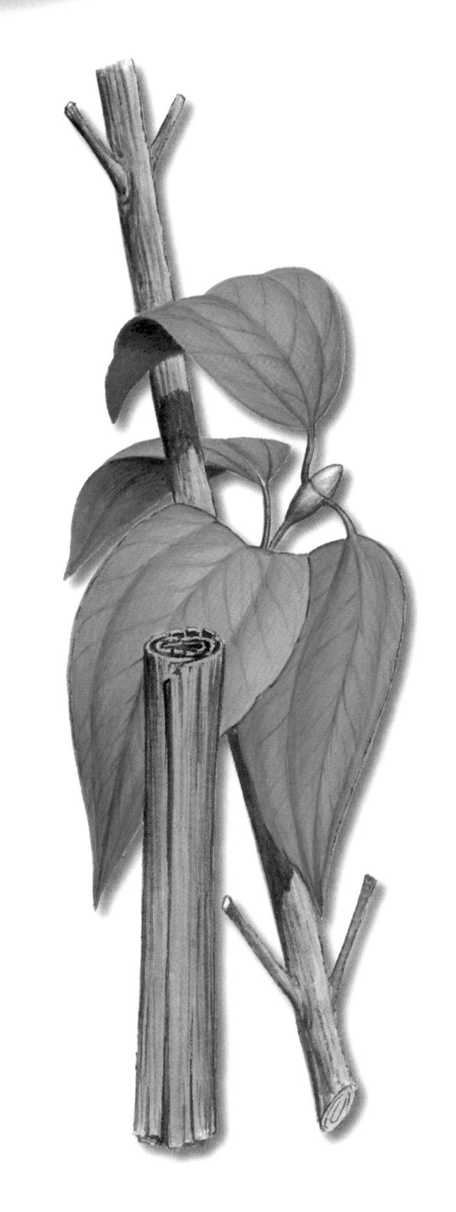

Description. *Tree of the Lauraceae family, growing up to 10 m high, from whose young branches an inner dun bark is obtained. It has large, oval-shaped leaves, and white or yellow flowers. The whole plant has a pleasant scent.*

Parts used. *The inner bark of young branches, which once fermented is known as cinnamon.*

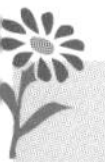

Chinese Cinnamon

Besides true Ceylon cinnamon, there is Chinese cinnamon *(Cinnamomum aromaticum* Nees = *Cinnamomun cassia* Blume), which is obtained from the bark of a similar tree, the Chinese cinnamon tree, with a more spicy, less delicate flavor. However, it has **the same medicinal properties** as Ceylon cinnamon. John Russell wrote in his book *Book of Nature,* published in the fifteenth century: "Cinnamon is for noble classes, and Chinese cinnamon for village people."

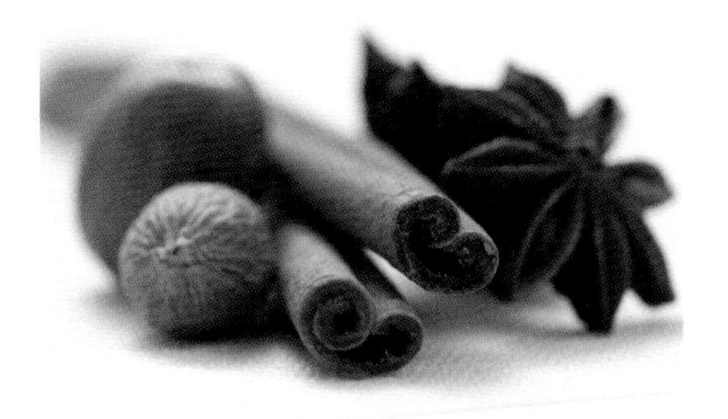

Some people consider it an aphrodisiac. However, having no scientific evidence of this fact, we think that cinnamon acts by suggestion.

PROPERTIES AND INDICATIONS. The bark of the cinnamon tree contains essential oils, cinnamal dehide, tannin, terpenes, calcium oxalate, starch, and traces of mucilage. The combined action of all these substances gives the bark **digestive, stomachic invigorating, and appetizer** properties. It increases the secretion of gastric and intestinal juices, as well as stomach motility.

As a result of this invigorating action of cinnamon on the body, an increase in appetite, and an enhancement of the whole digestive functioning is produced. Its use is especially recommended for people suffering from **lack of appetite, bloated stomach** caused by gastric atony (dilated stomach), and **flatulence** caused by lack of gastric juice **[❶,❷]**.

On the other hand, its use is ***advised for against*** **gastro-duodenal ulcer sufferers,** since a feature of this ailment is an excess of gastric juice, which is determinant for ulcer formation.

Its content in tannin gives cinnamon a mild **astringent** effect.

Cinnamon can produce skin allergies in sensitive people.

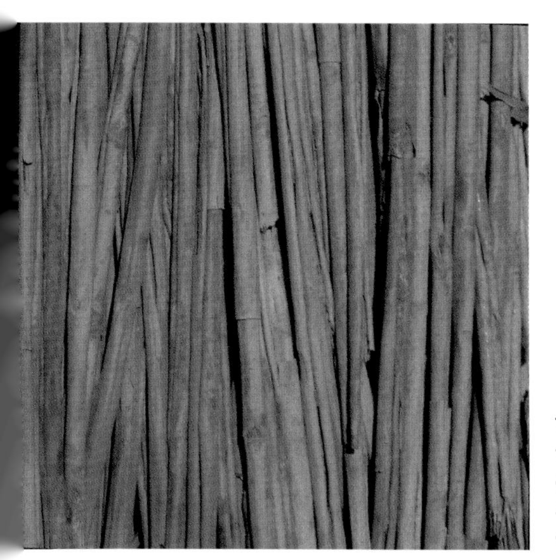

The bark of the cinnamon tree, in the form of cinnamon sticks or ground cinnamon, is an indispensable seasoning for rice with milk dishes, as well as in custard.

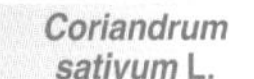

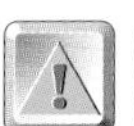
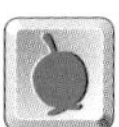
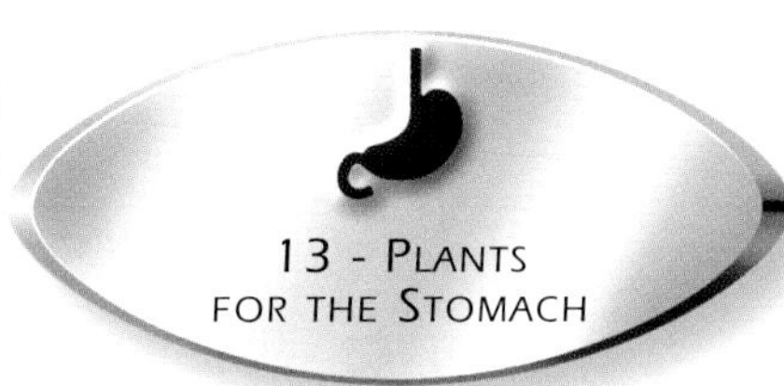

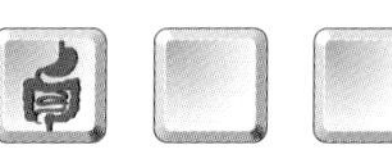

Coriander

Eupeptic and stimulant

EVEN THOUGH coriander is one of the medicinal plants which have been used for a very long time, and both the Assyrians and the Egyptians used it, the plant can provoke toxic effects on the nervous system (drunkenness) when taken in high doses. Coriander is highly appreciated as a seasoning.

PROPERTIES AND INDICATIONS. The fruits of coriander contain an essential oil rich in linalool, the active component to which the plant owes its properties.

- **Eupeptic.** It promotes digestion.
- **Carminative.** Eliminates gas.
- Mild **invigorator** of the nervous system, when taken in small doses.

In any of its methods of use [❶,❷,❸,❹], coriander is recommended for:

- **Digestive disorders.** Gastritis, pancreatic insufficiency, bloated stomach, lack of appetite, flatulence.

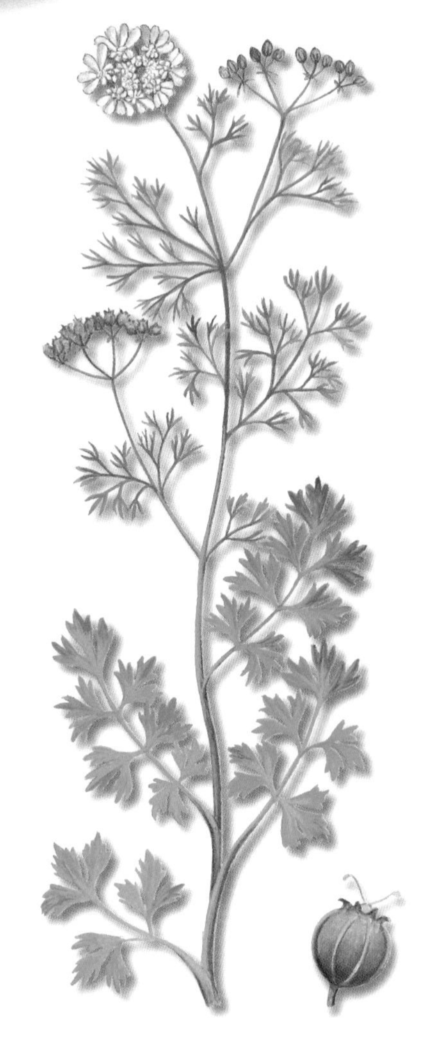

Description. Herbaceous plant of the Umbelliferae family, which grows from 20 to 60 cm high, with white or pink flowers. Its round fruits are from 3 to 5 mm in diameter.

Parts used. Only ripe fruits.

- **Convalescence** from infectious diseases, as an invigorator and stimulant of the appetite.
- **Halitosis** (bad breath) of people who consume garlic or onion, and of smokers.

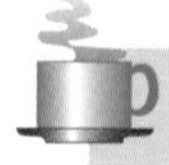

Preparation and Use

INTERNAL USE

❶ **Seasoning.** In diverse meals.

❷ **Infusion** with 30 g of fruits per liter of water. Drink a cup after each meal.

❸ Dry fruits **powder.** Take a teaspoonful (5 g) mixed with honey, after each meal.

❹ **Essence.** From one to three drops, three times a day.

Saffron

Appetizer and emmenagogue

SAFFRON ROSES, as its flowers are called, are pleasant colorful spots in any autumn landscape. The Egyptians, Israelites, and Greeks, highly valued saffron because of its medicinal properties. Later on, its properties were exaggerated to the point that Hetodt, a German physician of the seventeenth century, recommended saffron to heal any ailment, from toothache to the plague.

At present, it is more often used as a seasoning than as a remedy. It is the ***most expensive spice*** known.

PROPERTIES AND INDICATIONS. Saffron contains a bitter component (picrocine), a coloring substance (crocine), and an essential oil. It has **digestive, appetizer, and carminative** properties. Moreover, it is **emmenagogue** and can heal menstrual pain [❶].

When ***externally applied,*** a concentrated infusion [❷] is used to rub the gums of children, thus alleviating teething discomforts.

Preparation and Use

INTERNAL USE

❶ **Infusion** with some saffron strands per cup of water. Sweeten with honey, brown sugar or molasses (sugar cane honey).

EXTERNAL USE

❷ **Concentrated infusion** prepared with saffron enough to give a dark brown color to the water.

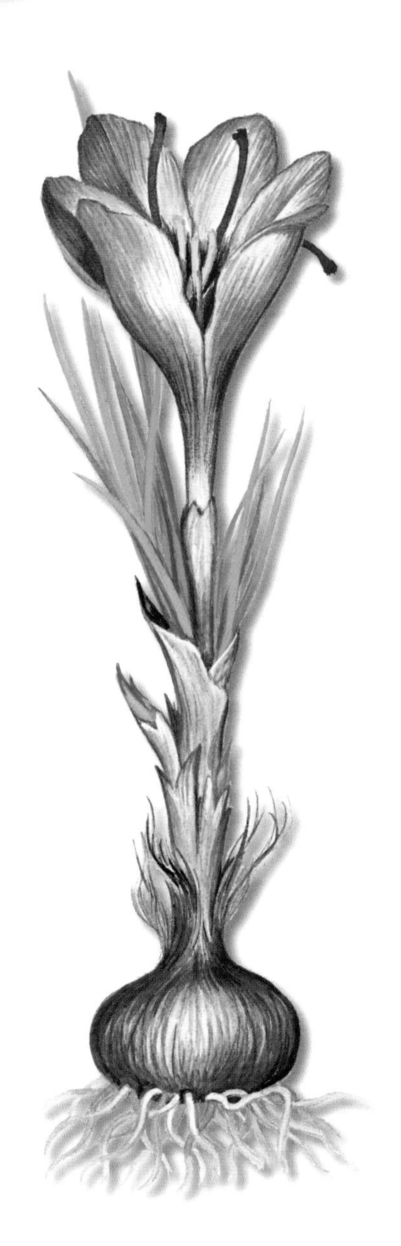

Description. *Bulbous plant of the Iridaceae family, growing from 10 to 15 cm high, with beautiful lilac-colored flowers, in the center of which there are three orange stigmas. These stigmas are the spice called saffron.*

Parts used. *The stigmas of its flowers.*

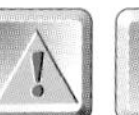
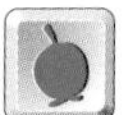
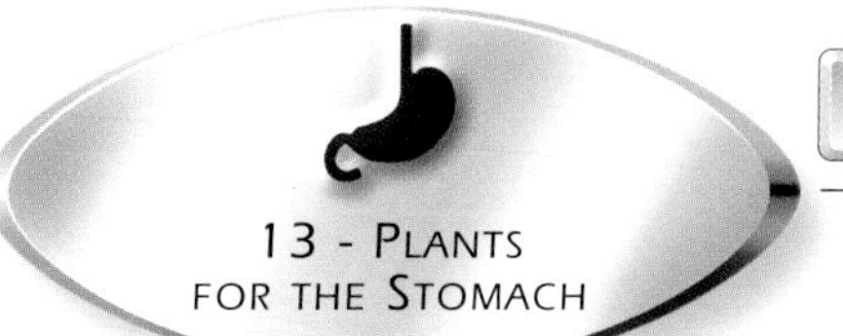

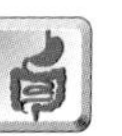
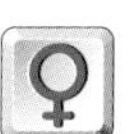
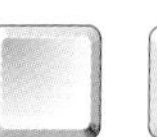
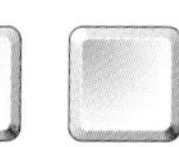

Cumin

Invigorates digestive organs

CUMIN was already used as seasoning or medicine by ancient Egyptians, as deduced from the fruits found in some tombs. In later centuries, its fruit has been substituted by the caraway, with similar properties though a milder flavor. However, cumin is still an excellent medicine and seasoning. Salads dressed with cumin have an exquisite aroma, and are able to satisfy the most discriminate taste.

PROPERTIES AND INDICATIONS. Cumins contain 10 % of ethereal oil, and an essence whose most important active component is cuminic aldehyde or cuminal. They have **appetizer, digestive, and carminative** (eliminate intestinal gas) properties **[❶,❷,❸]**.

Cumin also has a mild **galactogenic** effect, which means they promote the secretion of milk for breast-feeding women **[❶,❷,❸]**.

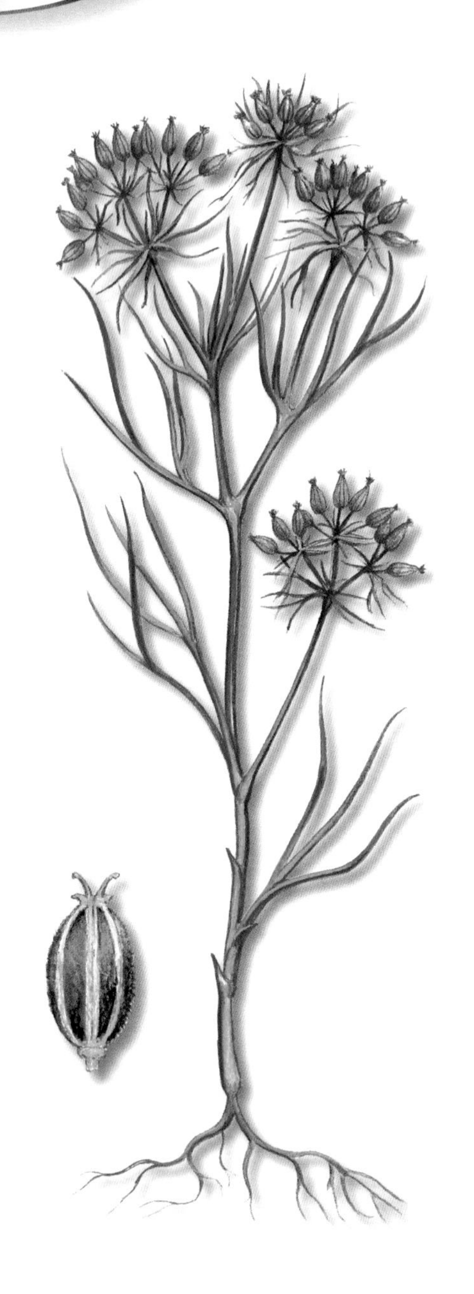

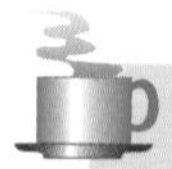

Preparation and Use

INTERNAL USE

❶ **Infusion** with 2 g of whole or slightly ground cumins (the tip of a teaspoonful) per cup of water. Drink a cup after lunch, and another after supper. Babies can have two or three spoonfuls of this infusion after each meal.

❷ **Powder.** The recommended dose is one gram after each meal, dissolved in water or milk.

❸ **Essence.** Take from one to three drops, three times a day.

Description. *Annual herbaceous plant of the Umbelliferae family, which grows up to 50 cm high, with very fine leaves. Its fruits, 5-6 mm large, grow on the tip of the umbels radii, and have marked, rough haired stretches.*

Parts used. *The fruits.*

Turmeric

A eupeptic hot spice

IT MAY SEEM strange, but hot spices and sauces play a very important role in tropical diet, since the preservation and digestion of food in warm climates would be difficult. Good use of spices proves popular wisdom once more.

Turmeric is one of the most important ingredients of curry, a hot sauce which consists of turmeric, pepper, coriander, ginger, cloves, cardamom, cumin, and nutmeg. This makes an explosive mixture for unaccustomed stomachs!

PROPERTIES AND INDICATIONS. The rhizome of turmeric contains an essential oil, coloring substances, a bitter component, organic acids, resin, and starch.

It is a **stomachic invigorator** similar to ginger. Turmeric increases the production of gastric juice, thus easing digestion for **lack of appetite or dyspepsia.** It is also used for chronic **gastritis** and **hypochloridria** (lack of hydrochloric acid in the stomach).

It also has **cholagogue [❶,❷]** (promotes the emptying of the gall bladder), and **carminative** (eliminates intestinal gas) **[❶,❷]** properties.

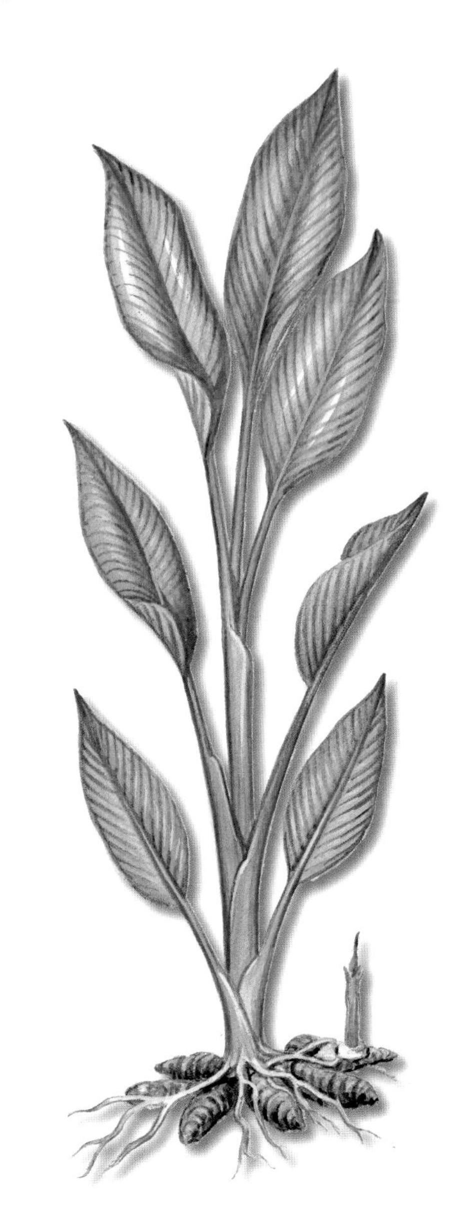

Description. *Vivacious plant of the Zingiberaceae family, which grows up to one meter high. It has from five to ten large leaves, with long petiole. Its flowers are white or yellowish, and its rhizome is gross, up to 10 cm in diameter.*

Parts used. *The rhizome (underground stem).*

Preparation and Use

INTERNAL USE

❶ **Infusion** with 15-20 g of rhizome per liter of water. Drink a cup during meals.

❷ **Powder.** One gram a day, distributed into three intakes.

Gentian

Excellent digestive invigorator

"LOOK WHAT a straight and beautiful plant!" a walker says to his companions.

"Look! It is a gentian!" said a member of the group who knew botany basics. "Its root is highly appreciated because of its medicinal properties."

"Let us pull it up and take it home!"

"No!" says the botanist."You may not believe it, but this plant grows so slowly that it takes ten years to bloom, and can live up to more than fifty years. Leave it here. If we need it later, this gentian will be here to offer its virtues. Perhaps it will live longer than any of us!"

This behavior could be an example for people fond of nature. Some greedy plant-gatherers have brought gentian to the edge of extinction. It is a pity when its huge root, which can weigh up to six kg, has been systematically gathered in order to give its aroma to alcoholic beverages.

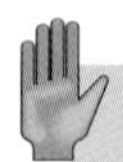

Warning

Gentian ***must not be mistaken*** *with* ***white hellebore*** (Veratrum album *L.), a* ***toxic plant*** *which grows near gentian. The difference is that the former has alternate leaves (which grow singly from the stem), hairy on the underside, as well as white flowers with a quite unpleasant smell.*

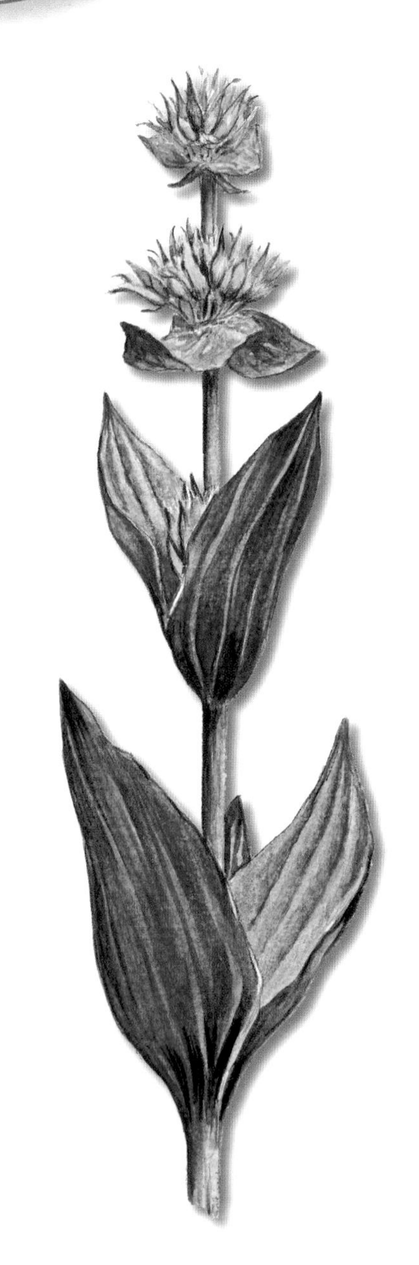

Description. *Vivacious plant of the Gentianaceae family, growing from 60 to 100 cm high, with a smooth, upright stem from which large, oval-shaped flowers grow opposite one another. Its flowers are bright yellow and grow in clusters.*

Parts used. *The root.*

Preparation and Use

INTERNAL USE

❶ **Cold extract.** Put a piece of gentian root (the size of a hazelnut: around 10 g) in a liter of cold water. Steep for four or five hours. Drink three cups daily before meals. Some anise seeds can be added during the process so as to reduce its intensely bitter flavor; however sweetening is advised against.

❷ **Decoction** with 10 g per liter of water. Boil for an hour. Drink half a cup before each meal.

❸ **Powder or dry extract.** The recommended dose is 0.5-1 g before each meal.

Dioscorides, the great Greek physician and botanist of the first century, wrote in his *De Materia Medica:* "The root of gentian, when drunk with water, helps people suffering from liver and stomach disorders." At present, some twenty centuries later, the observation of that Greek scholar is still valid, and gentian is ***one of the most appreciated appetizer and digestive plants.***

PROPERTIES AND INDICATIONS. The root of gentian contains diverse bitter components, among which the most outstanding are gentiopicrin and amarogentin. The latter is the ***bitterest substance*** known. When dissolving a part of amarogentin in fifty million parts of dissolvent, its bitter flavor still is noticeable. Moreover, gentian contains diverse sugars, tannin, and pectin.

Its properties are as follow:

- **Stomachic invigorator.** The bitter components of the gentian root excite the secretion of all digestive glands, including saliva glands. Thus, they increase appetite (**appetizer** properties), and promote digestion (**eupeptic** or digestive properties). The gentian root is especially recommended for chronic gastritis with lack of gastric juice (hypochloridria), ptosis, or gastric atony, indigestion, vomiting, lack of appetite, and in convalescence from febrile diseases **[❶,❷,❸]**. According to Dr. Leclerc, ***"Invigorator but not irritant."***
- **Choleretic and cholagogue.** It stimulates the secretion of bile in the liver, and its emptying into the duodenum. It is recommended for liver congestion and biliary dysfunction. **[❶,❷,❸]**.
- **Febrifuge.** Gentian does not have strong febrifuge properties, however it is ***especially effective*** for **malaria.** It has been proven that gentian is able to destroy the protozoa that cause malaria, and which attack red blood corpuscles. It can be used in association with quinine, and is particularly recommended for quinine-resistant malaria **[❶,❷,❸]**.
- **Immunostimulant.** It stimulates defenses of the body. It has been proven that gentian root produces an increase of white blood corpuscle (leukocytes) production, thus a positive action in cases of immune system depression (lack of infectious resistance) is probable **[❶,❷,❸]**.

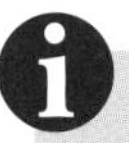

Gentian Liquor

We advise against the use of alcoholic preparations or liquors from gentian, since the negative effects of alcohol counteract the beneficial properties of the plant.

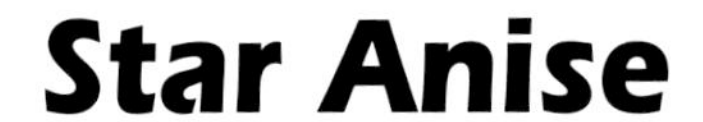

Star Anise

As digestive as anise, but more concentrated

THE TREE of the star anise resembles that of laurel in its beautiful appearance, and that of magnolia in its flowers. The whole tree has a pleasant aroma similar to that of anise, though more intense. The star anise was introduced in Europe in the late seventeenth century, when Eastern spices were most appreciated.

PROPERTIES AND INDICATIONS. The star anise, in spite of belonging to a different botanical family to that of common anise, has the same active component: an essence rich in anethole. Thus, its properties are similar to those of anise: **eupeptic** (promotes digestion) and **carminative** (eliminates intestinal gas and flatulence).

It is very useful [❶,❷] for heavy digestion, intestinal fermentation, and flatulence (excess of gas).

Due to its mild antispasmodic properties it alleviates the spasms of hollow internal organs (the stomach, the gall bladder, the intestine, the uterus, etc.).

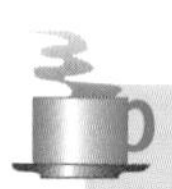

Preparation and Use

INTERNAL USE

❶ **Infusion.** The amount of plant needed is less than that of anise, since star anise is more concentrated. Two or three fruit per cup are enough. Drink two or three cups daily, after meals.

❷ **Dry extract.** The recommended dose goes from 100 to 300 mg a day.

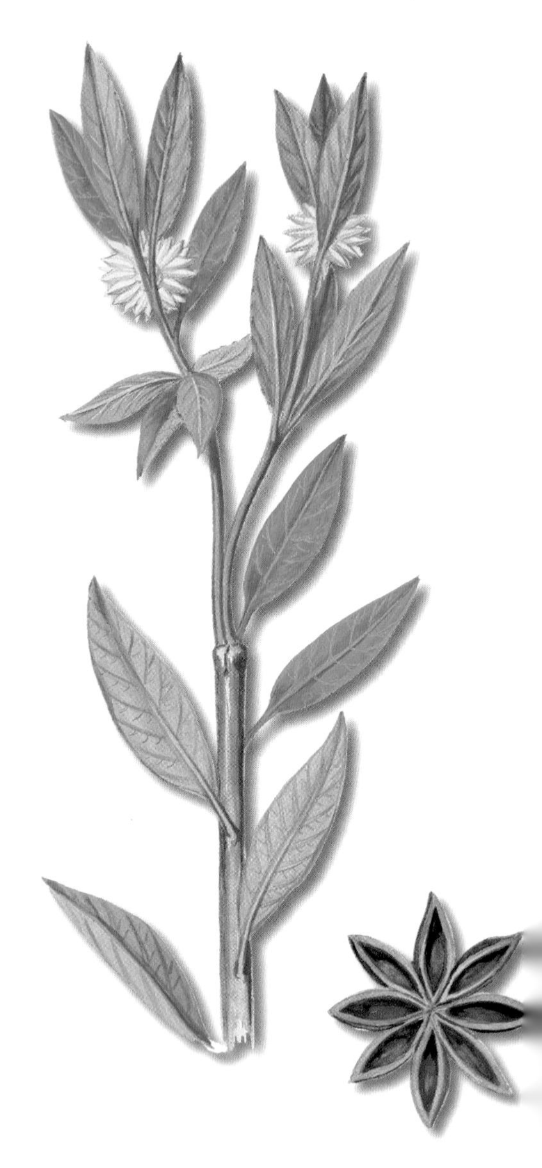

Description. *Evergreen tree of the Magnoliaceae family, which grows from two to five meters high, with white bark and spear-shaped leaves.*
The fruit is are star-shaped (eight or twelve points) and brown in color.

Parts used. *The fruit.*

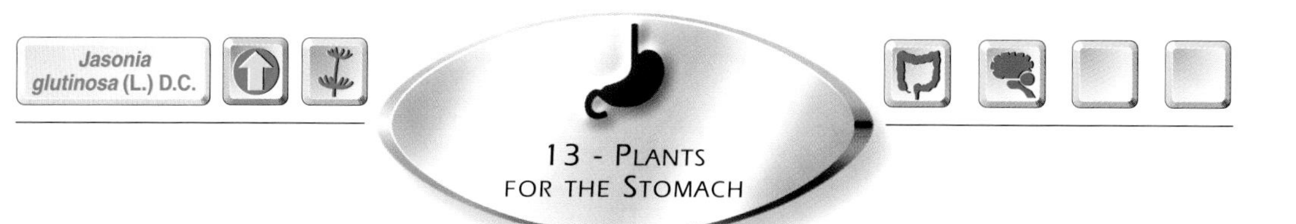

Rock's Tea

Stomachic and invigorating

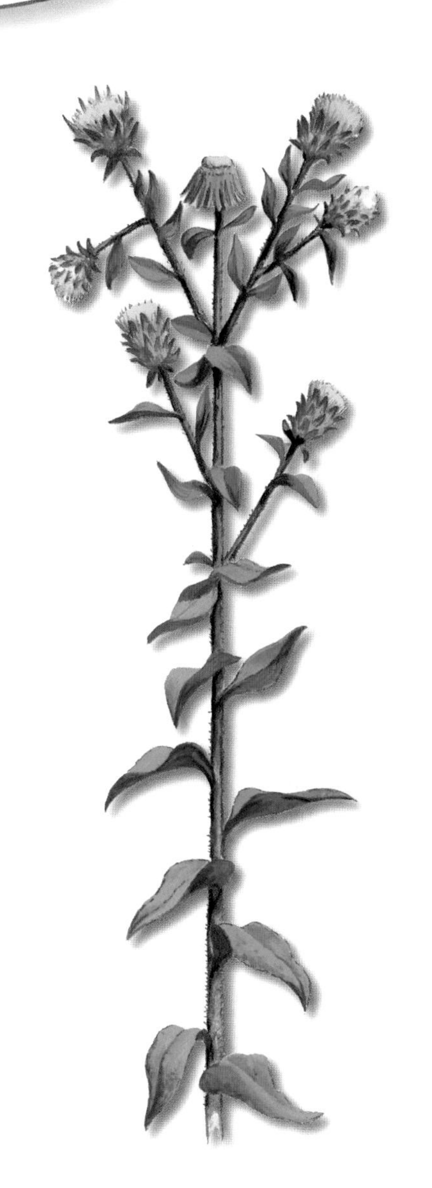

THE USE OF this tea is quite widespread in the Spanish region of Aragón. Herbal teas (infusions) made with this plant are highly valued, and have a slight camphor aroma, with a mildly bitter flavor. It can substitute common tea, and is better than the latter.

Dioscorides and other classic authors did not know about rock's tea, since it does not grow in eastern Mediterranean regions.

Properties and indications. Its composition is not well-known; however it has been proven that it does not contain caffeine or teaine. It contains an essence which gives the plant **digestive properties,** as well as abundant tannins which have **antidiarrheic properties [❶].**

- **Digestive problems.** Rock's tea is popularly used for upset stomach, indigestion, slow, heavy digestion, diarrhea, and intestinal fermentation [❶].
- **Nervous problems.** It also has an invigorating action, which lacks any irritant effects on the nervous system, unlike coffee or tea [❶].

Preparation and Use

Internal use

❶ **Infusion** with 20-40 g of plant per liter of water. Drink up to five cups daily after meals.

Description. *Vivacious plant of the Compositae family, which consists of a small woody base from which several stems grow from 20 to 40 cm high in the Spring every year. The whole plant is sticky and hairy. Its flowers are small, yellow, and gather in flower heads on the tip of the stems.*

Parts used. *The leaves and flower heads.*

Laurel

Promotes digestion and eases rheumatic aches

ROMAN EMPERORS, athletes, and victorious warriors wore laurel wreaths on their heads, which were supposed to protect them from lightning and evil forces.

PROPERTIES AND INDICATIONS. The active component which confers laurel its medicinal properties is the essential oil. The properties of laurel are as follows:

- **Appetizer, eupeptic** (promotes digestion) and **carminative** (eliminates gas in the digestive tract). It is thus recommended for people who suffer from lack of appetite, poor digestion, and bloated stomach **[❶]**.
- Mild **diuretic [❶].**
- **Emmenagogue** (stimulates menstruation) and **regulative of menstruation [❶]**.
- **Antirrheumatic and anti-inflammatory, very effective in external** applications. Laurel oil **[❷]** or laurel antirrheumatic balm **[❸]** prepared with its leaves are used for massaging in the case of stiff neck, lumbalgia, sciatic, ankle sprain, and other joint and muscle aches.

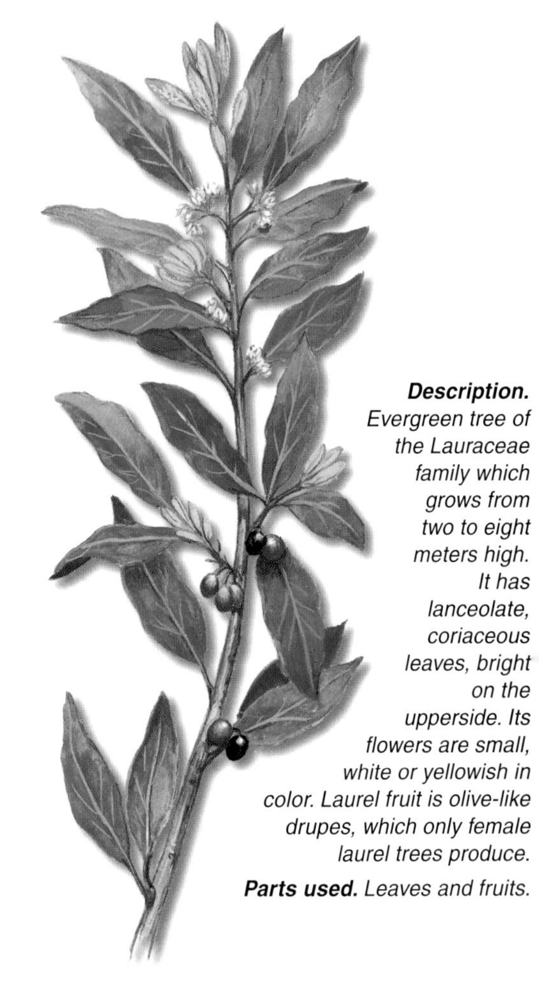

Description. *Evergreen tree of the Lauraceae family which grows from two to eight meters high. It has lanceolate, coriaceous leaves, bright on the upperside. Its flowers are small, white or yellowish in color. Laurel fruit is olive-like drupes, which only female laurel trees produce.*

Parts used. *Leaves and fruits.*

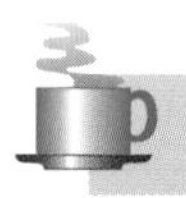

Preparation and Use

INTERNAL USE

❶ **Infusion** with 20-30 g of leaves per liter of water. A handful of ripe fruits can be added in order to achieve greater effectiveness. As an **appetizer,** drink a cup ten minutes before meals. As a **digestive,** drink a cup after each meal.

EXTERNAL USE

❷ **Laurel oil.** Put in cold extract for ten days under the sunlight, 30 g of laurel leaves per liter of olive oil. Apply as a lotion on the aching area. This oil is also effective as an insect repellent.

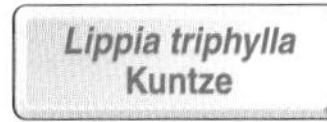

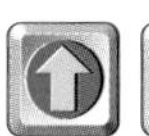
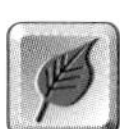
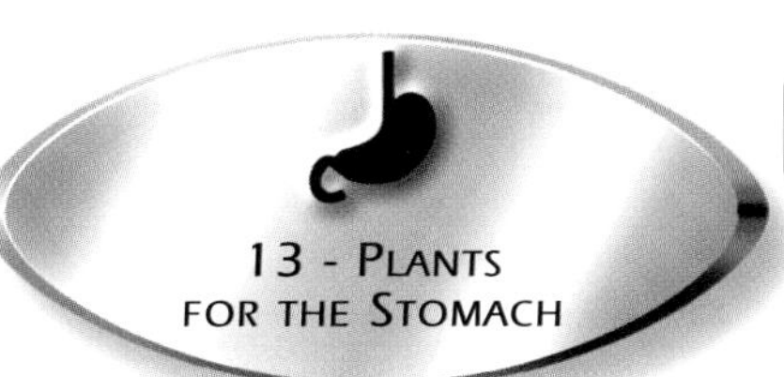

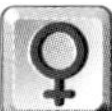
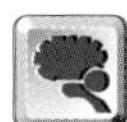
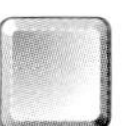
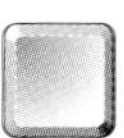

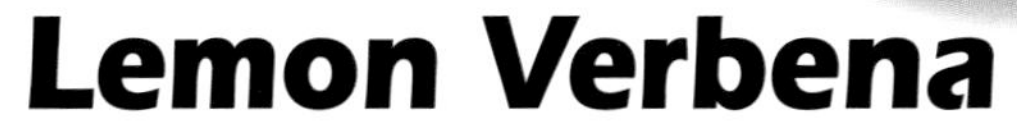

Lemon Verbena

Aromatic, stomachic, and sedative

LEMON VERBENA is another gift of the American flora, as well as tomato, potato, and many more. In Europe, lemon verbena has been cultivated since the eighteenth century.

Properties and indications. The whole plant, and especially its leaves, contain an essential oil which consists of more than one hundred substances, among which the most outstanding are citral, limonene, and caryophillene. This essence gives the plant **digestive, antispasmodic, and carminative** (promotes the expulsion of gas from the digestive system) properties.

Lemon verbena is recommended in the following cases:

• **Digestive disorders:** acute dyspepsia (indigestion or upset stomach) and chronic dyspepsia (slow digestion), and flatulence {❶}.

• **Menstrual pain** (dysmenorrhea), gall bladder and kidney **colic,** due to its antispasmodic properties {❶}.

• It is also recommended for different types of **nervous disorders, *especially*** for **anxiety** {❶}, since in many cases the results achieved are better than those of chemical tranquilizers, not causing side effects as the latter do.

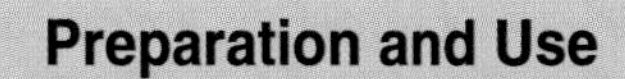

Preparation and Use

Internal use

❶ **Infusion** with 30 g of leaves per liter of water. Drink a hot cup after each meal. This infusion has a very pleasant flavor.

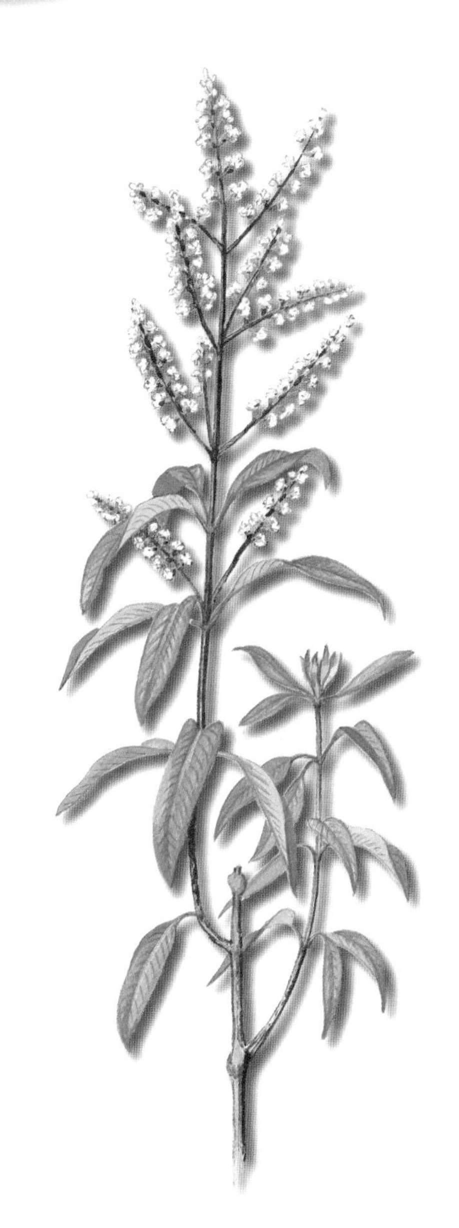

Description. *Small shrub of the Verbenaceae family, growing up to two meters high. It has lanceolate, rough leaves which have an intense lemon scent when rubbed. Its flowers are violet or lilac in color, and grow in bouquets.*

Parts used. *The leaves.*

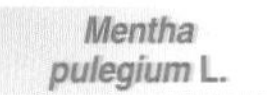

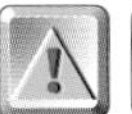
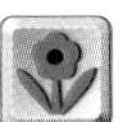
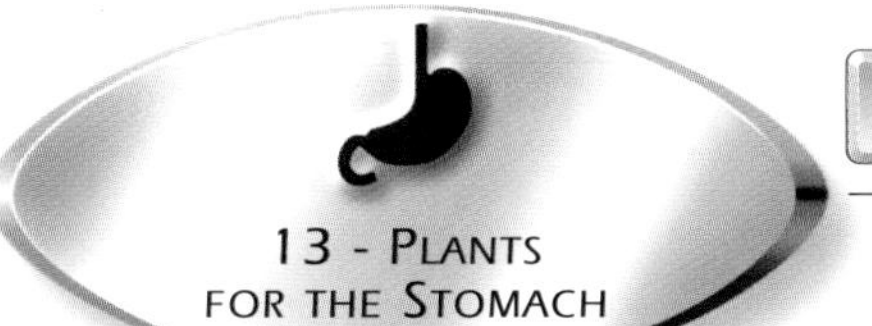

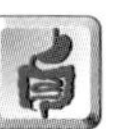
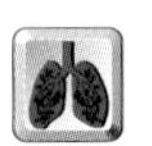
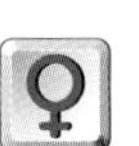
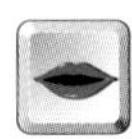

European Pennyroyal

A great friend of digestion

MANY YEARS before spray insecticide appeared, popular wisdom used pennyroyal sprays as insect repellents. Its name *pulegium* is a Latin word which means flea. Ancient Romans and Greeks already used the vapors of this plant to kill fleas.

The pennyroyal medicinal properties have been known for thousands of years. Dioscorides, the great Greek physician and botanist of the first century, said of this plant that "it has strength to heat, to achieve weight loss, and to digest."

"I am full up! I will have a cup of pennyroyal to help my digestion," a man in a restaurant said after an excellent meal.

"I will have one too. Pennyroyal helps 'clear' the head when one drinks alcohol...."

Indeed, pennyroyal helps in these cases. However, it would be better not to have to use it to treat the symptoms. Avoiding excess is wiser than healing the consequences, even with a natural remedy like herbal tea.

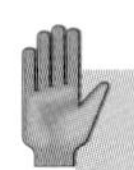

Warning

*Although pennyroyal is not advised against for **gastro-duodenal ulcer,** it must be used **with caution** and never in a period with ulcer attacks.*

The use of the plant, and particularly its essence in very high doses, may be dangerous.

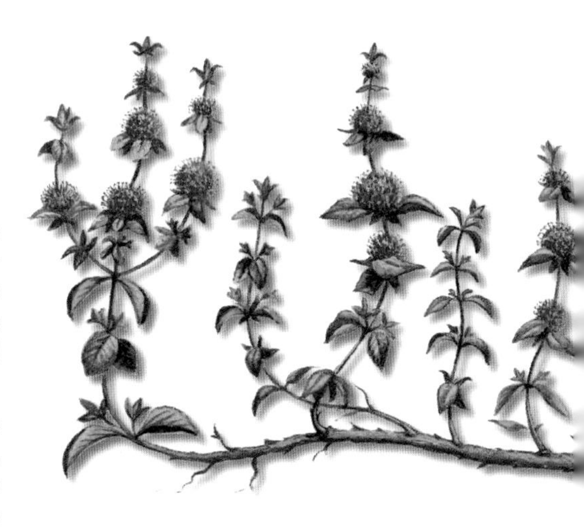

Description. *Vivacious plant of the Labiatae family, very aromatic, which grows from 25 to 40 cm high. Its flowers grow in the axils of the leaves, and are lilac, pink or white in color. Their aroma resembles those of lemon rind and peppermint.*

Parts used. *The whole plant.*

PROPERTIES AND INDICATIONS. The whole plant contains an essential oil (0.5%-1%) based on pulegone, an unsaturated ketone. It also contains menthone, limonene, and other ketones. Its properties are the following:

- **Digestive and stomachic invigorator.** Pennyroyal promotes digestive processes, increases the production of juices (gastric, pancreatic, intestinal), and stimulates the stomach and the small intestine action. It has **carminative** (eliminates excess of gas) properties, combats intestinal fermentation, and eases **headaches** caused by digestive disorders [❶]. It also increases bile secretion (**cholagogue** properties).

Its use is thus recommended whenever pro-

Preparation and Use

INTERNAL USE

❶ **Infusion.** After boiling a liter of water, add 10-20 g of pennyroyal and steep for some minutes. It may be sweetened with honey.

As **digestive invigorator,** drink a cup after every meal. For **bronchial afflictions or menstrual disorders,** drink a hot cup every other hour.

EXTERNAL USE

❷ **Mouth rinses** with a more concentrated infusion (30 g per liter).

❸ **Cleansings** with the aforementioned infusion.

moting digestive processes is required, such as for hypochloridria (lack of stomach juice), heavy digestion, excess of gas, and also gall bladder disorders (biliary dyskinesia).

- **Expectorant and antitussive.** It is useful for colds and whooping cough [❶].
- **Emmenagogue and antispasmodic.** It promotes menstruation and eases the pain which may accompany it [❶].
- **Vermifuge.** In order to expel intestinal parasites, drink a cup daily, with empty stomach, for five days [❶].
- **Antiseptic.** It is very useful in mouth rinses for bad breath or pyorrhea [❷], and also to wash skin wounds [❸].
- **Insecticide.** Put in your wardrobe some small bags with pennyroyal to repel moths. You can also kill pet fur parasites by rubbing pet hair with a pennyroyal concentrated infusion.

Besides promoting digestion, pennyroyal calms menstrual pains, especially in young women.

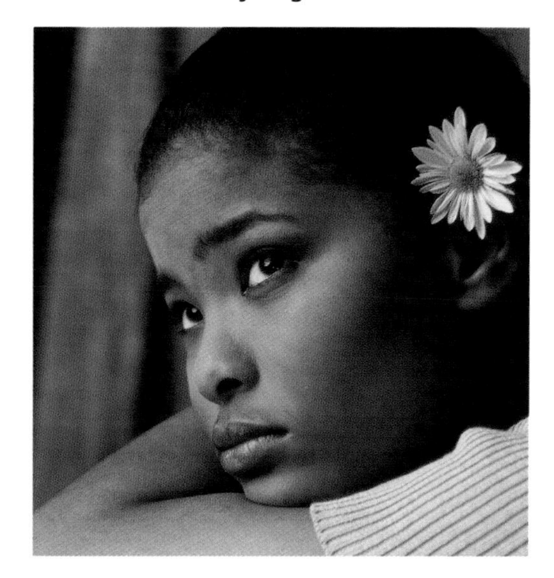

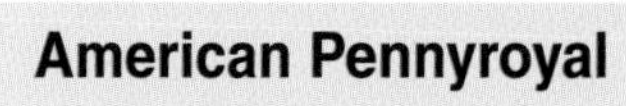

American Pennyroyal

American pennyroyal (*Hedeoma pulegioides* Pers.) grows in North America, and is **very similar** to common pennyroyal both in appearance and in **properties.**

North American natives used this plant to ease headaches and menstrual pains, as well as to heal wounds.

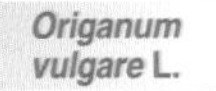

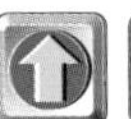
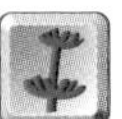
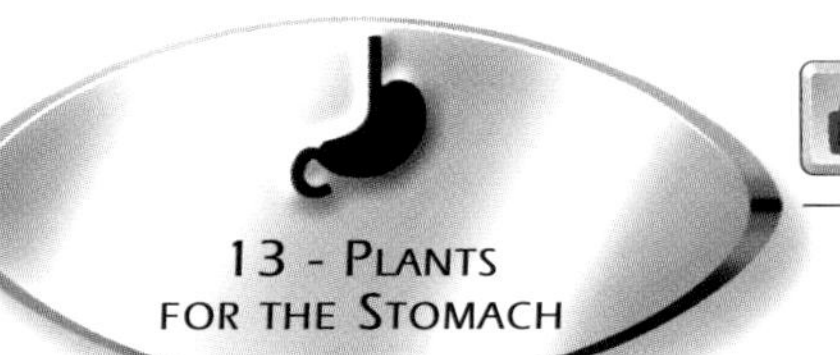

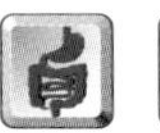
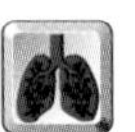
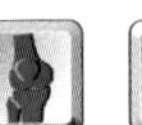
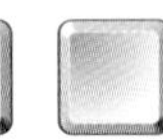

Wild Marjoram

Digestive and antirheumati

WILD MARJORAM is quite similar to marjoram, though unlike the latter, it grows wild as it name points out.

PROPERTIES AND INDICATIONS. The whole plant is rich in an essential oil which contains thymol and carvacrol, with **sedative, antispasmodic, and carminative** properties. Wild marjoram also contains flavonic substances and ursolic acid, which have antirheumatic properties. Its use is recommended for:

- **Digestive disorders:** dyspepsia (bad digestion) of nervous causes, flatulence, spasm or colic of the digestive organs [❶,❸]. Because of its carminative (combats intestinal gas) properties, it is a good seasoning in legume dishes, as well as pizza and soups [❶].
- **Respiratory afflictions** with dry or irritating cough, such as laryngitis (throat irritation) or whooping cough. Wild marjoram also has **expectorant, bechic, and antitussive** properties, both internally [❶,❷,❸] and externally [❹] used.
- **Muscular aches,** stiff neck, and lumbago, ***externally*** applied as poultices [❺] and in skin massage [❻].

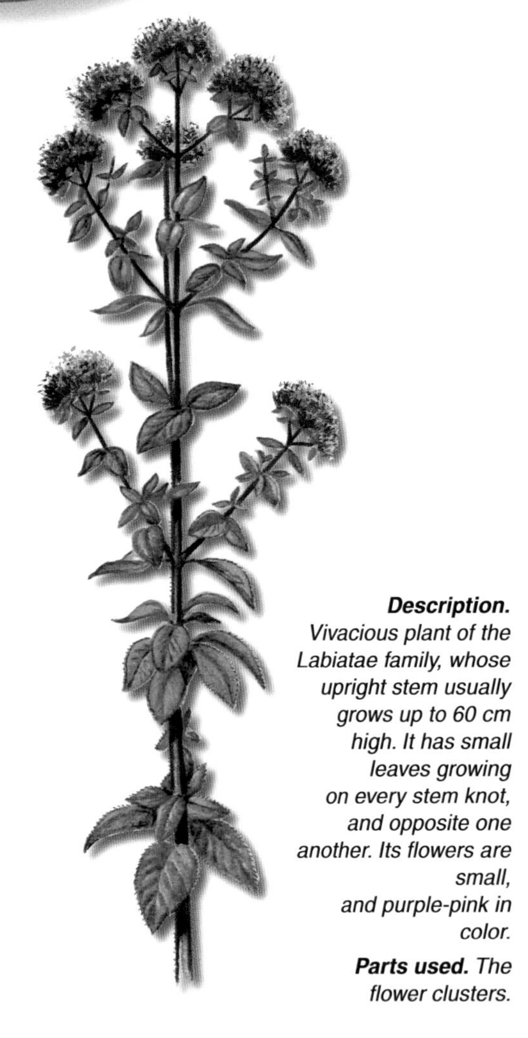

Description. *Vivacious plant of the Labiatae family, whose upright stem usually grows up to 60 cm high. It has small leaves growing on every stem knot, and opposite one another. Its flowers are small, and purple-pink in color.*

Parts used. *The flower clusters.*

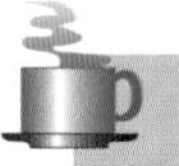

Preparation and Use

INTERNAL USE

❶ **Seasoning.** Dry leaves of wild marjoram are used in diverse cuisine recipes.

❷ **Infusion** with 15-20 g per liter of water. Drink one cup after each meal.

❸ **Essence.** The recommended dose is three intakes daily, of 4-6 drop each.

EXTERNAL USE

❹ **Steam inhalations,** for respiratory afflictions, with a handful of plant into the boiling water.

❺ **Poultices.** The mashed plant is heated in a bowl, then applied wrapped in a cloth on the aching or inflamed area.

❻ **Massage.** With some drops of essence directly applied to the affected area.

Quassia

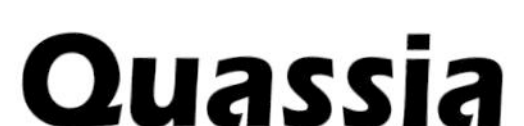

Digestive and febrifuge

QUASSI was the name of a Guyana native slave who, in 1756, revealed his secret for healing fever to a Dutch officer who protected him. That secret was quassia, a Guyanese shrub.

PROPERTIES AND INDICATIONS. The plant contains resin, mucilage, pectin, tannin, and an alkaloid called quassine, with a bitter flavor. This is its most important active component to which the plant owes its properties and indications.

- **Stomachic invigorator, digestive, and appetizer.** It increases the secretion of gastric juice, and promotes the functioning of the gall bladder **(cholagogue** action) **[❶]**. The quassia renders ***very good results*** for **dyspepsia** (difficult or slow digestion).
- **Febrifuge.** This plant is very useful in treating of tropical fever **[❶]**.
- **Vermifuge.** When applied as an enema it eliminates oxyuridae (parasites) which are usually located in the anus and rectum, where orally taken medicines cannot act **[❷]**.

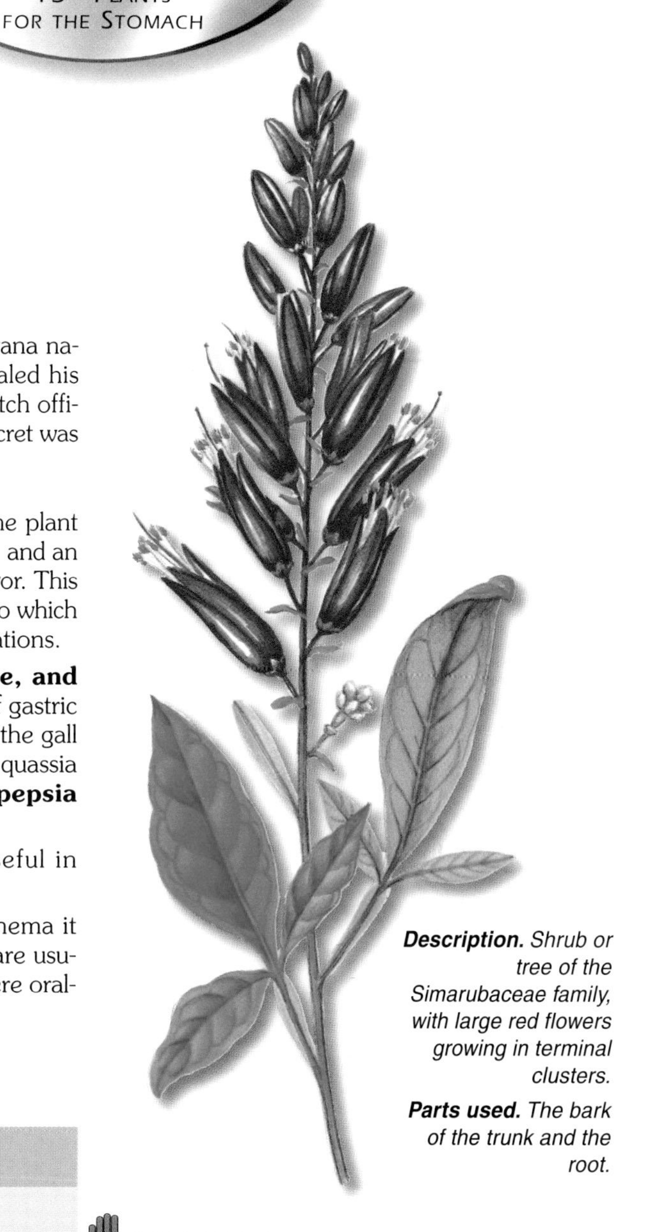

Description. *Shrub or tree of the Simarubaceae family, with large red flowers growing in terminal clusters.*

Parts used. *The bark of the trunk and the root.*

Preparation and Use

INTERNAL USE

❶ **Decoction** or cold extract with 5-10 g of bark and/or wood per liter of water. Drink a cup before each meal.

EXTERNAL USE

❷ **Enema.** With the same decoction used internally, apply an enema once a day as a **vermifuge.**

Warning

In high doses *this plant can produce* ***vomiting.*** *It should be* ***avoided*** *in the case of gastro-duodenal* ***ulcer*** *and during* ***menstruation*** *(it provokes uterine colic).*

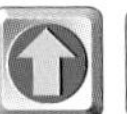
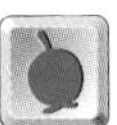
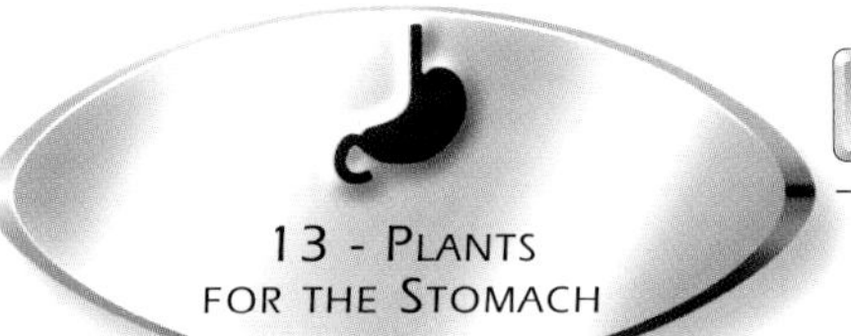

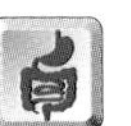
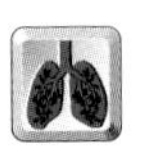
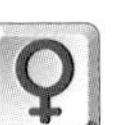
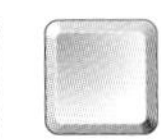

Anise

Digestive and galactogenic

ANISE WAS ALSO CALLED *"husbands-are-back,"* since those husbands who leave home due to the bad breath of their wives, when the latter take anise, the former are back.... That's another application of the plant which can be still used.

PROPERTIES AND INDICATIONS. Many properties of this plant are due to its essence, anethole, which when isolated from the rest of the active components of the plant, and then concentrated, loses its healing virtues and can even become toxic (it provokes convulsions). Anise liquors made with this essence have no medicinal properties but toxic effects because of both alcohol and anethole.

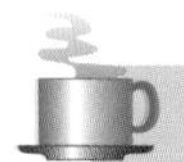

Preparation and Use

INTERNAL USE

❶ **Infusion** with a teaspoon (3 g) of fruits per cup of water. Drink up to three hot cups daily, preferably after meals. They may be sweetened with honey.

❷ **Infusion for babies on a milk diet.** This infusion is prepared with 1-2 tablespoonfuls of dry fruits (3-6 g) in a quarter of liter of water (250 ml). Sweeten with a teaspoonful of sugar (honey is not well tolerated by babies on a milk diet). Administer during the whole day.

❸ **Essence.** The recommended dose is 1-5 drops, two or three times a day.

❹ **Powder.** Up to two grams a day.

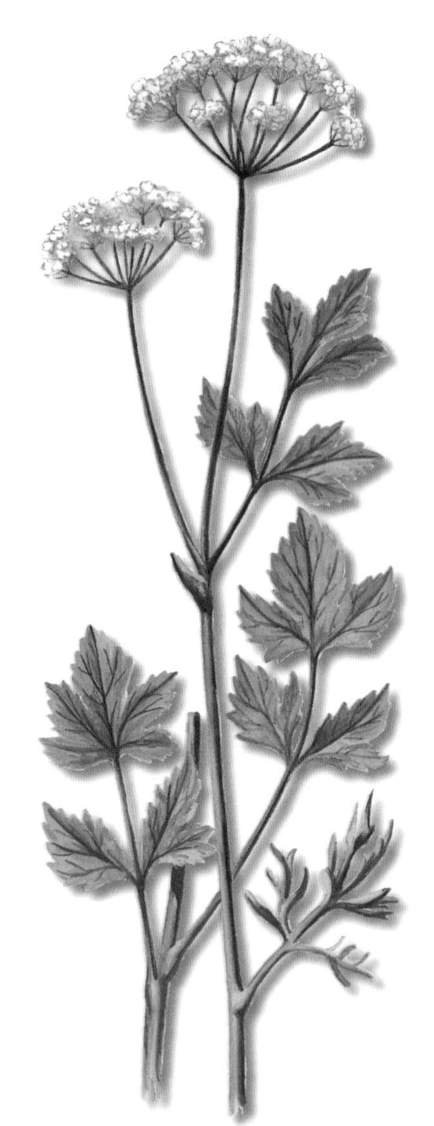

Description. *Plant of the Umbelliferae family, growing from 50 to 80 cm high, with grooved stem and whitish flowers growing in umbels. Its fruit is an oval grain which has a pleasant aroma. Though anise belongs to the same botanical family as poison parsley, both plants are difficult to mistake, since anise has a pleasant aroma and peculiar features.*

Part used. *The fruit.*

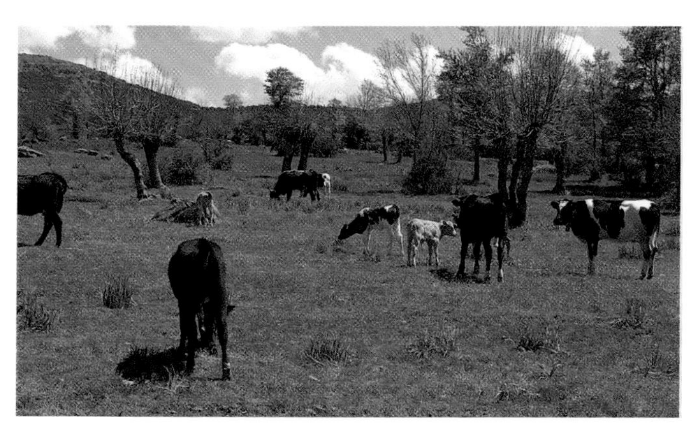

Cattle, in general, increase their milk production when eating anise mixed with their forage. Breast-feeding women can also take advantage of the galactogenic properties of this plant. Moreover, as anise passes to women's milk, this becomes easier to be digested, as well as acquiring antiflatulent properties.

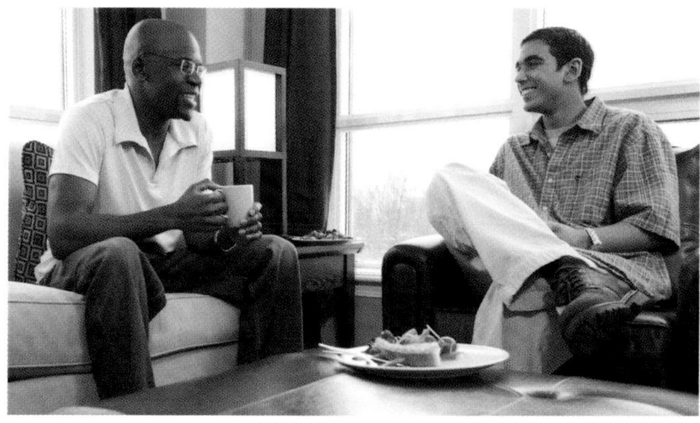

With the small fruits of anise both an infusion and an essence are recommended, which have antiflatulent and digestive properties. However, anise liquors, due to their high alcohol content, are advised against.

On the other hand, anise fruits as offered by nature practically lack any of its toxic essence effect. The fruits contain other substances such as phenol, malic acid, sugars, and choline, besides anethole.

Their properties are as follow:

• On the **digestive system:** Anise is the ***archetype of plants*** with **carminative, appetizer, digestive, and stomach invigorating** properties. It cleans fermentation and putrefaction from the intestine **[❶,❸,❹]**. With caraway, fennel, and coriander, it makes the "herbal tea of the four seeds", of which Font Quer said that no flatulence can resist it.

For children and babies on a milk diet, an infusion of anise is very useful for gas or diarrhea **[❷]**. Giving anise infusions to babies **on a milk diet** as a soft drink is a ***good habit.***

• On the **respiratory system,** anise has **expectorant** properties. It promotes the elimination of bronchial mucous, by making it more fluid. It is recommended for people suffering from **asthma and bronchial disorders,** and especially for those who want to give up smoking, since it acts as a true **antidote for nicotine** and tar, cleaning the irritating mucus of the bronchi, and promoting the regeneration of the mucosal cells **[❶,❸,❹]**. Moreover, tobacco-smelling breath is eliminated, giving a cool aroma.

• On **mammary glands,** it has **galactogenic** properties, which means it increases milk production **[❶,❸,❹]**. Cattle breeders give anise to their cows and sheep, mixing it with forage. Because anise is eliminated through the milk, ***breast-feeding women*** will help their babies by taking anise.

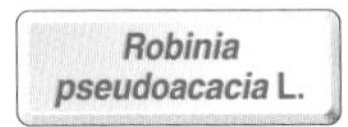

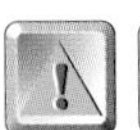

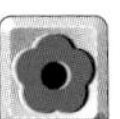

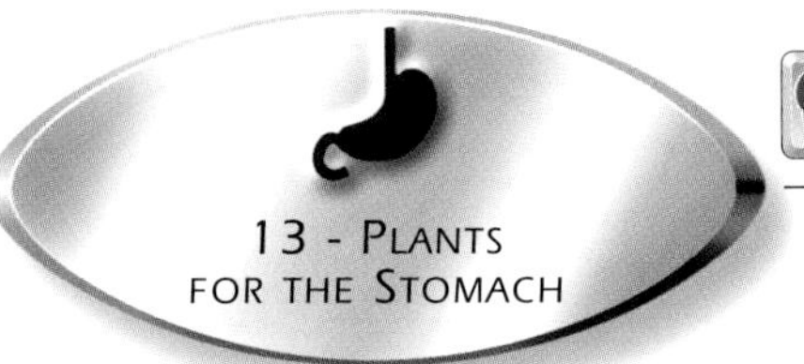

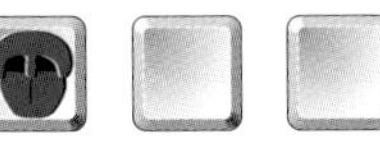

False Acacia

Useful against stomach acidity

FALSE ACACIA was introduced to Europe in 1601 by Jean Robin, gardener of the King of France. Thus, its scientific name (Robinia) and one of its common names, too. Though used as an ornamental plant, it has interesting medicinal properties. With the nectar of its flowers, bees produce a highly desired honey.

PROPERTIES AND INDICATIONS. The flowers and the leaves contain flavonoids, glycosides (robinine), tannin, and an essential oil. They have **antispasmodic** (alleviate the spasms of hollow organs), **cholagogue** (ease the emptying of bile), and **emollient** (soothe skin and mucosa) properties. They are used as **stomachic** for dyspepsia and gall bladder disorders. Due to their **emollient** properties, they protect the esophagus and stomach mucous membranes from an excess of acidity. They are recommended for pyrosis (acidity), esophagitis, and gastro-duodenal ulcer **[❶]**.

When taken in gargles, they alleviate **throat irritation [❷].**

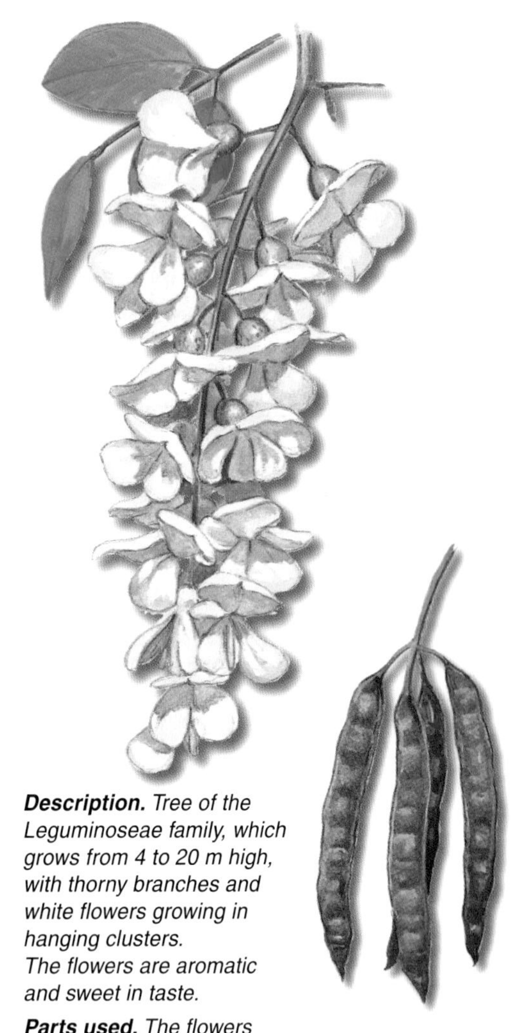

Description. *Tree of the Leguminoseae family, which grows from 4 to 20 m high, with thorny branches and white flowers growing in hanging clusters.*
The flowers are aromatic and sweet in taste.

Parts used. *The flowers and the leaves.*

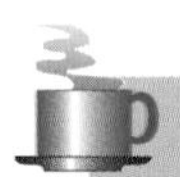

Preparation and Use

INTERNAL USE

❶ **Infusion** with 15-30 g of flowers per liter of water. The recommended intake is one cup after each meal.

EXTERNAL USE

❷ **Gargles** with the aforementioned infusion.

Warning

*The **seeds,** the **bark,** and the **root,** in spite of their sweet flavor, are toxic and cause vomiting.*

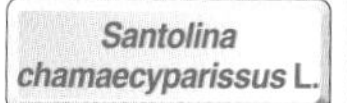

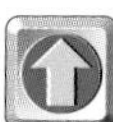
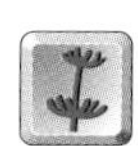
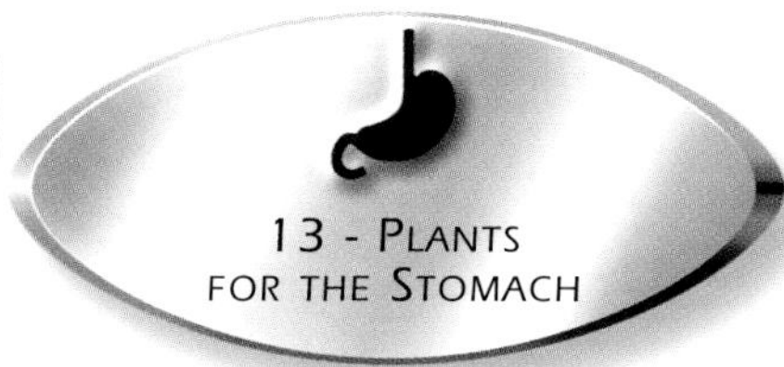

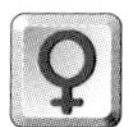
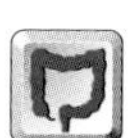
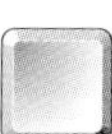
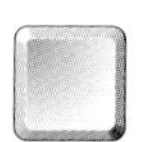

Lavender Cotton

Digestive and vermifuge

THIS PLANT, which likes the Mediterranean sunny climate, is a good substance for preserving clothes, since when putting its flower bouquets into the wardrobe it repels moths and other insects.

PROPERTIES AND INDICATIONS. The whole plant, and especially its flower heads, contain up to 1% of essence, which is composed of a ketone (santolinone) and an phenolic ester. Other components are tannin, resin, and a bitter component.

- **Stomachic tonic, digestive, and antispasmodic.** This is an ideal plant to ease digestion for those people suffering from stomach disorders **[❶,❷]**.
- **Vermifuge.** Very useful against intestinal parasites (oxyuridae, ascarides) which children usually have **[❸,❹]**.
- Mild **emmenagogue:** it produces menstruation **[❶,❷]**.

Preparation and Use

INTERNAL USE

As a digestive and emmenagogue substance:

❶ **Infusion** with six or seven flower heads per cup of water. Drink a cup after each meal.

❷ **Essence.** The recommended dose is 3-5 drops, three times a day.

As a vermifuge:

❸ **Infusion** with a teaspoonful of seeds per cup of water. Drink a cup every morning for a week. After one month, repeat the intakes.

❹ Seeds **powder:** 2-4 g, mixed with honey or fruit juice.

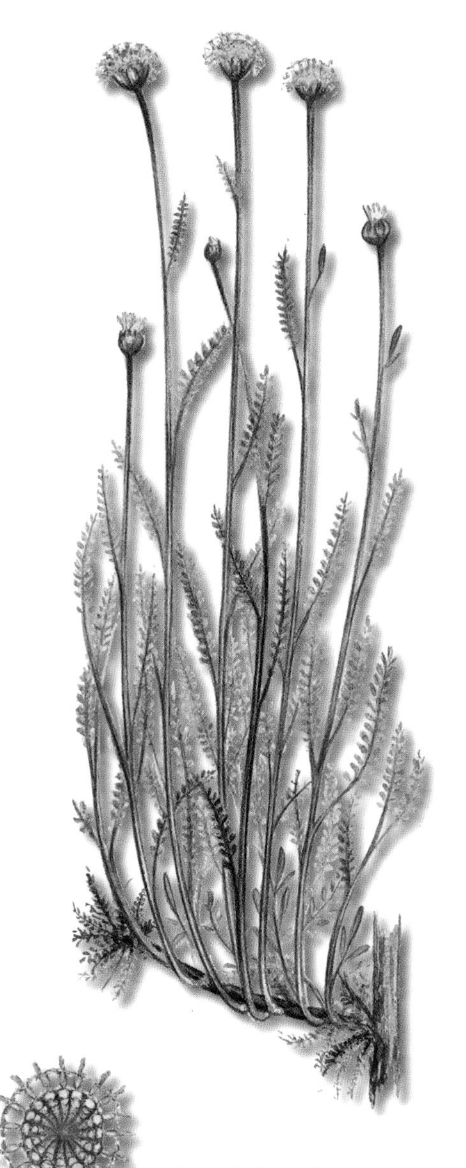

Description. *Vivacious plant of the Compositae family, growing from 20 to 50 cm high, with hairy, finely divided leaves resembling those of cypress. Its flowers are golden yellow in color, growing in terminal heads, with strong aroma and sour flavor.*

Parts used. *The seeds and the flower heads.*

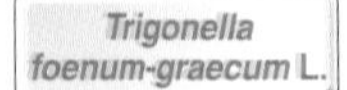

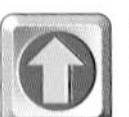
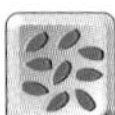
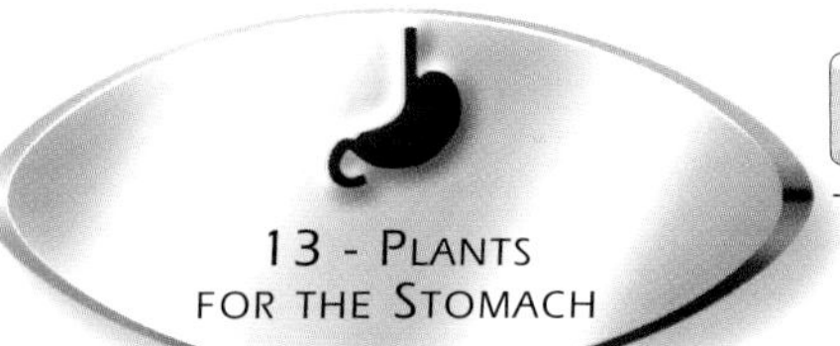

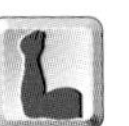
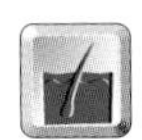
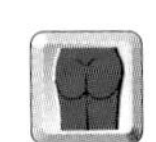
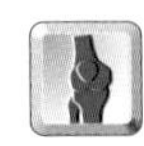

Fenugreek

Reduces inflammation and is a good food

FENUGREEK is one of the most ancient medicinal herbs. The Ebers Papyrus, an Egyptian medical document dated in the fifteenth century B.C., recommended fenugreek as a burn healing plant. Hippocrates remarked on the healing properties of its flour mucilage.

PROPERTIES AND INDICATIONS. The seeds of fenugreek are rich in mucilage and protein. When ***internally used*** they have a mild **laxative** action, besides reducing inflammation and protecting all digestive mucosa (an **emollient** property of mucilages) **[❶,❷]**. This fact makes all digestive processes more active, promoting a better metabolism of other foods.

Though at present there are many invigorating substances, fenugreek seed ***FLOUR*** is still a highly recommended remedy for people suffering from **lack of appetite or anemia,** and for those who want to gain weight **[❶].** It produces an increase of appetite and natural weight gain.

Maybe the ***most known application*** of fenugreek is in ***external use.***

Decoctions of fenugreek seeds produce a paste rich in mucilage, which is highly effective in case of hemorrhoids, skin afflictions or aching joints.

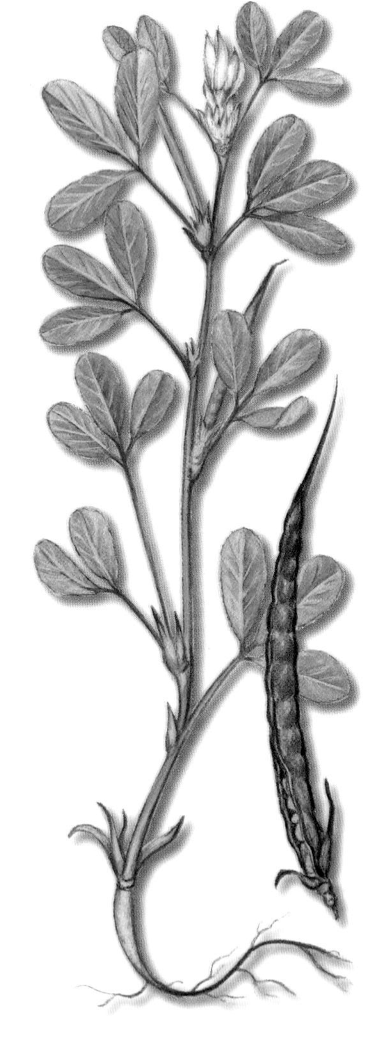
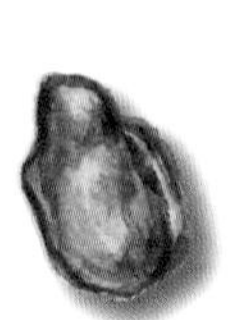

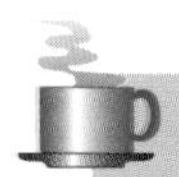

Preparation and Use

INTERNAL USE

❶ **Decoction** with a spoonful of seed flour per cup of water. Take as a purée. Honey or brown sugar can be added to this purée.

❷ **Dry extract.** The recommended dose is one gram in each of all three daily meals.

Description. *Plant of the Leguminoseae family, growing up to 50 cm high. The seeds (10-20) are contained in large, narrow pods. The whole plant has a typical aroma, not very pleasant.*

Parts used. *The seeds.*

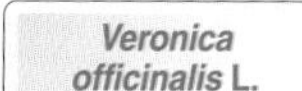

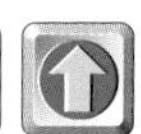
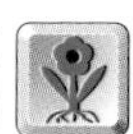
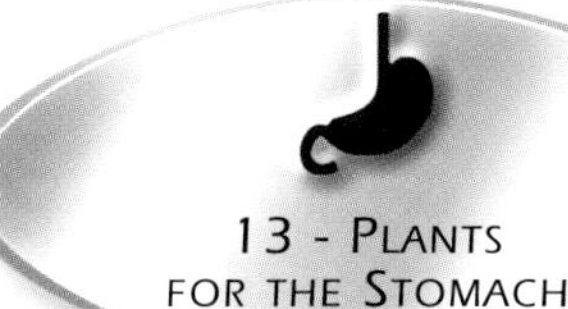

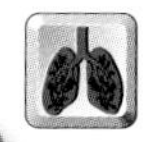
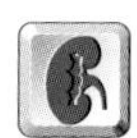
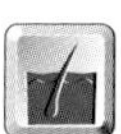
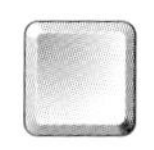

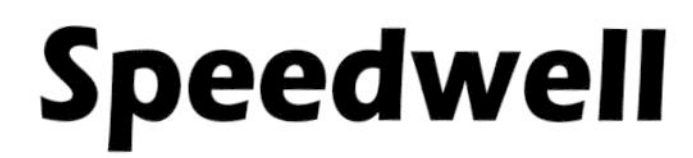

Speedwell

Cosmetic and tea substitute

IN NORTHERN European countries, a speedwell infusion substitutes tea. It has natural invigorating properties, and lacks any undesirable effects.

PROPERTIES AND INDICATIONS. The plant contains tannin and a bitter substance (aucubosid), which give it **astringent, invigorating, appetizer, and digestive** properties; saponins and mineral salts, with **expectorant, diuretic, and depurative** properties; and resin, manitol, and organic acids to which the plant probably owes its **emollient** properties on the skin. Its applications are as follow:

- **Digestive afflictions.** Lack of appetite, bloated stomach. Speedwell renders good results for migraines caused by bad digestion **[❶,❷]**.
- **Respiratory afflictions.** Pharyngitis, catarrh, cough, bronchitis, and asthma (it prevents its crises). It also has **antitussive and bechic** (throat soothing) properties **[❶,❷]**.
- **Diuretic, depurative, natural stimulant.** The plant provides a sensation of well-being **[❶,❷]**.
- **Skin.** Speedwell is used to wash eczema, to calm itching, to soothe cold-dried skin in cold climates, and as a **cosmetic [❸,❹]**.

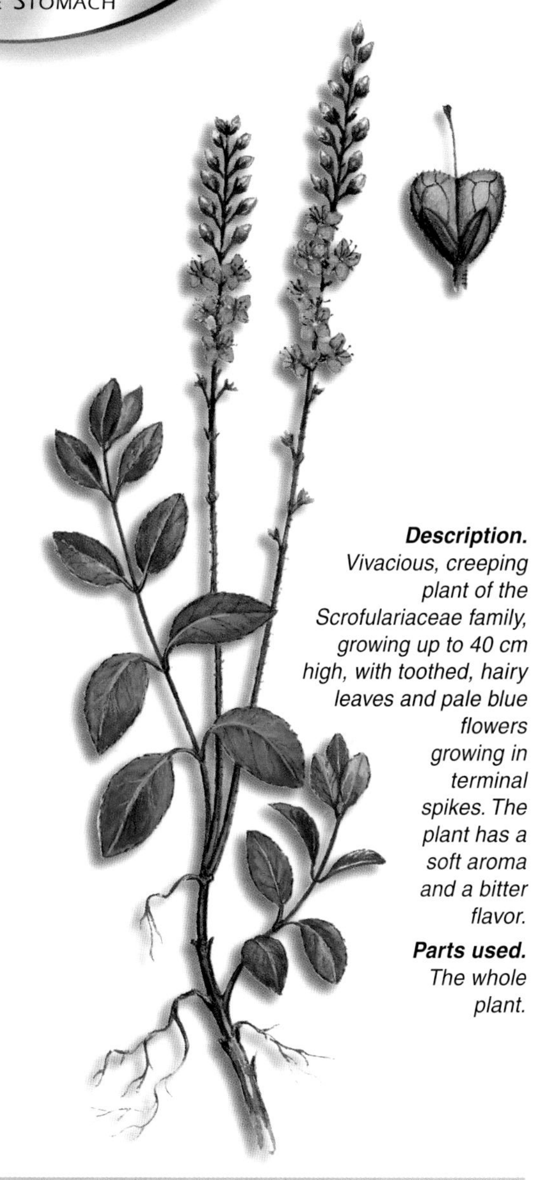

Description. *Vivacious, creeping plant of the Scrofulariaceae family, growing up to 40 cm high, with toothed, hairy leaves and pale blue flowers growing in terminal spikes. The plant has a soft aroma and a bitter flavor.*

Parts used. *The whole plant.*

Preparation and Use

INTERNAL USE

❶ **Infusion** with 30-40 g of plant per liter of water. Drink three or four cups daily. When used as an **appetizer** it must be drunk before meals.

❷ Fresh plant **juice.** Take two or three spoonfuls before each meal.

EXTERNAL USE

❸ **Compresses,** prepared with a decoction of 30-40 g of plant per liter of water. Boil for ten minutes. Apply directly on the skin.

❹ **Lotion** with the aforementioned decoction.

14

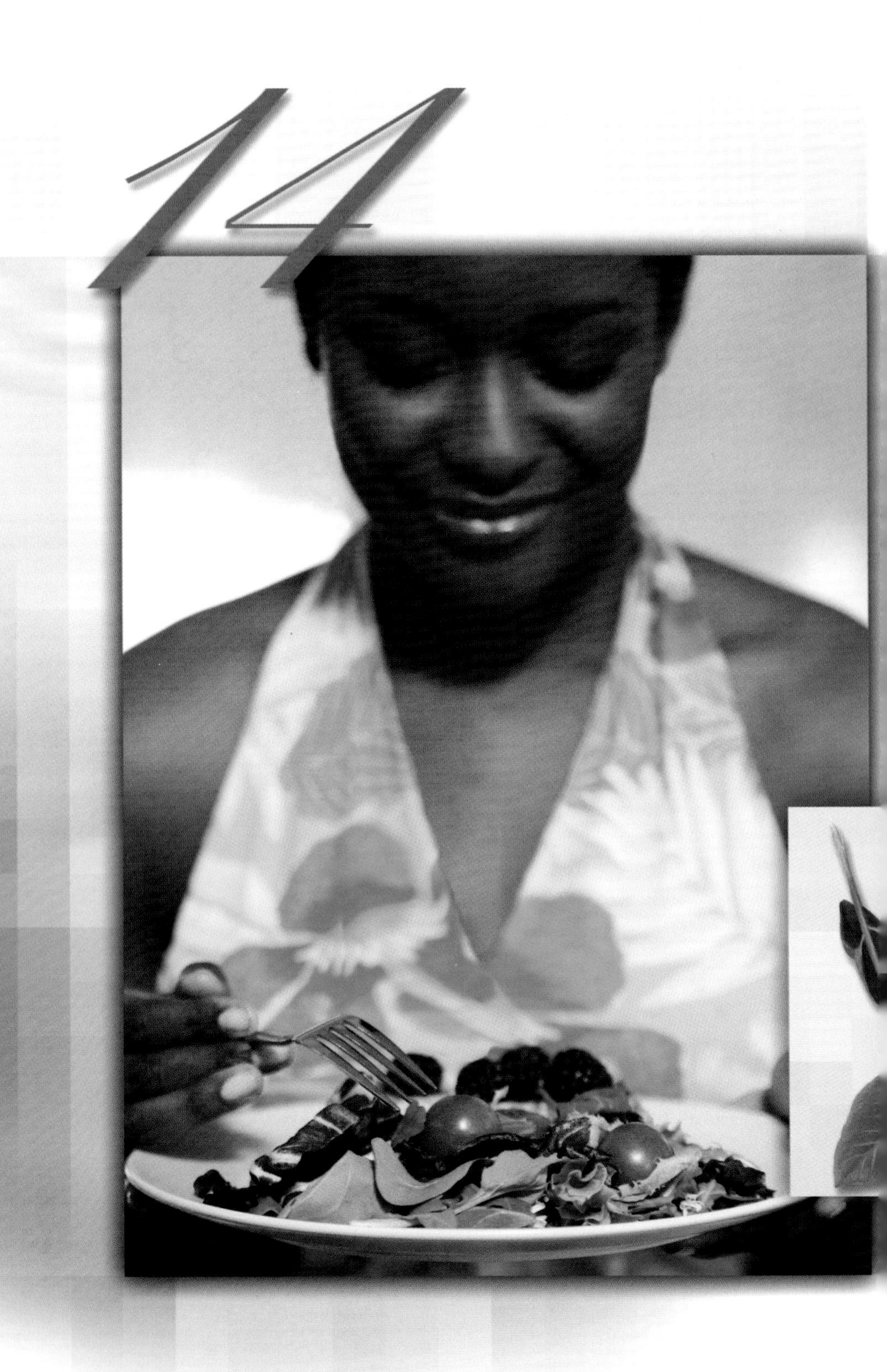

Plants for the Intestine

DISEASES	PAGES
Colitis	240
Constipation	241
Diarrhea, see Gastroenteritis	240
Fermentation, intestinal	239
Gas, intestinal	238
Gastroenteritis	240
Intestinal atony	240
Intestinal colic	240
Intestinal dysbacteriosis	239
Intestinal fermentation	239
Intestinal flora, alterations, see Intestinal dysbacteriosis	239
Intestinal gas	238
Intestinal parasites	241
Intestinal spasm, see Intestinal colic	240
Irritable bowel syndrome	239
Parasites, intestinal	241
Spasm, intestinal, see Intestinal colic	240

PLANTS	PAGES
Alder buckthorn	258
Beech tree	247
Bramble	264
Carob tree	245
Cascara sagrada	260
Castor bean	262
Early purple orchid	253
Flax	250
High mallow	252
Psyllium	254
Purging cassia	244
Purslane	256
Rhubarb	261
Tamarind	263
Tinnevelly senna	242
Tormentil	257
Walnut tree	248
Willowherb	246

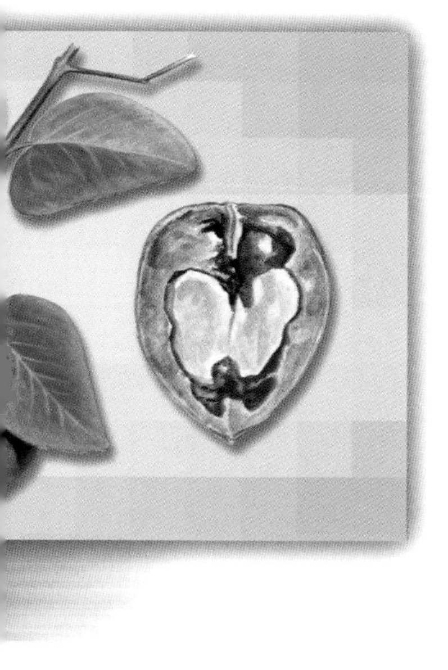

THE WHOLE intestinal tract is sensitive to the action of medicinal herbs. They exert two main effects on the intestinal mucosa:

- **Laxative:** Medicinal herbs promote or accelerate intestinal transit. Moreover, laxative plants are also **emollient,** that is to say, they soothe the intestinal mucosa.
- **Astringent:** Medicinal herbs dry and constrict the skin and mucous membranes. By diminishing the mucous secretion, they exert an **antidiarrheic** action. They also coagulate the bleeding of tiny blood vessels (antihemorrhagic action).

Almost all astringent plants owe their properties to the ***tannin*** they contain. Tannins clot proteins of the surface cells, thus drying, hardening, and reducing the inflammation of the skin and the mucosa.

Most medicinal herbs acting on the intestine are able to regulate intestinal transit, thus improving the body conditions so that healing will be complete, not only symptomatic. But we have to bear in mind that correct, ***healthy habits*** are required so that the treatment of intestinal afflictions will be effective.

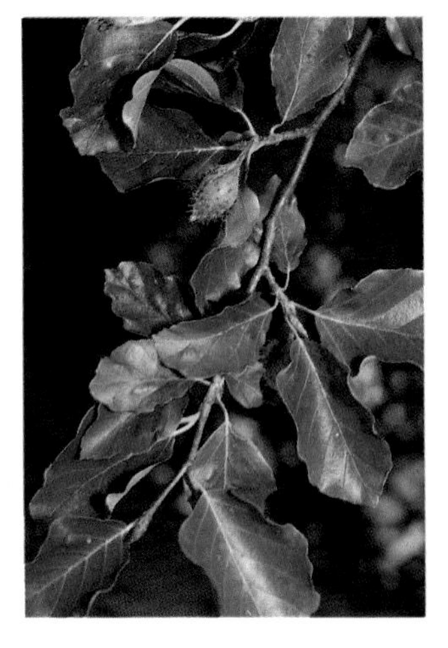

The beech tree provides a desired wood due to its charcoal, with antidiarrheic and antitoxic action.

INTESTINAL GAS

Causes

This is usually caused by intestinal fermentation produced by digestive intolerance to certain meals, or by alteration of the intestinal bacterial flora.

Phytotherapy

The plants here mentioned have ***carminative*** properties, thus promoting the expulsion of gas produced by intestinal fermentation. These carminative properties are usually a consequence of the aromatic essences plants contain.

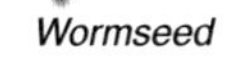

Wormseed

Charcoal, whether oak charcoal, poplar charcoal, or from other trees, also exerts a notable anti-flatulent action, however produced by other means. It adsorbs, that is to say,retains on its surface a high amount of toxins and intestinal gas.

Star anise

Treatment

Besides using one or several plants, treating an excess of intestinal gas demands ***changes in dietary habits,*** so that the products which cause flatulence will more be taken. Milk, legumes, white bread, and confectionery are usually the products which are more likely to lead to **flatulence.**

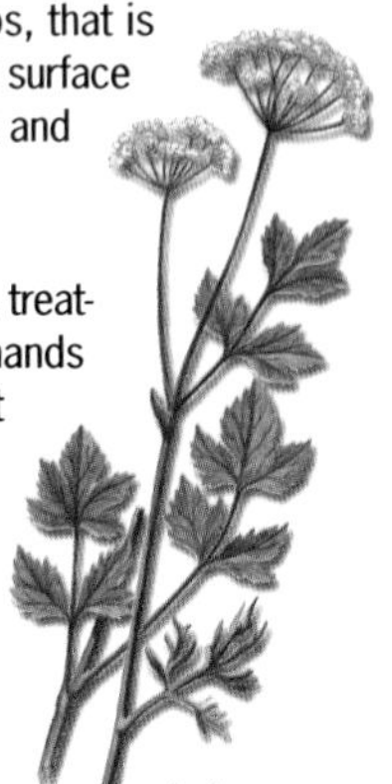

Anise

GARLIC	Eliminates from the colon the bacteria which cause flatulence
CARAWAY	Powerful antiflatulent
FENNEL	Promotes the expulsion of intestinal gas, stimulates peristaltic movements
GERMAN CAMOMILE	Regulates and normalizes intestinal functioning, carminative
PEPPERMINT	Eliminates intestinal gas and putrefaction
MARJORAM	Antispasmodic, digestive
WINTER SAVORY	Appetizer, antispasmodic, carminative
WORMSEED	Stomachic tonic, carminative
CUMIN	Appetizer, digestive, carminative
STAR ANISE	Promotes digestion, eliminates gas and flatulence
EUROPEAN PENNYROYAL	Eliminates gas, fights intestinal fermentation
WILD MARJORAM	Sedative, antispasmodic, carminative
ANISE	Carminative, appetizer, cleanses the intestine from fermentation and putrefaction
BEECH TREE	Adsorbent, disinfectant, fights intestinal fermentation and gas
MILFOIL	Digestive tonic, decreases intestinal fermentation

INTESTINAL FERMENTATION

Causes

It usually appears as a consequence of a lack of enzymes and digestive juice.

Food must usually be taken and absorbed into the blood flow inside the small intestine, so that only water and non-absorbable waste, such as vegetal bran, go to the larger intestine.

However, when this is not so, because of a lack of digestive juice, and undigested nutrients arrive in the large intestine unabsorbed, the high amount of bacteria in this part of the intestine ferment those nutrients. So, abundant **gas, intestine cramps,** and even **colitis** appear.

Thyme

Phytotherapy

These plants reduce intestinal fermentation by diverse ways, contributing to a good intestinal function.

Meat, and animal products are the main causative agents of intestinal fermentations.

LAVENDER	Antiseptic, prevents intestinal putrefaction
EUCALYPTUS	Adsorbs intestinal toxins
STAR ANISE	Promotes digestion, eliminates gas and flatulence
ANISE	Carminative, appetizer, cleanses the intestine from fermentation and putrefaction
BEECH TREE	Adsorbent, disinfectant, fights intestinal gas and fermentation
LINEN	Regenerates intestinal flora, regulates putrefaction and fermentation processes
MILFOIL	Digestive tonic, decreases intestinal fermentation
CINCHONA	Appetizer, invigorator, fights intestinal fermentation
THYME	Fights intestinal putrefaction caused by an imbalance of the intestinal flora

INTESTINAL DYSBACTERIOSIS

Definition

The large intestine usually houses a great amount of microorganisms, which form the intestinal flora. These bacteria play several indispensable roles in the digestive process, besides producing several vitamins, such as vitamin K.

Causes

The action of **antibiotics,** especially when taken orally, and also **colitis,** produce an alteration of the intestinal flora. Some types of bacteria increase, and other types diminish or even disappear.

This alteration of the intestinal flora is known as **intestinal dysbacteriosis,** and can be treated with the help of the listed medicinal herbs.

GARLIC	Balances intestinal flora, respecting normal saprophytes
EUCALYPTUS	Adsorbs intestinal toxins
BEECH TREE	Adsorbent, disinfectant, fights intestinal fermentation and gas
THYME	Fights intestinal putrefaction caused by imbalance of the intestinal flora

IRRITABLE BOWEL SYNDROME

Definition

This is a colon ailment with **nervous causes,** whose symptoms are functional disorders such as sudden changes between **constipation and diarrhea, spasms and flatulence.**

Phytotherapy

Besides these plants, all those listed on the table titled "Nervousness and Anxiety" can be used.

VALERIAN	Balances the autonomic nervous system
BLACKTHORN	Mild laxative, antispasmodic, relaxes muscles of the large intestine
ROSE	Calms stress and nervous imbalance

COLITIS

This is an **inflammation of the colon,** usually produced by noxious micro-organisms, but also by certain medicines such as antibiotics, and toxic substances such as coffee.

Repeated use of irritant laxative substances can also cause colitis. Alterations of the intestinal flora, and certain imbalances of the nervous system can also be accompanied by colitis (see "irritable bowel syndrome").

GARLIC	Balances intestinal flora. Respects normal saprophyte flora
EUCALYPTUS	Adsorbs intestinal toxins
BEECH TREE	Adsorbent, disinfectant, fights intestinal fermentation and gas
WALNUT	Powerful astringent, digestive invigorator
BRAMBLE	Astringent, antidiarrheic
THYME	Fights intestinal putrefactions caused by imbalance of the intestinal flora
NONI	Anti-infectious

INTESTINAL ATONY

Phytotherapy

Besides exerting a mild laxative action, the plants here mentioned stimulate the peristaltic movements of the intestine, which cause feces to pass through the tract.

All these plants are especially recommended in the case of **chronic constipation,** with long evolution, which cannot be treated with any other means. The results are slow, but effective.

Treatment

Any phytotherapeutical treatment must be accompanied by ***physical measures*** (exercise, abdominal showers, etc.), and a ***change*** of toilet habits.

Fennel	Promotes the expulsion of intestinal gas, stimulates peristaltic movements
German camomile	Stimulates digestive tract activity
Dandelion	Mildly laxative and depurative, useful for intestinal laziness or atony
Cascara sagrada	Invigorates the intestine, well tolerated purgative

GASTROENTERITIS

Definition

It consists of an **inflammation of the stomach and intestine.** It is usually caused by several noxious micro-organisms which affect the digestive tract. Gastroenteritis manifests itself with **vomiting, diarrhea,** and sometimes **fever.**

Treatment

A ***dietary treatment*** consists in abstaining from any solid food during the first days. Any of the infusions or decoctions we mention here can be taken as a ***drink*** when suffering from the acute phase of this disease, until **solid food** such as apple, carrot purée, or tapioca can be taken again.

ALTHEA	Anti-inflammatory and soothing
RHATANY	Astringent, anti-inflammatory. Recommended for children
WALNUT	Powerful astringent, digestive invigorator
EARLY PURPLE ORCHID	Intestinal emollient. Very useful for children's diarrhea
BRAMBLE	Astringent, antidiarrheic
ROSE	Mildly astringent, antiseptic
NONI	Anti-infectious

INTESTINAL COLIC

This is a **spasm** of the muscles covering the intestine, which usually goes with gastroenteritis, colitis, irritable bowel, spastic constipation, and other intestinal afflictions. The plants here listed here relax the walls of the intestine (antispasmodic action), and stop any excessive motility of the digestive tract.

BALM	Antispasmodic, sedative, digestive
PASSION FLOWER	Relaxes hollow organs suffering from spasms
GERMAN CAMOMILE	Sedative, antispasmodic, digestive
CATNIP	Calms diarrhea and the colic spasm usually associated with it
FLAX	Calms colic aches
TORMENTIL	Astringent, calms colic pain and spasm
RUE	Antispasmodic, antiseptic

CONSTIPATION

Most constipation cases have a functional reason, this is to say, they are not caused by organic lesions in the intestine. The plants we recommend have specific actions for **functional constipation,** due to their ***mild physiological laxative properties.***

Constipation can be caused by **atony** of the intestine walls. In this case, the plants listed on the lower part of the table must be taken.

When constipation does not disappear after administering any laxative substance for three or four days, a **physician consultation** is required.

BOLDO	Normalizes gall bladder function, mild laxative
DANDELION	Mild laxative and diuretic
CHICORY	Activates motility and fights intestinal laziness
TINNEVELLY SENNA	When taken in low doses, laxative promotes emission of soft feces, without colic
PURGING CASSIA	Mild laxative, non-irritant on the intestine
FLAX	Lubricates the digestive tract, regenerates intestinal flora
HIGH MALLOW	Non-aggressive laxative. Useful for children and elderly people
PSYLLIUM	Increases fecal volume, mild and safe laxative
ALDER BUCKTHORN	Mild laxative. Does not provoke addiction
CÁSCARA SAGRADA	Strong purgative, though well tolerated

Flax is a highly desirable plant because of the fabric obtained from it.

Its seeds are rich in pectin and mucilage, as well as in mineral salts and essential fatty acids. They are taken in the form of decoction or cold extract, but they can also be ingested raw. They are an effective and appreciated laxative, since besides promoting the transit of feces, they prevent intestinal fermentation and putrefaction processes.

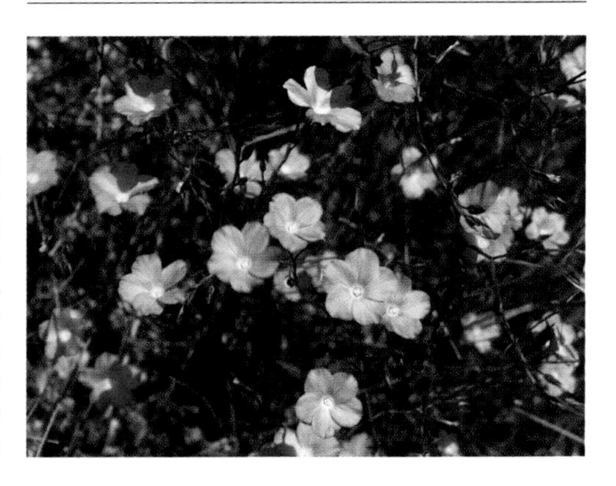

INTESTINAL PARASITES

Definition

Several types of worms can attack the intestine, especially that of children. The most common are:

Oxiures: white, small roundworms, difficult to see, which cause anal itching.

Ascaris: roundworms, bigger than oxiures, which can produce abdominal pain, nausea, and lack of appetite.

Taeniae: There are several types of taeniae, the most frequent being pig tapeworm (which can be up to five meters large), and hydatic cyst taenia.

Intestinal parasites live inside the human intestine, and stick to its walls with a kind of sucker they have on their head.

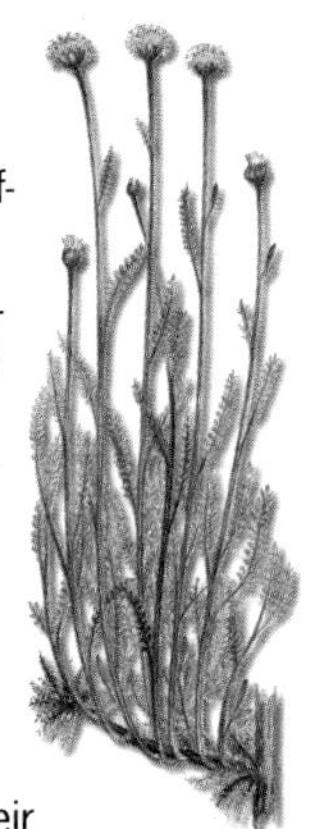

Lavender cotton

Phytotherapy

Plants with ***vermifuge*** properties loosen parasites, therefore promoting their elimination if a ***laxative*** substance is then administered.

GARLIC	Vermifuge especially active against roundworms and oxiures (small white worms)
WORMSEED	Destroys intestinal parasites, especially roundworms
EUROPEAN PENNYROYAL	Vermifuge, digestive
LAVENDER COTTON	Vermifuge. Useful for children
MUGWORT	Vermifuge, useful against oxiures
THYME	Vermifuge, especially active against taeniae

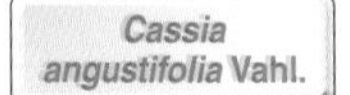

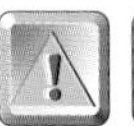
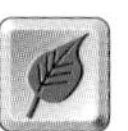
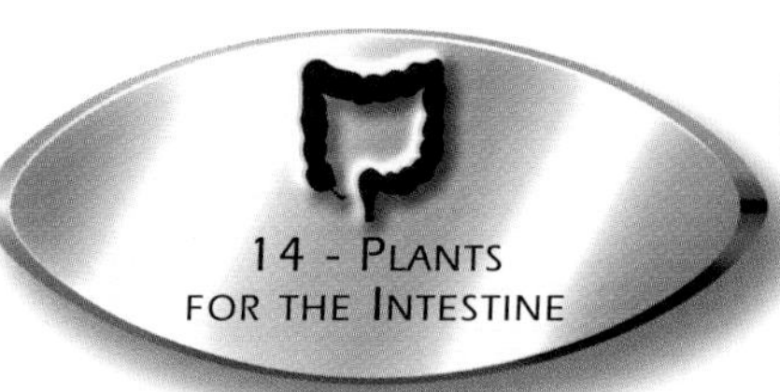

Tinnevelly Senna

The laxative par excellence

"I THINK YOU look melancholy and sad. You'd better have a purge with an ounce of tinnevelly senna."

"Purge? Me? You know, I visit regularly the closet, and defecate normally!"

"Understand the science Galen left to us: purges keep us away from inadequate humors, and mainly from that black, tetric humour called alterbile, which provokes all anxiety and sadness."

"So would I be free from this sadness which is depressing me?"

"Be sure of that. When you are purged with tinnevelly senna, your spirit will awake, and you will be joyful and happy again."

A physician and his patient talked this way, well into the sixteenth century. In those times, when the theories of Galen, the Greek physician of the second century, still ruled medicine, purgatives were widely used to eliminate any "excess of humors." With purgative substances, physicians pretended to heal multiple diseases.

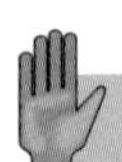

Warning

Due to its stimulant action on the hollow abdominal organs, which are covered by smooth muscle fibers (especially the uterus and the bladder) ***it must not be used*** *during* ***pregnancy,*** *nor* ***menstruation.*** *It must not be used for* ***colitis or cystitis.***

In the case of ***anal and rectal afflictions*** *(fissure, hemorrhoids, etc.) it must be used* ***with care,*** *and always in* ***low doses.***

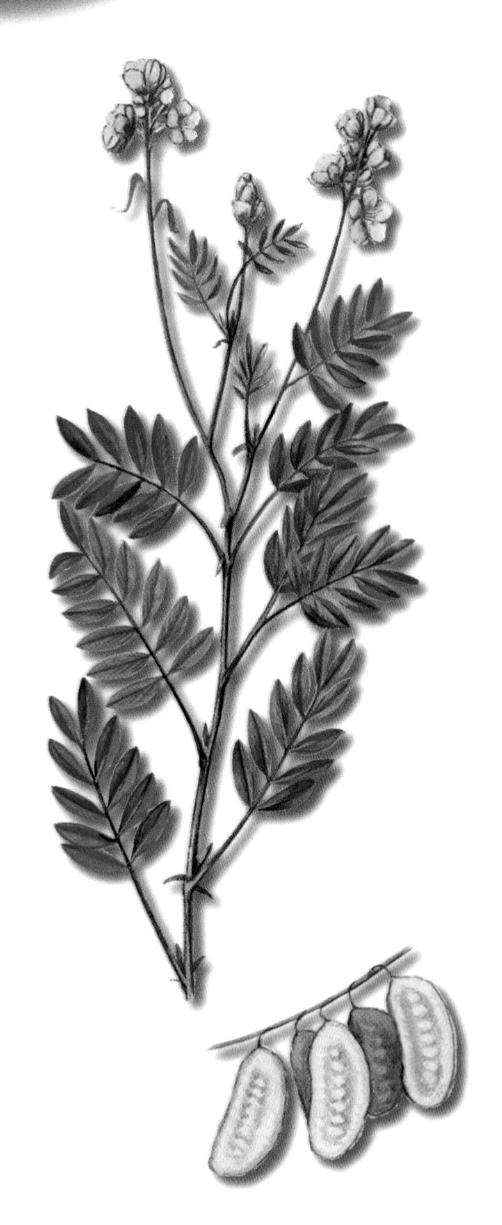

Description. *Shrub of the Leguminoseae family, growing from 0.5 to 1 m high. It has composed leaves, with five to eight pairs of oval folioles. Flowers are yellow, and the fruit is a plain-shaped legume, containing from six to eight seeds.*

Parts used. *The folioles (leaves) and the seeds.*

Preparation and Use

INTERNAL USE

❶ **Infusion.** The powder of ground tinnevelly senna lobules is used in doses ranging from 1 to 8 g, taken in infusion at night. Two or three grams are usually enough to achieve a laxative effect. Children have enough with half this dose. It should not be taken for more than seven days consecutively.

In order to avoid the irritant effects of its resin, which in large doses can provoke nausea and vomiting, we recommend you place tinnevelly senna leaves in **alcoholic cold extract** for 24-48 hours. After this time, throw away the alcohol, and prepare an infusion with these leaves.

❷ **Tinnevelly senna extract.** Recently, pharmaceutical industries have introduced to the market dried senosids, which are presented in the form of different **pharmaceutical preparations.** These substances lack any of the irritant effects of the resin, being thus especially appropriate for children and older people.

EXTERNAL USE

❸ **Enema.** With 20-30 g of tinnevelly senna per liter of water, prepare an infusion which will be administered as an enema. Effects are immediate.

Tinnevelly senna, which was introduced to Europe in the eleventh century by the Arabs, was one of the most appreciated purgative plants. With it, lunatics were drastically purged, with results not as successful as expected. In this way, with energetic diarrhea and bleeding, ancient physicians exercised their art.

At present, tinnevelly senna is one of the most commonly used medicinal herbs, however not being employed to "purge noxious humors," but as an ***effective and safe laxative.***

PROPERTIES AND INDICATIONS. The leaves and seeds of tinnevelly senna contain 2-3% of anthraquinonic glycosides, known as senosid A and B; they also contain mucilage and flavonoids, which help in the plant's laxative properties, and a resin with irritant action which, when taken in large doses, can provoke vomiting and nausea.

Senosids are inactive in their natural condition. They pass through the stomach with no alteration, then being partially absorbed in the small intestine, are eliminated with the bile. When arriving in the colon, senosids are chemically transformed by means of some enzymes produced by intestinal bacteria (glycosidase), which liberate the genine (aglycon), the active component of the senosid molecules. The chemical reaction produced goes as follow: ***senosid*** (glycoside) + **enzyme = genin** (active component) + ***sugar.***

Active derivatives of senosids exert their laxative action by means of two mechanisms:

1st By stimulating the action of the large intestine, increasing peristaltic movements. They also increase, though with a lesser intensity, the muscular tone of the urinary system and the uterus.

2nd By decreasing permeability of the intestinal mucosa, thus making the normal absorption of water which takes place in the large intestine more difficult.

Depending on the dose, tinnevelly senna produces two effects:

- **Laxative:** It eases the emission of soft feces, with no colic.
- **Purgative:** It causes evacuation of liquid, diarrheic feces, accompanied by cramps (colic).

The purgative or laxative effects manifest themselves six or seven hours after taking the plant. These effects may last for one or two days, and are never followed by reactive constipation.

The use of tinnevelly senna is recommended for constipation caused by journeys, changes of diet, child birth, and after surgical operations [❶,❷,❸]. It is very useful to prevent straining during defecation, in the case of patients suffering from high blood pressure or angina pectoris.

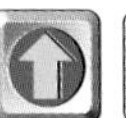
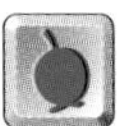
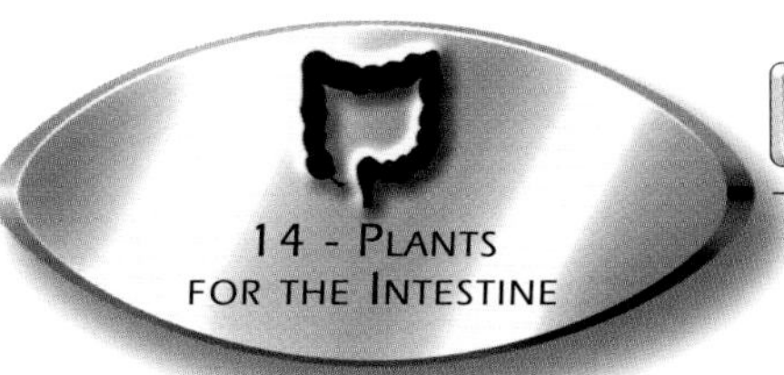
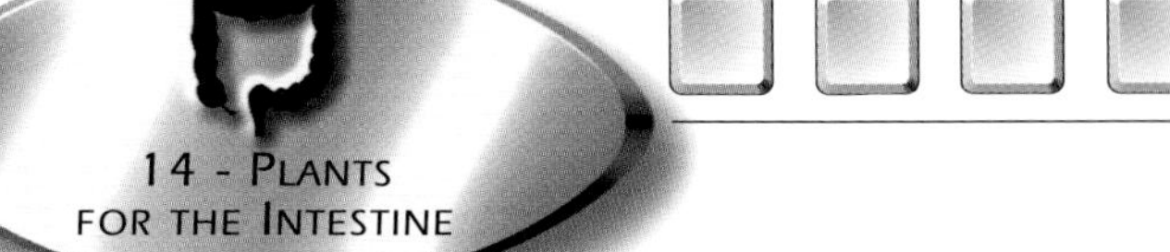

Purging Cassia

A mild and appreciated laxative

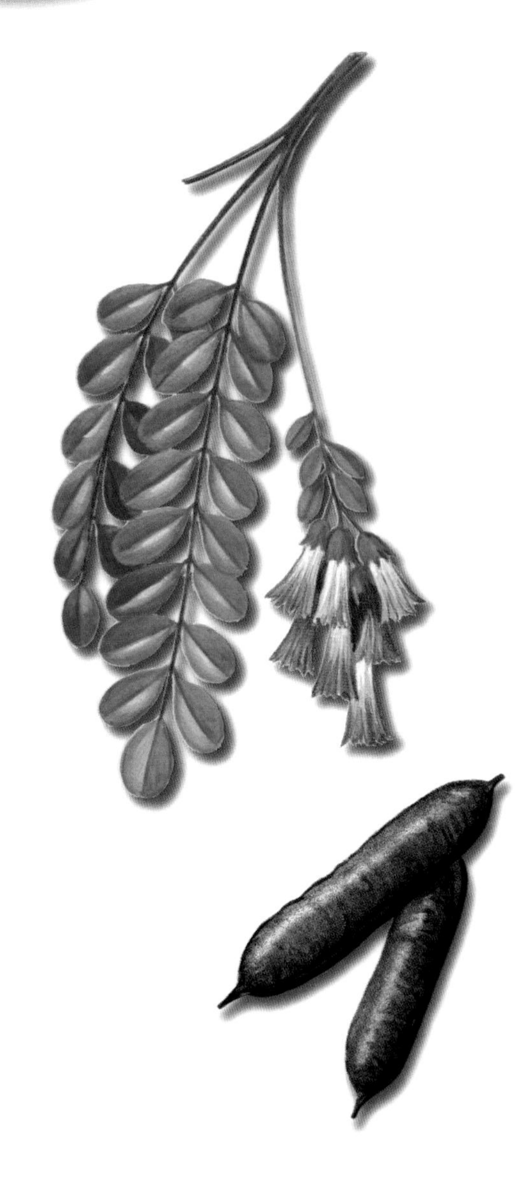

THIS TREE decorates the tropical areas of America. It is very common in the Mexican regions of Tierra Caliente, from Morelos and Guerrero to Tabasco and Chiapas. Its medicinal properties as a laxative are highly appreciated, and ***almost irreplaceable,*** thus being part of ***several laxative*** substances used ***world-wide.***

PROPERTIES AND INDICATIONS. The thick and sweet black flesh of the purging cassia fruit contains, besides several sugars and mucilage, a small amount of anthraquinonic derivatives, among which the most important is rein.

This mixture of active components gives the plant **mild laxative** properties, which ***lack any purgative or irritant effect*** on the intestine. It is thus very useful for constipation, and especially due to the mildness of its action, for children and elderly people with diseases [❶,❷].

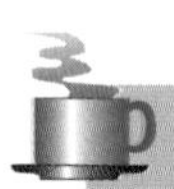

Preparation and Use

INTERNAL USE

❶ **Dissolved flesh.** From 30 to 60 g of flesh per liter of boiling water. Strain and drink one or two cups in the morning.

❷ **Flesh.** Directly eat the flesh. Five grams are enough to produce a laxative effect.

Description. *Tree of the Leguminoseae family, growing from 12 to 15 m high, with yellow flowers hanging in clusters. Its fruit is a cylindrical pod, ochre or black in color, which contains a black flesh with sweet flavor besides the seeds.*

Parts used. *The flesh of the fruit.*

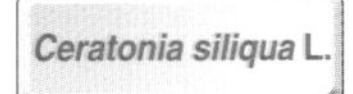

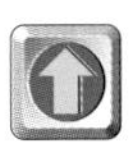
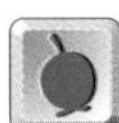
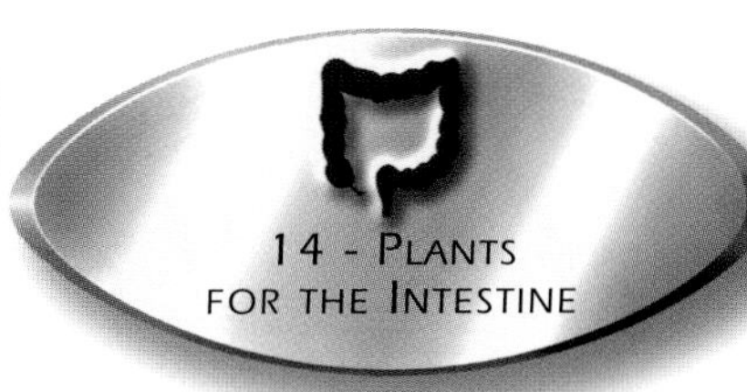

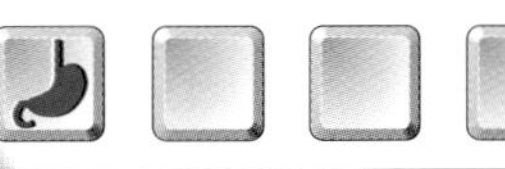

Carob Tree

An excellent antidiarrheic for children

THOUGH THE CAROB tree has been cultivated as forage for thousands of years in all Mediterranean countries, its notable medicinal properties were discovered only some decades ago.

PROPERTIES AND INDICATIONS. The flesh of its fruit, ***CAROB,*** contains a high amount of sugars (mainly saccharose) and pectin, as well as starch (3.8%), proteins (4%), fats (0.5%), cellulose, and mineral salts. ***Fresh*** carob has **laxative** properties. However, ***CAROB FLOUR*** when ***dried*** has **antidiarrheic** properties, besides having the ability to absorb toxins in the digestive system. It renders excellent results for children's diarrhea, up to the point that it is ***one of the most widely employed treatments for gastroenteritis*** of children still on a milk diet **[❶]**.

The seeds are rich in mucilage. From them, the carob gum is obtained. Once inside the stomach, this substance forms a kind of viscous gel, which because of its great increase in volume by means of adsorption of liquids, provides a sensation of being full, being thus used in **weight-loss diets [❷]**. When in the intestine, carob gum has **emollient** (soothing) and **laxative** properties.

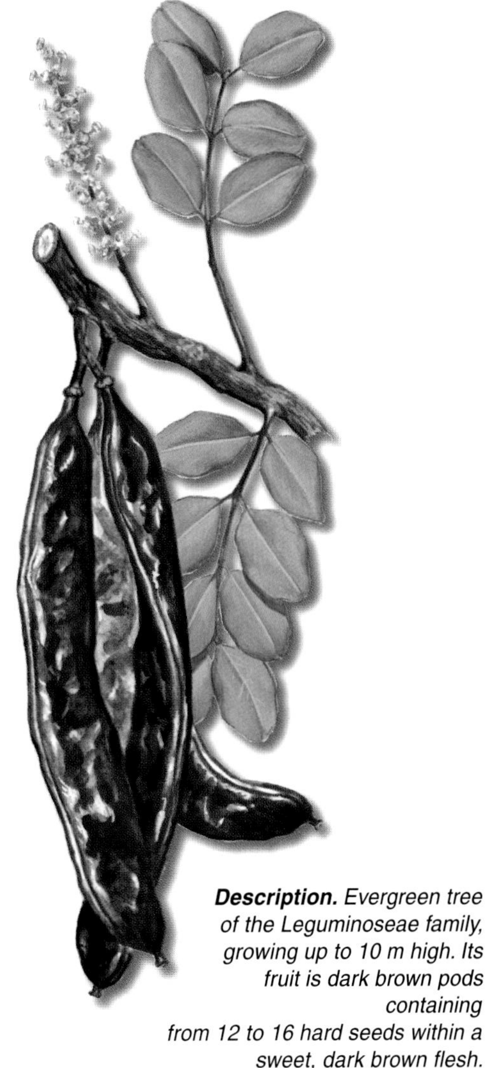

Description. *Evergreen tree of the Leguminoseae family, growing up to 10 m high. Its fruit is dark brown pods containing from 12 to 16 hard seeds within a sweet, dark brown flesh.*

Parts used. *The fruit (carob), and the seeds.*

Preparation and Use

INTERNAL USE

❶ **Flour.** Carob flour is sold in pharmacies, and with it a purée of pleasant flavor is prepared. This food, besides stopping **diarrhea,** is very nutritious.

❷ **Gum.** It is also sold in pharmacies, in the form of **capsules or bags.** The common dose (except when otherwise recommended by a physician, or in the pharmaceutical preparation) to produce a **full result** is 0.5 to 1.5 g, half an hour before each meal, together with a glass of water.

Willowherb

Antidiarrheic and anti-inflammatory

THIS BEAUTIFUL plant of the European mountains, besides making us joyful with its beautiful colors, sweetens all herbal teas in which it is present. In northern Europe it is highly appreciated, and its young buds are often consumed in salad dishes.

PROPERTIES AND INDICATIONS. The whole plant contains tannin, pectin, and mucilage. It has **astringent** properties, due to its content in tannin, and **emollient** properties (reduces the inflammation of the skin and the mucosa) due to its content in mucilage and pectin. Its most common applications are the following:

• **Diarrhea, gastroenteritis,** and, as a rule, all **inflammations of the digestive mucosa.** Besides its astringent properties, willowherb also has **anti-inflammatory** properties. It stops diarrhea and eliminates abdominal discomfort [❶].

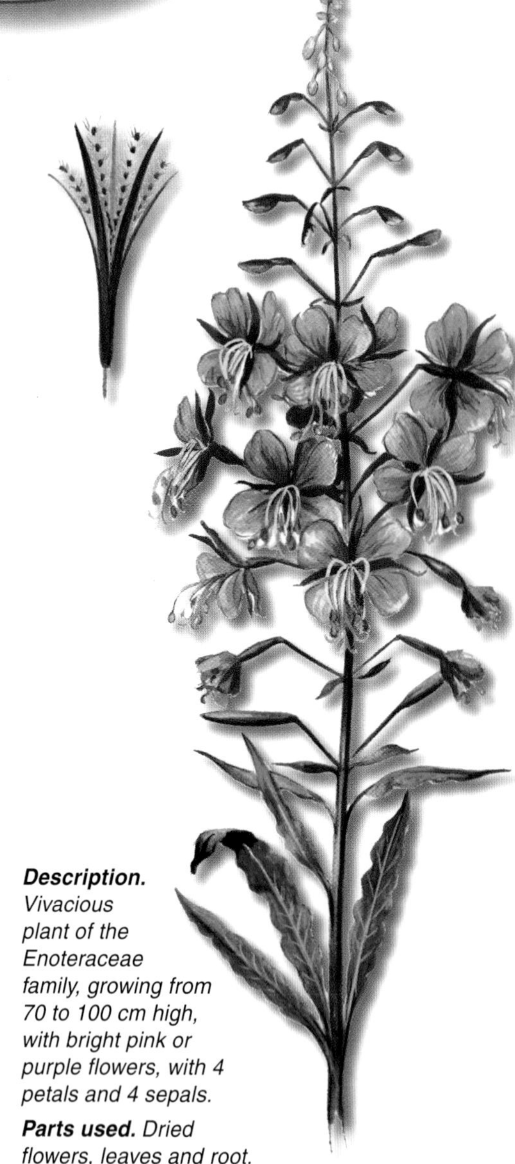

Description. *Vivacious plant of the Enoteraceae family, growing from 70 to 100 cm high, with bright pink or purple flowers, with 4 petals and 4 sepals.*

Parts used. *Dried flowers, leaves and root.*

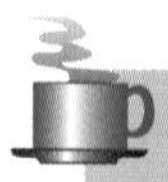

Preparation and Use

INTERNAL USE

❶ **Infusion** with 50 g of dry root, flowers and leaves. Fresh flowers should be avoided. Drink four of five cups daily.

EXTERNAL USE

❷ **Mouth rinsings and gargles.** With the aforementioned infusion.

• **Stomatitis** (inflammation of the oral mucosa), **gingivitis, and pharyngitis:** when applied in mouth rinses and gargles, it has **anti-inflammatory** properties and produces a pleasant cool sensation in the mouth [❷].

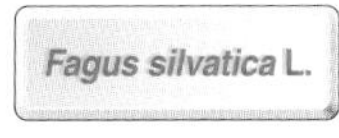

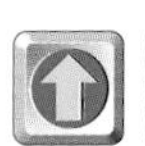
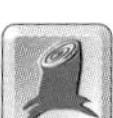
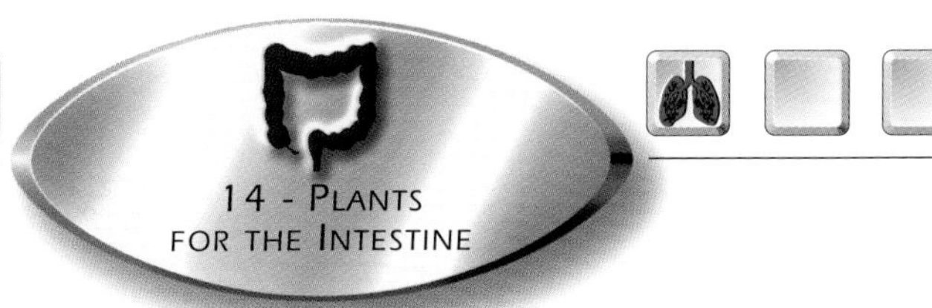

Beech Tree

Beech tree charcoal is very medicinal

BEECH NUTS must not be consumed in large amounts, since in the bark there seems to be a substance, mildly toxic, which can produce headaches.

PROPERTIES AND INDICATIONS. The ***CHARCOAL*** obtained from beech tree wood is excellent in combating intestinal **fermentation and gas, colitis and diarrhea,** due to its powerful adsorbent and disinfectant properties **[❶]**. It is also useful as a ***toothpaste*** and as ***universal antidote*** against any kind of **poisoning**.

From its ***WOOD, creosote*** is also extracted: an **expectorant and antiseptic** substance, rich in guaiacol, which is used in ***many syrups.***

The ***BARK*** contains high amounts of tannin. It has **astringent** (recommended for diarrhea and dysentery), **vermifuge** (expulses intestinal parasites), and **invigorating** properties **[❷].**

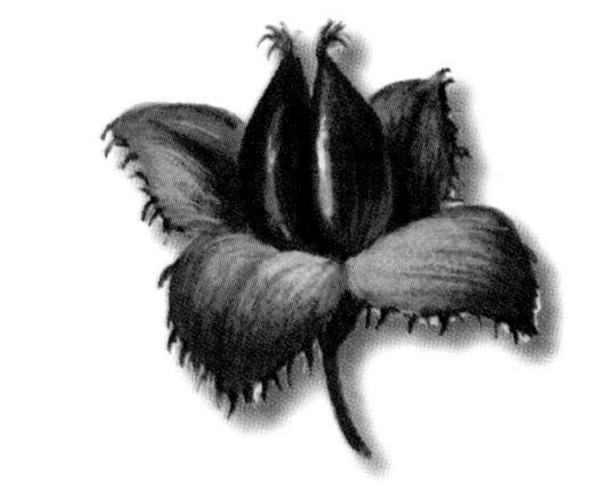

Preparation and Use

INTERNAL USE

❶ **Charcoal.** Take 10-20 g up to five times daily, dissolved into water or chewed as is. In severe cases, the dose can be raised up to 100 g in a once-only intake.

❷ **Decoction** of bark, with 60 g per liter of water. Boil until the liquid reduces to a half. Drink two or three cups a day. As a vermifuge, take for five consecutive days, two cups daily on an empty stomach.

Description. *Big tree of the Fagaceae family, growing up to 40 m high. The borders of its leaves are covered with fine hair. The fruit is similar to the chestnut.*

Parts used. *The wood and the bark of its branches.*

Walnut Tree

Reduces the inflammation of the skin and the mucosa

FROM THE EIGHTEENTH century onwards, chemical and nutritional research proved that the walnut tree, as well as walnuts, has many healing properties. At present, we know that walnuts have a high nutritional value, with a content in proteins similar to that of meat, to which they overcome in regards to the quality of fats contained, and to the amount of vitamins and minerals they contain.

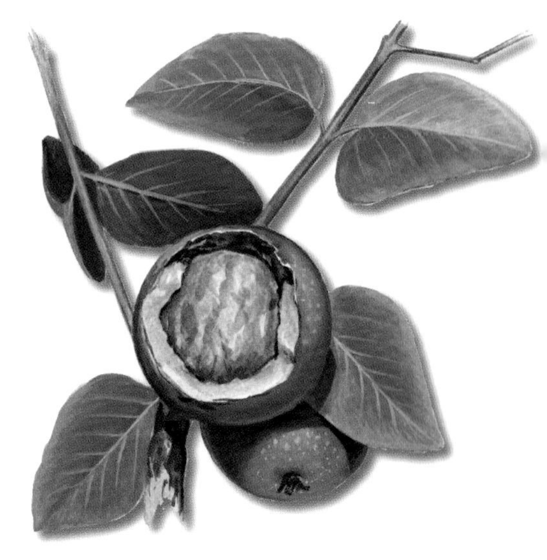

Description. *Tree of the Juglandaceae family, growing up to 30 m high, with grayish bark and long-petioled leaves. It has two types of flowers, male and female. The fruit are drupes (walnuts) .*

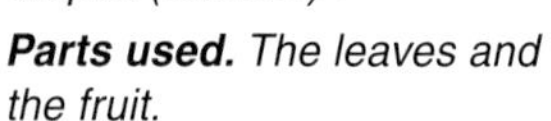

Parts used. *The leaves and the fruit.*

PROPERTIES AND INDICATIONS. Both the ***LEAVES*** and the ***GREEN COVERING*** of fruit contain a high amount of tannins of the gallic and the catechin types (9-11%), which give the ***strong* astringent** properties of walnut; they also contain anthraquinonic derivatives, the most important of which is juglone, a bitter substance which, along with vitamin C and organic acids, explains the **antiseptic, cicatrizant, invigorating, vermifuge,** and **hypoglycemic** properties. Its main applications are the following:

- **Digestive disorders.** Its powerful astringent properties make the walnut leaves and green rinds useful in all cases of diarrhea, gastroenteritis, colitis, stomach upset, and flatulence (❶). Its invigorating action on the digestive organs manifests itself by means of an increase of appetite, a speeding up of food passing through the stomach, and of secretion of bile and pancreatic juice. People suffering from dyspepsia, lack of appetite, and those convalescing from any disease will improve their health conditions with the use of walnut.

- **Gynecological disorders.** Leukorrhea (white flux), cervicitis or colpitis (inflammation of the womb neck), and ulceration on the womb neck are the ailments for which walnut has ***most important applications.*** Its **anti-inflammatory and antiseptic** actions are ***quite effective*** when administered in the form of vaginal irrigation (❸). But caution! Before applying any treatment for such female ailments, a ***gynecologist must check and evaluate*** the case, so that it can be ascertained whether these ailments are caused by malignant or cancerous reasons. Vaginal irrigations must ***never*** be applied ***during pregnancy.*** In order to achieve a more intense effect, we recommend taking an infusion (❶), as well as irrigations.

- **Urethritis** (inflammation of the urethra, or urinary tract), and cystitis: Apply a decoction of leaves and/or green rind (❸) through a urinary catheter. This will heal the itching and irritation

Preparation and Use

INTERNAL USE

❶ **Infusion** with 10-20 g of leaves and/or rind of green fruit per liter of water. Drink three or four cups daily. This infusion must not be taken with other plants or pharmaceutical preparations containing iron salts, jelly, mucilage, or alkaloids, which could neutralize its effects. Take it **alone** or if preferred, sweetened with honey.

❷ **Decoction** with 20 g of rind of green fruit per liter of water. As a **vermifuge,** drink two cups daily.

EXTERNAL USE

❸ **Decoction** made with 100 g of leaves and or rind of green fruits per liter of water, boiling for 15 minutes. Apply in vaginal **irrigations,** urethral **cleansing,** eye **baths** (conjunctivitis), **sitz baths** (hemorrhoids), in **compresses or baths** on the skin, or in **gargles** (pharyngitis). We recommend taking two or three applications daily.

felt when urinating, as well as reduce the inflammation of the urinary mucosa.

• **Skin and mucosal afflictions.** The application of a decoction of walnut leaves or green rind on the skin is good whenever an astringent, wound healing, and anti-inflammatory action is required: eczema, impetigo, folliculitis, ringworm, and wounds and sores that will not heal. Chilblains, tonsillitis, pharyngitis, conjunctivitis, and hemorrhoids, are some of the many afflictions which will be notably improved with the application of this decoction [❸].

• **Intestinal parasites.** The vermifuge action is more intense with green rinds than with leaves [❷].

• **Diabetes.** Both the leaves and the green rind of walnut have proven to possess a mild hypoglycemic effect (decrease the level of sugar in blood) [❶]. Though these substances alone are not enough to treat diabetes, they can be a useful ***complement*** to other dietary measures, since they allow you to reduce the dosage of antidiabetic medicines.

The ***SEEDS*** of fruit, that is to say, the walnuts, contain 15% of proteins with a high biologic value, 60% of fats, composed by linoleic and linolenic acids, and important amounts of calcium, phosphorus, and vitamins A, B_1, B_2, and B_6. Well-chewed, they make a very nutritive food, ideal for sportsmen, students, and teenagers. They are recommended for people suffering from **tiredness, asthenia, or nervous system disorders.** As has been proven, such habitual consumption of walnuts decreases the level of cholesterol in the blood.

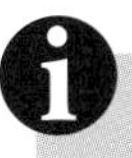

Walnuts and Cholesterol

On March, 4th, 1993, the prestigious medical magazine "New England Journal of Medicine" published the results of some research conducted by Dr. Joan Sabaté at the School of Public Health at Loma Linda University (USA), in which he proved that regular consumption of walnuts can reduce the level of cholesterol in blood. So, some diets against cholesterol, which forbid the consumption of walnuts and dried fruits, were shown to be wrong.

Despite walnuts containing up to 60% fat, these substances are mainly formed by polyunsaturated fatty acids (especially linoleic and linolenic acids), in a proportion seven times higher than that of saturated fatty acids.

*Latest research proves that unsaturated fatty acids, which are mainly found in vegetables, exert a reducing effect on the cholesterol production. Hence, the consumption of walnuts and other **dried fruits** not only does not produce cholesterol, but even reduces its production.*

Flax

Soothes the skin and the mucosa

FOUR THOUSAND years ago, flax was already cultivated in Mediterranean countries in order to obtain textile fibers, and 2500 years ago as a medicinal herb. Hippocrates recommended it as an emollient in the fifth century B.C.

PROPERTIES AND INDICATIONS. Flax seeds contain high amounts of mucilage and pectin, which give the plant **emollient and laxative** properties, as well as mineral salts and fats with a high biological value (essential unsaturated fatty acids). Its applications and indications are the following:

- **Chronic constipation.** Flax lubricates the digestive tract, making the feces softer. Moreover, it **regenerates the intestinal flora,** regulating the putrefaction and fermentation processes [❶,❷,❸]. Its effect is thus evident, since in the case of intestinal putrefaction, feces lose their putrid odor.
- **Gastritis, duodenitis, and gastro-duodenal ulcer.** It presents an anti-inflammatory and emollient action, which promotes the regeneration of the harmed digestive mucosa. Flax

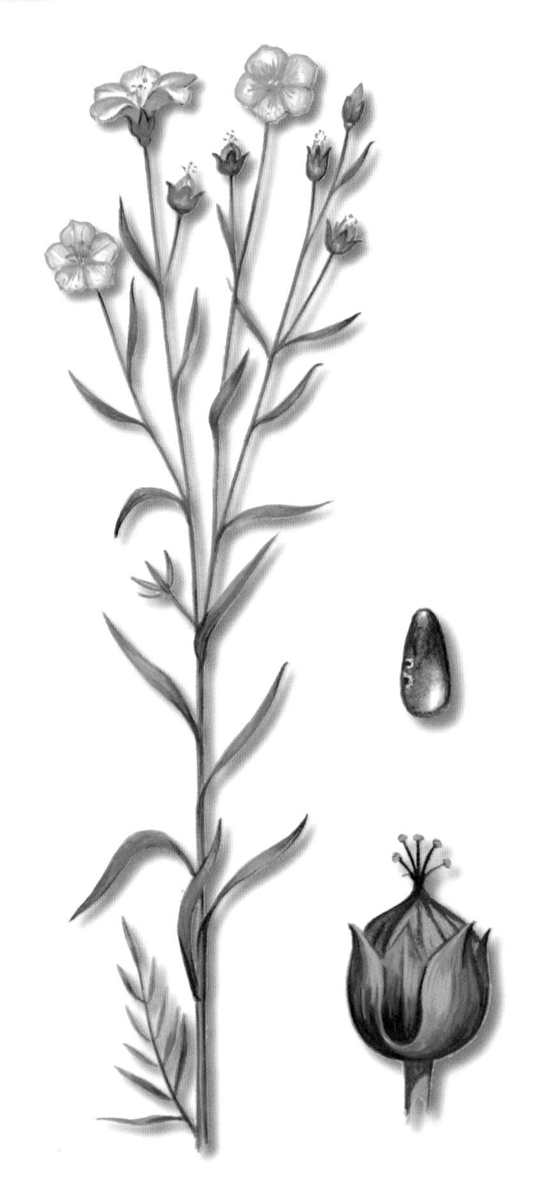

__Description.__ Herbaceous plant of the Linaceae family, growing from 40 to 80 cm high, with an upright stem and elongated, narrow leaves. Its flowers are light blue in color, with five petals, and its fruit is a globe-like capsule with ten brown seeds.

__Parts used.__ The linseed (flax seeds).

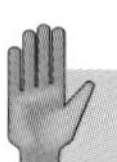

Warning

The __oil__ contained in linseed flour becomes __rancid__ quite easily, then produces __skin irritation.__ Therefore, __recently prepared flour__ is better for preparing the poultices.

Preparation and Use

INTERNAL USE

❶ **Decoction** of 30 g of seeds per liter of water, boiling for five minutes. Drink two or three cups daily, sweetened with honey if desired.

❷ **Cold extract.** Steep for 12 hours a spoonful of seeds per glass of water. Drink two or three glasses of the liquid every day.

❸ **Seeds.** Whole seeds can be taken, chewed (a spoonful every 12 hours).

EXTERNAL USE

❹ **Poultices.** Ground linseed (linseed flour) is added to boiling water until forming a thick paste. From 30 to 40 g of linseed flour are usually required per liter of water. When applying the poultice, it is advisable to protect the skin with a cold cloth to avoid burns.

❺ **Lotions with linseed oil.** Apply directly on the affected skin area.

seeds should be taken in a decoction as ***complement*** of any specific treatment for these processes.

• **Inflammation** of the **respiratory and urinary ways:** especially bronchitis and cystitis, due to its emollient and soothing effect on the mucosa **[❶,❷,❸]**.

Flax ***SEEDS*** (linseed) can also be used as a ***food.*** They are especially recommended for **diabetes,** due to their low content in sugars, and its high content in proteins and fats. Linseed must be consumed by those people wanting to **gain weight** or those suffering from **malnutrition** **[❸]**.

Poultices of linseed flour are applied whenever constant heat is required: colds and bronchitis, menstrual pain, chronic aches of the abdomen (whether kidney or gall bladder aches), intestinal spasms, insect bites, abscesses, and furuncles **[❹]**. They have **resolvent, antispasmodic, sedative, and anti-inflammatory** properties, besides **retaining heat** for a long time.

Linseed oil is used as a **skin soothing product** for eczema, dried skin, mild burns, and dermatosis **[❺]**.

Hot poultices of linseed flour are a traditional remedy which has proven its resolvent, sedative, and anti-inflammatory properties. They are very useful in treating abscesses, furuncles, and insect bites. They are also employed for of painful menstruation, kidney or intestinal colic, and bronchitis.

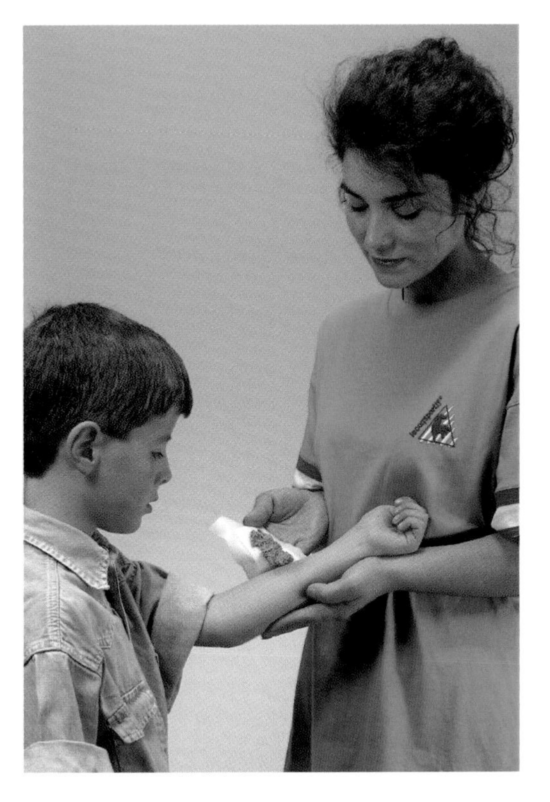

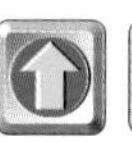

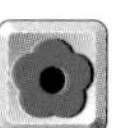

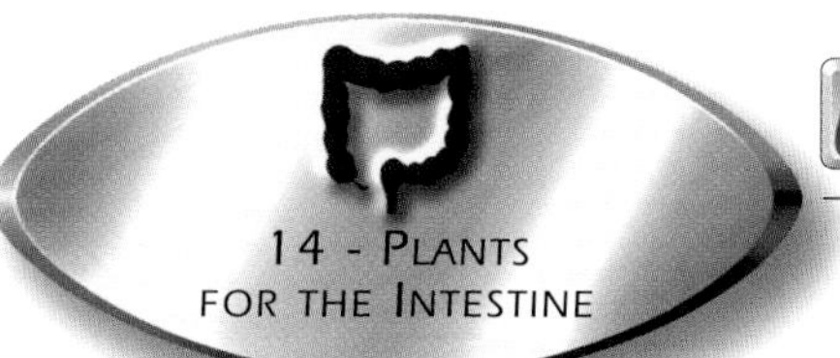

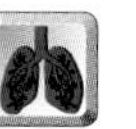

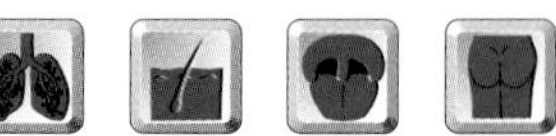

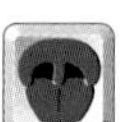

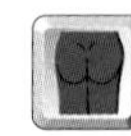

High Mallow

Soothes and reduces inflammation

HIPPOCRATES recommended it as an emollient and laxative herb, two properties which have been proven, and which at present are still used.

PROPERTIES AND INDICATIONS. The whole plant, and especially its flowers and leaves, contain a high amount of mucilage.

The use of high mallow is recommended in the following cases:

- **Chronic constipation.** It acts as a non-aggressive laxative, even when taken in large doses, which lubricates the intestinal tract. It is especially recommended for children and elderly people **[❶]**.
- **Respiratory afflictions.** It has **antitussive and expectorant** properties, thus being prescribed for colds, influenza, bronchitis, irritative or dry cough, and asthma **[❶]**.
- **Afflictions of the skin and the mucosa.** When applied ***locally,*** it helps heal pharyngitis, vaginitis, anal and rectal inflammation, eczema, acne, furuncles, and as a rule, all ***superficial irritation*** **[❷].**

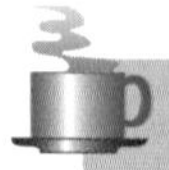

Preparation and Use

INTERNAL USE

❶ **Infusion or decoction** with 30 g of flowers and/or leaves per liter of water. Drink three or four hot cups daily.

EXTERNAL USE

❷ **Infusion or decoction.** The same one used internally, but slightly more concentrated, is also used externally in **gargles, vaginal irrigation, enema, and compresses** on the affected skin area.

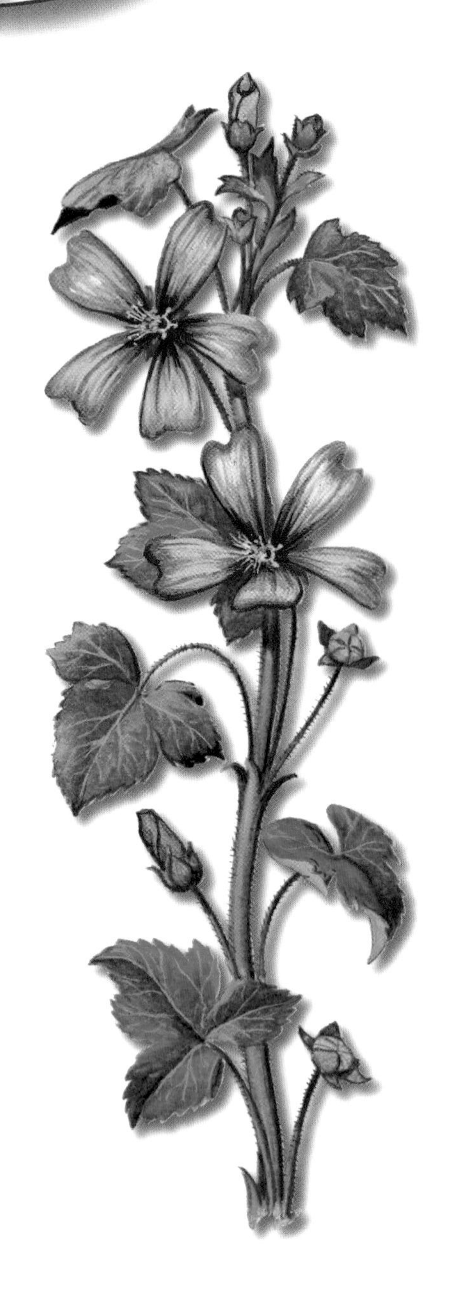

Description. *Biennial plant of the Mauvaceae family, growing from 20 to 70 cm high, with bright purple flowers with five petals.*

Parts used. *The flowers and leaves.*

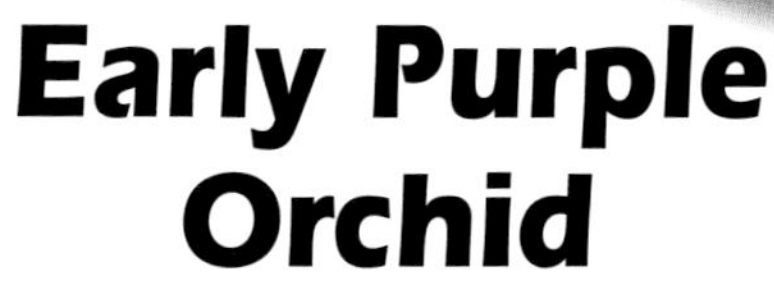

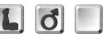

Early Purple Orchid

An antidiarrheic for children

ORCHIDS ARE the most numerous family of the Vegetal Kingdom, with more than 20,000 species spread all over the world. Their beautiful flowers and their botanical peculiarities make them a very desirable species.

Their two underground tubers gave birth, from ancient times on, to the idea of testicles. The name orchid is derived from the Latin word *orquis* (testicle).

PROPERTIES AND INDICATIONS. In Arab countries, a kind of flour is extracted from the early purple orchid tubers, as well as from those of other orchid species. This flour is called *salep.* The genesis of this word is the Arabic expression *djosa ataleb* (fox testicles).

Salep contains 50% of mucilage, 25% of starch, 5% of proteins, and 1% of sugar. It is highly effective as an **intestinal emollient, antidiarrheic, and invigorating.** It is recommended for of gastroenteritis, colitis, and dyspepsia. Salep is a good **food** for **children's diarrhea [❶].**

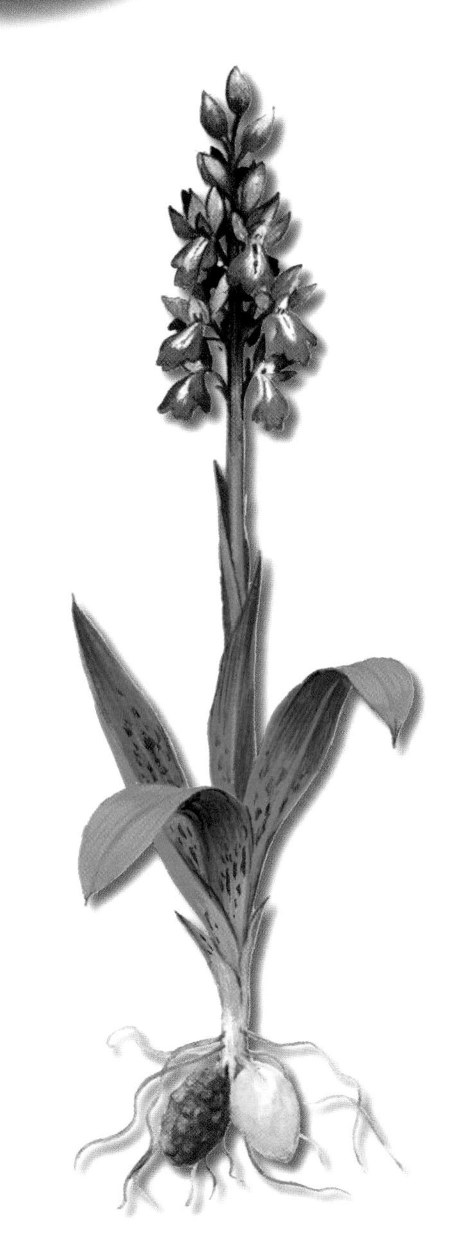

Description. *Vivacious plant of the Orchidaceae family, which grows from 15 to 30 cm high. Its elongated leaves have reddish brown stains. Its root is a tuber, with two unequal bulbs.*

Parts used. *The tubers.*

Preparation and Use

INTERNAL USE

❶ *Salep* is prepared in the form of **herbal tea, purée, or soup.** At present, it comes from Eastern countries, since orchids are protected species in almost all Western countries.

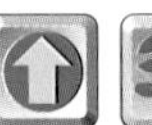
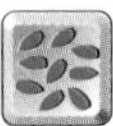
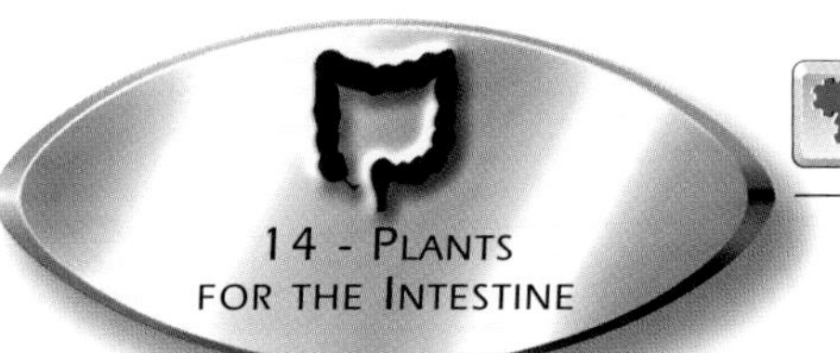

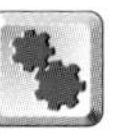
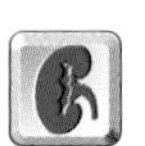
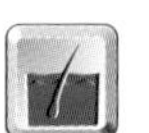
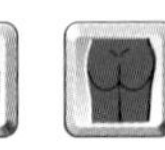

Psyllium

A laxative plant which protects the digestive tube

ANCIENT PEOPLE saw in this plant seeds a similarity to fleas (Greek *psyla*). Dioscorides recommended it in the first century A.D. as an emollient (soothing), and it has been used this way from that time until the mid-twentieth century, when it was found to have also mild laxative effects. At present, psyllium is part of several ***pharmaceutical preparations*** for **constipation.**

PROPERTIES AND INDICATIONS. The seeds of this plant contain a high amount of mucilage (up to 15%) which gives them laxative, emollient, and anti-inflammatory properties. Psyllium is ***one of the plants with a higher amount of mucilage*** known, even higher than flax seeds. It also contains fats with plant steroids (sitosterols), potassium salts and trace elements. These are its properties:

• **Digestive afflictions: Mucilage** acts as a hydrophilous colloidal substance, that is, its molecules become surrounded by many water molecules, which make it increase its volume and become a soft mass of gelatinous appearance. This way, mucilage achieves two effects:

— It creates a protective viscous layer which covers the whole interior of the digestive tract, from the stomach to the large intestine. With this, it offers a **soothing and anti-inflammatory** action on the **digestive mucosa,** which is highly beneficial for **gastritis, gastric or duodenal ulcer, and colitis.** It eases pyrosis **(acidity)** and **stomach ache,** and stops **colic pains** and **diarrhea** from colitis.

— It increases the volume of feces, and makes them softer, thus these substances pass more easily through the digestive tract, demanding less peristaltic effort from the colon. All

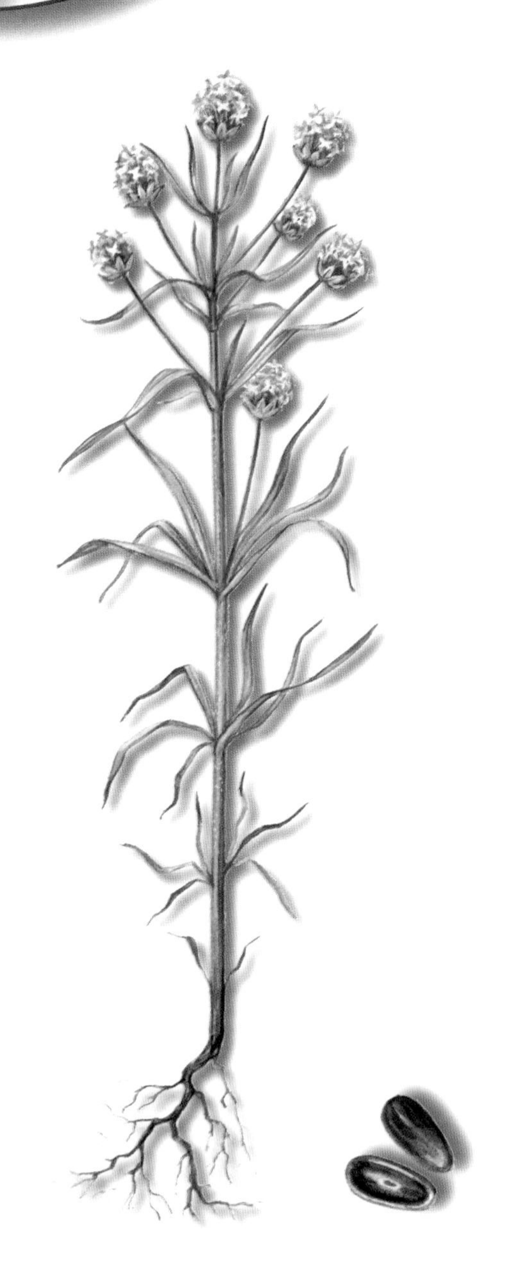

Description. *Annual plant of the Plantaginaceae family, with an herbaceous, upright stem growing up to 30 cm high. Its flowers are small, white, and grow in oval spikes. The fruits contain two 3 mm sized seeds, smooth and brown in color.*

Parts used. *The seeds.*

Preparation and Use

INTERNAL USE

➊ **Seeds cold extract.** Grind or mash the seeds and steep them for one or two hours (a spoonful of seeds per glass of water). Then take the resulting mucilage by straining the liquid. If desired add a teaspoonful of anise seeds to improve the flavor. Drink a glass in the morning and another at night, before going to bed.

EXTERNAL USE

➋ **Seed poultices.** After cold extract, heat the seeds and prepare a poultice, which should be put on the affected area for at least 15 minutes, two or three times daily.

➌ **Enema.** It is done with the liquid resulting from the cold extract. From 100 to 250 ml are enough for each application. Administer up to three enemas daily.

these facts result in a **mild laxative effect,** with no cramps or irritation, without creating addiction or producing potassium or mineral salts loss, that is to say, without undesirable side effects. The mucilage psyllium contains ***can be continuously used*** for months or even years. It is very useful in treating chronic constipation and its consequences, such as **hemorrhoids** or **colon diverticulosis.** It also prevents such consequences.

Diverticulosis results from excessive pressure exerted by the colon to make hard or dry feces progress through it. Meat-rich diets lacking in vegetables, fruits, and integral grains, produce heavy, scant feces which demand great efforts from the large intestine. The result is constipation and its complications, the most severe of which is cancer of the colon.

Treatment with mucilage must be accompanied by a ***change in dietari habits.***

Laxative properties of mucilage [➊] are enhanced by those of the hemicellulose, a fiber which forms the seed covering.

The beneficial effects of mucilage on the intestine can be also obtained when administering it in enemas, which are recommended for anal and rectal inflammations [➌]. It reduces the inflammation of hemorrhoids and eases discomfort caused by anal fissures. It is also recommended for proctitis (rectal inflammation), and colitis, even ulcerative colitis. In this last case it is used to ***complement*** the specific treatment.

• **Obesity treatment.** Psyllium seed intake with plenty of water, during meals, produces a full sensation in the stomach, decreasing the appetite [➊]. This action is due to the hydrophilous ability of mucilage, which swells and increases its volume with the water.

This effect also contributes to the weight loss achieved when taking psyllium.

Moreover, it has been proven that mucilage decreases the **cholesterol** and **triglyceride** levels in the blood [➊], This is likely due to its interference with the fat absorption process on the small intestine.

• **Urine afflictions.** Psyllium mucilage also acts as an **anti-inflammatory** substance on the urinary mucosa. It helps ease cystitis discomforts and promotes the regeneration of irritated mucosa [➊]. It is usually employed ***in combination*** with other treatments.

• **Skin afflictions.** When applied ***locally*** as poultices, it protects and reduces the inflammation of the skin when it has been irritated from eczema, dermatosis, or rashes. It has wound healing properties when used on burns, wounds, or varicose ulceration [➋]. It is also used in ***cosmetics*** to improve skin beauty.

Purslane

Laxative and eye calmant

PURSLANE WAS cultivated in ancient times as a vegetable to be consumed in salads, though at present there are peasants who regard it as a weed. Its medicinal applications are still used.

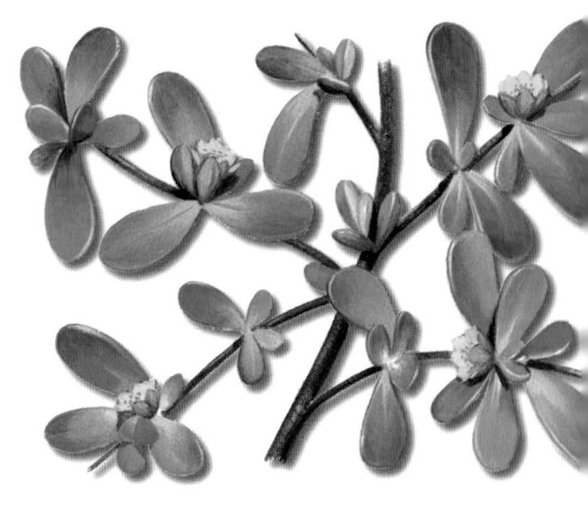

PROPERTIES AND INDICATIONS. The whole plant contains a high amount of mucilage, which is its most important active components, and give the plant **emollient, anti-inflammatory, and laxative** properties. It also contains vitamin C, to which it owes its antiscorbutic properties. Purslane has **diuretic and depurative** properties, though the causative active component is still not known.

This plant is applied for chronic **constipation.** As a diuretic and depurative plant, it is recommended for **obesity** or rich diets. Due to its soothing and anti-inflammatory properties, it is very useful for **cystitis** and kidney **stones** **[❶,❷]**.

In ***external application,*** it is used in poultices for **blepharitis** (eyelid inflammation) and **conjunctivitis [❸].**

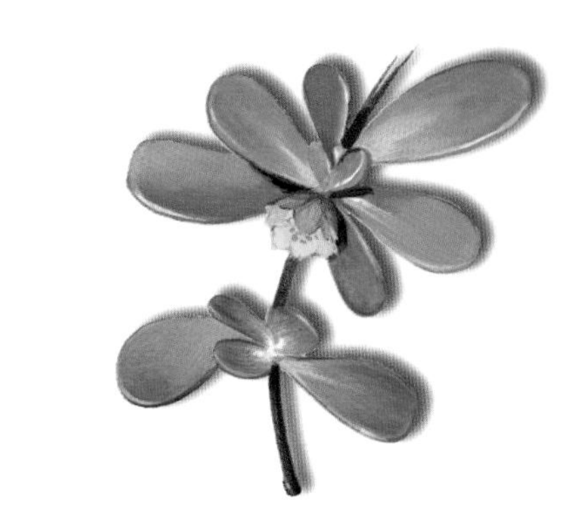

__Description.__ Annual, creeping plant of the Portulaceae family, with thick, juicy stems and small, oval-shaped, fleshy leaves, white on their underside. Its flowers are small, yellow in color.

__Parts used.__ The leaves, and fresh stems.

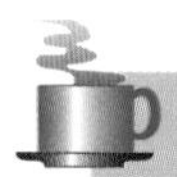

Preparation and Use

INTERNAL USE

❶ As a vegetable in salads, dressed with oil, salt, and lemon juice.

❷ **Decoction** with 100 g of fresh plant per liter of water. Drink up to five cups daily.

EXTERNAL USE

❸ **Poultices** with the fresh plant, mashed.

Tormentil

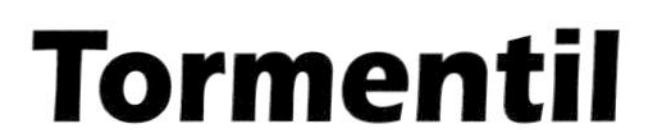

THIS PLANT has been used since the Middle Ages to ease what in that time was known as "torments" (intestinal colic). Its name originates from that fact. And, due to its intense effects, it is called *Potentilla* in Latin, which comes from *potentem* (powerful).

PROPERTIES AND INDICATIONS. The main component of the tormentil rhizome is tannin, which makes up 15% of its weight. It also contains a glycoside (tormentilline) and bitter chinovic acid. It has ***strong* astringent and antidiarrheic** properties, as well as **hemostatic** (stops hemorrhages) properties. It is recommended for the following cases:

- **Infectious diarrhea** of all types. It calms colic aches caused by intestinal spasms which usually go together with diarrhea [❶,❷].
- **Hemorrhoids.** When ***locally applied*** (sitz baths) it reduces the inflammation of hemorrhoids and stops bleeding [❸].
- **Stomatitis and pharyngitis.** Used in mouth rinsings and gargles [❹].
- **Epistaxis** (nasal hemorrhages). Applied as irrigation or by soaking a gauze packing [❺].

Description. *Plant of the Rosaceae family, growing from 10 to 40 cm high, with weak stems, leaves with three toothed segments, and flowers with four petals, unlike other Potentilla species such as silverweed and five-finger grass which have five petals.*

Parts used. *The rhizome (underground stem) when fresh.*

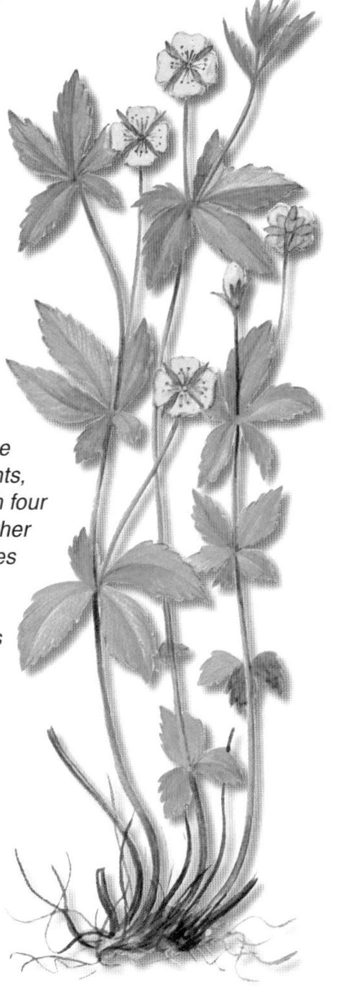

Preparation and Use

INTERNAL USE

❶ **Decoction** with 30 g of rhizome per liter of water. Drink three or four cups daily, until diarrhea stops.

❷ **Powder.** The recommended dose is 2-4 g daily, in capsules.

EXTERNAL USE

❸ **Sitz baths.** Add to the bath water 1-2 liters of a decoction more concentrated than that used internally (60-100 g per liter).

❹ **Mouth rinses and gargles.** With the aforementioned decoction.

❺ **Irrigation and nasal packing,** with the same decoction.

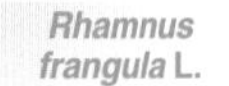
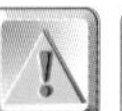
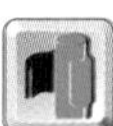
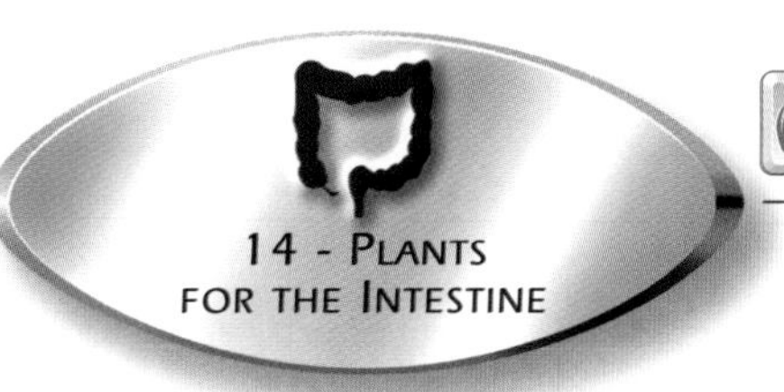
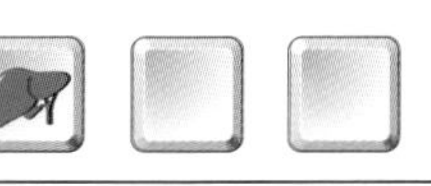

Alder Buckthorn

Ideal laxative for chronic constipation

THE GREAT Renaissance botanist Andrea Mattioli published in 1554 a commentary edition of Dioscorides' *De Materia Medica,* in which he said, according to Font Quer's quote, that the "alder buckthorn bark is a mild purgative, which cleanses the liver [...]. But it must be only used when dry. When fresh, it causes vomiting."

This scholar botanist noticed the curious process which takes place in the alder buckthorn bark: when ***fresh it is toxic*** and has an intensive vomiting effects. However, as times goes by, it loses toxicity spontaneously, and acquires notable medicinal properties. After ***one year drying,*** the alder buckthorn bark becomes a highly appreciated remedy against constipation.

At present, we know one of the enzymes contained in the alder buckthorn bark, ramnodiase, slowly oxidizes its anthraquinonic glycosides with vomitive properties, thus becoming franguloemodine and rhamnose, two medicinal active components. This process takes about one year when spontaneous, but dry artificial heat can make it quicker.

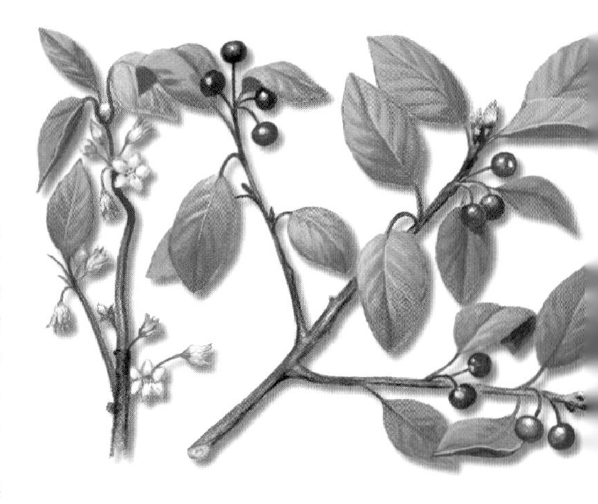

Description. *Shrub of the Rhamnaceae family, growing from 2 to 3 m high, without thorns, with small five-petals flowers. Its berries are red colored in Summer and bright black colored in Fall, when ripe.*

Parts used. *Dry trunk and branches bark.*

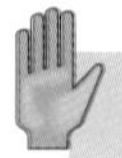

Warning

*Alder buckthorn **bark** must **never be consumed with** sodium bicarbonate, magnesium milk, or any other alkaline substance, as its effects would be decreased.*

*We **advise against** its use **in the case** of pregnancy, breast-feeding, menstruation, and inflamed hemorrhoids).*

Who was the first one to observe this interesting transformation taking place in the alder buckthorn bark? Thanks to his or her persistence, and to that of many other anonymous researchers, we can currently enjoy the healing properties of medicinal herbs.

PROPERTIES AND INDICATIONS. As we mentioned, the active components of the alder buckthorn bark are anthraquinonic glycosides, which give the plant the following properties:

• Mild **laxative,** however effective **[❶]**. It does not produce cramps, liquid defecation, or any

Preparation and Use

INTERNAL USE

❶ Decoction with 20-30 g of ground bark, aged (at least one year), in half a liter of water. Boil for 20 minutes. If steeped for some hours, its effectiveness increases. Strain and drink one or two cups, preferably at night, so that it has results the morning after.

other side effects relative to irritant laxatives. It does not cause loss of potassium or any mineral salts, nor right lower side colitis; facts which are often observed in the case of chemical laxatives. And the intestine does not become accustomed to its use, so its effects are constant even when it is taken for long periods of time. The alder buckthorn is thus ideal for those suffering from **intestinal laziness** that lasts for ***years,*** and have tried diverse laxative substances with no success, sometimes with undesirable side effects. These patients, usually women, should have a ***diet rich in*** bran to overcome this uncomfortable ailment.

• **Choleretic.** According to Mattioli, the alder buckthorn bark also promotes the good function of the liver due to its choleretic properties. People suffering from acute and chronic hepatitis, diverse liver dysfunction, and even cirrhosis, should take advantage of its use **[❶]**.

The alder buckthorn is a shrub whose bark has a mild and effective laxative action. It is recommended for chronic constipation which young women usually suffer from.

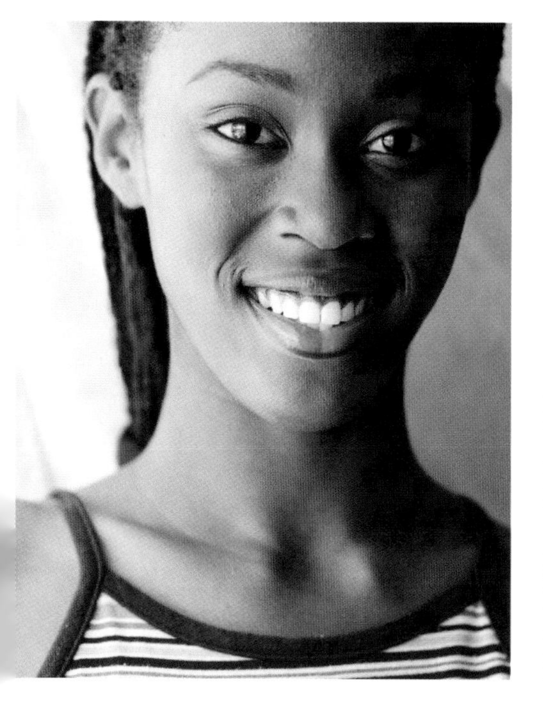

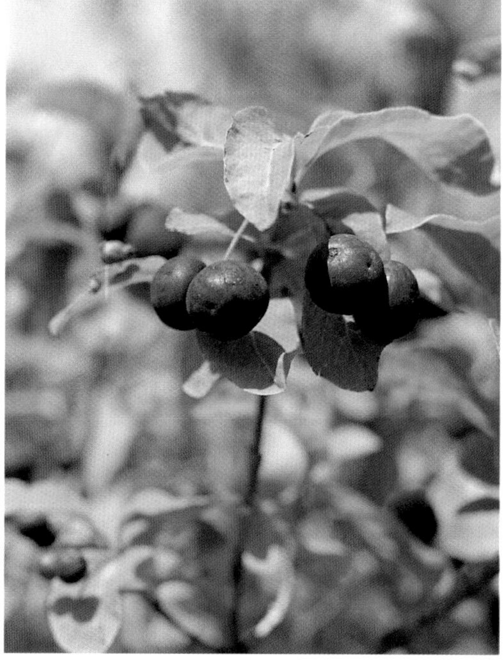

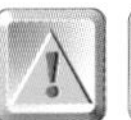

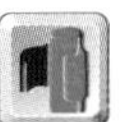

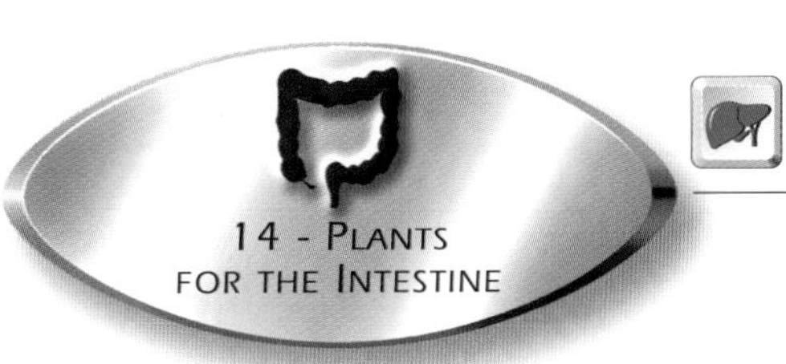

Cascara Sagrada

A powerful, recommended laxative

LIKE THE BARK of the alder buckthorn (*Rhamnus frangula* L.), a similar species which grows in Europe, cascara sagrada must not be consumed until it has been dried for ***one year,*** since ***when fresh it has toxic effects.***

PROPERTIES AND INDICATIONS. The bark of this tree contains anthraquinonic glycosides (emodine, chrysophine), similar to those of the alder buckthorn, as well as other glycosides (aloin, chrysaloin). Its intense purgative effect, more drastic than that of the alder buckthorn, is due to the combined action of all these active components.

Though being a ***potent*** **purgative,** in therapeutic doses it is ***quite well tolerated,*** and does not produce cramps or colitis. It can be used for ***long periods*** of time, unlike chemical laxatives. This plant is thus ideal for chronic constipation or intestinal atony, especially for elderly people [❶,❷].

It also has mild **cholagogue and eupeptic** properties, thus promoting the emptying of the gall bladder, and easing digestion [❶,❷].

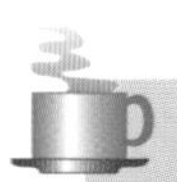

Preparation and Use

INTERNAL USE

❶ Bark **powder.** The recommended dose is 0.2-0.3 g, twice a day.

❷ **Infusion,** with 3 g of bark per cup of water. Drink up to three cups daily, on an empty stomach.

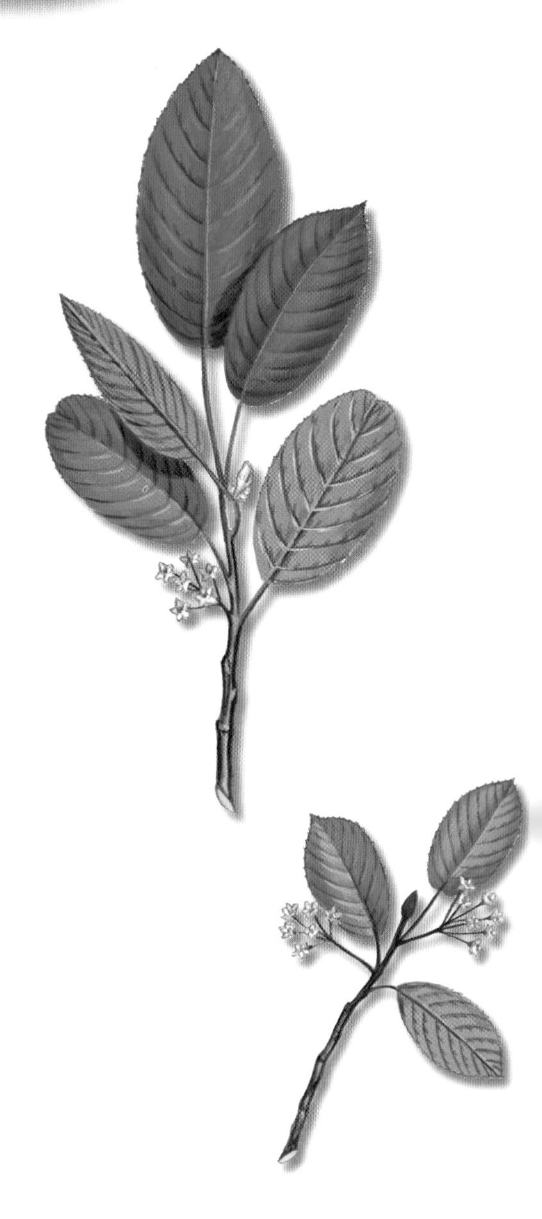

Description. *Tree or shrub of the Rhamnaceae family, growing from 2 to 6 m high, with oval leaves which have prominent nerves. Its bark is greyish, and is often covered by lichen.*

Parts used. *The bark of the trunk and branches, when dry.*

Rhubarb

Laxative and invigorator

RHUBARB is one of the plants which has been used since ancient times with medicinal aims. It was mentioned in the writings of Chen-Nung, a Chinese Emperor, 2700 years B.C. Dioscorides, in the first century A.D., introduced its use to Europe.

PROPERTIES AND INDICATIONS. The rhubarb root contains anthraquinonic derivatives to which the plant owes its laxative and purgative properties, as well as tannin, which give it astringent, invigorating, and digestive properties. Its effects depend on the dose taken:

- **Low doses** (0.1-0.5 g of root powder **[❶]** or half a cup of infusion **[❷]**): **Astringent** properties of tannin predominate. It stops diarrhea, increases appetite, and stimulates the functions of the stomach **(eupeptic:** it promotes digestion) and of the liver **(choleretic:** relieves liver congestion and promotes bile secretion). In short, it invigorates and regulates the digestive system.
- **Medium doses** (0.5-1 g of root powder **[❶]** or a cup of infusion **[❷]**): **Laxative** properties of anthraquinones predominate. It produces a defecation with no colic some 8-10 hours after its intake. It presents a strong congestion-relieving effect on the liver.
- **High doses** (1-3 g of root powder **[❶]** or 2-3 cups of infusion **[❷]**): **Effective purgative and vermifuge.**

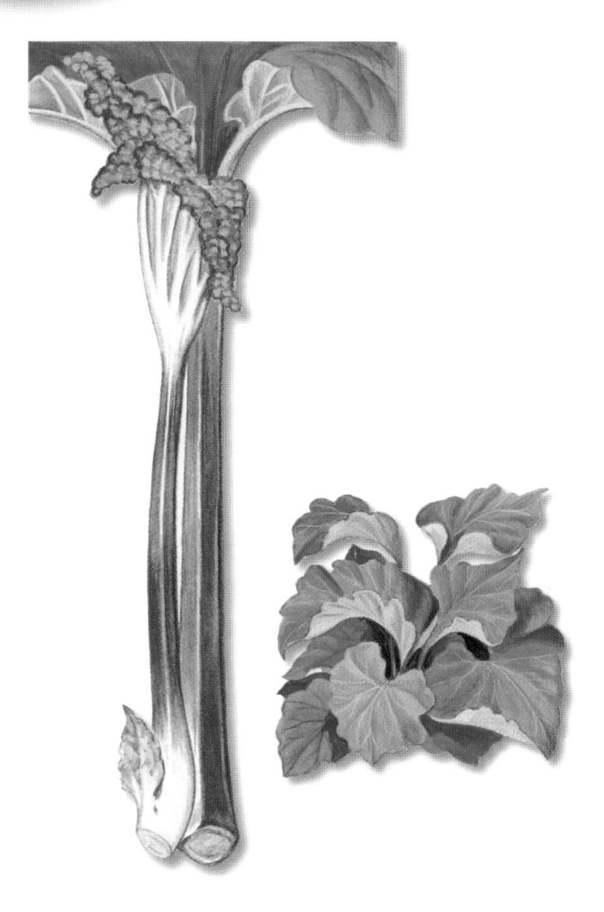

Description. *Vivacious plant of the Polygonaceae family, growing from 1 to 2 m high, with large, palm-shaped leaves, and a large rhizome with a characteristic smell.*

Parts used. *The root.*

Preparation and Use

INTERNAL USE

❶ **Root powder.** It usually comes in the form of pills. The doses are those recommended in the text, see section "Properties and Indications". We recommend that you begin treatment by trying low doses. Maximum dose for adults: 3 g per day; for children, never exceed 0.05 g per year of age.

❷ **Infusion of root,** with 5-10 g per liter of water. Drink from a half to three cups at night before going to bed. One cup approximately equates to 1 g of root powder.

Castor Bean

Classic and safe purgative

DIOSCORIDES, in the first century A.D., already knew the purgative properties of castor bean oil, however until the eighteenth century, it was not used in Europe.

PROPERTIES AND INDICATIONS. Castor bean seeds contain around 50% of oil, ricinine (an alkaloid), and ricin, a very toxic glycoprotein which agglutinates red blood cells, but remains in the flesh of the seed after extracting its oil.

At the recommended doses, castor bean oil produces a mild **purgative** effect some two hours after its intake. It is non irritant, with no colic or cramps. It effectively heals any constipation case, even those in children [❶]. However, if the case of **habitual constipation,** we recommend adopting ***dietary measures*** as well as employing ***milder laxative substances.*** It is also useful to expel **intestinal parasites.**

Externally used, both the ***OIL*** and the ***SEEDS*** of the plant have **emollient and healing** properties. They are applied for eczema, herpes, wounds, burns, skin rashes, and to fight hair loss, both in the form of lotions and in poultices [❷,❸].

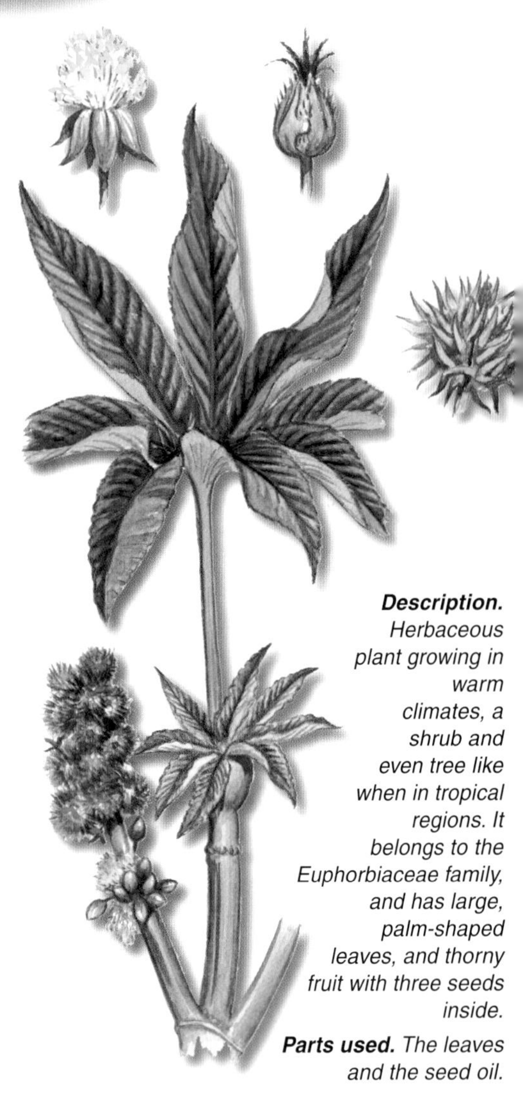

Description. *Herbaceous plant growing in warm climates, a shrub and even tree like when in tropical regions. It belongs to the Euphorbiaceae family, and has large, palm-shaped leaves, and thorny fruit with three seeds inside.*

Parts used. *The leaves and the seed oil.*

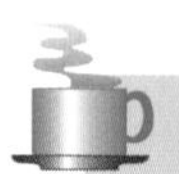

Preparation and Use

INTERNAL USE

❶ As a **purgative,** the dose is 5-10 g of oil for children, and 15-30 g for adults, taken in the morning, on an empty stomach.

EXTERNAL USE

❷ **Lotion** with the oil on the affected skin area.

❸ **Poultices** with mashed fresh leaves.

Warning

*An intake of three **seeds** can cause **death** to a child, and 10-15 seeds, to an adult person.*

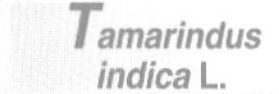

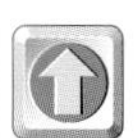
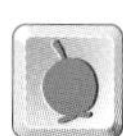
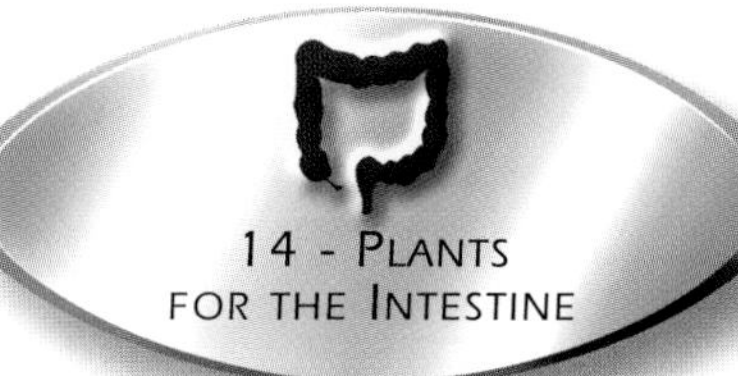

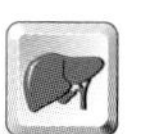
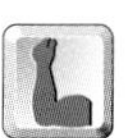
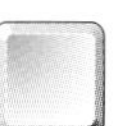
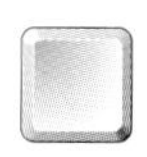

Tamarind

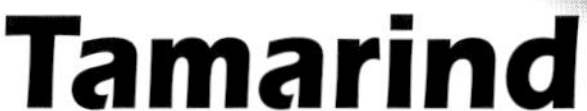

Refreshing and a mild laxative

IN CARIBBEAN and Central American countries, soft drinks based on tamarind flesh are very common, and have a sweet and sour flavor at the same time. Besides its pleasant flavor, this plant has several medicinal properties.

PROPERTIES AND INDICATIONS. The flesh covering the seeds of tamarind is rich in sugar (60%-65%) and organic acids (citric, malic, and tartaric). It also contains pectin.

The medicinal applications of this ***FLESH*** are as follows:

- **Mild laxative,** because of the sugars and pectin it contains. It is usually associated with tinnevelly senna (p. 492) in order to enhance its action. It produces soft defecation with no colic **[❶]**.
- **Mild choleretic and cholagogue.** It is recommended for gall bladder and liver disorders, since it can relieve liver congestion and promote the emptying of the gall bladder **[❶]**.
- **Refreshing and invigorating.** Its use is recommended for febrile afflictions and during sports training **[❶,❷]**.
- Its ***LEAVES*** have **anthelmintic and vermifuge** properties (destroy intestinal parasites), as well as **astringent [❷].**

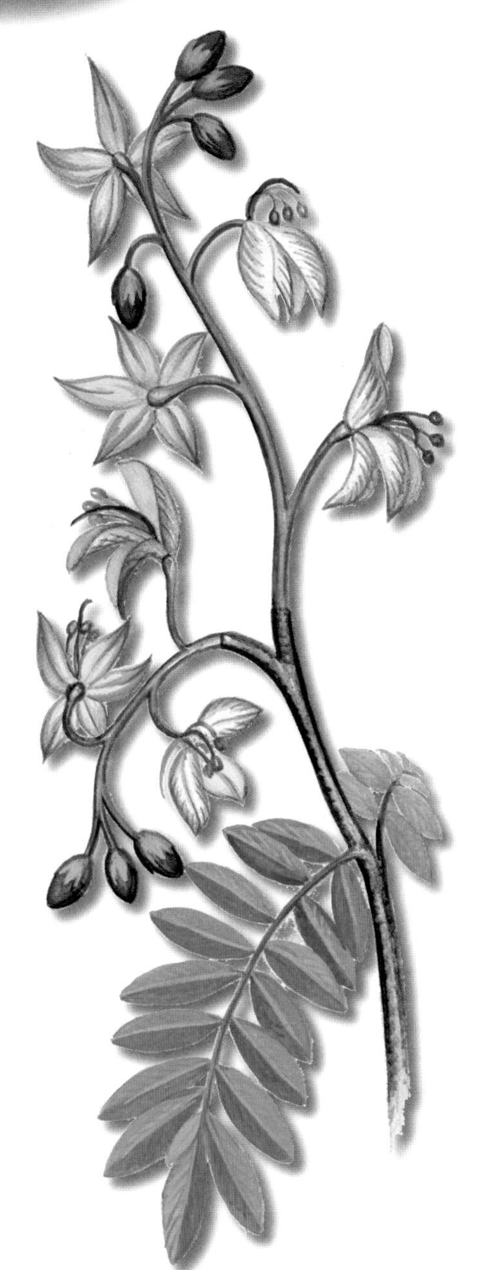

__Description.__ Evergreen tree of the Leguminoseae family, growing up to 25 m high. Its fruit are hanging pods, 15-20 cm long, whose interior have a yellow flesh covering the seeds.

__Parts used.__ The flesh of the fruit and the leaves.

Preparation and Use

INTERNAL USE

❶ **Flesh.** Take from 20 to 40 g, dissolved in water, up to three times a day.

❷ **Infusion** with 30 g of leaves per liter of water. Drink three cups daily.

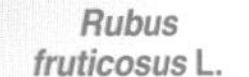
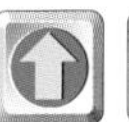
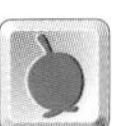
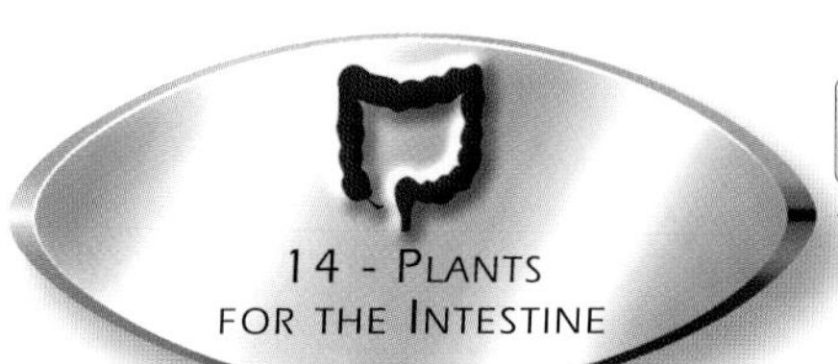

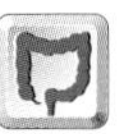
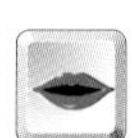
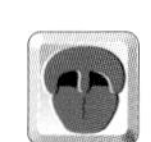
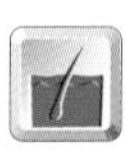

Bramble

Improves hemorrhoids and stops diarrhea

DIOSCORIDES recommended bramble leaves for the treatment of hemorrhoids many years ago. Its fruit, blackberries, have been used for many ages as food, being an excellent natural sweet for both children and adults.

Around one hundred varieties of brambles are known, all of them with the same properties.

PROPERTIES AND INDICATIONS. Leaves and young buds of brambles contain a high amount of tannin, which give the plant astringent and hemostatic properties. The fruit contains, besides tannin, sugars, (glucose and levulose), provitamin A, vitamin C, and organic acids (citric, lactic, succinic, oxalic, and salicylic). Their indications are as follows:

• **Hemorrhoids.** A decoction of both ***LEAVES*** and ***YOUNG BUDS*** of brambles is applied ***lo-***

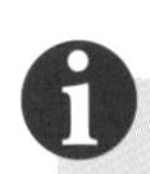

Bramble Buds Against Tobacco

*Smokers wanting to give up their noxious habit may try a new way to stop smoking. Put between your lips a **young bud** of bramble, and slowly suck it.*

The slightly sweet and sour flavor of these buds creates a certain aversion towards tobacco, and decreases the desire for a cigarette, at least while the bud is held in your mouth.

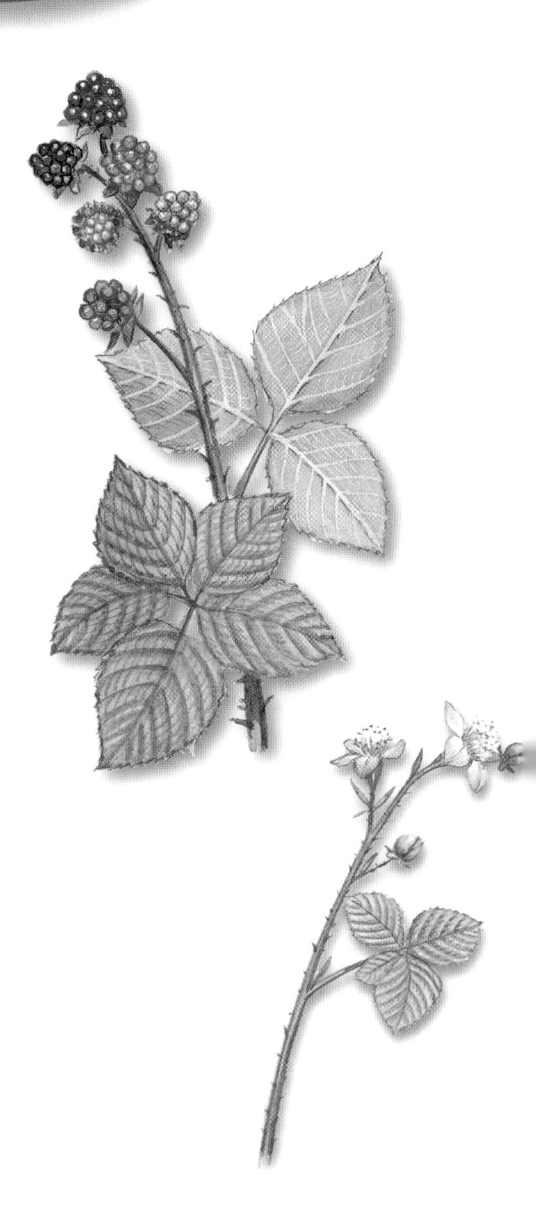

Description. *Thorny shrub of the Rosaceae family, growing up to 4 m high, with white or pink flowers, 5 petals each. The fruit consists of several small drupes, dark purple or black in color, with a seed inside each one.*

Parts used. *The leaves, young buds, and the fruit (blackberries).*

Preparation and Use

INTERNAL USE

❶ **Decoction** with 30-50 g of young buds and/or leaves per liter of water, boiling for ten minutes. Drink up to three cups daily.

❷ **Young buds** in Spring. They can be directly eaten, and provide a healing action when touching the oral mucosa.

❸ **blackberry juice.** Drink it freshly made, the dose being from one to three glasses daily.

❹ **Syrup.** Prepared by adding to the juice, two times its weight of sugar, preferably brown sugar, then heating until it is completely dissolved.

Both blackberry juice and syrup are usually mixed with the decoction in order to improve the effects and enhance the latter's flavor.

EXTERNAL USE

❺ **Decoction** slightly more concentrated (50-80 g per liter) than the internally used one. Apply it in the form of **compresses, sitz baths, rinses, and gargles.**

❻ **Poultices** made with mashed leaves. Apply them on the affected skin area.

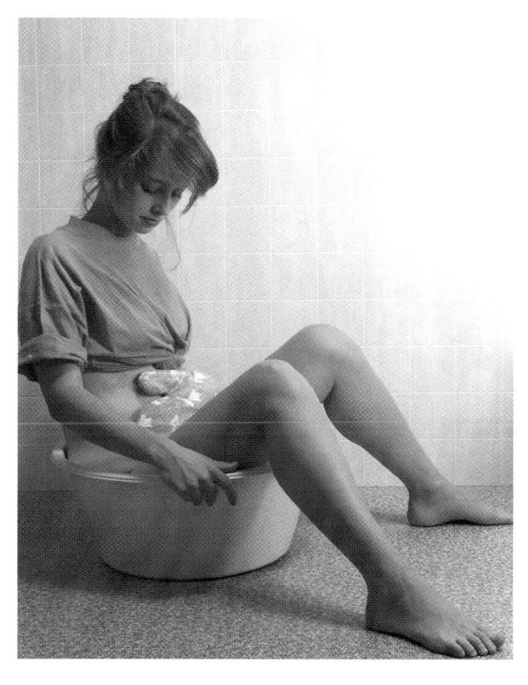

The upper picture clearly shows the right way to take a sitz bath for hemorrhoids, with a decoction made from leaves and buds of bramble.

Gentle massage with a bath glove on the lower stomach helps improve blood circulation in the pelvis, which also helps heal hemorrhoids.

The lower picture shows the delicious blackberries which are so attractive to children and adults.

cally in sitz baths or compresses in order to reduce their inflammation and prevent them from bleeding [❺].

• **Diarrhea, gastroenteritis, and colitis,** because of their notable astringent properties. The ***YOUNG BUDS*** and ***LEAVES*** [❶] are more astringent than the ***FRUIT*** [❸,❹], however all of them are usually ***consumed*** together to enhance their effects and take advantage of the flavor of the fruit. **Children** suffering from diarrhea can take blackberry juice in spoonfuls [❸], or the syrup made with this juice [❹].

• **Febrile diseases.** The juice of the ***FRUIT*** (blackberries) is refreshing and invigorating, thus being recommended for weakened people or those suffering from febrile diseases [❸].

• **Oral and pharyngeal afflictions.** Both a decoction of ***LEAVES*** and ***YOUNG BUDS*** [❶], young green buds [❷] and the ***FRUITS*** [❸], have beneficial effects on mouth sores, as well as for gingivitis (gum inflammation), stomatitis (inflammation of the oral mucosa), pharyngitis, and tonsillitis.

• **Skin wounds, ulcers, and furuncles.** Apply compresses or baths with the decoction [❺], or poultices with mashed ***LEAVES*** [❻]. These will help with healing.

15

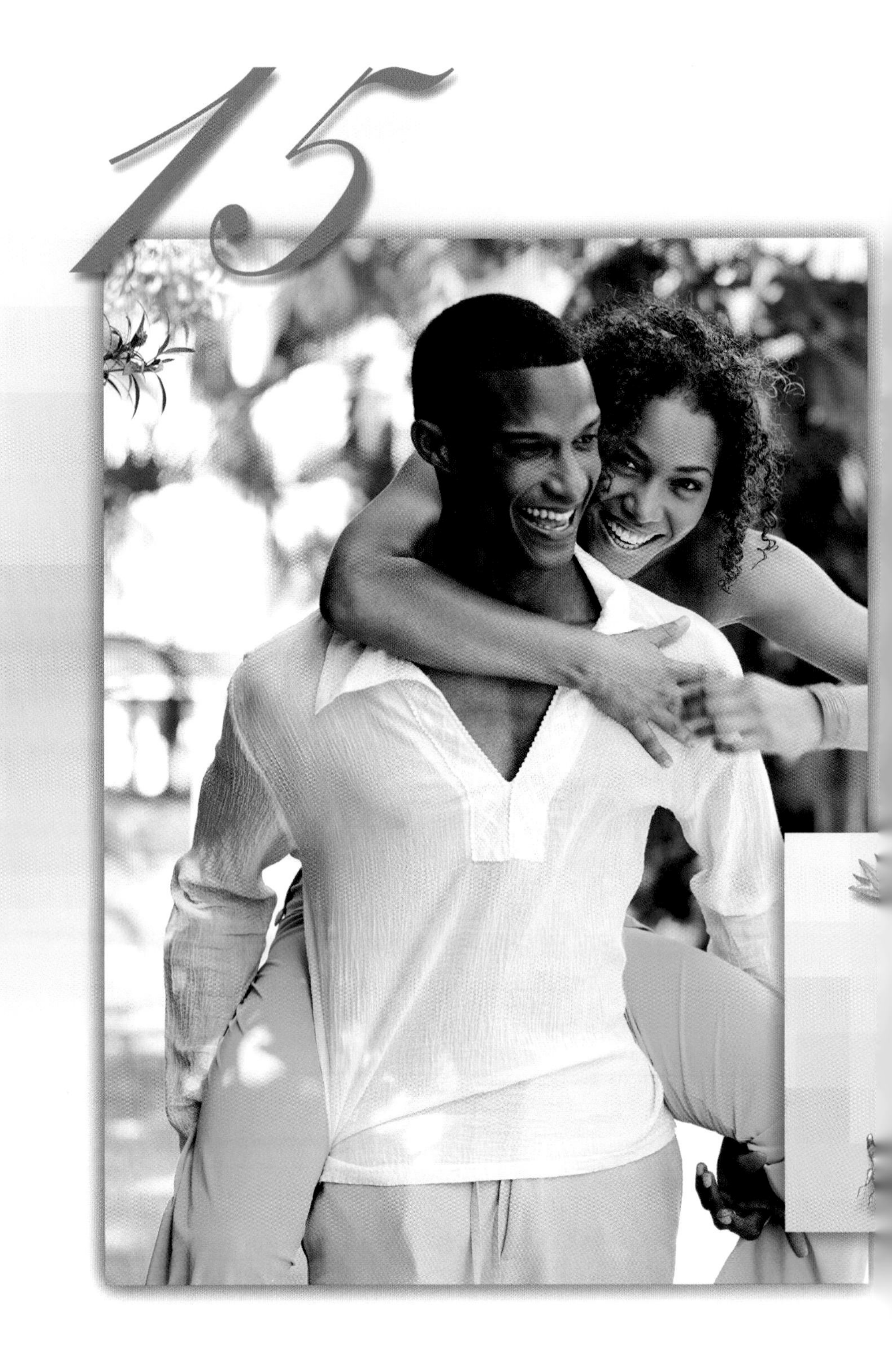

Plants for the Urinary System

DISEASES	PAGES
Calculi, urine, see Urinary lithiasis	268
Colic, kidney	269
Cystitis	271
Dropsy	269
Edema	269
Enuresis	270
Incontinence, urinary	271
Infection, kidney, see Pyelonephritis	270
Infection, urinary	270
Kidney colic	269
Lithiasis, urinary	268
Nephritis and nephrosis	270
Pyelonephritis	270
Stones in the urine, see Urinary lithiasis	268
Urethritis	271
Urinary calculi, see Urinary lithiasis	268
Urinary incontinence	271
Urinary lithiasis	268

PLANTS	PAGES
Agave	272
Bearberry	274
Buchu	277
Cane	276
Copaiba	280
Eryngo	281
Golden-rod	286
Juniper	282
Madder	284
Pellitory of the wall	283
Saxifrage	285
White birch	278
Witch grass	273

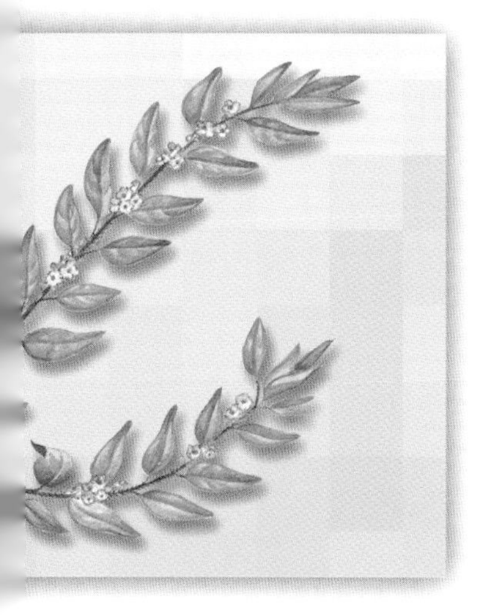

ALMOST ALL medicinal herbs act on the kidneys, causing an increase in the amount of urine. These diuretic properties of plants are enhanced by the water with which herbal teas are prepared.

By increasing urine volume, plants promote the function of **eliminating waste substances** which kidneys perform. Hence, they help cleanse the blood and purify the whole body.

Uric acid and **urea** are two of the most toxic substances our body continuously produces, and they must be eliminated through urine. There are many effective plants which promote the elimination of both metabolic waste substances.

Plants are highly effective in increasing the solubility of mineral salts which usually are dissolved into the urine. When they are not dissolved, these salts form precipitations in the kidneys, called **kidney stones** or **calculi.** There are plants which can even dissolve kidney stones (unlike gall bladder stones).

Since many active components of plants are eliminated through the urine, when these active components have antiseptic or antibiotic properties, they successfully combat **infections** of the urinary system, from the kidneys to the urethra.

There are plants which improve the muscle tone of the urinary bladder, and promote its functioning, thus the cases of enuresis and urine incontinence will improve.

URINARY LITHIASIS

Definition

Lithiasis is the formation of **calculi** in a liquid environment, in this case, urine. Calculi form because of precipitation or solidification of substances which are usually dissolved. Due to any physical or chemical reason, these dissolved substances form a solid core, called calculus.

The size of calculi varies widely, from that of sand grains, easy to eliminate, to larger calculi.

Phytotherapy

These plants exert a ***preventive action*** which is notable on calculi formation. They even can dissolve, in some cases, already formed calculi.

These plants require to be taken during ***certain periods*** of time in order to exert their effects: between one and six months, and stopping one week per month.

White birch

NETTLE	Promotes elimination of metabolic acid waste which form sands
WHITE BIRCH	Promotes elimination of sand, prevents formation of kidney stones
MADDER	Sedative for pain, antiseptic, promotes calculi dissolution
SAXIFRAGE	Promotes dissolution and expulsion of urinary calculi
MEADOWSWEET	Promotes dissolution and elimination of calculi
HORSETAIL	Diuretic and depurative, eliminates toxic waste from the body

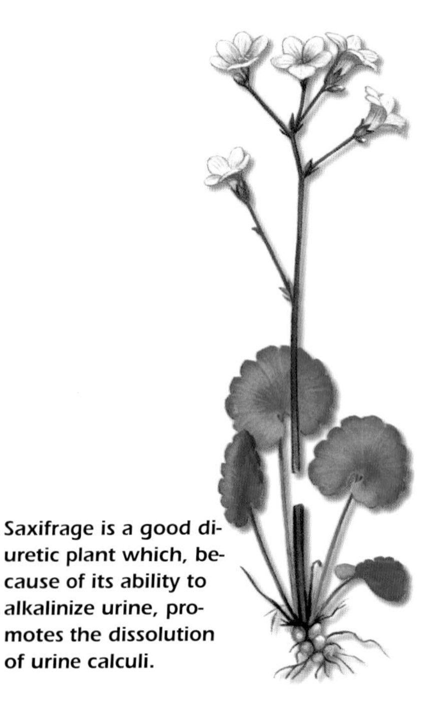

Saxifrage is a good diuretic plant which, because of its ability to alkalinize urine, promotes the dissolution of urine calculi.

KIDNEY COLIC

Definition

Also called **renal or nephritic colic,** this ailment manifests itself as a very intense pain which starts in one or both kidneys and goes towards its groin area.

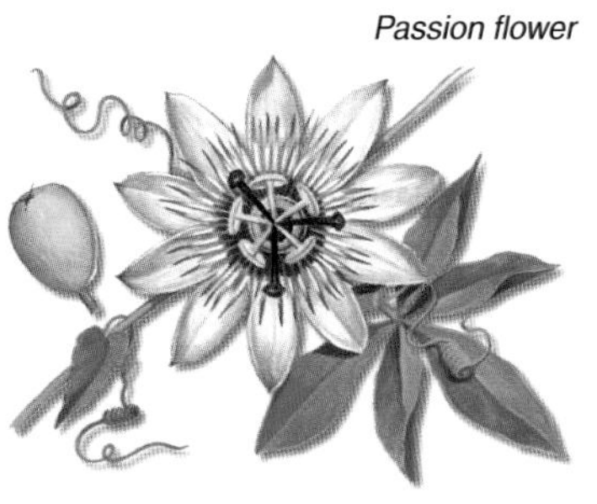
Passion flower

It is produced when a calculus becomes blocked within the urethra, a fine duct which joins the kidneys with the urine bladder. The pain is caused by **spasms** of the tiny muscle which forms the walls of the urethra, with which it is trying to expel the calculus inside it.

Phytotherapy

Phytotherapeutical treatment is based on **antispasmodic and diuretic plants,** able to relax the spasms of the urethra, and to increase the production of urine. In ***external applications*** hot **poultices** of linseed flour are very useful.

PASSION FLOWER	Antispasmodic, sedative, calms cholic pain
VERVAIN	Calms kidney cholic pain
GERMAN CAMOMILE	Sedative, antispasmodic
LEMON VERBENA	Antispasmodic
FLAX	Sedative and anti-inflammatory
WHITE BIRCH	Diuretic, promotes elimination of sands
PELLITORY OF THE WALL	Diuretic, anti-inflammatory, helps eliminating calculi
MADDER	Pain sedative, antiseptic, helps dissolving calculi
SAXIFRAGE	Promotes dissolution and expulsion of urinary calculi

EDEMA

Definition

An excessive accumulation of liquid in tissues. It may be caused for **renal** reasons, when kidneys are inflamed (nephritis) and do not produce enough urine, or for **circulatory** reasons. In both cases, a passing of water and sodium chlorine from blood to tissues occurs.

When there is edema, an increase of body weight and a decrease of the volume of urine take place.

Plants recommended here have a ***mild and safe diuretic*** effect, which will eliminate liquids retained in the tissues.

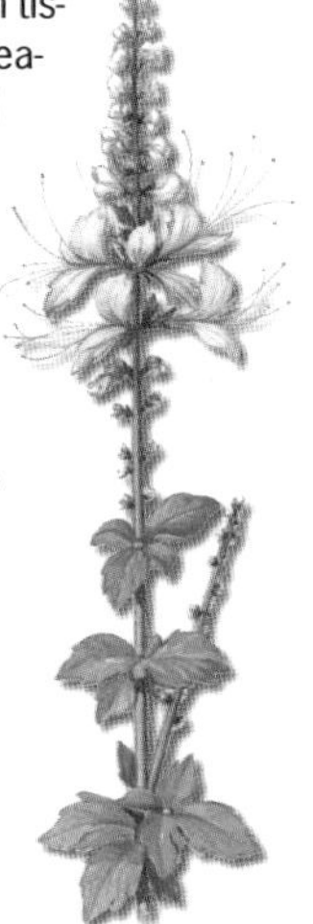
Javan tea

WHITE BIRCH	Diuretic, regenerates and reduces the inflammation of kidney tissues
GOLDEN-ROD	Increases urine production, reduces kidney inflammation
JAVAN TEA	Diuretic, promotes elimination of fluids
HORSETAIL	Diuretic and depurative, eliminates toxic waste from the body

DROPSY

Definition

A **general edema,** which manifests itself by total body swelling. It is usually due to heart insufficiency or to severe metabolic disorders.

Phytotherapy

Phytotherapeutical treatment, which must be applied **under medical control,** is based on plants with ***diuretic and sudorific*** properties, which promote the elimination of liquids, as well as on ***cardiotonic*** plants which improve heart performance.

FOXGLOVE	Increases heart efficiency, diuretic
BLACK ELDER	Diuretic, purgative, prevents retention of liquids

NEPHRITIS AND NEPHROSIS

Nephritis, also called **glomerulonephritis,** is an inflammation of kidneys, usually with autoimmune causes, which manifests itself by means of a lack of urine, and the little passed is bloody. Other symptoms are facial edema (swollen face), and blood high pressure.

Nephrosis is another kind of kidney affliction which manifests itself with the emission of important amounts of proteins into the urine.

In both cases, **medical assistance** is required. These plants can, however, promote the regeneration of the afflicted renal tissues.

Golden-rod

WHITE BIRCH	Diuretic, regenerates and reduces inflammation of kidney tissues
GOLDEN-ROD	Diuretic, promotes good functioning of kidneys

ENURESIS

Definition

This is an **involuntary emission of urine,** especially when sleeping. This ailment is quite frequent in children and teenagers.

Phytotherapy

Phytotherapy provides plants such as cypress, which are quite useful in ***improving the muscular tone*** of the urinary bladder, thus its ability to retain urine. ***Invigorating and balancing*** plants for the nervous system are also useful, such as St. Johnswort.

CYPRESS	Increases the tone of the urinary bladder and allows a better control of the nervous system of this organ
ST. JOHNSWORT	Invigorator and balancer of the nervous system

URINARY INFECTION

Germs causing urinary infections are sensitive to chemically synthesized antibiotics; however, they quickly become resistant to these substances.

Antiseptic and antibiotic substances contained in medicinal herbs have less intense action than synthesized antibiotics, but they undergo ***fewer resistance reactions*** from germs, ***do not suppress body defenses,*** and reduce the **inflammation** of urinary organs. When correctly used, these plants can solve urinary infections of several types, especially in **chronic** repetitive cases.

GARLIC	Antibiotic against bacteria causing urinary infection, such as E. coli
WITCH GRASS	Urinary antiseptic and anti-inflammatory
BEARBERRY	Powerful urinary antiseptic
ECHINACEA	Increases organic defenses
THYME	Diuretic and antiseptic
NASTURTIUM	Natural antibiotic, it is eliminated via urine

PYELONEPHRITIS

Definition

An **infection** of the pelvis and renal tissues, usually caused by diverse micro-organisms. Its symptoms are high fever and kidney pain.

Phytotherapy

Phytotherapeutical treatment is based on plants with ***antibiotic, antiseptic,*** and ***anti-inflammatory*** properties on the urinary organs, especially kidneys.

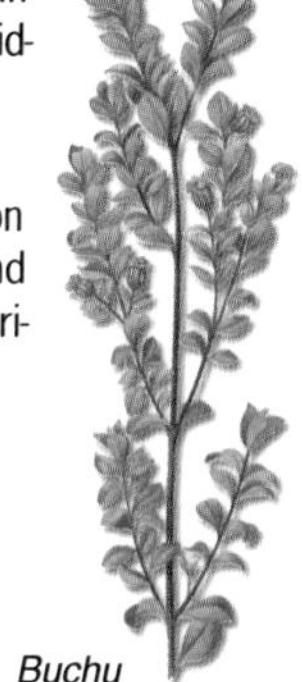

Buchu

BEARBERRY	Powerful antiseptic and urinary anti-inflammatory
BUCHU	Diuretic, antiseptic, and anti-inflammatory on the urinary organs
NASTURTIUM	Antibiotic, very effective on the urinary pathways

URETHRITIS

Definition

This is the **inflammation of the urethra,** the tract which joins the urinary bladder and the exterior. It is usually caused by bacteria, and in many cases it appears with **cystitis**.

Phytotherapy

Medicinal herbs which fight urethritis are taken ***orally and/or in washings*** with a urethral catheter.

Copaiba

WALNUT	Astringent, antiseptic, reduces urethral inflammation
WITCH GRASS	Antiseptic and urinary anti-inflammatory
BEARBERRY	Powerful urinary antiseptic
BUCHU	Antiseptic, regenerates urinary mucosa and makes its discomfort disappear
COPAIBA	Urinary antiseptic and anti-inflammatory, effective in the case of blenorrhage

URINARY INCONTINENCE

It is usually caused by mechanical reasons, such as a detachment of the urinary bladder in women, as a consequence of labor. Men can experience the same as a result of prostate surgery. Cypress is effective taken both in infusions and applied in sitz baths.

CYPRESS	Increases the tone of the urinary bladder and allows a better control of the nerves of this organ

CYSTITIS

Definition

The **inflammation of the urinary bladder,** usually caused by bacteria ascending through the urethra, from the exterior.

It tends to repeat itself, especially in women.

Phytotherapy

Medicinal herbs mainly exert a **preventive** action on these cases, and they must be taken from one to three weeks after the acute phase has passed.

GARDEN VIOLET	Supplies mucilage with emollient and anti-inflammatory action
FLAX	Antispasmodic, sedative, anti-inflammatory
PSYLLIUM	Calms cystitis discomforts, promotes regeneration of the irritated mucosa
BEARBERRY	Powerful urinary antiseptic, calms burning sensation
BUCHU	Diuretic and urinary antiseptic, alleviates pain and rashes caused when urinating
PELLITORY OF THE WALL	Increases urine production, sedative and anti-inflammatory on the urinary organs
GOLDENROD	Diuretic, anti-inflammatory, calms discomforts when urinating

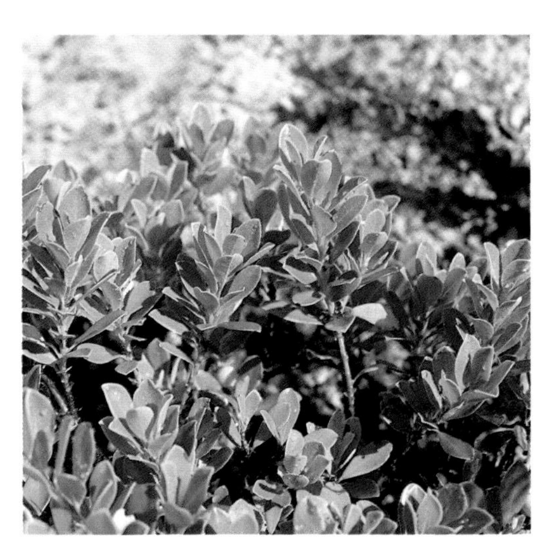

Bearberry is a powerful urinary antiseptic.

Agave

Depurative and diuretic

MORE THAN 150 agave species are known, all of them quite similar in appearance and properties, and spread all over Mexico and Central America. These plants were used by ancient Aztecs for medicinal purposes. They were introduced to Spain in the sixteenth century, and quickly spread all over the Mediterranean coastline.

PROPERTIES AND INDICATIONS. All plants of the Agave genus contain steroid glycosides, among which the most outstanding is hecogenin, as well as saponins. The ***ROOT*** and the ***LEAVES*** obtain from these substances their **diuretic** and blood **depurative** properties, and are successfully used for edema and retention of liquids **[❶]**.

In Mexico and Central American countries, agave is traditionally used for infectious diseases, **digestive disorders, jaundice,** and **hepatitis.**

Externally applied, the juice or ***SAP*** flowing from the stem has **vulnerary** and **wound-healing** properties. It is applied in compresses for bruises and skin wounds **[❷]**.

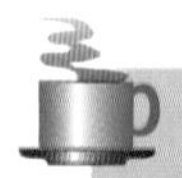

Preparation and Use

INTERNAL USE

❶ **Infusion** with 30 g of root or ground dry leaves per liter of water. Drink three or four cups daily, sweetened with honey.

EXTERNAL USE

❷ **Compresses** with the juice or sap of the leaves, applied on the affected skin area.

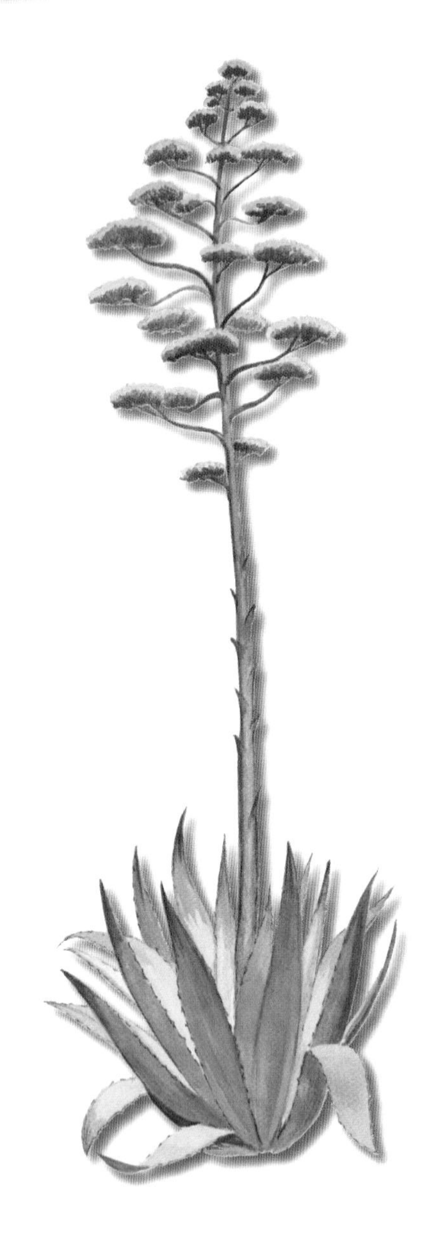

Description. *Plant of the Amarillidaceae family, with large, fleshy, point-tipped, spiked basal leaves (up to one meter large). Its flowers grow on the tip of a 6 m high stem.*

Parts used. *The root, the leaves, and the sap.*

Witch Grass

Diuretic and emollient

WITH THE FIBROUS roots of this plant, which some peasants regard as a weed, some brooms are made. However witch grass performs the most efficient sweeping in the blood and the kidneys.

PROPERTIES AND INDICATIONS. The rhizome of this plant contains a mucilaginous substance, triticene, as well as an antibiotic, potassium, silicon, and several sugars. It has diuretic, antiseptic, and emollient properties. Hence, it is used in the following ways:

- **Antiseptic and anti-inflammatory** for cystitis, urethritis, and urinary infections in general **[❶]**.
- **Diuretic and depurative,** for kidney stones, gout, arthritis, and cellulitis **[❶]**.
- **Sudorific** for infectious diseases with fever (influenza, cold, measles, scarlet fever, etc.) **[❶]**.

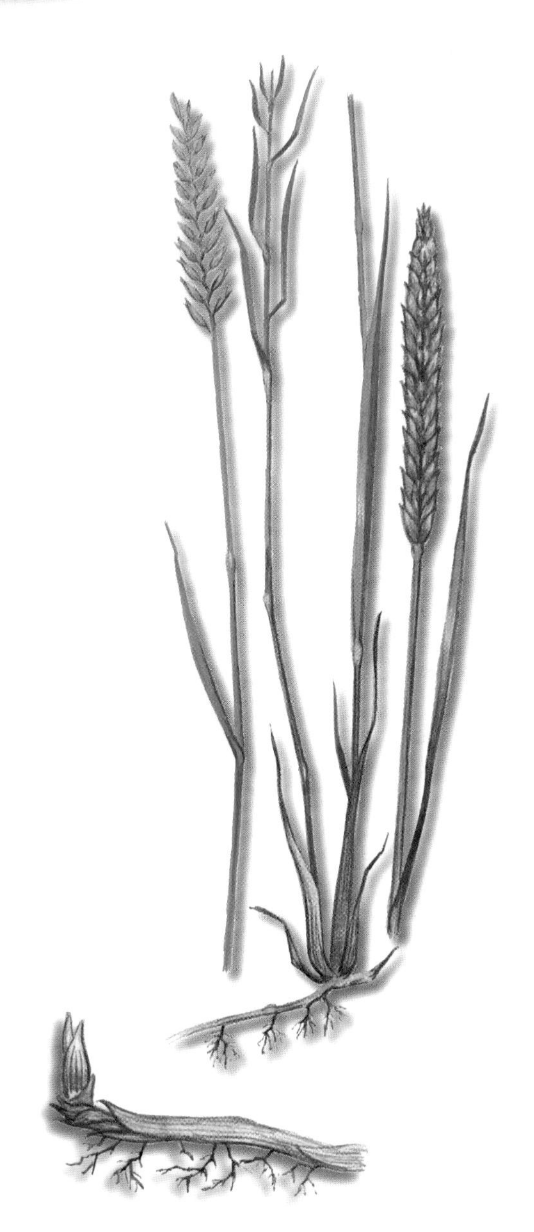

__Description.__ Vivacious plant of the Graminaceae family, growing from 40 to 100 cm high, with large creeping rhizomes with knots, from which small roots grow.

__Parts used.__ The rhizome.

Preparation and Use

INTERNAL USE

❶ **Decoction** with 30-50 g of dry rhizome per liter of water. Boil for 10 minutes. Drink from two to four cups a day.

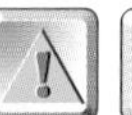
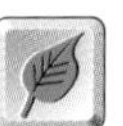
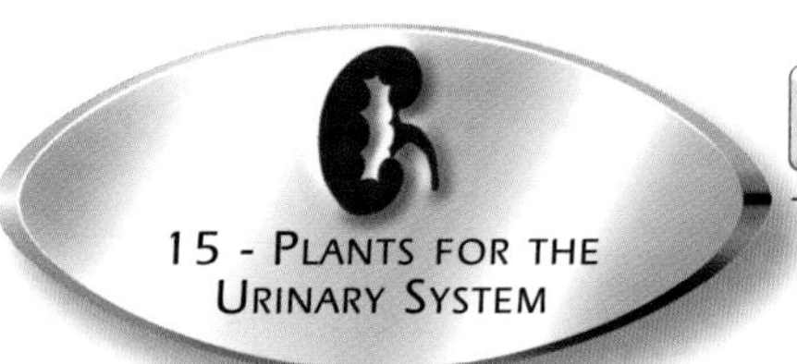

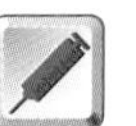
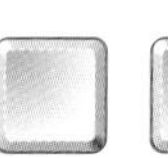
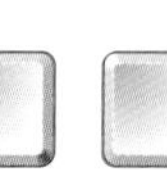

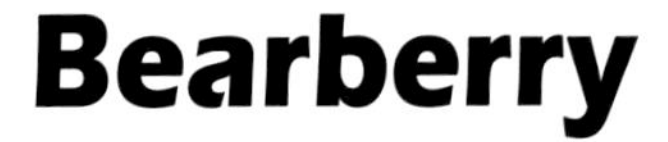

Bearberry

Powerful urinary antiseptic

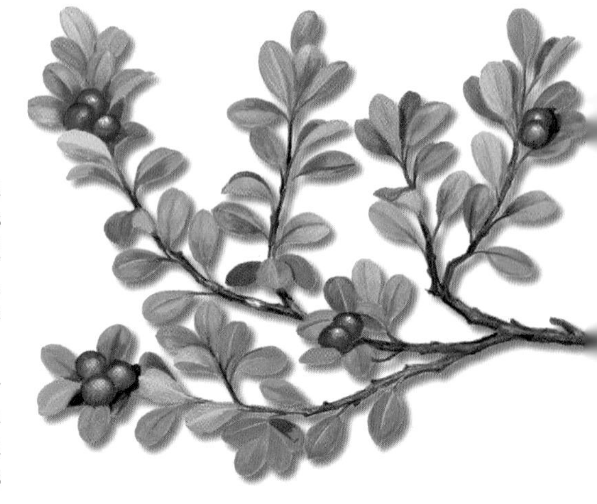

Description. *Woody shrub of the Ericaceae family, growing from 15 to 30 cm high, with long, creeping stems, and evergreen, small, fleshy leaves dark green in color. Its flowers are round, white or pink in color, and its fruit are bright red berries.*

Parts used. *The leaves.*

WHEN BEARS still lived in the European mountains, they enjoyed bearberries whose shape and flavor resembled those of small apples. These berries are edible, though the medicinal properties of this plant lie mainly in its leaves.

The use of bearberry began long ago in northern European countries, but classical Roman and Greek botanists did not know this plant. In the eighteenth century, the excellent properties of this plant to treat urinary ailments were already known all over Europe and America.

At present, its properties have been proven by scientific research, and it is a valuable remedy for people suffering from urinary ailments. Hence several ***pharmaceutical preparations*** are made from bearberry extract.

PROPERTIES AND INDICATIONS. The leaves of bearberry contain high amounts of tannin, which give the plant **astringent** properties, flavonoid glycosides, to which bearberry owes its mildly **diuretic** properties, and fatty and resinous substances. However, its most important active component is arbutin, a phenol glycoside whose genine is ***hydroquinone.*** This substance provides a ***powerful* antiseptic and anti-inflammatory *action*** on the **urinary organs,** and is eliminated through the urine.

In order for the hydroquinone to exert its action, the **urine** must have **alkaline** reaction, since the alkaloid is neutralized in acid pH environments. This is no problem for those who have vegetarian diets, as they have alkaline urine. However, those people with diets is rich in meat and shellfish produce acid urine, and bearberry cannot exert its beneficial action.

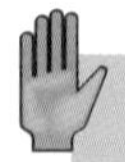

Warning

*Treatments with bearberry must not last longer than **10 days** or **15 as a maximum.** If needed, they could be repeated after a few weeks.*

*Some people with **delicate stomachs** may present digestive intolerance to the **tannin** the bearberry leaves contain. In such cases, we recommend that you make herbal teas less concentrated (only 20-30 g of leaves) and take charcoal at the same time, which absorbs tannin.*

Preparation and Use

INTERNAL USE

❶ **Decoction** with 50-60 g of dry ground leaves, previously soaked for 3-4 hours, per liter of water. Boil for 15 minutes and drink a cup every 3-4 hours. Intake should be close together, since bearberry's active principles are quickly eliminated through urine.

❷ **Cold extract** with 50-60 g of leaves in a liter of water. Steep for 24 hours, then strain and drink three cups daily, gently heated. This is a good way to take bearberry which lacks undesirable side effects of tannin, though the effects are less intense than those of the decoction.

❸ There are several **pharmaceutical preparations** based on bearberry extract which doctors can prescribe depending on the patient's condition.

Therefore, we recommend a ***vegetarian diet*** to be followed when a ***treatment*** of bearberry is intended. This diet must be rich in fruits and vegetables, and besides causing the urine to become alkaline and allowing bearberry to act, it will have a positive effect on urinary afflictions.

The urine can also become temporary alkaline by taking sodium bicarbonate, though the action of this substance does not last for long and has several side effects.

Since the germs which cause urinary infections usually become resistant to habitual antibiotics and antiseptic substances, bearberry offers a valid alternative to treat such afflictions, though for **urinary infection** you should always ***see the doctor.***

Bearberry, alone or combined with other treatments, is recommended in the following cases [❶,❷,❸]:

- **Pyelonephritis.** This is the infection of the renal pelvis (a cavity inside the kidneys), in which the urine that is produced collects. This affliction manifests itself with intermittent high fever, cloudy urine, and kidney pain. By eliminating its active components through urine, bearberry acts as an antiseptic and anti-inflammatory substance.
- **Cystitis** (infection and inflammation of the urinary bladder). Bearberry eases the sensation of burning and pain suffered when urinating. It is ***especially effective*** for **chronic cystitis** which has been proven resistant to other treatments.
- **Urethritis.** An infection of the urethra, which in some cases can be caused by sexually transmitted diseases.
- **Prostatitis.** Almost always caused by urinary infections.
- **Kidney sand and stones.** Though according to some people bearberry dissolves kidney stones, this fact has not been proven. In any case, it has a beneficial action on these afflictions, since it prevents the urine infections which usually go with them.

Bearberry gives a greenish color to urine, which shows the treatment is effective.

Bearberry is a notably effective plant in treating any kind of urinary infections, when urine is alkaline, not acid. An alkalization of urine is achieved by following a vegetarian diet, with predominance of fruit and vegetables.

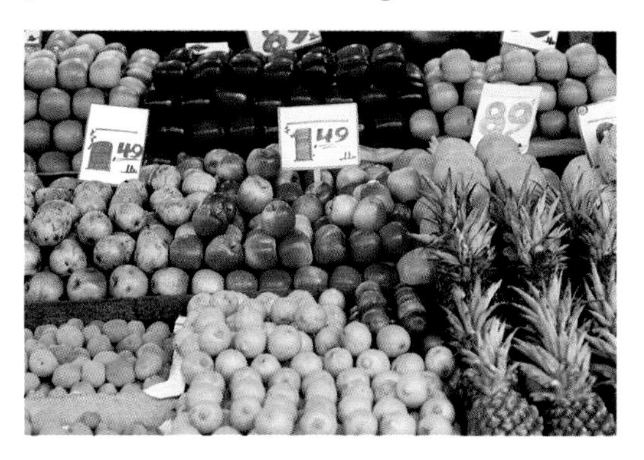

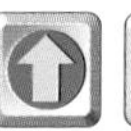
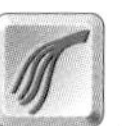
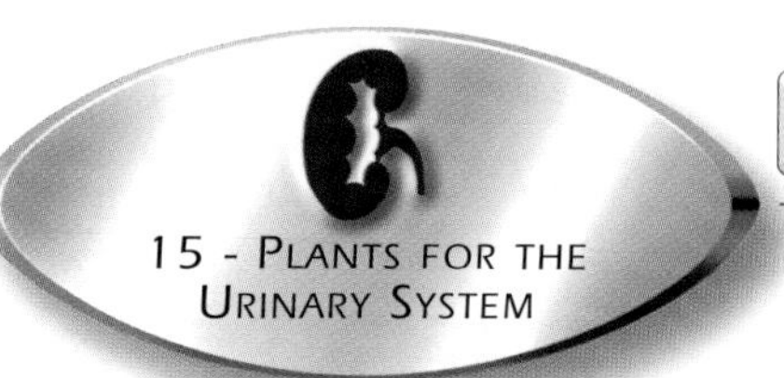

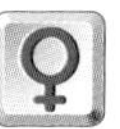
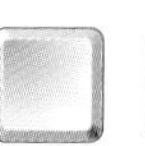
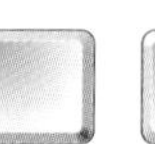
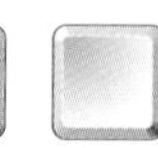

Cane

Increases urine production and stops breast-feeding

DIOSCORIDES, the great Greek botanist and physician of the first century A.D. recommended the use of cane to increase urine production. This plant was probably used in ancient times with these aims, because grows near streams.

PROPERTIES AND INDICATIONS. The rhizome (underground stem) and the root of cane contain a sugar (saccharose) and many silicon derivatives. It has two main properties:

- **Diuretic.** It produces a mild increase of urine production, promoting the elimination of uric acid and other waste substances. It is recommended for people suffering from kidney colic and also for those who want to take a depurative treatment [❶].
- **Galactofuge.** When taken for some days, cane stops milk production on breast-feeding women. It is useful for all those women who, for any reason, want to give up breast-feeding [❶].

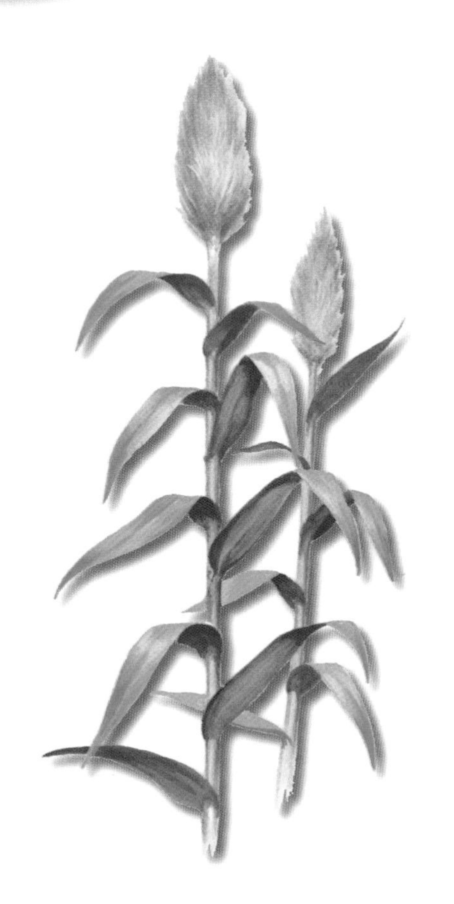

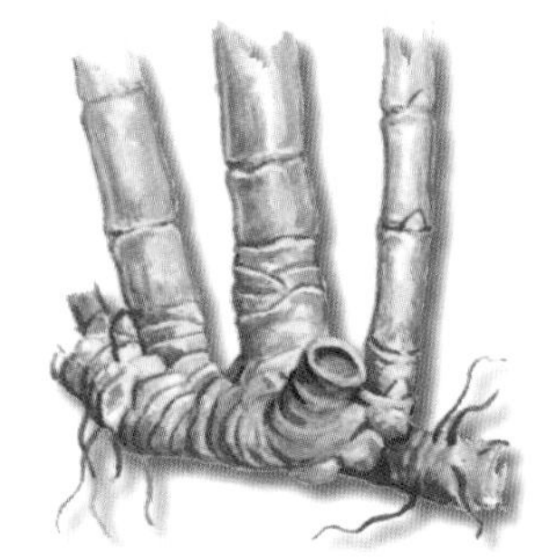

Description. Plant of the Gramineae family, growing up to 5 m high. It should not be mistaken for bamboo, since on every stem knot of cane only one leaf grows.

Parts used.
The rhizome (underground stem) and the root.

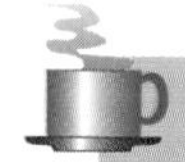

Preparation and Use

INTERNAL USE

❶ **Decoction** with the rhizome or root of the plant, sliced or ground, in a proportion of 50 g per liter of water. Boil for 15 minutes and drink from two to four cups daily.

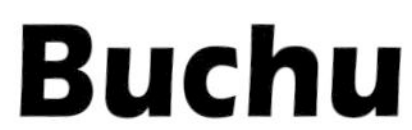

Buchu

An excellent remedy for urinary organs

ITS EXCELLENT virtues to combat urinary organ inflammation have led it to becoming spread world-wide. Now it can be found used by many herbalists and in a lot of phytotherapeutical preparations.

PREPARATION AND USE. The leaves of buchu contain an essential oil (diosphenol), which is its most important active component. It acts as:

- Diuretic.
- Urinary antiseptic.
- Genital and urinary organs anti-inflammatory, especially of urine bladder and prostate.

Buchu, as well as bearberry is ***one of the most effective plants*** known to successfully fight **inflammatory diseases of urinary organs.** It is especially recommended in the following cases:

- **Pyelonephritis** (inflammation of the renal pelvis and kidneys) [❶].
- **Cystitis** (inflammation of the urinary bladder): it alleviates with great success the pain and burning felt when urinating [❶].
- **Urethritis** (inflammation of the urethra), whether or not it is caused by sexually transmitted germs (blennorrhagia). It regenerates the urinary mucosa, and makes discomfort disappear. It is useful both taken in infusion [❶], and applied in urethral cleansing [❷].

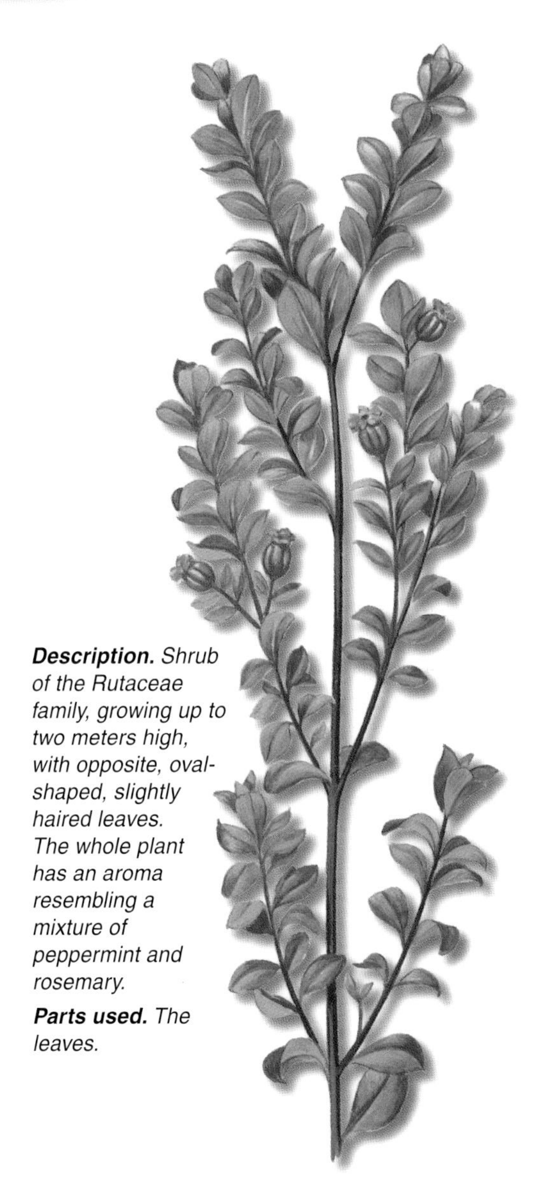

Description. *Shrub of the Rutaceae family, growing up to two meters high, with opposite, oval-shaped, slightly haired leaves. The whole plant has an aroma resembling a mixture of peppermint and rosemary.*

Parts used. *The leaves.*

Preparation and Use

INTERNAL USE

❶ **Infusion** with around 50 g of leaves per liter of water. Drink three cups a day.

EXTERNAL USE

❷ **Urethral** washings with the same infusion used internally, in the case of urethritis.

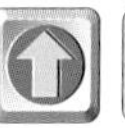

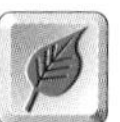

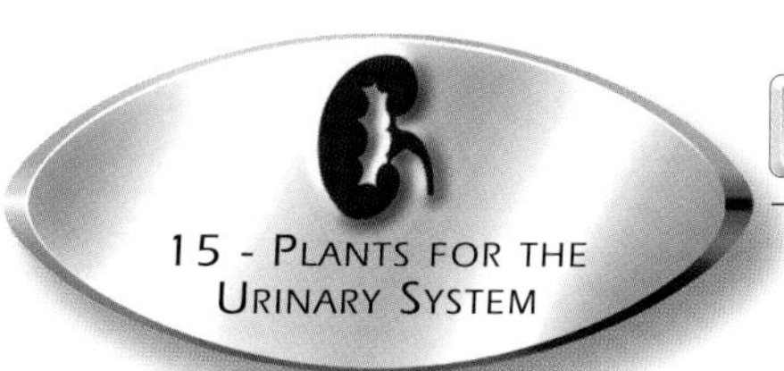

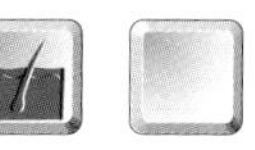

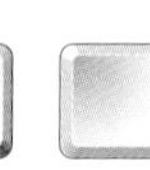

White Birch

A good remedy for kidney colic

THIS TREE has many applications. Its wood, and especially its charcoal, is excellent. Its bark is waterproof, and with it, ancient shepherds made jars and even covers for snowshoes.

Properties and indications. The ***leaves*** and the ***buds*** of the white birch tree contain mainly flavonoids (miricitrine and hyperoside), which give them ***notable* diuretic *properties*** (elimination of liquids); as well as bitter com-

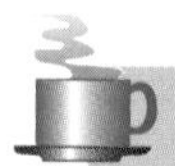

Preparation and Use

Internal use

❶ **Infusion** with 20-50 g of leaves and/or buds per liter of water. Drink up to one liter daily. As its flavor is slightly sour, it can be sweetened with honey or brown sugar. When adding 1 g of **sodium bicarbonate** the effectiveness of white birch herbal teas is enhanced, since its active components are better dissolved in alkaline environments.

❷ **Decoction** of bark, with 50-80 g per liter of water. Boil until the liquid reduces to a half. Drink two or three cups daily, sweetened with honey.

❸ **Sap.** Take it after dissolved in water (in a proportion of 50 %) as a soft drink. Avoid its fermentation.

External use

❹ **Compresses** on the skin, with the same infusion described for internal use.

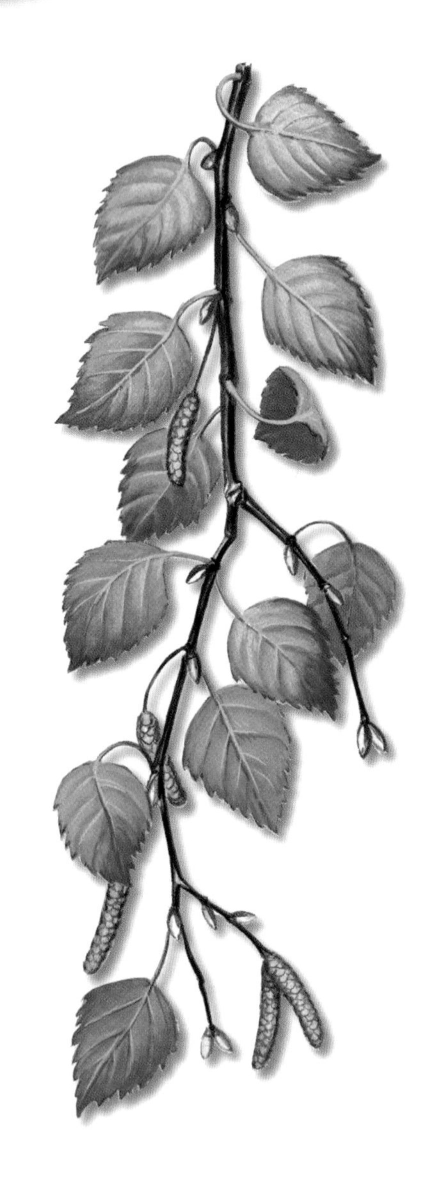

Description. *Fine deciduous tree of the Betulaceae family. The whiteness of its bark, which comes off in fine sheets, is the main feature of this tree. It has young hanging branches (after those it is named* Betula pendula*), with small nodes which gave birth to other of its scientific names:* Betula verrucosa. *Male and female flowers grow on the same tree.*

Parts used. *The leaves, the buds, the sap, and the bark.*

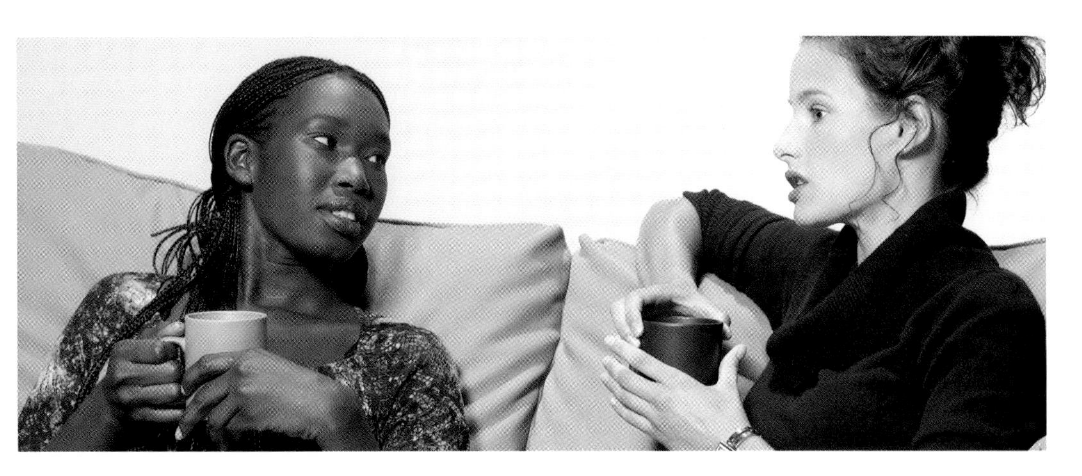

Many women, prior to menstruation, suffer from fluid retention, which causes swollen legs, abdomen, and breasts. Infusions made with leaves and buds of the white birch tree, with diuretic properties but not de-mineralizing, are an ideal remedy to heal this discomfort.

ponents, catechic tannins, and essential oils. Their applications are as follow:

- **Edema.** They help to eliminate liquids retained in the body, especially for renal or heart insufficiency {❶}.Unlike other chemical diuretic substances, white birch leaf infusions do not provoke the loss of huge amounts of mineral salts via urine, nor do they irritate kidney tissues. On the contrary, they are able to regenerate it and reduce its inflammation, producing a decrease of the amount of albumin eliminated through urine for nephrosis and renal insufficiency.

- They are also successfully used for **pre-menstrual syndrome {❶}**. When taking this herbal tea some days before menstruation, the volume of urine increases, and the swelling of tissues decreases, especially that of the legs, the abdomen, and breasts.

- **Kidney calculi.** Infusions made with leaves and buds of the white birch tree promote the elimination of urine sands and prevent the formation of kidney stones {❶}. It has been proven that in some cases, these herbal teas can even dissolve calculi. The use of infusion is recommended both for nephritic colic attack (kidney colic) and, in a ongoing way, to avoid the formation of calculi.

- **Depurative.** Leaves and buds of the white birch tree have depurative properties on the toxic substances on the blood, such as uric acid. Hence, herbal teas made with them are recommended for **gout or arthritis {❶}**.

- **Skin afflictions.** Due to their depurative properties, when ***internally used*** they are recommended to cleanse the skin from impurities in the case of chronic eczema and cellulitis {❶}.

- **Wounds and sores. *Externally applied,*** as compresses, these leaves and buds have **antiseptic and healing** properties for **wounds and sores,** due to the amount of tannin they contain {❹}.

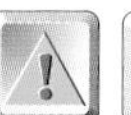

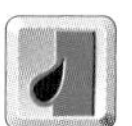

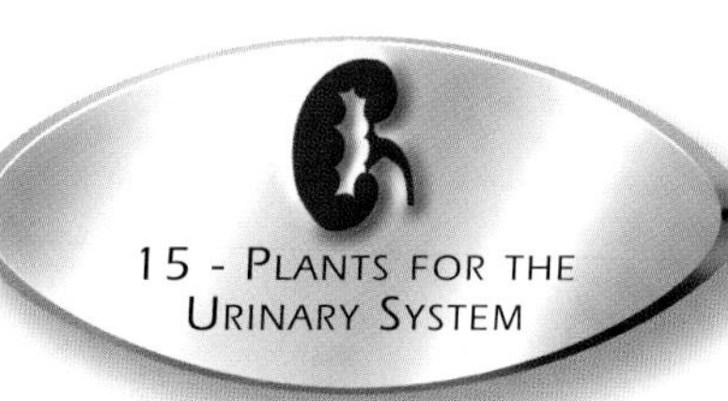

Copaiba

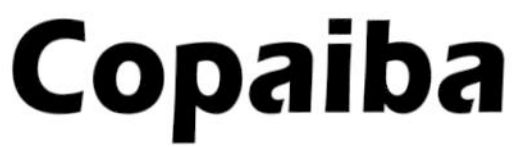

Very effective against blennorrhagia

IN THE BASINS of the rivers Orinoco and Amazon there are several species of trees belonging to the genus Copaifera, which exude resin when suffering an incision of perforation on their trunk. By distilling this resin the so-called "wood oil" or "copaiba balm" is obtained. This substance was already used in the seventeenth century as a remedy against sexually transmitted diseases.

PROPERTIES AND INDICATIONS. ***Copaiba balm* [❶]** contains an essential oil and a resin, in whose composition copaibic acid predominates. This acid is eliminated through urine (kidneys) and acts as an **antiseptic and anti-inflammatory** substance on the genital and urinary mucosa. It is effective for **blennorrhagia** in both males and females. This is a sexually transmitted disease which manifests itself by inflammation and irritation of the urethra (the tract through which urine flows outside the body). It also has been used as a **balm** for **bronchitis.**

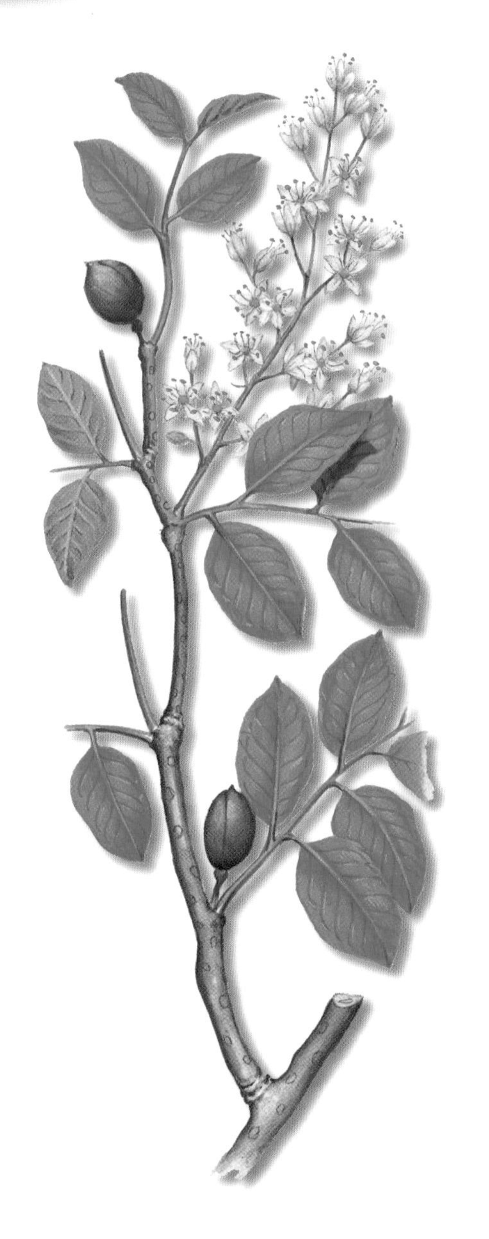

__Description.__ Magnificent tree of the Leguminoseae family, growing from 15 to 20 m high. Its flowers are white and form spikes. The fruit is an oval-shaped pod containing an single seed covered by flesh.

__Parts used.__ The resin which is extracted from the trunk.

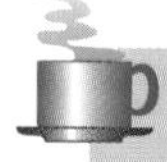

Preparation and Use

INTERNAL USE

❶ **Copaiba balm.** Take a teaspoonful (5 g) one or two times a day.

Eryngo

An effective diuretic and appetizer

ERYNGO is a plant of the Umbelliferae family that, however, looks like a thistle. It is sometimes called "watling street" thistle as in Fall, when wind blows, its dry stems and leaves are blown with the wind and carried away to populate other soils.

Properties and indications. Eryngo root contains saponins, tannin, sugar, and an essential oil. These substances give eryngo notable **diuretic** properties. Therefore, its use is recommended in the following cases:

- **Edema** (retention of liquids), especially those occurring on legs and ankles [❶,❷].
- Excess of **uric acid** (arthritis) and **sand** in urine, when cleansing kidneys is recommended [❶,❷].

We have to remark that the diuretic properties of eryngo saponins are quite intense, but not constant and decreasing day after day. In one week they will practically disappear. Thus, it is not recommended that it be used for ***more than two or three days.*** After resting some days, it once again becomes effective.

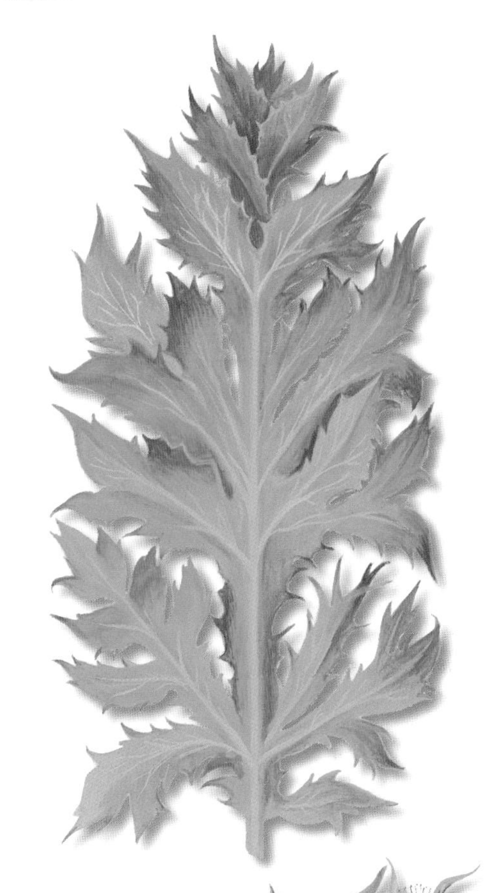

__Description.__ Plant of the Umbelliferae family, growing from 40 to 60 cm high, with slim stems and prickly leaves. Its flower chapters are formed by many small, white greenish flowers. The whole plant gives a smell similar to that of carrot, except its root, which is a bit sour.

__Parts used.__ The root (which is gathered in Spring or Fall), young buds and leaves (which are gathered in Summer).

Preparation and Use

Internal use

❶ **Salad.** Its buds and young leaves are highly appreciated by people fond of wild vegetables.

❷ **Infusion** with a handful of ground root (30-40 g) per liter of water. Steep until cold, and drink two or three cups daily. Do not keep this infusion more than twenty-four hours, since it loses its properties.

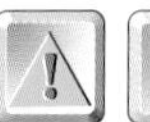

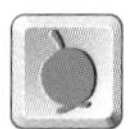

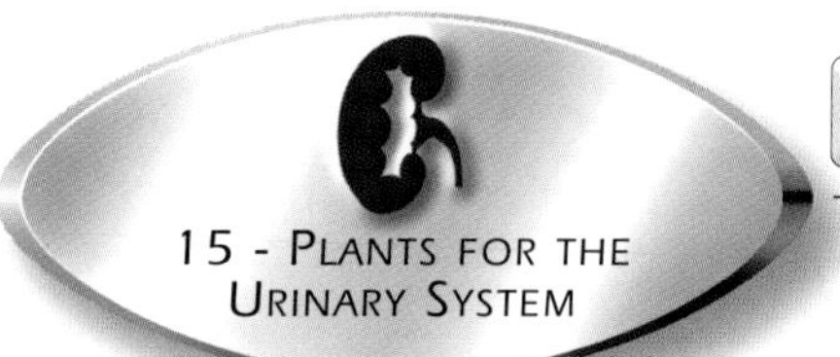

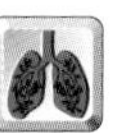

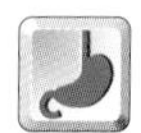

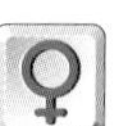

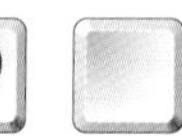

Juniper

Diuretic and expectorant

DIOSCORIDES, who lived in the first century A.D., knew the medicinal properties of juniper fruit, which of course have more applications than simply giving their aroma to some alcoholic beverages.

PROPERTIES AND INDICATIONS. The whole plant, and especially its leaves, contain an essential oil rich in terpenic substances with the following properties:

- **Diuretic.** The essential oil of juniper increases glomerules strain on kidneys, thus increasing urine production. However, ***high doses*** of this plant when continuously taken induce the straining capabilities of kidneys, and can even produce **nephritis.** The use of juniper is recommended for **edema** caused by coronary insufficiency, and also as a depurative substance to eliminate excess **uric acid [❶,❷,❸].**
- **Expectorant and bronchial antiseptic.** Since a great part of its essence is eliminated via the lung airways, its berries have been used as a complementary treatment of any kind of bronchial and lung diseases, even in the case of tuberculosis [❶,❷,❸].
- **Appetizer,** stomach **invigorator,** and **carminative [❶,❷].**

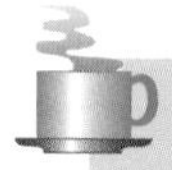

Preparation and Use

INTERNAL USE

❶ **Ripe berries.** They can be taken whole as if they were pills, six after every meal, three times a day.

❷ **Infusion** with 30 g of berries per liter of water. Drink up to three cups daily.

❸ **Essence.** The recommended dose is two drops, three times a day.

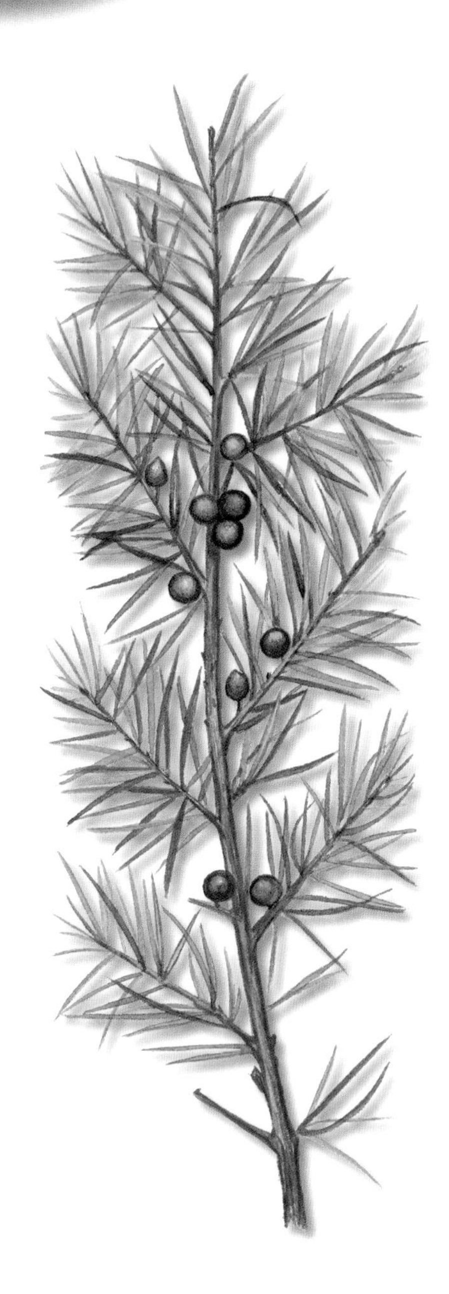

Description. *Evergreen shrub of the Cupresaceae family, growing from 1 to 3 m high, with short, sharp-pointed leaves. Its fruit are small balls, blue or black in color, with a resinous, sweet flavor.*

Parts used. *The fruit.*

Pellitory of the Wall

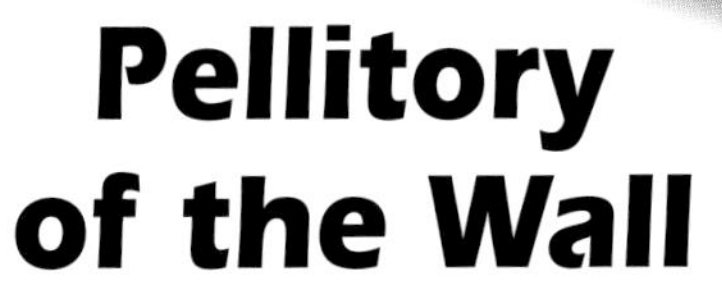

It alleviates renal colic

IN CLASSICAL botanical literature, this plant was given the Greek name of *helxine,* and also the Latin name of *muralis herba* (grass of the wall). It not only grows on walls, but also near streams.

PROPERTIES AND INDICATIONS. Its active components are potassium nitrate and flavonoids, which give this plant diuretic properties, and mucilages, to which it owes its **anti-inflammatory and emollient** properties.

• When ***internally used,*** the main application of pellitory of the wall is for **urinary tract afflictions:** renal colic (it helps eliminate calculi), cystitis, and oliguris (lack of urine) **[❶,❷]**. It has interesting effects, since besides increasing urine production, it relaxes, sedates, and reduces the inflammation of urinary organs.

• It is used ***externally*** with good results to heal **wounds, burns, stretches** on the lips, the skin, and the nipples, as well as **anal fissures [❸].**

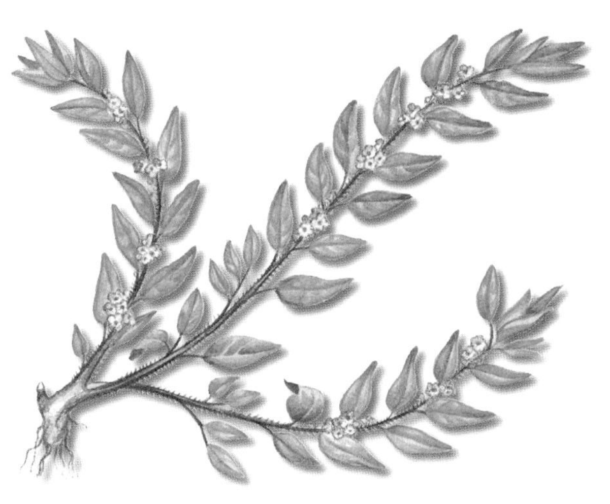

Description. *Vivacious plant of the Uricaceae family, growing up `to 30 cm high. Its leaves are covered by non-urticant hair.*

Parts used. *The stem and the leaves.*

Preparation and Use

INTERNAL USE

❶ **Infusion** with 40-60 g of dry plant (better if fresh) per liter of water. Drink four or five cups daily.

❷ **Fresh juice.** Drink half a glass, three times a day. It can be flavored with lemon juice or lemon rind.

EXTERNAL USE

❸ **Poultices** with the plant fresh and mashed, applied on the affected area.

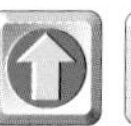
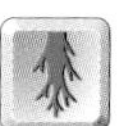
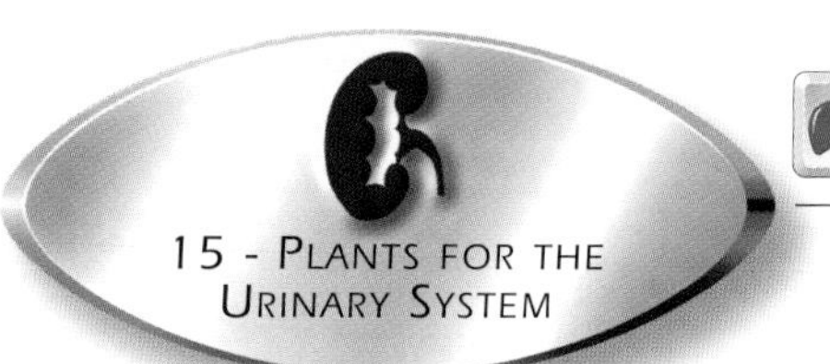

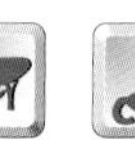
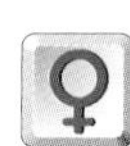
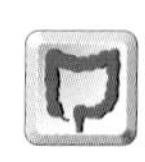

Madder

Diuretic and sedative

HIPPOCRATES already used it as a diuretic, a property which is still taken advantage of at present.

PROPERTIES AND INDICATIONS. The root of madder contains anthraquinonic glycosides to which the plant owes its coloring and diuretic properties, as well as alkaline citrates, and malic and tartaric acids. Its more outstanding properties are the following:

- **Diuretic.** It is recommended for all kind of renal afflictions (calculi, colic, infections) as well as for cystitis [❶,❷].
- It **relieves** aches and has **antiseptic** properties on the **urinary pathways,** which make it very useful for colic [❶,❷]. It has been proven that this plant is able to dissolve certain types of **renal calculi** (kidney stones).
- **Appetizer:** it increases appetite [❶,❷].
- **Choleretic.** Recommended for gall bladder disorders [❶,❷].
- **Emmenagogue.** It promotes menstruation and ease pain [❶,❷].
- **Laxative.** It promotes intestinal evacuation [❶,❷].

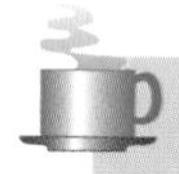

Preparation and Use

INTERNAL USE

❶ **Decoction** with 30-40 g of ground root per liter of water. Boil for ten minutes. Drink from four to six cups daily.

❷ **Root powder.** The recommended dose is 2-4 g daily, distributed into three intakes.

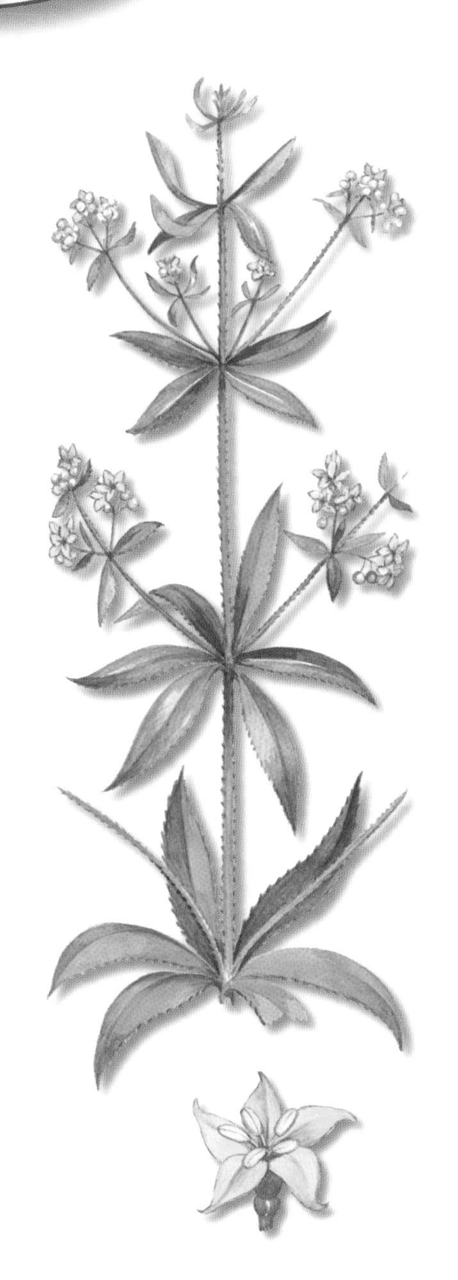

Description. *Vivacious plant of the Rubiaceae family, growing up to one meter high. Its stem is quadrangular, reddish in color, and covered by thorny hooks. The root is large, winding, red in color.*

Parts used. *The root.*

Saxifrage

Very effective against urine calculi

WHEN THIS plant is uprooted, at the base of its stem we can see some small bulbs which gave it the Latin denomination *granulata*. Since these bulbs resemble some kind of urinary calculi, from ancient times onwards it was supposed that the use of saxifrage could recommended to heal the "stone disease" or urinary lithiasis. "It breaks up stones," said Andrés de Laguna in the sixteenth century, when commenting on the works of Dioscorides.

At present, saxifrage is still used with the same aims, and it is highly appreciated in rural environments of southern Europe.

PROPERTIES AND INDICATIONS. The whole plant, and especially its root, contains tannin, resin, glycosides, and vitamin C. It has notable **diuretic** properties, and perhaps since it has the ability of **alkalinizing** urine, it promotes the expulsion and dissolution of urine calculi.

Its use is recommended to promote the elimination of urine, especially in the case of urinary lithiasis (kidney stones), sand in urine, and renal colic **[❶]**.

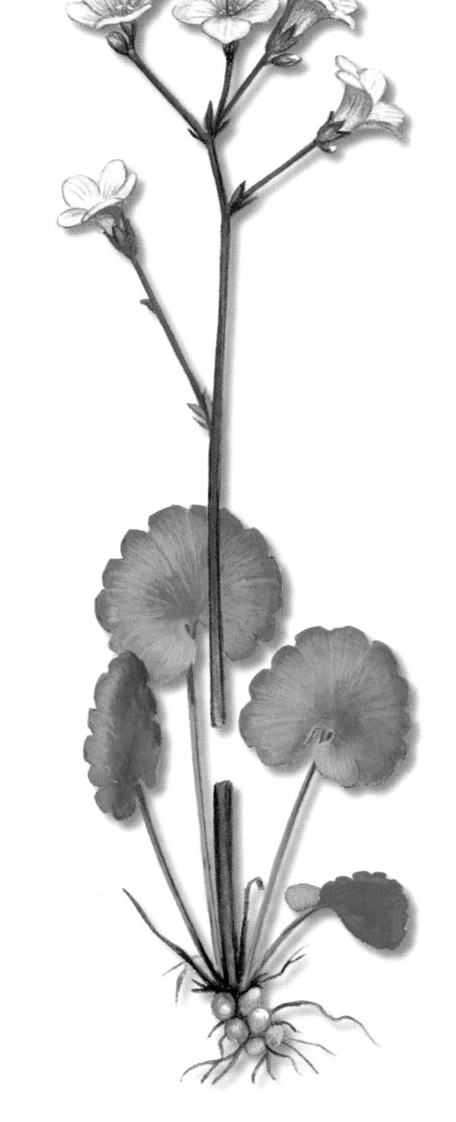

Description. *Herbaceous plant of the Saxifragaceae family, growing up to 50 cm high, with toothed, long-petioled leaves, and white flowers growing in terminal clusters.*

Parts used. *The root, the flowers, and the leaves.*

Preparation and Use

INTERNAL USE

❶ **Infusion or decoction** with 40-60 g of plant per liter of water. Drink two or three cups daily.

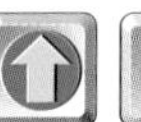
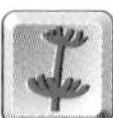
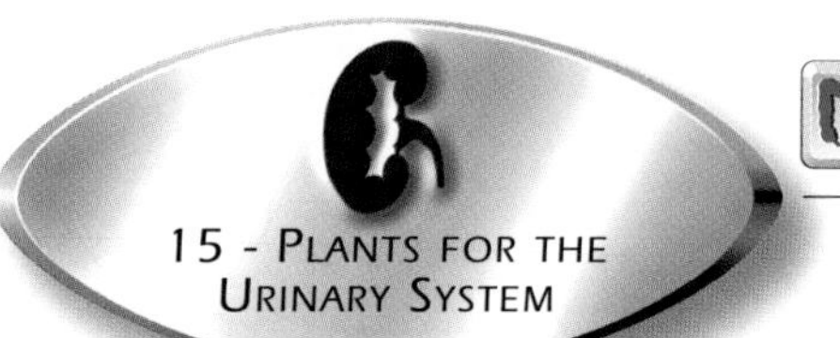

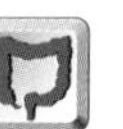
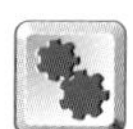
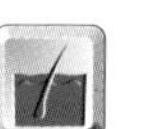
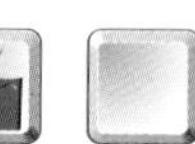

Goldenrod

A good friend of kidneys

ARNAU DE Vilanova (Valencia, Spain, 1240- Genova, Italy, 1311), a great Middle Age physician among whose patients were kings and popes, and one of the most credited professors of the ancient Medicine College of the University of Montpellier, was first to describe the medicinal properties of this plant, saying that it was "admirable in producing urine and breaking up kidney stones." More than seven centuries after him, at present, goldenrod is still used with the same aims, and its properties have been scientifically proven.

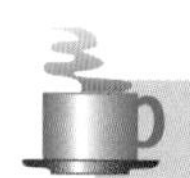

Preparation and Use

INTERNAL USE

➊ **Decoction** with 30-40 g of flower clusters per liter of water, boiling for 5-10 minutes. Drink up to five cups daily.

➋ **Syrup.** In order to treat children's **diarrhea,** we recommend increasing decoction time until the liquid reduces by a half, then add brown sugar or honey to prepare a syrup, which will be taken by the spoonful.

EXTERNAL USE

➌ **Compresses** soaked in a more concentrated decoction (50-100 g per liter) than that used internally.

➍ **Lotions** with the concentrated decoction.

➎ **Poultices** with the plant, mashed, directly applied on the skin for 15 minutes, two or three times a day.

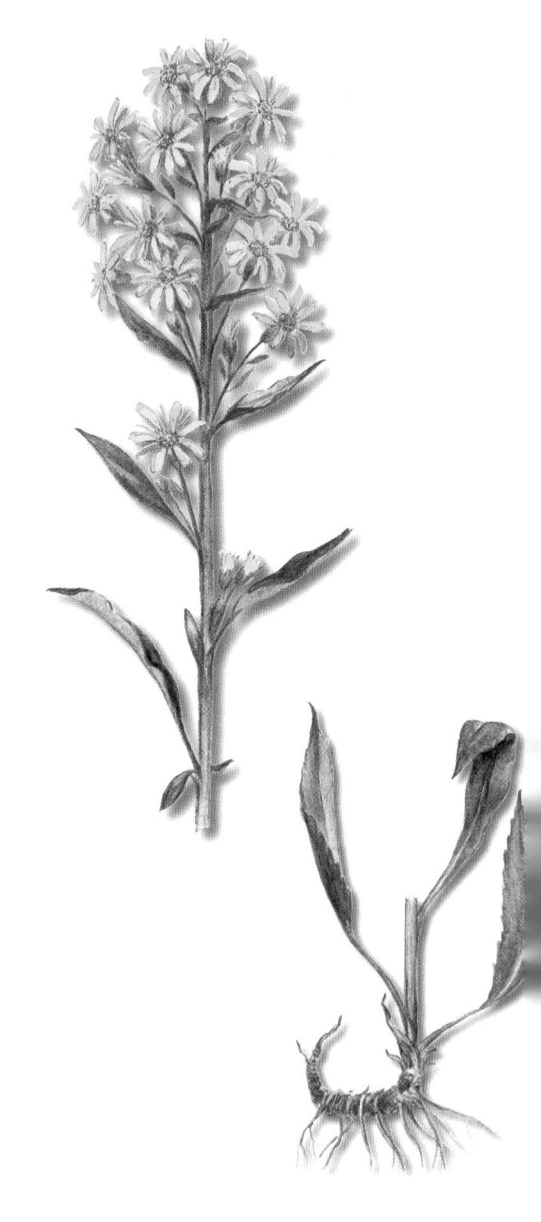

Description. *Vivacious plant of the Compositae family, with upright stems growing up to one meter high. It has yellow flowers which gather in terminal chapters.*

Parts used. *The flowering tops.*

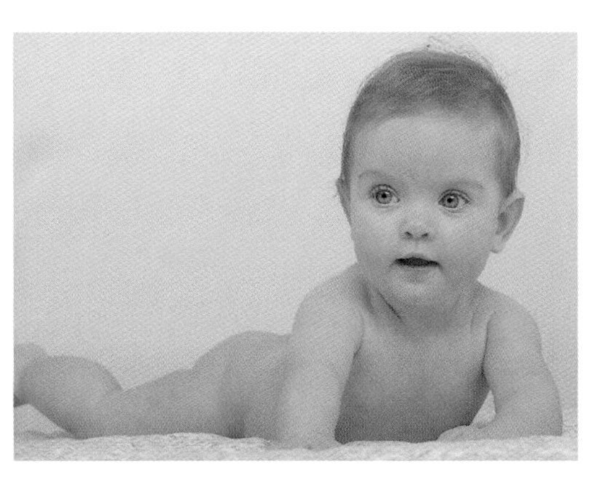

An infusion of goldenrod has been traditionally used in Spain to stop children's diarrhea, especially those occurring in Summer or during teething.

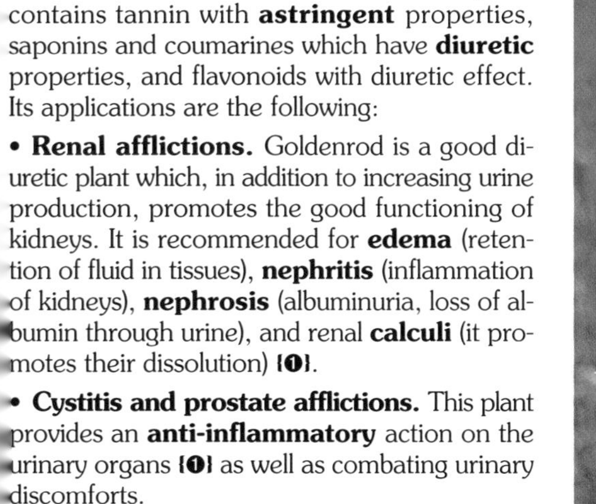

PROPERTIES AND INDICATIONS. This plant contains tannin with **astringent** properties, saponins and coumarines which have **diuretic** properties, and flavonoids with diuretic effect. Its applications are the following:

• **Renal afflictions.** Goldenrod is a good diuretic plant which, in addition to increasing urine production, promotes the good functioning of kidneys. It is recommended for **edema** (retention of fluid in tissues), **nephritis** (inflammation of kidneys), **nephrosis** (albuminuria, loss of albumin through urine), and renal **calculi** (it promotes their dissolution) {❶}.

• **Cystitis and prostate afflictions.** This plant provides an **anti-inflammatory** action on the urinary organs {❶} as well as combating urinary discomforts.

• **Depurative treatments.** It promotes the elimination of metabolic waste substances such as uric acid. It is recommended for **arthritis, gout, eczema,** and as a rule whenever the blood should be cleansed of toxic substances {❶}.

• **Obesity.** Due to its diuretic and depurative properties, goldenrod is a good ***complement*** in treating obesity {❶}.

• **Diarrhea and colitis.** Because of its astringent properties, in many places in Spain this plant is used to stop children's diarrhea, especially those occurring in Summer and those which seem to be caused by teething {❷}.

• **Astringent and vulnerary.** In ***external applications,*** it is employed to heal **wounds** and heal torpid **ulcers** (sores), whether it is applied as compresses {❸}, lotions {❹} or poultices {❺}.

The beautiful flowers of this plant justify its name of goldenrod.

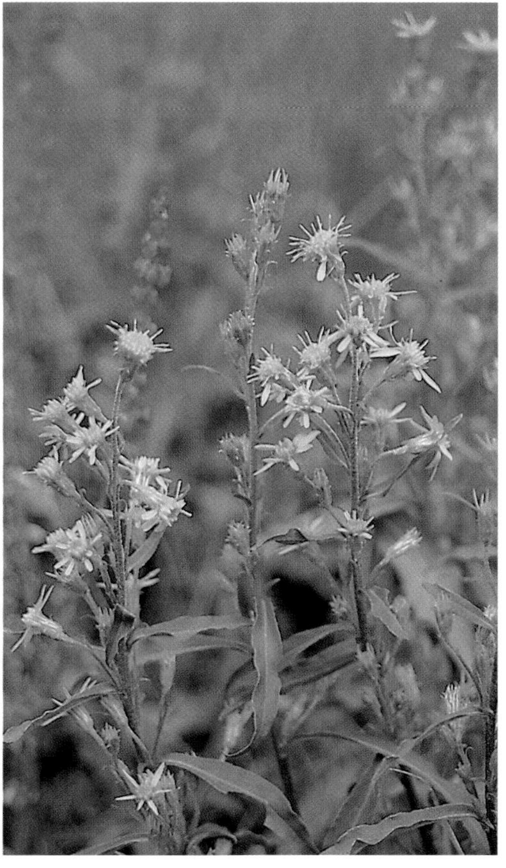

16

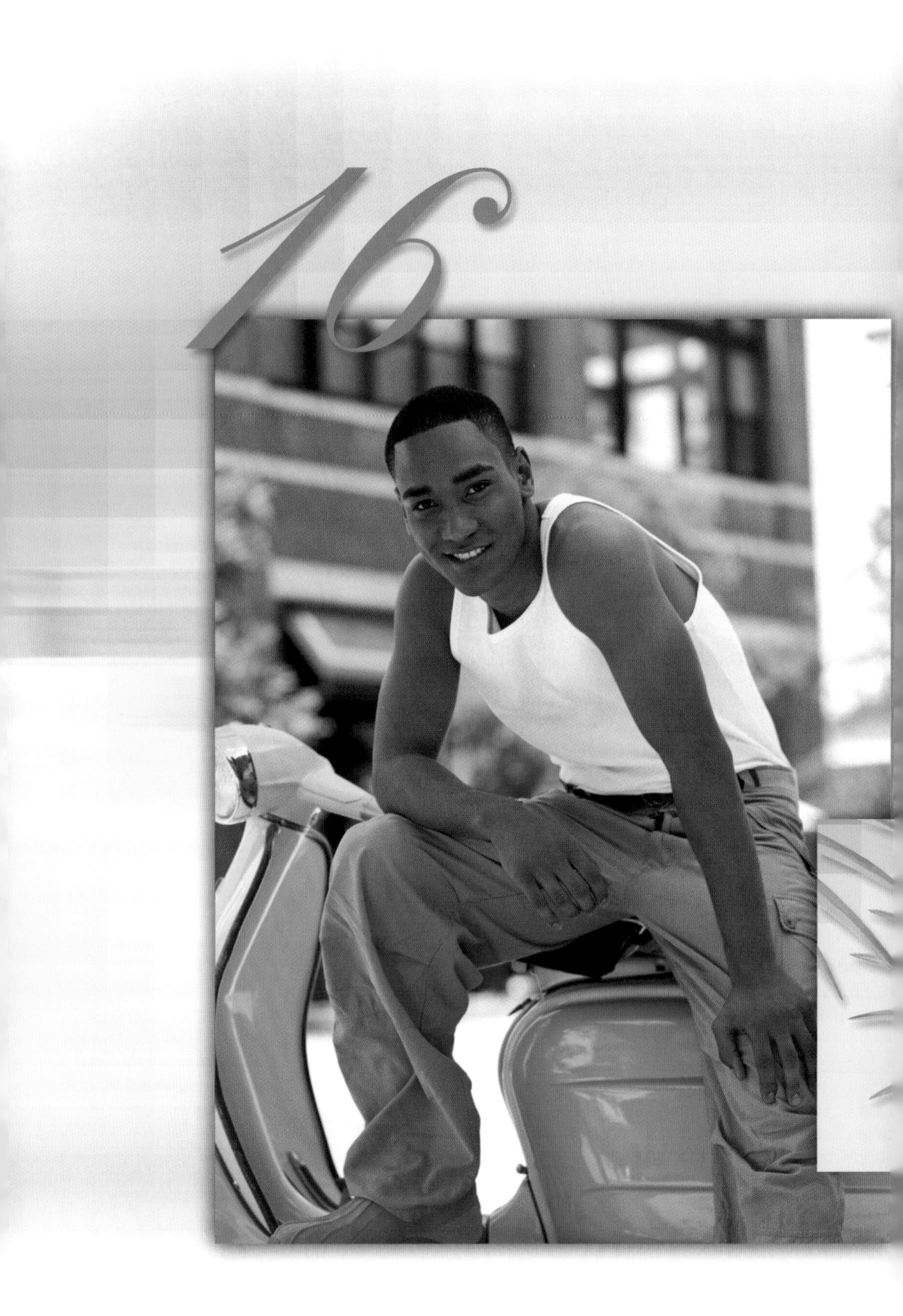

Plants for the Sexual Organs

DISEASES	PAGES
Cervicitis	293
Dysmenorrhea	292
Female sterility	291
Leukorrhea	293
Male sterility	291
Menopause	292
Menstruation, excessive	293
Menstruation, irregular	293
Menstruation, retention of fluids	291
Nipple sores	291
Ovary, insufficiency	291
Pregnancy	291
Premature ejaculation	291
Prostate, afflictions	290
Sexual excitation, excessive	290
Sexual impotence	290
Vaginitis, see Leukorrhea	293

PLANTS	PAGES
Calendula	296
Damiana	307
Ginseng	300
Mugwort	294
Rose	302
Rue	303
Sage	304
Shepherd's purse	298
Shrub palmetto	306

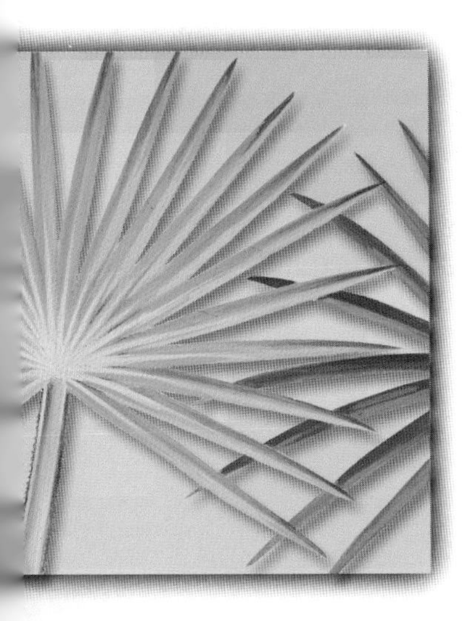

MEDICINAL HERBS can do a lot of good for women's health and well-being. Many plants can alleviate menstruation **pain** (dysmenorrhea), **balance menstrual cycle** when irregular, and **reduce hemorrhaging** during excessive menstruation.

State of mind, emotions, and even character depend to a certain degree on **hormonal balance.** A woman's body experiences cyclic oscillations of its sexual hormone level, which can provoke emotional imbalances more or less frequently.

These plants **do not only exert a symptomatic action,** easing pain or menstrual disorders, but they can even produce a true readjustment on the delicate hormone mechanism which periodically gives birth to menstruation. As in other phytotherapeutical fields, in this way medicinal herbs have a true ***preventive action*** on many of women's disorders and diseases.

When applied locally as a ***vaginal irrigation,*** medicinal herbs act successfully against infections of the vagina and the neck of the uterus. During **pregnancy** and especially during **breast-feeding,** plants can also serve women well. Some plants increase milk production, and others decrease it. In natural breast-feeding disorders, such as nipple sores and mammary gland inflammation (mastitis), phytotherapy can also provide practical solutions.

Actually, most plants regarded as aphrodisiac have a **revitalizing and invigorating** action on the body. Aphrodisiac properties are just a consequence of the increasing general vitality these plants provide.

PROSTATE, AFFLICTIONS

For young or middle aged males, the most usual prostate affliction is **prostatitis** caused by infections, while in males over the age of 50, the most common affection is **hypertrophy** or enlargement of prostate.

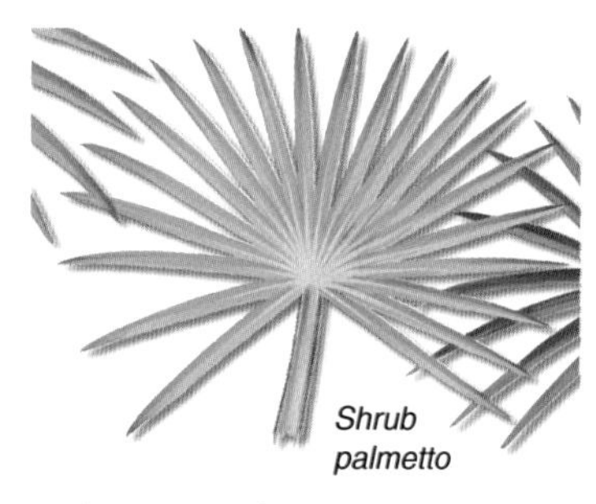
Shrub palmetto

Phytotherapy provides some very effective plants for treating both afflictions.

HORSE CHESTNUT	Reduces the size of prostate and promotes urine emptying
CYPRESS	Increases the tone of the urinary bladder
BEARBERRY	Powerful urinary antiseptic, effective in the case of prostatitis
BUCHU	Antiseptic and anti-inflammatory on the urinary and genital organs
GOLDENROD	Urinary anti-inflammatory, calms discomforts when urinating
SHRUB PALMETTO	Stops growth of prostate and reduces urinary discomforts
ECHINACEA	Stimulates defenses, reduces the congestion of prostate

SEXUAL IMPOTENCE

Definition

The inability to finish sexual intercourse due to lack of penile erection.

Causes

Apart from psychological reasons, the most usual organic causes are severe **diabetes** and **arteriosclerosis** of the iliac arteries.

Treatment

Not forgetting to treat the psychological and organic causes of impotence, the following plants improve penis erection.

WINTER SAVORY	Mild aphrodisiac, though progressive
GINSENG	Stimulates sexual glands, increases sexual performance
DAMIANA	Nervous system invigorator, revitalizer, aphrodisiac

EXCESSIVE SEXUAL EXCITATION

The following plants provide **anaphrodisiac or antiaphrodisiac** properties (they decrease sexual desire). They can be useful for over-sexed teenagers, or in the case of psychological disabilities.

HOPS	Sedative, calms sexual excitation
WHITE WILLOW	Calms nervousness, anxiety, and sexual hyperexcitation

MALE STERILITY

Inability of semen to fertilize female ovule.

Besides enhancing sexual ability and performance, these plants can increase the amount and vitality of spermatozoa.

GINSENG	Increases production of spermatozoa, stimulates sexual glands
DAMIANA	Increases the number and vitality of spermatozoa

FEMALE STERILITY

Definition

The inability of women of fertile age to conceive.

Causes

It can have ***organic*** causes, such as obstruction of the fallopian tubes, or have ***functional*** causes.

Phytotherapy

Medicinal herbs assist only in the latter case, by ***stimulating*** ovary functions, and ***balancing*** the hormonal system.

Evening primrose

EVENING PRIMROSE	Balances the hormonal system
GINSENG	Stimulates sexual glands (ovaries)
DAMIANA	Nervous invigorating, revitalizing, aphrodisiac
SAGE	Promotes female hormonal balance

OVARY, INSUFFICIENCY

Ovaries are the female sex glands. They have a double function: produce sex**hormones** (estrogens and progesterone), and produce **ovules** or germinal cells which will join with spermatozoids to create a new being. The plants mentioned here can ***stimulate*** both ovary functions.

EVENING PRIMROSE	Balances hormonal system
DAMIANA	Regularizes menstruation and stimulates ovary function

NIPPLE SORES

These are **small skin ulcers** which occur on the nipples of breast-feeding women. The treatment consists of hygiene and the help of any of these plants.

Nipple scars or sores are the most important causative factor of **mastitis** (inflammation of the mammary glands) during breast-feeding. This inflammation can provoke an excess of pus, obliging then to give up natural breast-feeding. Therefore, it is important to pay enough attention and an adequate treatment to these sores.

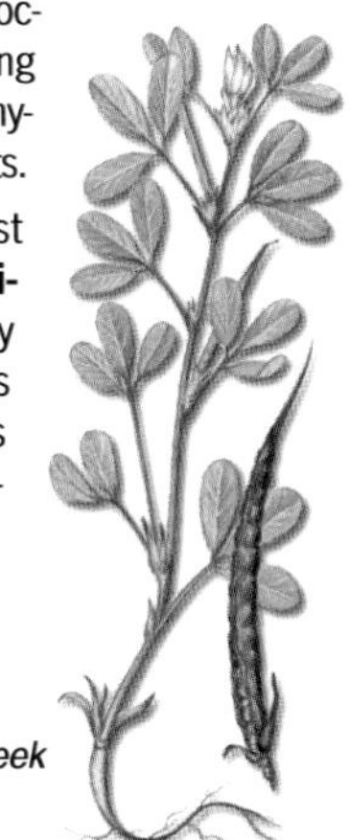

Fenugreek

FENUGREEK	Emollient (soothing), healing

PREGNANCY

The following plants are especially useful during pregnancy, due to their ***invigorating and nutritive*** properties.

Edema (retention of fluids), quite common during pregnancy, can be alleviated with safe and mild ***diuretic*** plants such as corn stigma.

During pregnancy, all ***oxytocic and emmenagogue*** plants must be ***avoided***, since they contract the uterus. Also, all plants mentioned on **page 100** must be avoided.

SPIRULIN	Nutritive, increases production of red blood red corpuscles

PREMATURE EJACULATION

Besides damiana, plants with **invigorating properties on the nervous system,** recommended for **exhaustion** and **asthenia** are also a valuable help.

DAMIANA	Nervous system invigorator, revitalizer, aphrodisiac

MENSTRUATION, RETENTION OF FLUIDS

See also plants recommended for **edema**.

WHITE BIRCH	Increases the volume of urine and reduces tissue swelling

DYSMENORRHEA

Definition

It could be defined as an **irregularity** of the **menstrual function,** which usually is accompanied by **pain** and general discomfort. **Secondary** dysmenorrhea is a consequence of diverse organic diseases of the genital organs. However, often one finds no organic pathology, and in this case we have to talk about **primary or essential** dysmenorrhea.

Pain suffered when dysmenorrhea occurs is caused by spasmodic contractions of the uterus.

Sage

Phytotherapy

Phytotherapeutic treatment provides ***antispasmodic*** plants, which relax the uterus (see more of these plants on page 621), as well as ***emmenagogue*** plants which balance menstruation (see more plants on page 621) and plants which ***regulate*** hormonal balance, such as evening primrose or borage.

Local applications of linseed flour in the form of hot poultices serve as complement to the antispasmodic properties of orally taken herbal teas.

ORANGE TREE	Antispasmodic, sedative
BALM	Balances the nervous system, antispasmodic
PASSION FLOWER	Relaxes spasm-suffering uterus, sedative
EVENING PRIMROSE	Balances the hormonal system
LICORICE	Antispasmodic, relaxes the uterus
GERMAN CAMOMILE	Normalizes menstruation, calms pain
BASIL	Promotes menstruation, decreases pain caused by uterine spasms
SAFFRON	Emmenagogue, alleviates menstrual pain
LEMON VERBENA	Antispasmodic, calms menstrual pain
EUROPEAN PENNYROYAL	Promotes menstruation, calms pain
FLAX	Antispasmodic, sedative, anti-inflammatory
MADDER	Promotes menstruation and calms pain
MUGWORT	Normalizes menstruation, calms menstrual pain
CALENDULA	Fights painful uterine spasms, sedative
SAGE	Stimulates and regulates menstruation, calms menstrual pain
WHITE WILLOW	Analgesic, anti-inflammatory, calms menstrual pain
MILFOIL	Antispasmodic, alleviates dysmenorrhea

MENOPAUSE

This is a period in a woman's life in which menstruation and reproductive activity cease. It is not a disease, but a time of hormonal change, during which time a woman's body must adapt to a decrease of ovarian functions.

Intake of **herbal teas** made with these plants can alleviate disorders which belong to this stage of women life.

CYPRESS	Vasoconstrictor, stops metrorrhagia of the menopause
WITCH HAZEL	Stops hemorrhages, strengthens capillary and veins walls
SAGE	Promotes female hormone balance

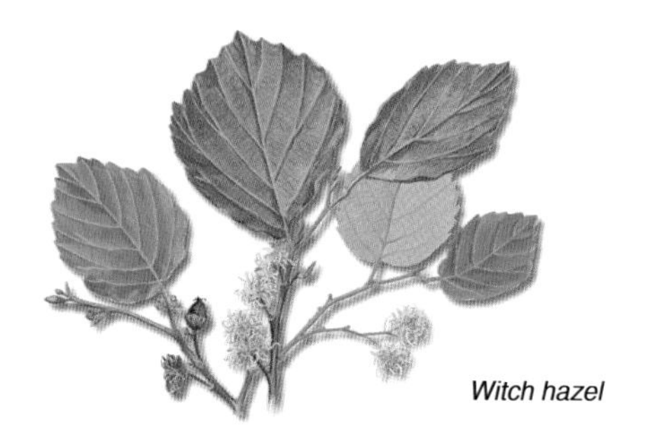

Witch hazel

EXCESSIVE MENSTRUATION

Once the causes of **hypermenorrhea** or excessive menstruation are ascertained, and whenever any ***organic cause has been discarded,*** these plants can help reduce the amount of menstrual blood or the duration of menstruation, due to their ***vasoconstrictor*** properties (contract small arteries and capillaries) and their ***hemostatic*** properties (promote blood coagulation) respectively. ***Oxytocic*** plants are also recommended.

All plants are taken orally, as infusion or decoction.

GOLDENSEAL	Contracts the uterus, hemostatic
WITCH HAZEL	Stops bleeding, strengthens venous and capillary walls
NETTLE	Vasoconstrictor, hemostatic
CALENDULA	Emmenagogue and menstrual regulator
MILENRAMA	Hemostatic, stops excessive menstruation and uterine bleeding
HORSETAIL	Heals bleeding tissues

IRREGULAR MENSTRUATION

Menstrual cycle depends on the hormones which are secreted by the hypophysis and the ovaries. At some point of women's life, such as ***teen years*** and ***menopause,*** menstrual cycle disorders are relatively frequent. As a rule, these disorders are caused by a **lack or an excess** of sexual hormones.

The following medicinal herbs have ***balancing*** properties on the endocrine glands which produce these hormones, and contribute in a good way to normalize menstrual cycle.

EVENING PRIMROSE	Balances hormonal system
LAUREL	Emmenagogue, regulates menstruation
MUGWORT	Emmenagogue, normalizes menstruation
CALENDULA	Emmenagogue and menstrual regulator
RUE	Contracts the uterus, emmenagogue
NASTURTIUM	Regulates and normalizes menstruation

LEUKORRHEA

Definition

This is the flow of a **thick, whitish fluid** through the vagina, fluid secreted by the vagina itself or by the uterus. It is usually caused by **infections,** though it can also be related to any imbalance in the usual **bacterial flora** of the vagina, or to **hormonal** alterations.

Phytotherapy

Phytotherapy provides several useful plants to make ***vaginal irrigations***. All of them have ***astringent*** (dry and reduce the inflammation of mucosa) properties, and some of them also have ***antiseptic*** properties.

RHATANY	Astringent, anti-inflammatory
GOLDENSEAL	Astringent, anti-inflammatory
WALNUT	Astringent, anti-inflammatory
ROSE	Astringent, anti-inflammatory, antiseptic. Very appropriate for intimate hygiene
WHITE WILLOW	Astringent, reduces infection

CERVICITIS

Definition

The **inflammation of the cervix**, which is usually caused by diverse bacteria or virus. It manifests itself by means of mucus or pus flowing (leukorrhea), and pain, during the days of menstruation, or during intercourse.

Phytotherapy

Both plants mentioned here, which are also used for **leukorrhea,** are the most important for cervicitis, since they have ***astringent, antiseptic, and anti-inflammatory*** properties.

Walnut tree

As we note on page 73, vaginal ***irrigations must never be applied during pregnancy.***

WALNUT	Astringent, anti-inflammatory
ROSE	Astringent, anti-inflammatory, antiseptic. Appropriate for intimate hygiene

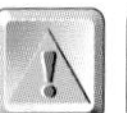

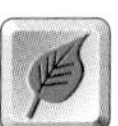

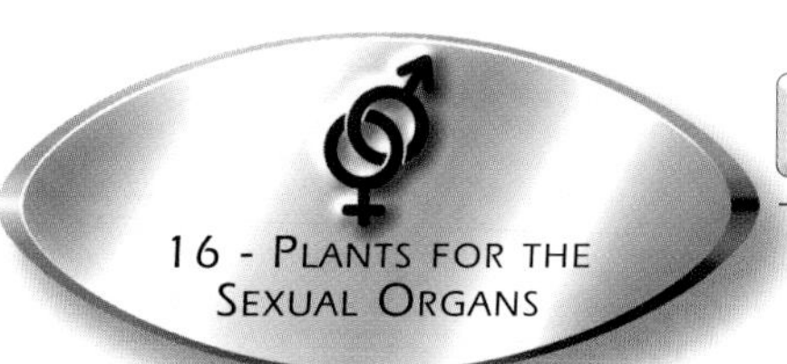

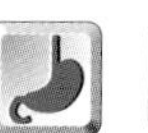

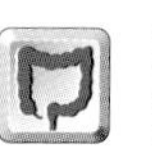

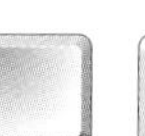

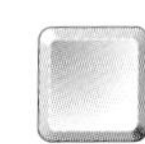

Mugwort

Regulates menstruation and increases appetite

MUGWORT WAS already used by the ancient Greeks. Dioscorides, the father of phytotherapy, talked about this plant in the first century A.D. Andrés de Laguna, a famous Spanish physician of the sixteenth century, who worked in the Netherlands, Bologna, Rome, and Venice, said of this plant that "it is called *Artemisia*, from the name of the goddess Artemis, also called Diana, since like the goddess, the plant helps women in labor, without ever failing ."

Mugwort has always been a plant used because of its effects on the female genitals.The French medical school, with its characteristic finesse, said as early as during the Renaissance that "mugwort turns women into flowers again," meaning the effects of the plant on menstruation.

PROPERTIES AND INDICATIONS. The whole plant contains an essence whose main component is eucalyptol or cyneole, as well as small

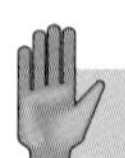

Warning

*Like wormwood, mugwort can have undesirable effects on the nervous system when the recommended **doses** are widely **exceeded,** or when it is taken for more than **ten days.***

***Pregnant** women must **abstain** from taking mugwort, since it is likely to have abortifacient properties. **Breast-feeding women** must also abstain from taking this plant because it gives milk a bitter flavor.*

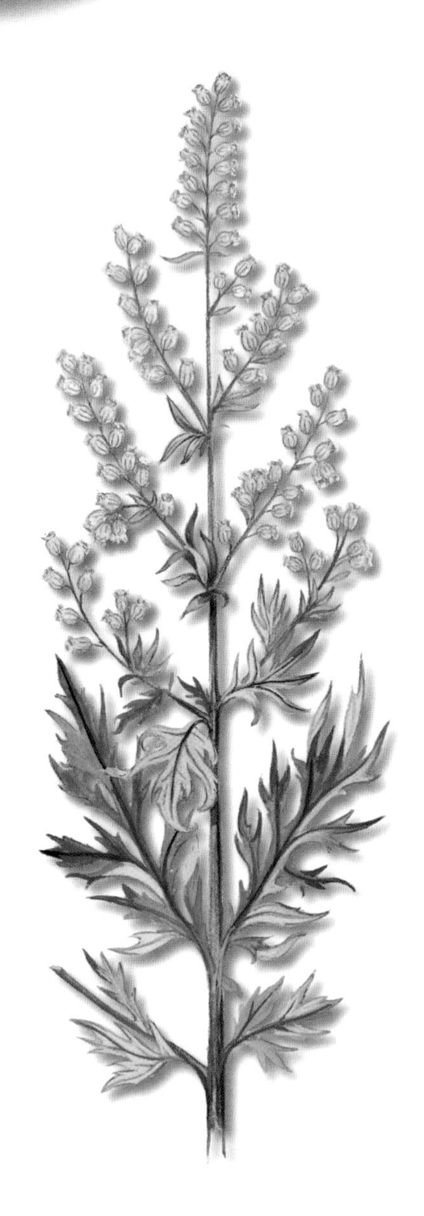

***Description.** Vivacious plant of the Compositae family, similar to wormwood but taller (60-120 cm high). Its stem is reddish in color, and its leaves are silver on their undersides. Each flower chapter is formed by 10-12 small flowers, yellow or reddish in color.*

***Parts used.** The leaves and the flower clusters, in summer, and the root in Fall.*

Preparation and Use

INTERNAL USE

❶ **Infusion** with 20-30 g of flower clusters or ground root per liter of water. Drink from two to four cups daily.

❷ As a **vermifuge,** that is, when dealing with intestinal parasites, the patient must drink a cup on an empty stomach, and two more before every meal, for three days. Repeat another cycle one week later.

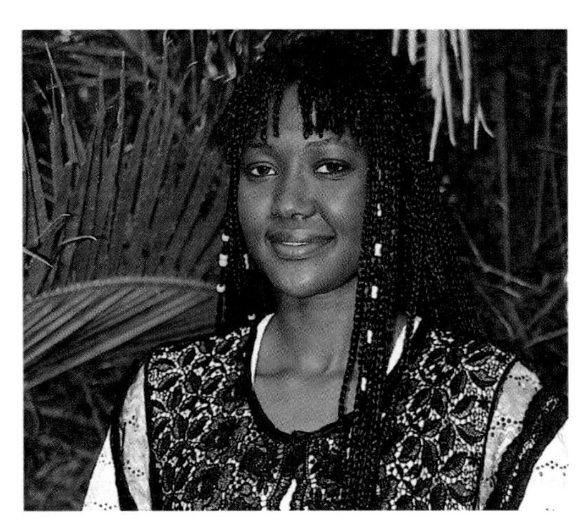

Mugwort promotes menstruation, in some cases of amenorrhea (lack of menstruation) caused by functional reasons.This plant is especially recommended for women suffering from irregular menstruation or dysmenorrhea (menstrual pain), since it helps normalize the menstrual cycle.

amounts of thujone, tannin, mucilage, and a bitter component. Its properties are as follows:

• **Emmenagogue.** It can produce menstruation in the case of **amenorrhea** (lack of menstruation) due to functional disorders. The plant also has the properties of normalizing menstrual cycle and easing menstrual pain (**dysmenorrhea**) [❶].

In ancient times it was applied as poultices on the stomach of women suffering from difficult or prolonged labor. At present, fortunately we have better remedies to accelerate labor.

• **Appetizer and cholagogue.** Because of its bitter component, it has the following properties: increases **appetite,** stimulates the emptying of the stomach (recommended for gastric ptosis) promotes **digestion,** and normalizes the function of the **gall bladder.** It also has mild **laxative** properties [❶].

• **Vermifuge.** It produces expulsion of intestinal parasites. It is especially effective against oxyuridae [❷]. In Central America, this plant is widely used because of this action.

This plant was formerly used as a sedative, to treat epilepsy and Parkinson's disease. However today it is no longer used. We have no proof of its effectiveness in these cases.

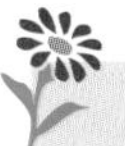

Other Artemisia Species

In tropical areas of the Americas there are several species and varieties, very similar to common mugwort, which have the **same properties,** such as the *Artemisia dracnculuoides* Pursh., which is cultivated in North America, where it is called false tarragon.

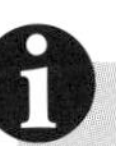

Mugwort Baths

*For **menstruation disorders,** it is useful to employ a combination of **oral intake** of this plant with hot water **baths** to which some handfuls of mugwort are added.*

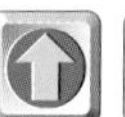
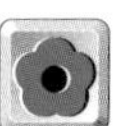
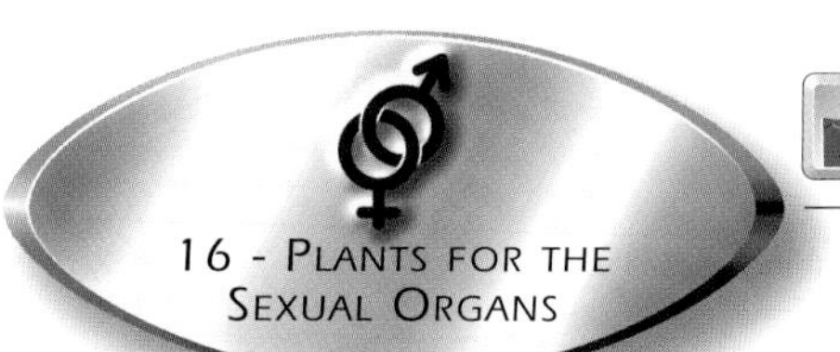

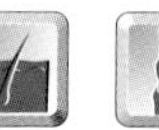
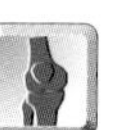
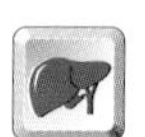
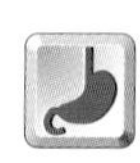

Calendula

Heals wounds and normalizes menstruation

CALENDULA, also called garden marigold, is a living example of how beauty and usefulness can go hand in hand. Its flowers open to the morning sun showing their wonderful colors. In the evening, they close the quietly until next morning.

People supporting the theory of signs, including Paracelsus and other Renaissance physicians, recommended calendula for jaundice and gall bladder disorders because of the bile-like color of its flowers. Those pioneers of medicine were not so wrong, since now we know its properties on a scientific basis, calendula is still used for the same purposes, and for other ones which have been also discovered.

PROPERTIES AND INDICATIONS. The flowers of calendula contain carotenoids (provitamin A), a bitter component (calendine), flavonoids, saponins, resin, essential oil, and small amounts of salicylic acid. All these substances combine themselves to turn this flower into a precious remedy. Its most outstanding properties are as follows:

• **Emmenagogue and menstrual regulator.** Calendula is useful both for scanty menstruation, due to its emmenagogue properties, and when there is excessive bleeding. Therefore, calendula normalizes both the frequency and the quality of menstruation. It also eases the pain caused by menstruation (**dysmenorrhea**), since it has spasmolytic (combats painful **spasms**) and mild sedative properties. It must be taken from one week before the menstruation period until it has ended **[❶]**. Results are noticeable.

• **Choleretic.** It increases bile production on

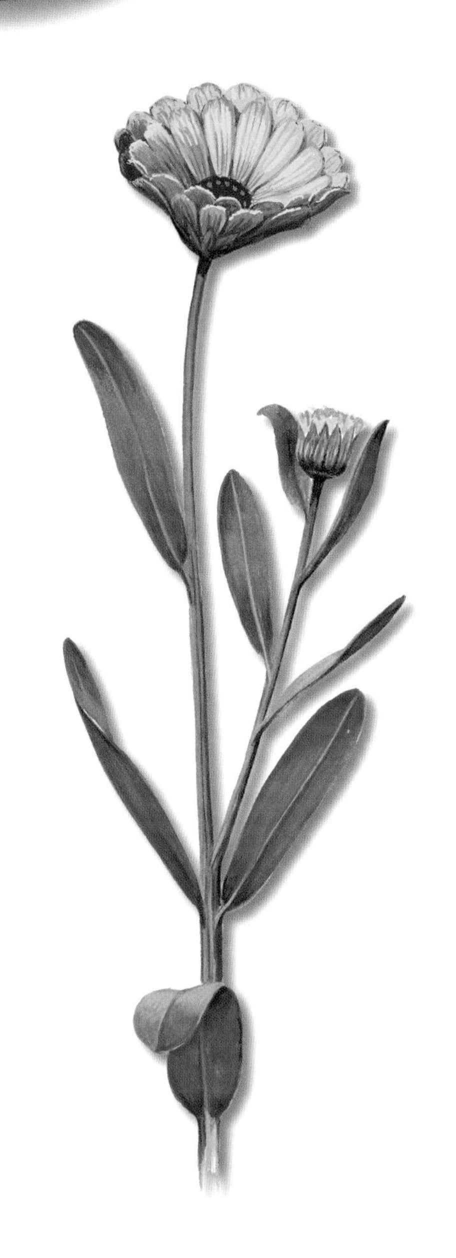

Description. *Herbaceous plant of the Compositae family, growing from 30 to 50 cm high, with elongated, toothed, fleshy leaves and exuberant, yellow or orange flowers.*

Parts used. *The flowers.*

Preparation and Use

INTERNAL USE

❶ **Infusion** with 1-2 flowers per cup of water. Drink two or three cups daily, which can be sweetened with honey.

EXTERNAL USE

❷ **Compresses and baths** with a decoction made with two handfuls of flowers per liter of water. Apply on the affected skin area.

❸ **Poultices** with fresh flower petals, applied wrapped on a fine cotton cloth.

❹ **Lotion with fresh juice** of flowers, applied in the affected skin area.

❺ **Oil.** It is directly applied on to the skin, but can also be added to the bath water to achieve a pleasant soothing effect on the skin. See picture bellow to find out how to obtain calendula oil by means of cold extract.

❻ **Cream.** It can be prepared by pressing 100 g of fresh flowers and mixing the resulting juice with 500 g of butter or other fatty substance.

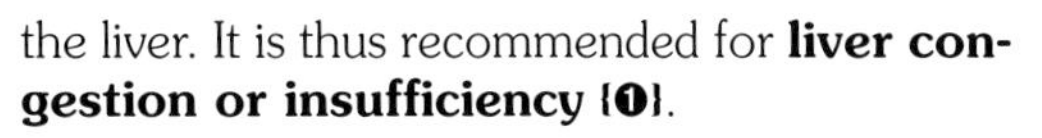

the liver. It is thus recommended for **liver congestion or insufficiency** (❶).

• **Antiulceration.** Calendula has the ability to heal stomach and duodenal ulcerations (❶). Its effects are more intense when taken in association with nettle and speedwell. Due to its healing and anti-inflammatory properties, it is also effective for **gastritis** (stomach inflammation), **gastroenteritis, and vomiting** (❶).

• **Anti-inflammatory, antiseptic, and healing.** This is ***one of the most outstanding plants*** for its **vulnerary** properties, that is to say, for healing wounds and bruises. When ***locally*** applied, it notably speeds up **wound** healing, even when these are infected, as well as skin **sores, burns, furuncles, and eczema** (❷,❸,❹). When applied to joints, it has **antirrheumatic** properties (❷,❸).

• **Wart remover.** In ***local applications*** it makes viral **warts** (common warts) of the skin disappear (❷,❹,❺). This effect is caused by the salicylic acid in it.

• **Emollient** (skin soothing). Calendula oil soothes and hydrates the skin (❺). It is recommended for dry or delicate skins, as well as for children. Both the oil (❺) and the cream (❻) render good results for treating **burns and eczema.**

Calendula oil is made by preparing a cold extract from its flowers in oil.
After some days, this oil, which would have become reddish in color, must be strained and kept in a glass jar.

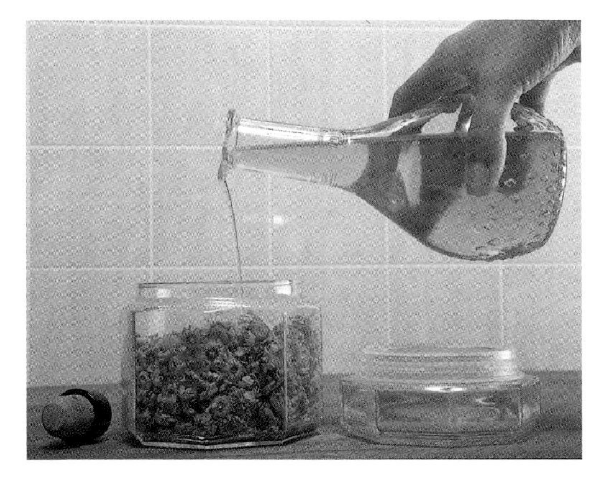

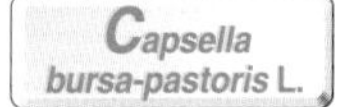
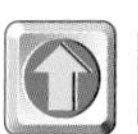
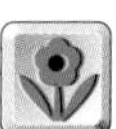
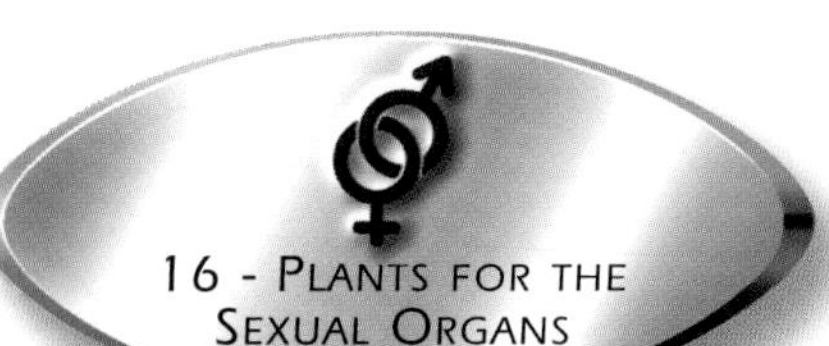

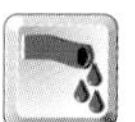
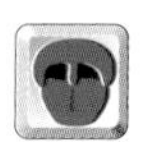
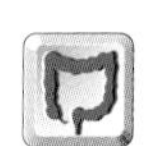
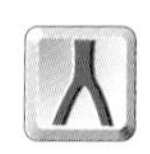

Shepherd's Purse

Stops hemorrhage and normalizes menstruation

THE FRUITS of this plant resemble the purses of shepherds in ancient times, and this fact is what has given the plant its name. Honoring what its name represents—a purse with which one travels—this plant is one of the most widespread known. It is found both along the coast and at 2000 meters high, in the mountains, both in cold climates of central and northern Europe and in tropical areas of the Americas and Asia.

It is regarded as a native of the Mediterranean countries; however the ability of its seeds to travel and adapt to any kind of soil have made this plant one of the most widespread in the world.

Properties and indications. The whole plant contains biogenic amines (choline, acetylcholine, and tyramine, among others), which act on the autonomic nervous system, producing contraction of arterioles, the uterus, the intestine, and other hollow organs. Its properties are the following:

- **Hemostatic** (stops hemorrhages). The substances this plant contains contract small bleeding arteries. Moreover, shepherd's purse is rich in flavonoids of the ***diosmin*** type (an active component of ***several pharmaceutical preparations***), which increases the endurance of the capillary walls and promotes returning venous blood flow.
- **Oxytocic.** It contracts the uterus and collapses blood vessels which cause bleeding in its interior.
- **Digestive tract invigorating.** Shepherd's purse causes the intestines to recover their muscular tone and peristaltic contractions (those which make the intestinal bolus progress inside the intestine).

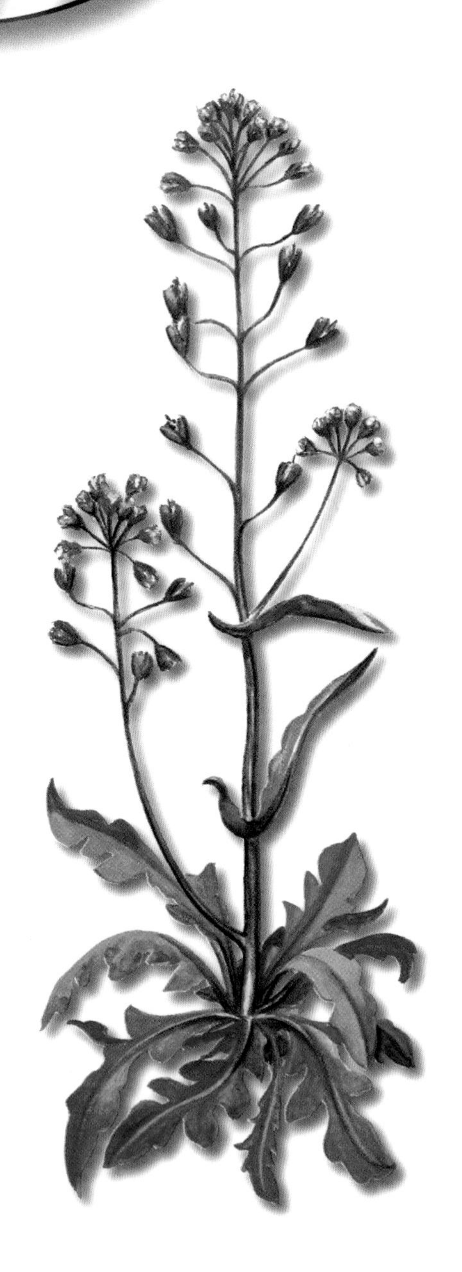

Description. *Annual plant of the Cruciferae family, growing up to 50 cm high. Its leaves grow in the form of a rose, near the soil, and it has small, white flowers. The fruit is triangle-shaped, flat, and has a slightly salty flavor.*

Parts used. *The whole plant.*

Preparation and Use

INTERNAL USE

❶ **Infusion** with 30-60 g of plant per liter of water, steeping for 10 minutes. Drink from three to five cups daily; not at meal time. In the case of **menstrual disorders,** this infusion must be first taken a week before the day menstruation is expected to occur.

EXTERNAL USE

❷ **Compresses** soaked in the same infusion used internally.

❸ **Gauze packing,** soaked in the aforementioned infusion, especially for nose bleeds.

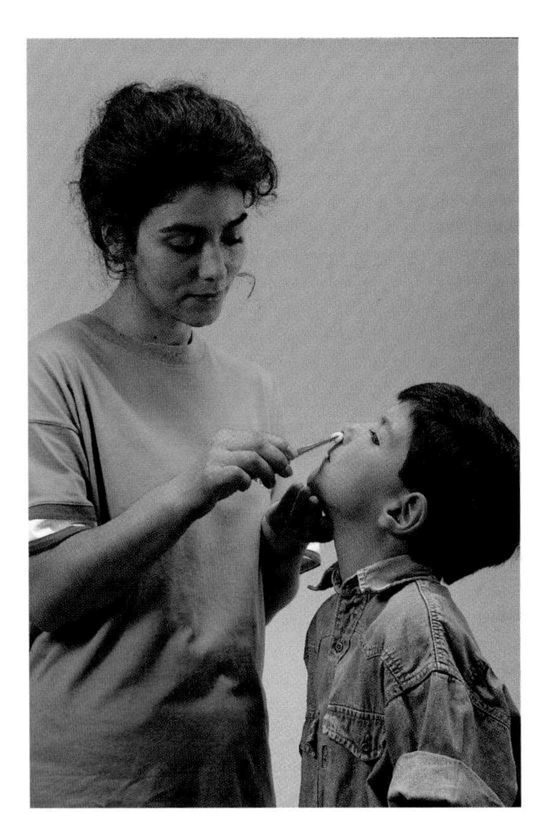

A cotton plug soaked in a shepherd's purse infusion is a good remedy to stop nose bleeding.

Because of these interesting therapeutic properties, shepherd's purse is a valued plant, useful for diverse diseases, as we note here:

- Uterine hemorrhages (**metrorrhage**). This is its ***most important application,*** since it stops both too abundant menstruation of some teenagers which appears soon after their first menstruation (menarche), and uterine bleeding which sometimes appears in menopause [❶]. That is to say, shepherd's purse is good for both mother and daughter. We have to remark, however, that it is necessary to undergo a ***gynecological examination*** in order to be sure that the causes of these disorders do not include tumors, anatomic alterations, or other uterine causes of bleeding.
- **Epistaxis** (nose bleeding). In this case, besides taking an infusion of this plant for some days, it can be ***locally*** applied. The method consists in applying a noseplug soaked in the infusion into the bleeding nostril [❸]. It can also be applied on skin wounds and bleeding sores [❷].
- **Labor acceleration,** for uterine atony or weakness [❶]. Its action is similar to that of ergotamine, an alkaloid which is extracted from the rye ergot, but with less side effects.
- **Intestinal atony.** Shepherd's purse is useful to combat intestinal atony produced during convalescence from fever or infectious diseases, as well as for the frequent cases of constipation caused by intestinal laziness [❶].
- **Low blood pressure.** It is recommended for those people suffering from low blood pressure, and especially thin women [❶].

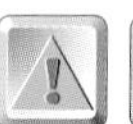
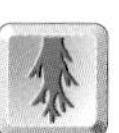
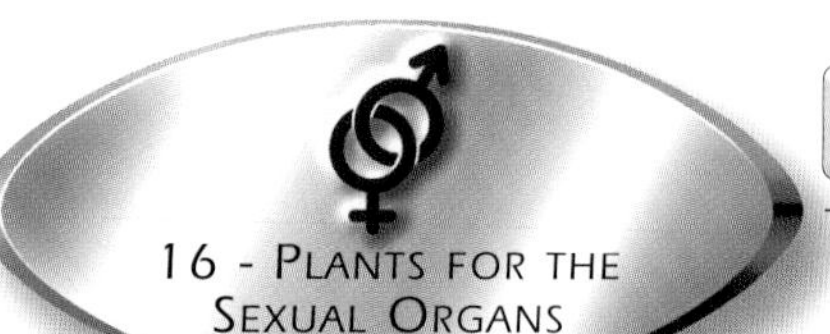

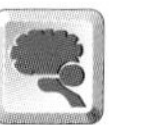
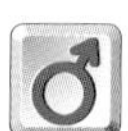
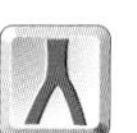
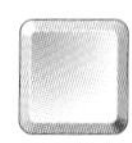

Ginseng

Not a dope... but it works!

ITS SCIENTIFIC name of *Panax* comes from the Greek words *pan* (all) and *axos* (healing). For Chinese people, ginseng is a true panacea, able to heal a wide range of afflictions. Its aphrodisiac effects have given it a wide popularity in Western countries, in which stress, tobacco, alcohol, and other drugs have become a continuous aggression to sexual performance.

PROPERTIES AND INDICATIONS. The active components of ginseng root are so chemically complex that it has not been possible to synthesize them up to now. They are called ginsenosides, and chemically these are steroid glycosides from the group of triterpenic saponins. Therapeutic properties of ginseng are due mainly to these substances, but are also enhanced by other components: minerals and trace elements, the most outstanding being sulphur, manganese, germanium, magnesium, calcium, and zinc; vitamins B_1, B_2, B_6, biotin, and pantothenic acid; phytosterol, enzymes, and other substances as well.

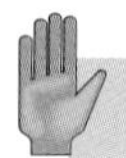

Warning

Excessive doses** can produce **nervousness.

***Do not associate** it with **coffee or tea,** since it can produce nervous excitation, nor with medicines containing **iron,** because this mineral interferes chemically with the active components of ginseng, decreasing its effects.*

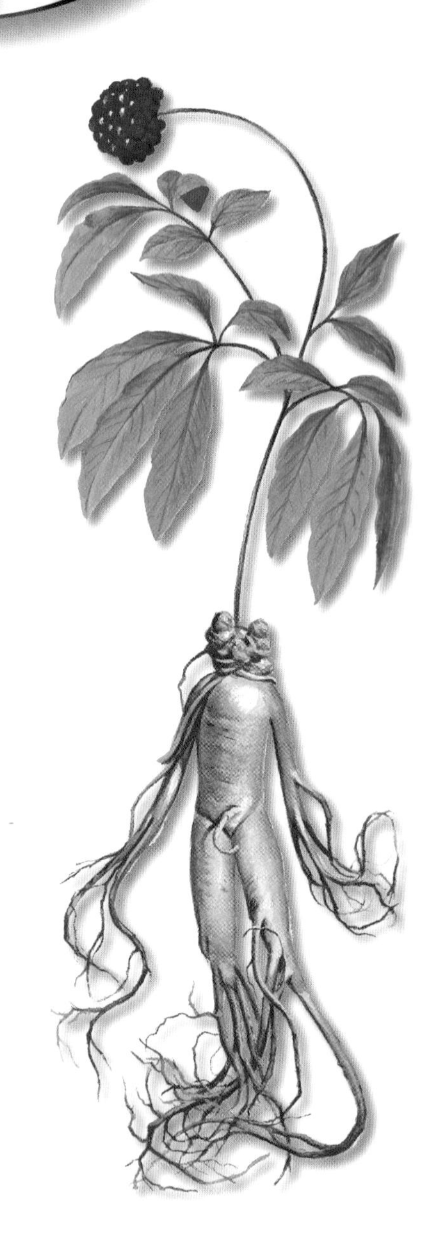

***Description.** Plant of the Araliaceae family, growing from 20 to 50 cm high. Its flowers grow in groups of five. It has purple flowers, which give birth to small fruits (berries). The root is fleshy, greyish or white in color, from 10 to 15 cm large, and an average of 200 g weight.*

***Parts used.** The root after five years of age.*

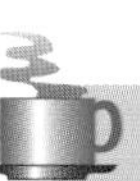

Preparation and Use

INTERNAL USE

❶ Ginseng is usually presented as **pharmaceutical preparations** (extract, capsules, liquid, etc.). The usual dose is 0.5-1.5 g of root powder per day, in a single or several intakes.

Ginseng action is slow but accumulative. Ginseng effects will be noticeable after two or three weeks of treatment.

We recommend that you take ginseng continuously for a period of time (a maximum of two or three months), and stop for one or two months before a starting a new treatment.

Ginseng has a wide range of effects on the body [❶].

- **Invigorator.** Ginsenosides increase physical performance and endurance. This is not due to any excitant properties, such as in cocaine, coffee, tea, or other drugs, but to an improvement of metabolic processes. Ginseng speeds up the enzymatic process of glycogenesis (production of glycogen on the liver from sugar), and glycogenolysis (production of sugar from the stored glycogen); decreases the concentration of lactic acid in muscles, which causes stiffness, because of a better sugar metabolism; increases the production of ATP (adenosine-triphosphate), a substance of great energetic capabilities for cells; enhances the use of oxygen by cells; increases protein synthesis (anabolic effect); stimulates hematopoiesis (blood production) in the bone medulla, especially after bleeding. All these biochemical effects have been experimentally proven. Therefore, ginseng ***invigorates but does not excite or provoke addiction,*** since it increases energy production on cells.
- **Nervous system.** It has **antidepressive and anxiolytic** properties (eliminates anxiety). Ginseng promotes mental performance, increasing **concentration and memory** capabilities.
- **Endocrine system.** Ginseng has **anti-stress** properties due to its "adaptogenic" properties, because it increases adaptation capabilities of the body to physical or psychological efforts. Research conducted on animals has proven that both hypophysis and suprarenal glands are stimulated with ginseng.
- **Cardiovascular system.** Ginseng has vasorregulating properties, balancing blood pressure.
- **Reproductive system.** Ginseng promotes spermatogenesis (increases the production of spermatozoids); stimulates sexual glands (both male and female) and increases hormone production; it **increases sexual capability,** improving both frequency and quality of male erection, and promoting female genital organs excitation. It is not a true aphrodisiac substance, since its action does not consist in arousing sexual desire, but in improving function and capabilities of genitalia.

Indications for using ginseng are the following:

- **Physical exhaustion.** Asthenia (weakness), easy fatigue, lack of energy, convalescence from diseases or surgery.
- **Sports training.** Ginseng is not one of the listed doping substances forbidden in sports.
- **Stress, psychosomatic disorders.** (Gastritis, colitis, migraine, asthma, palpitations).
- **Psychological exhaustion, depression, anxiety, insomnia.** Ginseng is very useful for students during examinations.
- **Premature aging, senility.**
- **High or low blood pressure.**
- **Anemia.** Ginseng is especially useful to recover blood loss after donation or bleeding.
- **Sexuality disorders.** Impotence, female frigidity, hormonal insufficiency, male or female sterility.

Rose

Soothes, reduces infection, and invigorates

FROM A MEDICINAL standpoint, the French rose or *Rosa gallica* is the one offering the best and most properties.

PROPERTIES AND INDICATIONS. Although rose ***PETALS*** have been celebrated by some people—maybe due more to a poetic than to a scientific meaning—as an almost universal remedy, they basically have **astringent, anti-inflammatory, and antiseptic** properties. They also provide **sedative** properties on the nervous system. Their medicinal applications are the following:

• **Gynecological afflictions.** An infusion of rose petals is used for vaginal irrigations for **leukorrhea** (increase of vaginal flow), **vaginitis, cervicitis** (inflammation of the uterine neck). It is highly recommended for the **hygiene** of the external female genitalia, applied as cleansing and irrigation [❹].

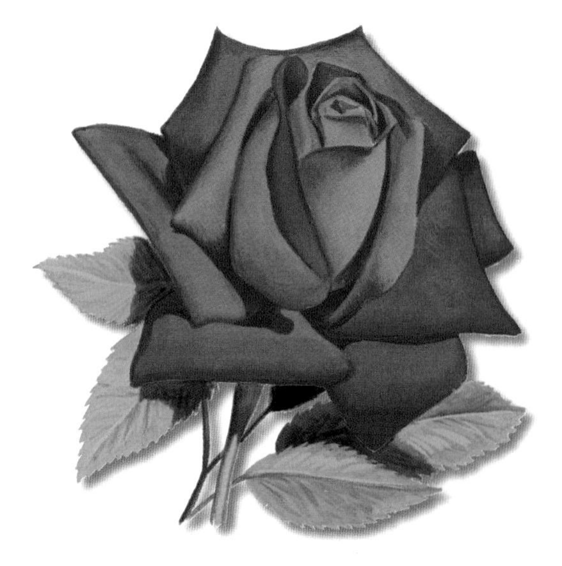

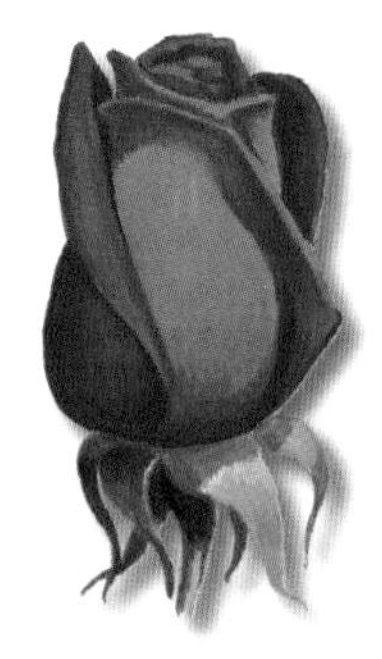

Description. *Shrub of the Rosaceae family, growing from 0.5 to 1.5 m high, with upright stems with spines, and single, big, red, velvet-like flowers.*

Parts used. *The petals of its flowers.*

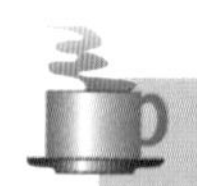

Preparation and Use

INTERNAL USE

❶ **Infusion** with 20-30 g of petals per liter of water. Drink from four to six cups daily (sweetened with honey).

EXTERNAL USE

The same infusion used internally can be employed as:

❷ **Gargles, mouth rinses, and nose irrigation.**

❸ **Eye irrigation.**

❹ **Vaginal irrigations.**

• **Digestive afflictions.** Rose petals are useful to stop several kinds of **diarrhea,** especially summer diarrhea [❶].

• **Respiratory affections of the upper airways.** Both drunk [❶], and applied as gargles, mouth rinses, and nasal irrigation [❷], infusions of rose petals, and rose water are effective for nasal catarrh, sinusitis, pharyngitis and hoarseness.

• **Eye afflictions.** Rose petal infusions are excellent to wash eyes for eye irritation and conjunctivitis, especially for children [❸].

Rue

Normalizes menstruation

DURING THE Middle Ages, it was cultivated in monastery cloisters since it was regarded to have antiaphrodisiac properties. At present it is still used for several female disorders.

PROPERTIES AND INDICATIONS.

- **Gynecological afflictions.** Rue contains an essence rich in methyl-n-nonylketone, with strong **oxytocic** activity (it contracts the uterus), and also **emmenagogue** properties. Thus, it is used for **amenorrhea** (lack of menstruation), once this lack is ascertained not to be caused by pregnancy; and also for weak, irregular, or painful menstruation (**dysmenorrhea**) [❶].
- **Antispasmodic and antiseptic.** Rue ***essence*** has both properties, and is thus administered to calm **colic abdominal** pain [❷].
- **Antihemorrhagic.** Rue contains rhutin or rhutosid (vitamin P) which increases the resistance of blood capillary vessels, and can stop some **internal hemorrhages** [❶,❷]. However, the cause of this hemorrhage must always ***be determined*** before taking rue.
- **Antirrheumatic.** ***Externally*** applied, rue has **revulsive** properties, and it is used as compresses to calm **rheumatic aches** [❸].
- **Skin afflictions.** Due to its revulsive action, it is recommended in certain skin affections: psoriasis, eczema, scabies [❸].

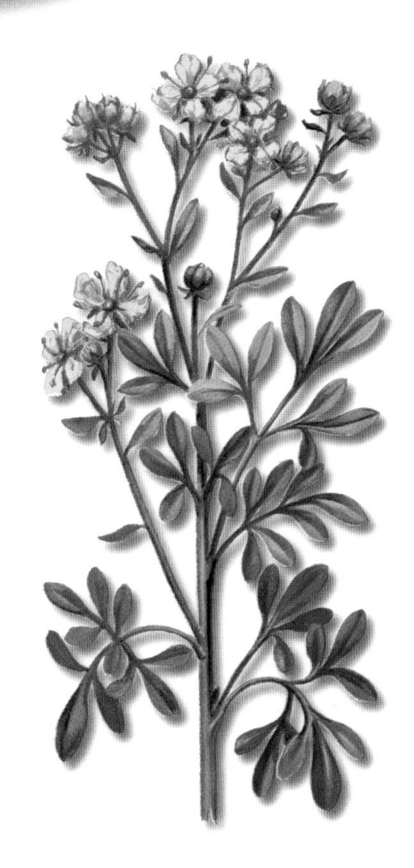

Description. *Vivacious, herbaceous plant of the Rutaceae family, growing up from 0.6 to 1 m high, with yellow-greenish flowers which gather in umbels. Rue has a very peculiar strong odor.*

Parts used. *The flower clusters.*

Preparation and Use

INTERNAL USE

❶ **Infusion** with 2-5 g of plant per liter of water. Drink two cups daily. For **menstrual disorders** drink it the week before menstruation is expected.

❷ **Essence.** The recommended dose is 2-3 drops per day.

EXTERNAL USE

❸ **Compresses** soaked in a concentrated infusion (10-20 g per liter of water) and applied directly on the affected skin area.

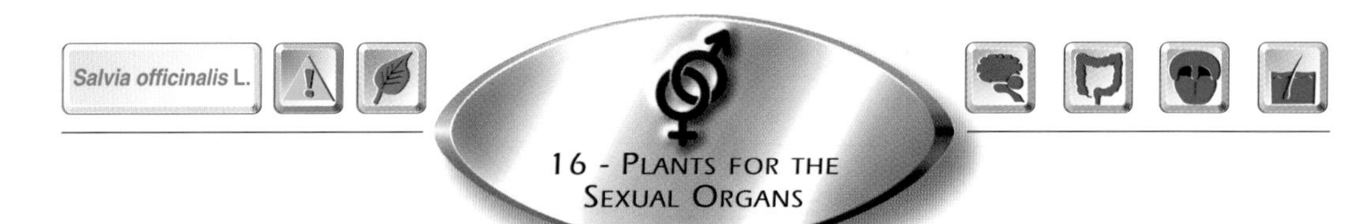

Sage

Ideally invigorating for women... and more!

THE SCIENTIFIC name of sage comes from the Latin word *salvare*, which means to save, since sage was believed to heal almost all diseases with the exception of death. Thanks to scientific research, we currently know its true properties, and we are able to use it correctly.

PROPERTIES AND INDICATIONS. The whole plant contains an essence (up to 2.5%) which is rich in thujone that explains its antiseptic, antiperspirant, and emmenagogue properties; catechic tannins, which give the plant astringent and invigorating properties; flavonoids and phenolic acids, with antispasmodic and choleretic properties, and substances with similar properties to those of foliculine, a estrogenic hormone which is secreted by the ovaries. The applications of sage are the following:

• **Gynecological afflictions.** Due to its **antispasmodic and emmenagogue** properties,

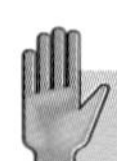

Warning

*When taken in **high doses,** sage **essence** is **toxic and produces convulsions.** Therefore, it is recommended to take sage for no longer than **one month.***

Internal use** of sage is totally **advised against,** for the following cases: **breast-feeding** (it stops it), **pregnancy,** except during the last month (it contracts the uterus), and states of irritability or great nervous **excitation.

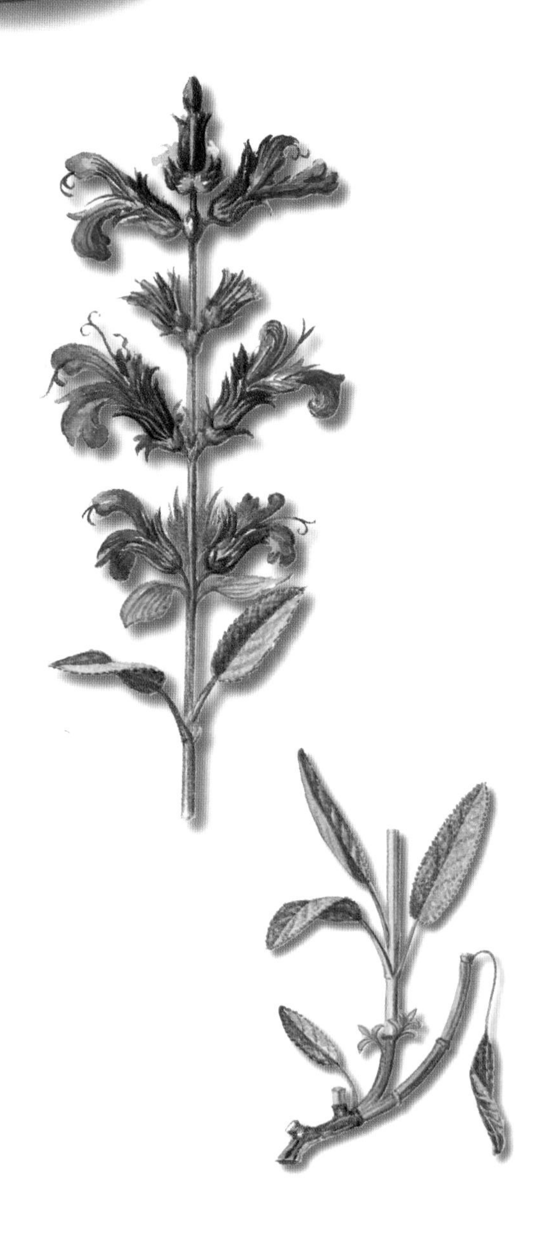

***Description.** Shrub of woody base of the Labiatae family, growing from 50 to 80 cm high. It has greyish green oval-shaped leaves, and bluish or violet flowers growing in spike clusters.*

***Parts used.** The leaves.*

it stimulates and at the same time regulates menstruation, eases menstrual pains, and fights menstrual disorders {❶,❷}. When taken the month before labor, it stimulates labor contractions and eases them. In short, sage **promotes hormonal balance** in women's bodies, thus it may also promote fertility. Its use is recommended to treat vaginism and frigidity. In the form of vaginal irrigations, it fights **leukorrhea** {❺}.

- **Nervous system invigorating.** Sage has a mild **stimulant** action on **suprarenal** glands. It is thus recommended for depression, asthenia, low blood pressure, shivers, vertigo, and other manifestations of autonomic nervous system imbalance {❶,❷}.
- **Sweating states.** Sage is perhaps ***the plant with strongest antiperspirant properties known.*** About two hours after taking it, sage reduces excessive perspiration, especially at night, for infectious diseases, tuberculosis, and certain degenerative afflictions {❶,❷}. Sage has also febrifuge properties (it makes fever decrease).
- **Diabetes.** This plant offers a proven hypoglycemic action which allows a reduction of the dose of antidiabetic medicines {❶,❷}.
- **Digestive afflictions.** Sage has **digestive and carminative** properties, as well as **antispasmodic and antiseptic** actions which help easing vomiting, **diarrhea,** and abdominal **colic** ache {❶}. Its **choleretic** properties (stimulates bile secretion) reduce the congestion of the liver and promote digestion {❶}.
- **Mouth and pharyngeal afflictions.** Due to its **astringent and antiseptic** properties, sage renders very good results for **gingivitis** (inflammation of the gums), mouth sores, **tonsillitis, and pharyngitis.** When used as gargles, it calms throat itching and smoker's cough {❹}.
- **Skin afflictions.** In this case, sage **reduces infection and heals.** It is useful for wounds, ulcers, abscess, furuncles, and **insect bites** {❸}. Baths with sage help keep the **facial skin beautiful** {❻}.

Preparation and Use

INTERNAL USE

❶ **Infusion** with 15-30 g of leaves and flower clusters per liter of water. Drink up to four cups daily. For **menstrual disorders,** sage is administered during the week previous to the expected menstruation date.

❷ **Essence.** The recommended dose is 2-4 drops, three times a day.

EXTERNAL USE

❸ **Compresses and lotions** with a decoction prepared with 80-100 of leaves per liter of water.

❹ **Mouth rinsings and gargles** with the aforementioned decoction.

❺ **Vaginal irrigations** with this decoction, well strained one time.

❻ **Baths.** The same decoction is added to the bath water to achieve a cosmetic effect on the skin and to make it more beautiful.

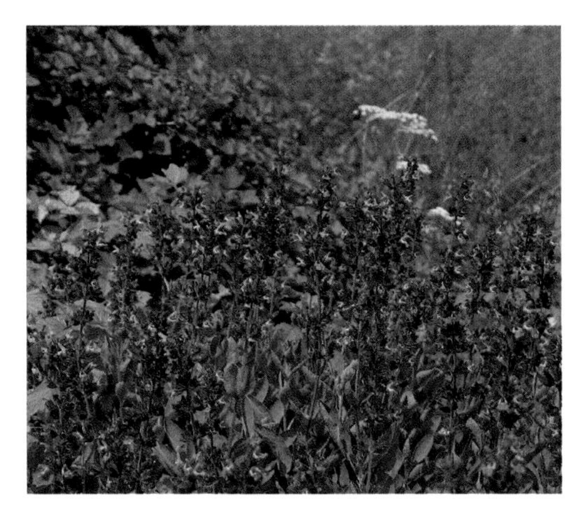

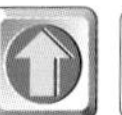
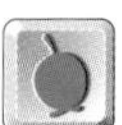
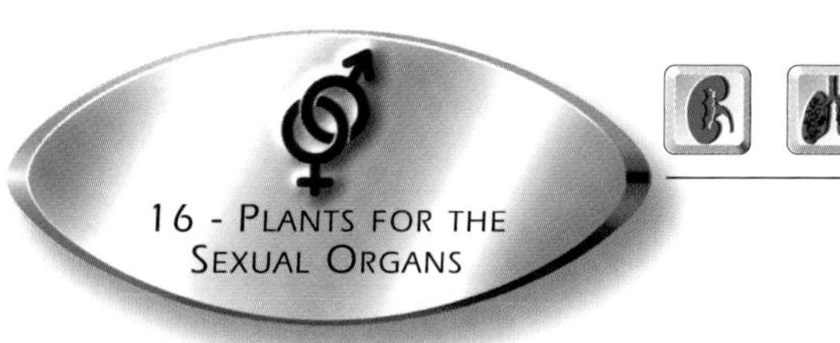

Shrub Palmetto

It stops prostate growth

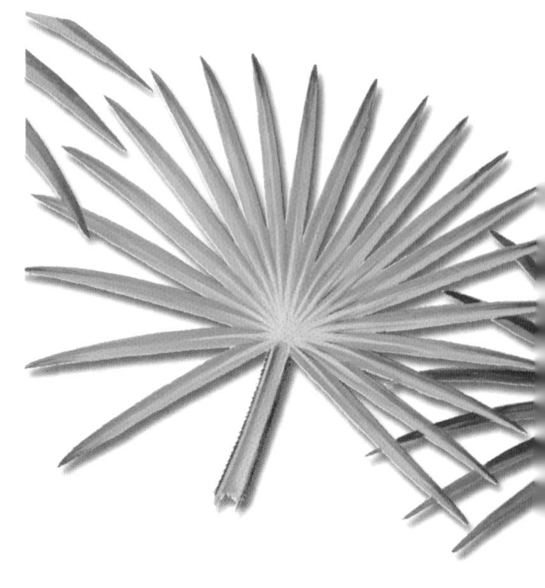

THE FRUIT of this small American palm is a kind of small dates which has been consumed for a long time in Georgia, Florida, Louisiana, and other states of southeastern America. Ancient native inhabitants of the region already knew the medicinal properties of this plant, and even used its fruit as an aphrodisiac. Recently some very interesting active components have been discovered in the fruit, which at present is part of several ***pharmaceutical preparations.***

Properties and indications. The fatty extract obtained from the fruit of shrub palmetto, after being dissolved in a fatty environment, contains several phytosterols, especially betasitosterol; a triterpenic alcohol (cycloartenol), and fatty aliphatic alcohols of high molecular weight, all of them with anti-inflammatory properties on the prostate. Their action mechanism is ***of hormonal type,*** and prevents a proliferation of androgens in prostate tissues.

Description. *Palm of the Palmaceae family, growing up to 3 m high, with ivory-colored flowers. The fruit is date-like, around 2 cm long, which are blackish in color when ripe.*

Parts used. *The fruit when ripe.*

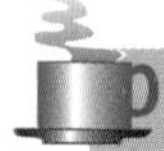

Preparation and Use

❶ Ripe fresh **fruit.** An amount of 50-100 g per day can be consumed.

❷ **Decoction** of fruit, 50-100 g per day.

❸ **Extracts** which are part of several pharmaceutical preparations.

• **Prostate.** The use of shrub or saw palmetto is useful for prostatic **hypertrophy** or **adenoma** [❶,❷,❸]. It stops prostate gland enlargement and notably reduces the major discomforts of the prostatic syndrome: dysuria (difficulty to urinate), pollakiuria (urge to urinate often), and vesicle tenesmus (permanent sensation of urge to urinate). It is also recommended for **prostatitis,** both acute and chronic.

• **Diuretic.** Besides its antiprostatic properties, this plant mildly promotes diuresis. It has also mild **pectoral** properties [❶,❷].

Damiana

Invigorator and aphrodisiac

THE LEAVES of this plant, which has a pleasant aromatic flavor, were used in Mexico as a substitute for tea, and enjoy a deserved fame as an aphrodisiac substance.

PROPERTIES AND INDICATIONS. The leaves contain an essential oil, a glycoside. Its medicinal properties are as follows:

- **Nervous invigorator.** The use of damiana renders good results for treating asthenia, weakness, physical or intellectual exhaustion, and stress [❶,❷]. Unlike other stimulant products, damiana has a mild action which does not lead to addiction.
- **Genitalia stimulant.** Damiana has been proven to produce an increase in the number and vitality of spermatozoids. In women, it regularizes menstrual cycles and stimulates ovary functions. For both sexes, it has **revitalizing and aphrodisiac** properties, which unlike other sexual stimulants, ***does not have any*** known ***side effect***. It is recommended for male impotence, premature ejaculation, and spermatorrhea (involuntary emission of semen) [❶,❷].
- Mild **diuretic** [❶].

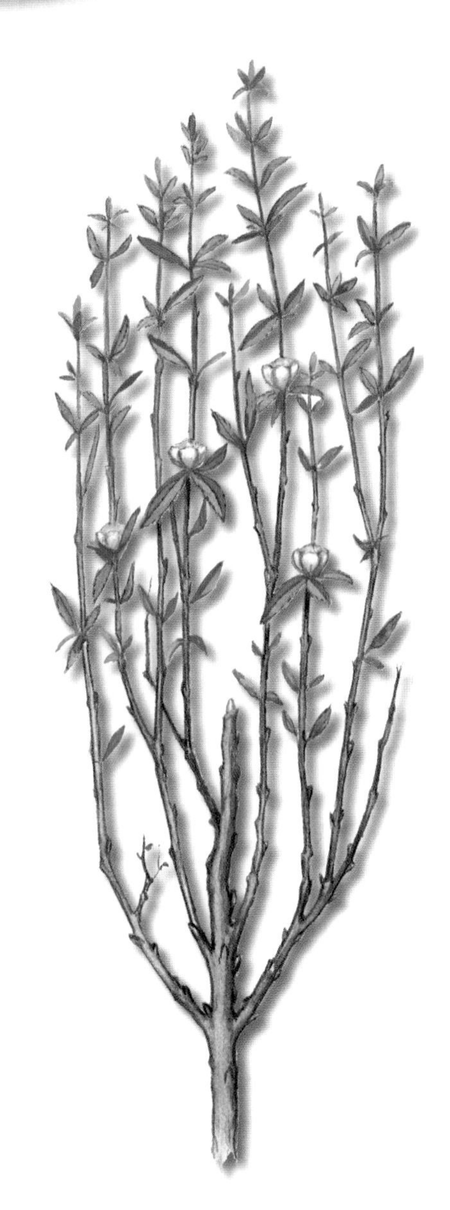

Description. *Shrub of the Turneraceae family, growing up to two meters high. It has small, toothed leaves, lighter in color on their undersides, and small, yellow flowers which grow in the upper leaf axils of the plant.*

Parts used. *The leaves.*

Preparation and Use

INTERNAL USE

❶ **Infusion** with 60-90 g of leaves per liter of water. Drink two or three cups daily.

❷ **Extracts.** These extracts are presented as diverse pharmaceutical preparations.

17

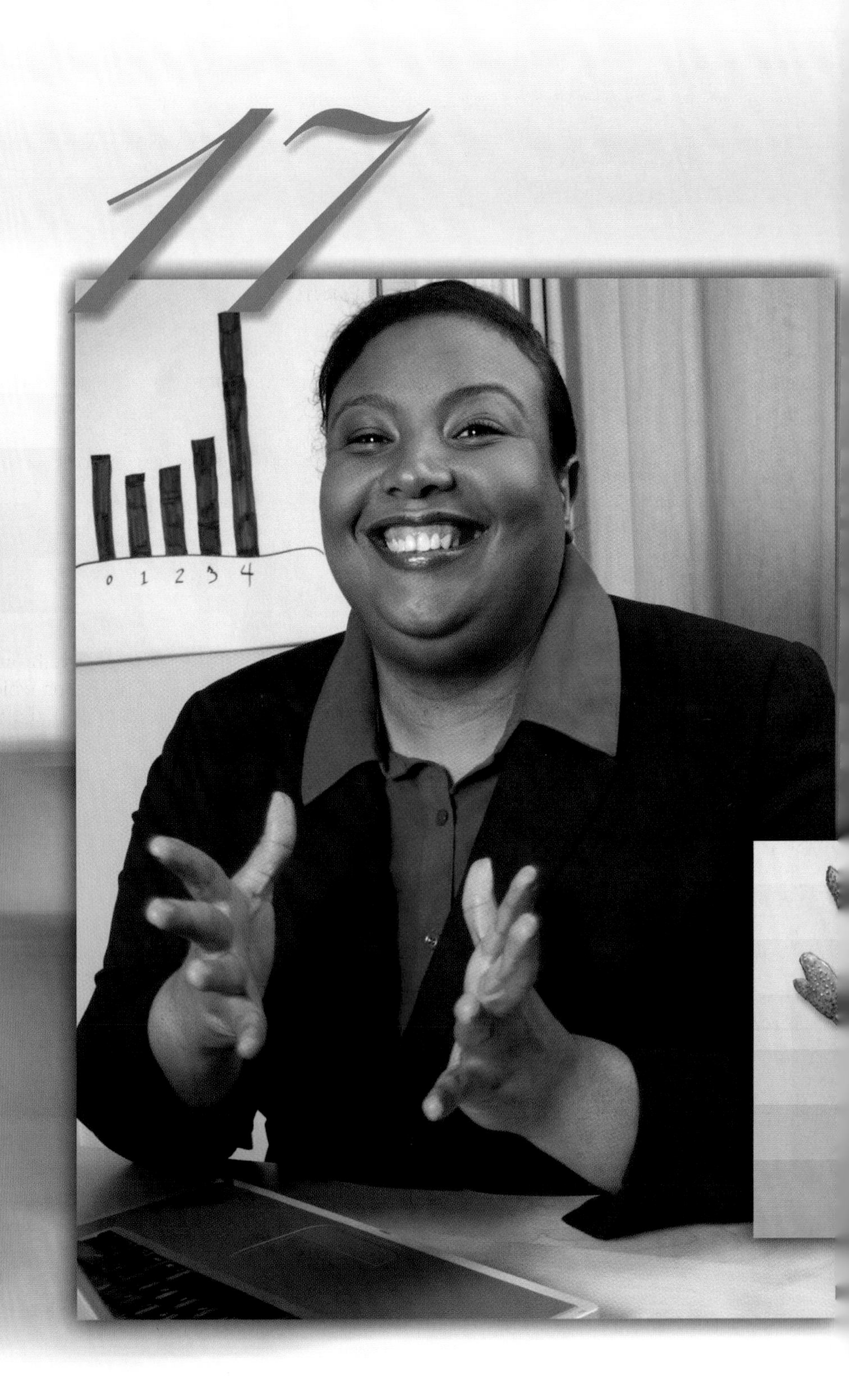

Plants for the Metabolism

DISEASES	PAGES
Acid, uric, excess of, see Gout	311
Appetite, excess of, see Bulimia	310
Bulimia	310
Diabetes	311
Excess of appetite, see Bulimia	310
Gout	311
Hyperuricemia, see Gout	311
Malnutrition	311
Obesity	310
Sugar in the blood, excess, see Diabetes	311
Uric acid, excess of, see Gout	311
Weight loss	310

PLANTS	PAGES
Fucus	312
Javan tea	315
Kelp	314

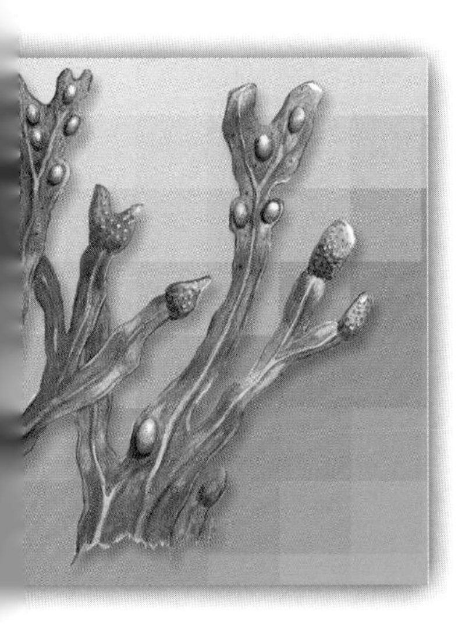

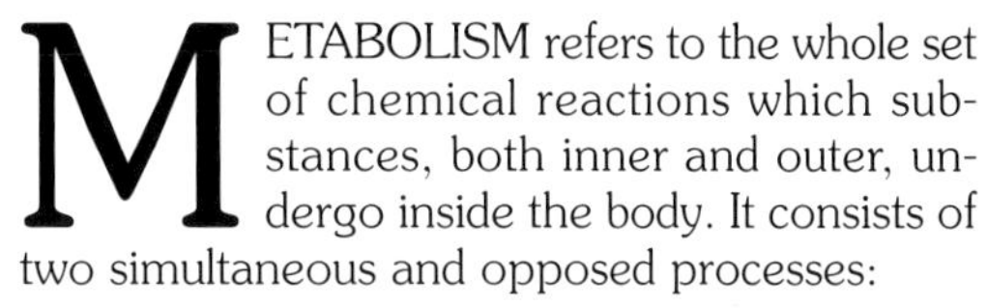

METABOLISM refers to the whole set of chemical reactions which substances, both inner and outer, undergo inside the body. It consists of two simultaneous and opposed processes:

- **Anabolism.** The synthesis of organic products to store reserves.
- **Catabolism.** Disintegration of the stored products to obtain the needed energy in order to keep life going.

Metabolic processes are regulated by **hormones,** especially by those produced by the thyroid gland and the pancreas. There are medicinal herbs which act on both endocrine glands: On the **thyroid,** by increasing or decreasing its activity; and on the **pancreas;** by enhancing insulin production, which reduces the level of sugar in the blood.

As a result of metabolic activity, a level of toxic substances is produced, and these substances must be eliminated. Most of them have an **acid reaction,** such as **uric acid** and **urea.** Depurative medicinal herbs help our body in the task of eliminating that important amount of metabolic waste substances which are continuously produced. These substances are mainly eliminated through **urine** and **sweat.**

OBESITY is one of the most common metabolic disorders, and can be treated with the following types of medicinal herbs:

- **Sedative,** which eliminate the anxiety which is usually related to obesity and produces the wish of eating in a non-controlled way.
- **Appetite reducers.** Plants with these properties ***lack any side effect*** like those of synthetic anorexigens which derive from ***amphetamines.*** These plants are rich in **mucilage,** such as algae, and are able to absorb a large amount of water in the stomach. This way, they increase their volume and produce a sensation of being full by using a purely physical mechanism. They are taken before meals, or whenever you want to eliminate the sensation of hunger.
- **Diuretic.** These plants avoid the retention of liquids which usually occurs in the case of obesity. ***It is not recommended to lose weight by*** eliminating fluids using ***chemical diuretic substances*** as some weight-loss treatments do. This causes imbalances in the composition of organic liquids and electrolytes. Fortunately, ***diuretic plants do not present any risk of*** electrolyte imbalance, and they can be used as part of weight-loss treatments. Besides eliminating water and making one lose weight, they promote the elimination of waste substances from the body.

OBESITY

Phytotherapy ***complements the dietetic treatment*** of obesity by means of plants which reduce ***appetite,*** activate the ***metabolism,*** then increasing the assimilation of ingested calories, and promote the elimination of retained liquids (**diuretic**).

VERVAIN	Sedative, mild diuretic
GARLIC	Activates metabolism, promotes elimination of waste substances
PSYLLIUM	Produces sensation of being full, reduces appetite
PURSLANE	Laxative, diuretic, depurative
GOLDENROD	Diuretic, depurative, cleans blood from waste substances
FUCUS	Provokes sensation of being full, reduces appetite
KELP	Stimulates metabolism, produces sensation of being full

BULIMIA

Definition

This is the case of an **endless hunger,** usually provoked by **anxiety** or other nervous disorders.

Phytotherapy

Phytotherapeutical treatment consists of ***sedative*** plants, as well as plants which produce ***a sensation of having a full*** stomach, such as fucus and kelp (algae).

PRICKLY LETTUCE	Sedative, calms nervous excitation
VALERIAN	Sedative, eases anxiety, recommended in autonomic nervous dysfunction
MARJORAM	Sedative, eases anxiety
FUCUS	Produces sensation of being full, decreases appetite
KELP	Stimulates metabolism, provokes sensation of being full

WEIGHT LOSS

Causes

Spontaneous weight loss, with **no definite reason,** is a worrying symptom which must ***always*** be a reason ***to consult with a doctor.***

Treatment

Once **the reason is known** for weight loss, one or several of these plants, which supply plenty of ***nutrients*** and promote their ***assimilation,*** can be administered.

FENUGREEK	Reconstituent, provokes increase of appetite and natural weight gain

DIABETES

Definition

A disorder on the metabolism of carbohydrates, caused by a **lack of insulin.** This hormone, which is produced in the pancreas, makes the sugar in the blood pass into the cells where it can be metabolized.

Treatment

These medicinal herbs ***complement*** the dietetic treatment of diabetes. Their action may enhance, and in some cases substitute, that of the antidiabetic medicines which are taken orally.

While taking hypoglycemic plants like these, the patient must undergo ***periodic controls*** regarding the level of blood sugar level, as happens with any other antidiabetic treatment.

GARLIC	Normalizes the blood sugar level
WALNUT	Mild hypoglycemic effect
SAGE	Hypoglycemic
BURDOCK	Contains inulin (carbohydrate ideal for diabetic people)
NONI	Balances glucose blood level, antioxidant

MALNUTRITION

Causes

This can be produced by a **minimal intake** of nutrients, a **lack of assimilation,** or an **excessive consumption** of them.

Treatment

Phytotherapy provides plants ***rich in nutrients,*** such as alfalfa or spirulina, and other ones which ***promote their assimilation*** using a general ***invigoration*** of the body and the digestive process, such as nettle or sea buckthorn.

SPIRULINA	Supplies essential nutrients, vitamin B_{12}, iron, and minerals
NETTLE	Reconstituent, invigorating, antianemic
FLAX	Supplies plenty of proteins and fats

GOUT

Definition

This is an ailment which results from an increase of uric acid in the blood, and its deposit on the joints (known as **uric arthritis or arthritis**) as well as in the renal tissues.

Gout only affects males, and its most characteristic symptom is a painful inflammation of the toe joint, though it can also affect other joints.

Phytotherapy

The following medicinal herbs are very effective in ***eliminating uric acid*** through urine, because of their ***uricosuric diuretic*** properties.

WATERCRESS	Blood depurative, diuretic. Recommended for gout
NETTLE	Depurative, diuretic, alkalinizant, promotes elimination of uric acid
DANDELION	Diuretic, depurative, promotes elimination of waste substances
WHITE BIRCH	Diuretic, depurative, eliminates uric acid
JUNIPER	Depurative, eliminates uric acid
MEADOWSWEET	Anti-inflammatory, analgesic, calms joint aches
ASH TREE	Diuretic, depurative, laxative, eliminates excess of uric acid
DEVIL'S CLAW	Anti-inflammatory, antirrheumatic, promotes elimination of uric acid
BURDOCK	Diuretic, depurative, sudorific, eliminates uric acid

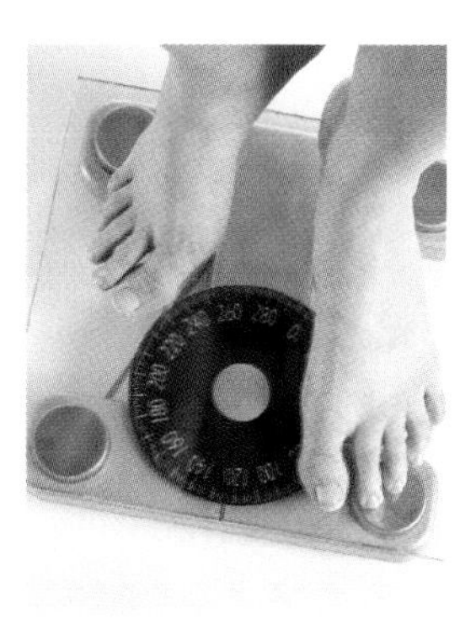

Phytotherapy renders good results for treating obesity, if complemented with an adequate diet regime.

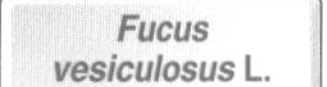

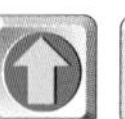
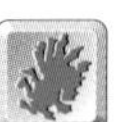
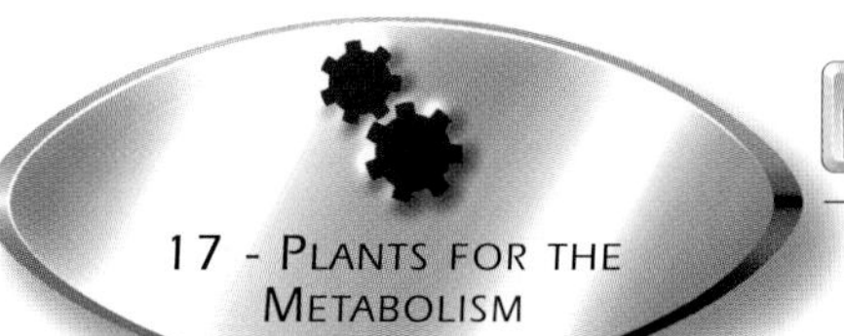

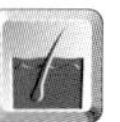
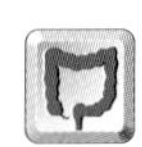
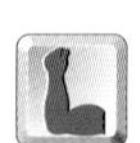
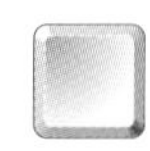

Fucus

Fights obesity and cellulitis

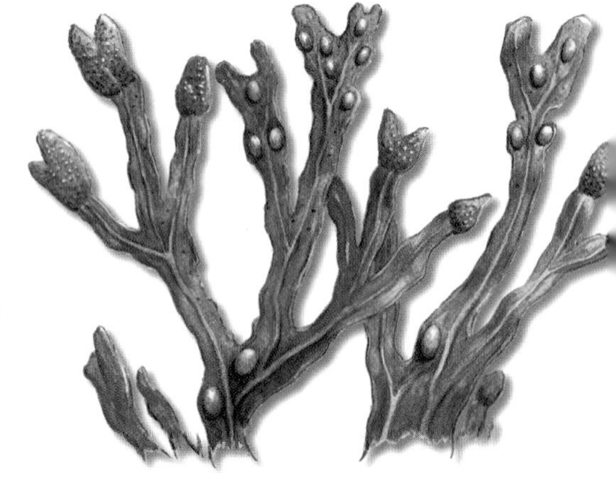

Description. *Algae of the Fucaceae family, brown in color, whose thallus is formed by tape-shaped sheets which stick by their base to underwater rocks. These sheets contain air bladders (aerocysts), which keep the plant upright. The reproductive system of the algae is located in its apex.*

Parts used. *The thallus (the body of the algae).*

ALGAE ARE water plants with chlorophyll or other coloring substances, whose size vary from micro-organisms (unicellular algae) to the size of an earth plant (multicellular algae). In China and Japan, algae have been used as food for many centuries.

Phytotherapists of past centuries, when observing the bladders of fucus, filled with air (floats), thought that, according to the theory of signs, it could be useful against diseases such as mumps and scrofula (an inflammation of neck ganglion, often caused by tuberculosis).

Modern scientific research has proven fucus usefulness in these afflictions, but the main discovery has been some interesting properties which make fucus a highly recommended algae when used against obesity and cellulitis, both ailments common among the inhabitants of the developed world.

PROPERTIES AND INDICATIONS. Fucus, or bladder fucus, when dry, contains 65% sugar, among which the alginic acid is remarkable (12-18%), as well as fucoidin (a mucilaginous polysaccharide). Fucus also contains 15% mineral salts, especially iodine, potassium, and bromine; 5% of proteins, and 1%-2% fat, as well as vitamins A, B, C, and E. Fucus is likely to contain small amounts of vitamin B_{12} since it is frequently polluted by microscopic algae which are the true producers of this vitamin. Therefore, fucus is very promising for people who want to follow a strict vegetarian diet.

Fucus has antiscurvy, nourishing, remineralizing, depurative, and mildly laxative properties, but it mainly acts as a weight loss plant, an anticellulite, and an invigorating of the thyroid. Its basic applications are the following:

• **Absorbent and anorexigen** (calms the sensation of hunger). Alginic acid and its salts (alginates), as well as the other mucilages contained in fucus, can absorb water up to six times their own weight. Because of this property, they increase in volume when in the stomach, and produce a full sensation. Therefore, fucus is a very useful remedy in treating **obesity** caused by **bulimia** (excess of appetite) **[❶,❷,❸]**.

• **Digestive.** Fucus absorbs gastric juices, decreasing **acidity.** It is recommended to treat **gastritis and** esophagic **reflux, hiatal hernia,** and other causes of pyrosis or hyperacidity **[❶,❷,❸]**.

• **Nourishing, remineralizing, and antiscurvy.** Bladder fucus provides mineral salts, vitamins, proteins, and other nourishing sub-

Preparation and Use

INTERNAL USE

❶ **Fresh alga.** It is taken as a vegetable, though its flavor is not enjoyable for everybody.

❷ **Decoction or infusion** of fucus dry extract, with 15-20 g per liter of water. Drink three or four cups daily.

❸ **Powder.** It is taken in the form of capsules. The usual dose is 0.5-2 g, 1-3 times a day.

In the case of **weight loss diets,** fucus must be taken in any of the listed ways, fifteen minutes **before meals.** This way, it exerts a greater anorexigen action (which reduces appetite).

In other cases, fucus can be taken with meals, or after them.

EXTERNAL USE

❹ **Compresses** soaked in the liquid resulting of the decoction, then applied hot on the affected areas, two or three times a day, during 10-15 minutes.

❺ **Poultices** prepared with the fresh alga, previously heated in a bowl with water. Apply hot on the affected skin area during 10-15 minutes, three or four times daily.

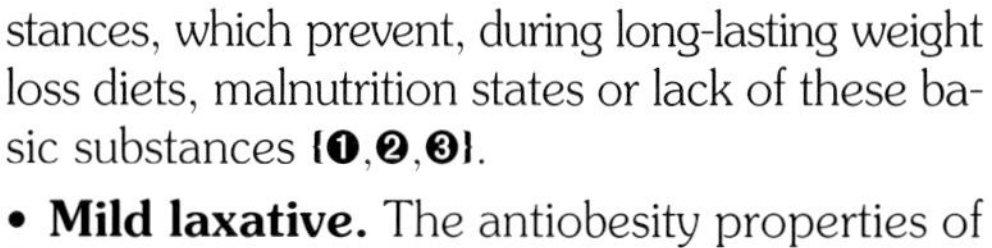

stances, which prevent, during long-lasting weight loss diets, malnutrition states or lack of these basic substances [❶,❷,❸].

- **Mild laxative.** The antiobesity properties of fucus are enhanced by its mild laxative and emollient effect due to its high content of mucilage [❶,❷,❸].

- **Thyroid invigorating.** This alga contains a ***high concentration of iodine*** and organic iodine salts: 150 mg per kilogram of algae (in order to obtain the same amount we would need 3,000 of seawater liters). Iodine is required by thyroid to produce tyrosine, a hormone which promotes the burning of the nourishing substances we eat, thus activating metabolism.

Because of its content in organic iodine, it is used as a ***complementary treatment*** **of hyperthyroidism,** whether associated or not with goiter. In these cases, ***medical advice*** is required. Fucus can be taken orally in any of its preparations [❶,❷,❸], and applied in compresses soaked in its decoction on the throat [❹].

- **Emollient.** ***Externally applied*** on the skin as compresses [❹] or poultices [❺], bladder fucus has soothing and anti-inflammatory properties, promotes the elimination of chlorine salts, and helps reduce the volume of adipose tissues. All these actions make fucus a very useful plant to treat cellulitis, wrinkles, stretch marks, and skin flaccidity [❹,❺].

By decreasing appetite, by its laxative properties, and by accelerating the metabolism, fucus achieves an effective weight-losing action which lacks any side effect.

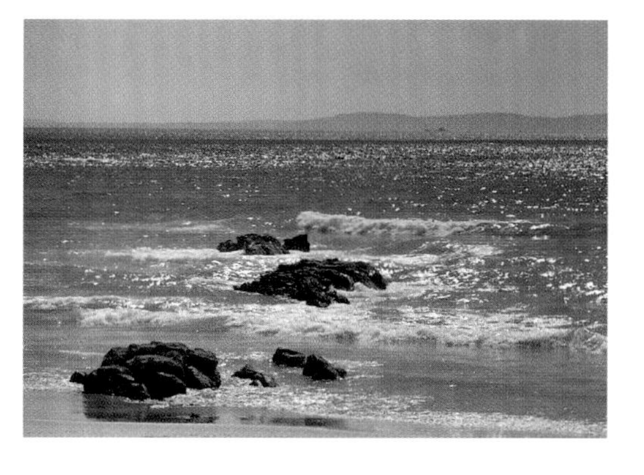

Kelp

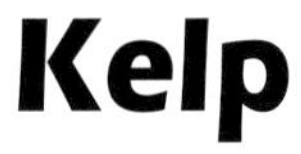

Stops hunger and invigorates

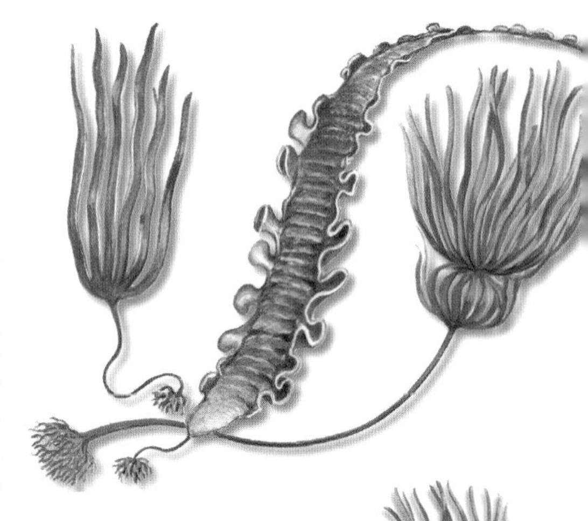

Description. Dun algae of the Laminariaceae family, growing up to 2-3 m large. It sticks to the rocks by means of a kind of root, called rhizoids. Its thallus is divided into tape-shaped (fronds) fragments, which vary in size and shape depending on the species it is.

Parts used. The thallus (the body of the alga).

ALGAE, an important ingredient of traditional Chinese and Japanese cuisine, are more and more commonly used in Western countries. There are several kelp species, all of them with similar properties (for instance, *Laminaria digitata* Lam., and *Laminaria hyperborea* Foslie.). A mixture of them all, pressed and dried, makes ***kombu,*** which is an ingredient in many oriental meals.

PROPERTIES AND INDICATIONS. Kelp contains alginates (vegetal jelly which is obtained from algae), sugars (carbon hydrates), minerals (especially iodine, phosphorus, calcium, and sodium), and vitamins A and B.

Alginates have the capability of increasing their volume up to six times by absorbing water. Thus, when in the stomach they produce sensation of being full, which is useful for calming the appetite in treatments against obesity. It is also used in gynecology to dilate the uterine neck, by putting a piece of algae, previously disinfected, inside of it.

Kelp, like other algae, has **invigorating and stimulant** properties for the metabolism, due to its content in iodine. Therefore, kelp is recommended for people suffering from **obesity** and **hypothyroidism [❶,❷,❸]**.

Alginates are also used in pharmacological and chemical industries as **excipients and thickeners.**

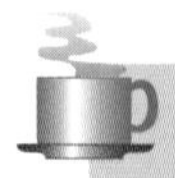

Preparation and Use

INTERNAL USE

❶ As a dressing or ingredient for **salads** and several **cooking recipes.**

❷ **Decoction** with 30 g of algae in 200 ml (a glass) of water, boiling for five minutes, and drinking before every meal. You can take the liquid alone, the algae, or both.

❸ Several **pharmaceutical preparations** are based on algae, whose use and dosage are clearly shown on their information leaflets.

Javan Tea

Reduces both weight and cholesterol

IT WAS INTRODUCED to Europe in the late nineteenth century by Dutch traders. Its pleasant aroma and notable medicinal properties have made it spread all over the world.

PROPERTIES AND INDICATIONS. Though the composition of this plant is still not well-known, it contains a high amount of potassium salts, to which it owes its diuretic properties, and a bitter component which explains its cholagogue properties. Moreover, it contains terpenic derivatives (orthosiphonol), saponins, choline, and an essential oil.

• **Energetic diuretic.** It promotes the elimination of nitrogenic organic waste (especially urea). It is recommended for renal insufficiency, retention of fluids (edema and ascitis), and renal lithiasis **[❶]**. Its ***main application,*** however, is as a **complement in weight-loss diets,** due to its **diuretic, depurative, and anticholesterol properties [❶]**. How it reduces the level of cholesterol in the blood is still unknown.

• **Cholagogue.** It is used for disorders of gall bladder dysfunction, generally caused by atony (laziness) of the gall bladder. Because of its cholagogue properties, it promotes the emptying of bile **[❶]**.

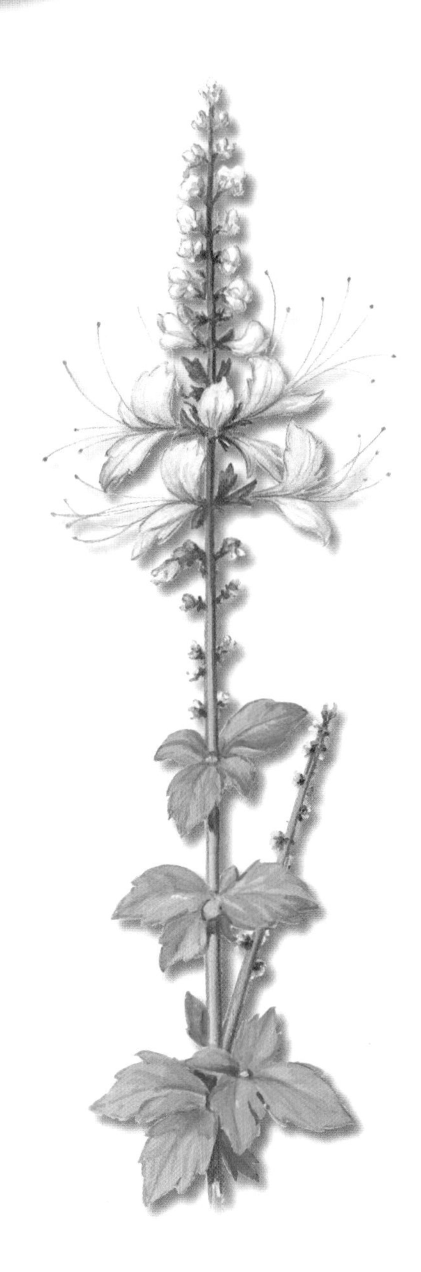

Description. *Vivacious plant of the Labiatae family, growing from 40 to 60 cm high, with a quadrangular stem, and spiked flower clusters, purple, bluish, or white in color.*

Parts used. *The leaves and the flowers.*

Preparation and Use

INTERNAL USE

❶ **Infusion** with 20-30 g of leaves and flowers per liter of water, drinking one cup before each meal.

18

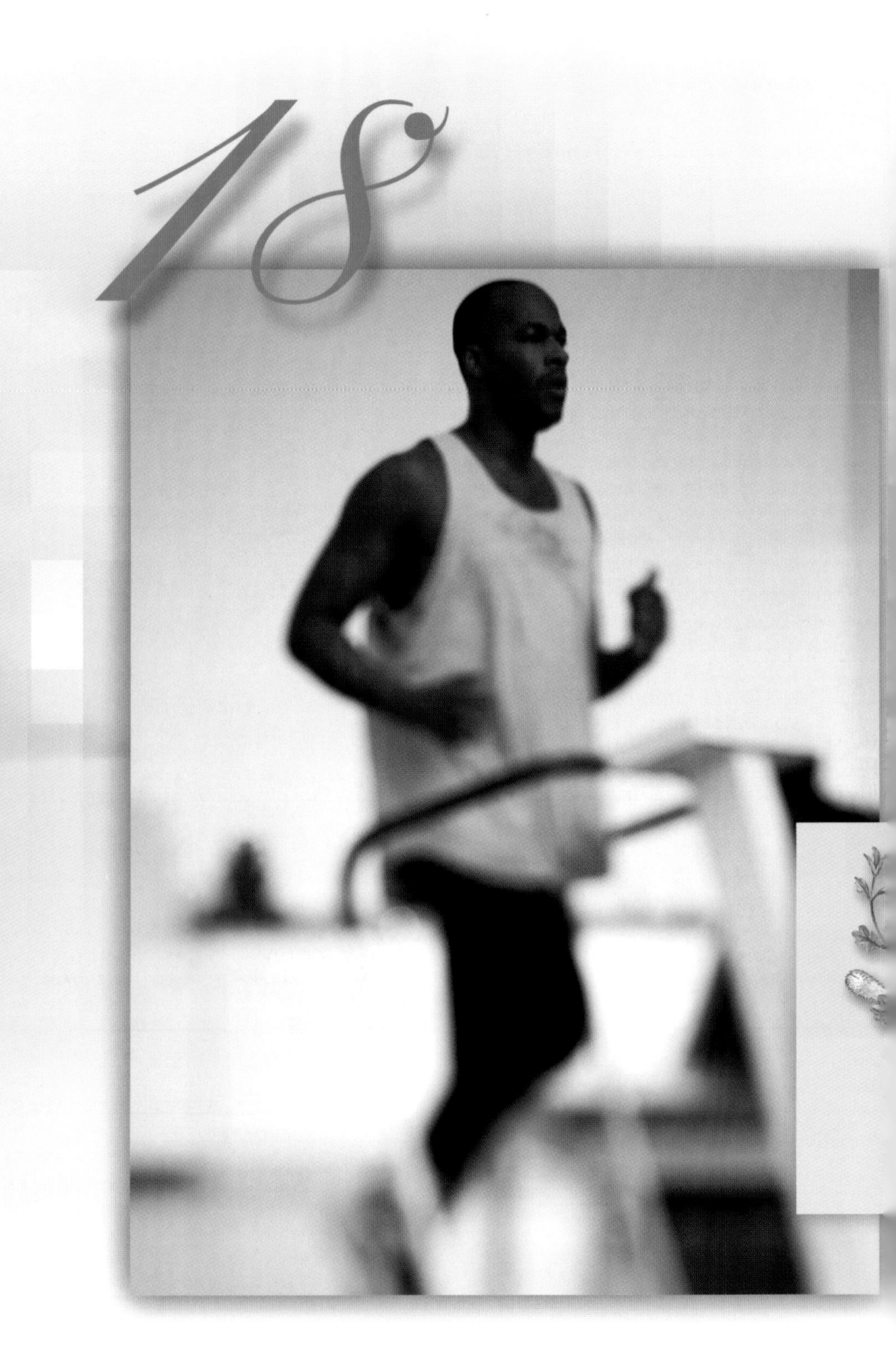

Plants for the Locomotive System

DISEASES	PAGES
Ache, kidney, see Lumbago	319
Ache, rheumatic, see Rheumatic pain	319
Arthritis, uric, see Gouty arthritis	319
Arthrosis	320
Back ache, see Lumbago	319
Bruises, see Contusion	318
Contusion	318
Foot disorders	320
Gouty arthritis	319
Lumbago	319
Osteoporosis	318
Pain, rheumatic	319
Rheumatic pain	319
Rickets	318
Sciatica	320
Sports	320
Sprain	318
Uric arthritis, see Gouty arthritis	319

PLANTS	PAGES
Arnica	321
Black mustard	322
Common Ash tree	326
Devil's claw	328
Kidney vetch	327
Meadow-sweet	324
Rosemary	330
White willow	332

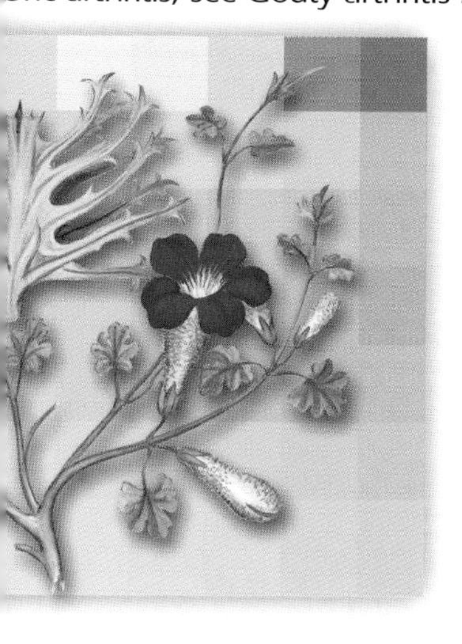

ANTIRRHEUMATIC plants act both ***internally*** and ***externally*** applied by producing a ***slow, but effective and harmless*** **anti-inflammatory and analgesic** action. Unlike anti-inflammatory medicines, which produce ***many side effects,*** the most important of which is **gastritis,** antirrheumatic plants are ***well*** **tolerated when taken orally.**

Revulsive plants also help to alleviate rheumatic aches. When applied on the skin, they produce irritation and reddening, which reduces the congestion and the inflammation of the internal tissues by attracting the blood which flows through them towards the skin.

CONTUSION

Definition

Contusions or bruises are **traumatic injuries** which generally affect the **skin** and **underskin tissues,** caused by a violent crashing with a flat surface. Bruises ***do not have open wounds*** on the skin, though in many traumas, bruises and wounds occur together.

Treatment

Besides ***physical measures,*** with application of cold, phytotherapeutic treatment consists of local application of ***vulnerary*** plants such as those mentioned here, which ***reduce** the **inflammation*** of tissues and ***easc pain.***

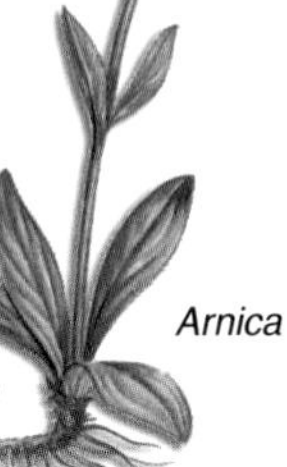
Arnica

LAVENDER	Antirrheumatic, anti-inflammatory
SILVER FIR	Antirrheumatic, reduces the inflammation of bruised tissues
LUNGWORT	Anti-inflammatory
AGAVE	Vulnerary, wound healing
ARNICA	Anti-inflammatory, traditional remedy against hits and bruises
MILFOIL	Vulnerary, heals wounds and bruises
PRICKLY PEAR	Heals wounds, bruises, and skin irritations

SPRAIN

Definition

A violent **twisting or distortion** of a joint, which may even break muscular fibers or ligaments.

Treatment

Besides ***immobilizing*** the affected joint, ***local applications*** of these plants in the form of lotions, massages, compresses, and poultices are highly effective. Any of these external treatments is ***better and more effective*** than an intake of analgesic or anti-inflammatory medicines which produce undesirable side effects.

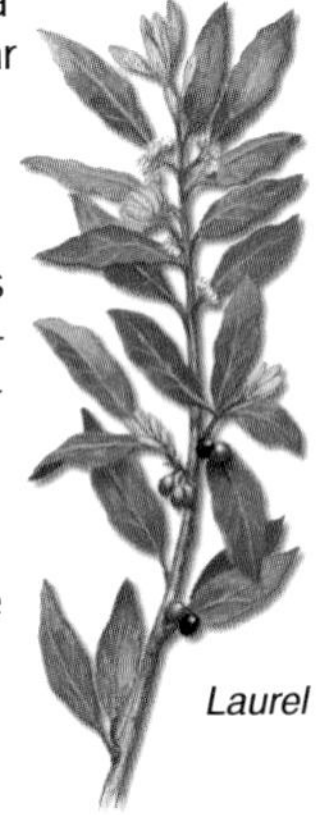
Laurel

LAVENDER	Antirrheumatic, anti-inflammatory
SILVER FIR	Antirrheumatic, reduces the inflammation of tissues affected by the sprain
LAUREL	Anti-inflammatory, alleviates osteo-muscular aches
ARNICA	Anti-inflammatory, traditional remedy against trauma and bruises
ROSEMARY	Vulnerary, antirrheumatic, relaxes muscles
WILD DAISY	Anti-inflammatory, wound healing

RICKETS

Child's ailment which is caused by lack of **vitamin D,** which is responsible for the absorption of calcium.

These plants are a ***complement*** for the treatment, since they improve the nutritional condition and also promote the assimilation of calcium.

HORSETAIL	Supplies silicon, promotes assimilation and fixing of calcium in the bone

OSTEOPOROSIS

Definition

This ailment consists of a loss of the consistency and mass of the bones, which makes them more likely to suffer **breaks and deformations.**

Causes

Osteoporosis is caused by hormonal and metabolic factors, which become more severe with a ***diet*** abundant in **proteins** or salt.

Phytotherapy

Plants rich in ***silicon*** are a ***complement*** to the general treatment.

HORSETAIL	Supplies silicon, stimulates the activity of bone-producing cells

RHEUMATIC PAIN

Definition

This is the pain or ache which afflicts any part of the **musculoskeletal system** (bones, muscles, ligaments, joints, tendons) with a certain degree of **inflammation.** The ailments which usually cause this kind of pain are **arthrosis** (degeneration of articular cartilages), **arthritis,** chronic **articular rheumatism,** and muscular afflictions such as **torticollis** (stiff neck).

Phytotherapy

These plants with ***antirrheumatic and revulsive*** properties ease pain and reduce inflammation, both when ***used internally*** and ***externally.***

Meadowsweet

LAVENDER	Calms rheumatic aches, either articular or muscular
VALERIAN	Analgesic, calms bone and muscle aches
PINE TREE	Revulsive, anti-inflammatory, alleviates rheumatic aches
GERMAN CAMOMILE	Antirrheumatic
PEPPERMINT	Alleviates rheumatic and muscular aches
MARJORAM	Calms rheumatic aches and muscular spasm
LAUREL	Antirrheumatic, alleviates bone and muscle aches
WILD MARJORAM	Antirrheumatic
MEADOWSWEET	Anti-inflammatory, analgesic, alleviates osteo-muscular aches
ROSEMARY	Vulnerary, antirrheumatic, relaxes muscles
NONI	Antirrheumatic, anti-inflammatory, calms aches

LUMBAGO

Definition

This is a ***rheumatic ache*** located in the bones and muscles of the **lumbar area,** that is to say, the lower back area. Sometimes it is called **kidney pain,** however it is not the kidneys which are aching, but the area of the body where they are located.

Treatment

Besides a ***physical and positional treatment,*** these medicinal plants, both ***internally*** and ***externally*** applied, significantly help alleviate lumbalgic pain and inflammation.

VALERIAN	Analgesic, calms bone muscle aches
SILVER FIR	Antirrheumatic, reduces the inflammation on lumbago-affected tissues
PINE TREE	Revulsive, anti-inflammatory, alleviates rheumatic aches
LAUREL	Antirrheumatic, alleviates joint and muscle aches
DEVIL'S CLAW	Anti-inflammatory, antirrheumatic, depurative
ROSEMARY	Vulnerary, antirrheumatic, relaxes muscles

GOUTY ARTHRITIS

Definition

This is the **inflammation of joints** caused by ***uric acid*** deposits.

Phytotherapy

The treatment comprises ***diuretic*** plants with uricosuric action, ***depurative***, and ***antirrheumatic*** plants, both ***internally*** *and* ***externally*** used.

GARLIC	Activates metabolism, promotes elimination of waste substances
NETTLE	Depurative, diuretic, alkalinizant, promotes elimination of uric acid
WHITE BIRCH	Diuretic, depurative, eliminates uric acid
MEADOWSWEET	Anti-inflammatory, analgesic, calms articular aches
DEVIL'S CLAW	Anti-inflammatory, antirrheumatic, promotes elimination of uric acid

SCIATICA

Definition

This is a painful **inflammation** of the **sciatic nerve.** It manifests itself with pain in the lower part of the back, which extends throughout the buttock and the back side of the thigh. It usually affects only one side of the body.

Phytotherapy

Both ***internally*** *and* ***externally applied,*** these plants alleviate **neuralgic** pain.

VALERIAN	Analgesic, calms bone and muscle aches
VERVAIN	Analgesic for rheumatic aches and neuralgia
CAMPHOR TREE	Alleviates rheumatic aches and neuralgia
LAUREL	Antirrheumatic, alleviates bone and muscle aches
BLACK MUSTARD	Revulsive, reduces the congestion of internal tissues
MEADOWSWEET	Analgesic and antirrheumatic osteo-muscular aches and neuralgia

ARTHROSIS

Definition

This is a **chronic ailment** which consists of a degeneration of articular cartilage, and mainly affects the **hips** and the **knees.**

Phytotherapy

Phytotherapeutic treatment not only alleviates pain, but also exerts a ***preventive*** action on articular degeneration. Though its effects are not immediately perceived, it is ***highly effective in the medium and long term.***

LAVENDER	Calms rheumatic aches, whether articular or muscular
FENUGREEK	Alleviates inflammation of joints caused by arthrosis or arthritis
MEADOWSWEET	Anti-inflammatory, analgesic, alleviates osteo-muscular aches
DEVIL'S CLAW	Anti-inflammatory, antirrheumatic, depurative
HORSETAIL	Supplies silicon, regenerates articular cartilage

FOOT, DISORDERS

These medicinal plants, when ***locally*** applied, can alleviate many of the common disorders of feet.

Hygiene and care of the feet is especially important for **diabetes** or **blood flow** disorders in the lower extremities. In these cases, a simple bruise or wound on feet can become a severe infection.

MILFOIL	Wound healer, antiseptic, fights bad odor and excess of perspiration

SPORTS

It is clear that sports are not included here as ailments; however the consequences of forced training can become severe ailments.

The following medicinal herbs can prepare our body for the **physical overload** of sports training, and are also an ***effective help*** for sportsmen.

WALNUT	Nutritive, energetic. Ideal food for sportsmen
GINSENG	Enhances physical performance and resistance to exhaustion

Rosemary alcohol is prepared by mashing a handful of green rosemary leaves, then putting them in a bottle with 100 ml of ethyl alcohol. After steeping for three days, strain the resulting liquid, which is rosemary alcohol.

When this alcohol is applied in frictions it alleviates rheumatic and muscular aches.

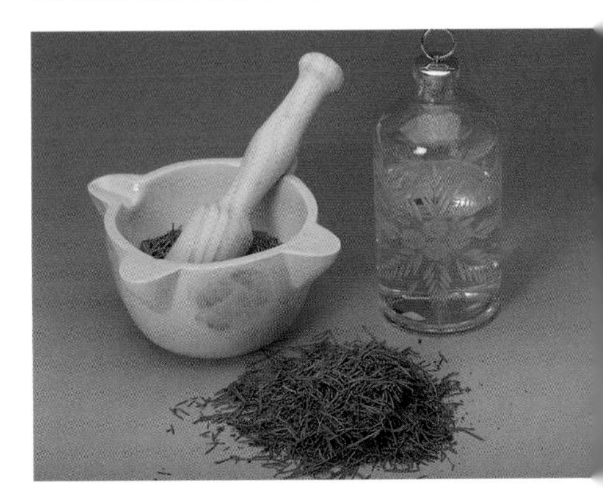

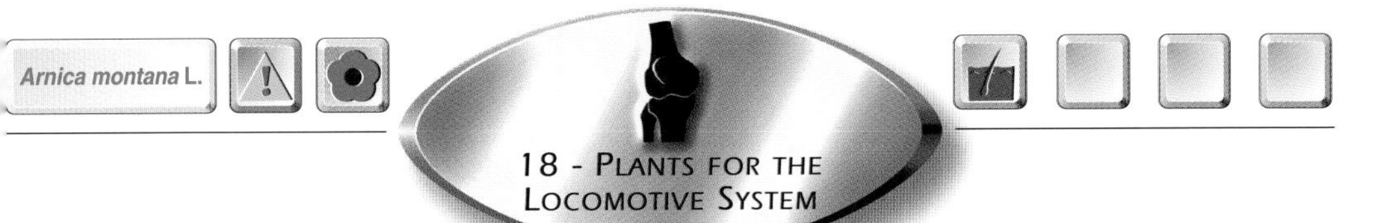

Arnica

Traditional remedy for bruises

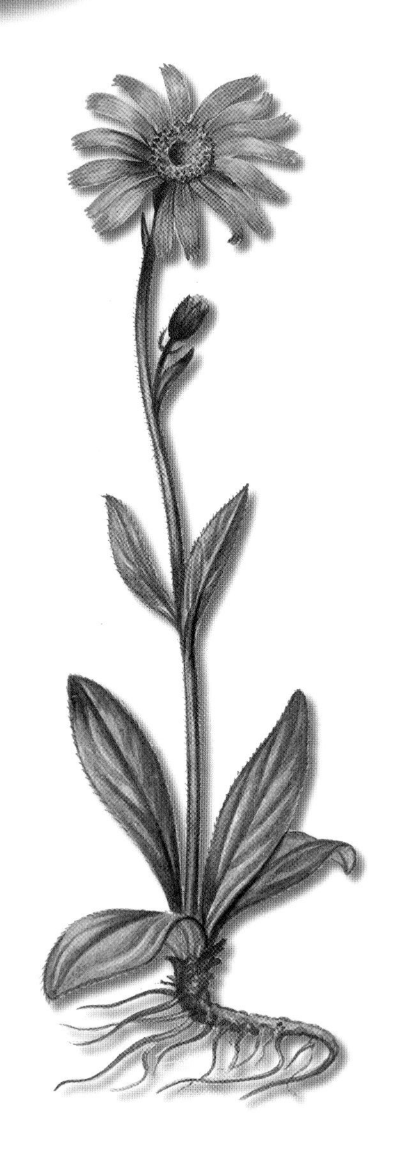

THE OUTSTANDING botanist Font Quer was impressed by "the fact that such a widely used plant as arnica, which has had such an unusual fame among physicians, as well as among common people [...] was not known by the great ancient pharmacists."

PROPERTIES AND INDICATIONS. The plant contains an essential oil, phenolic substances, flavonoids, and tannin. It has notable stimulating properties on the heart and the blood circulation. However, it is highly poisonous to the nervous system, and nowadays its ***internal use*** is no longer recommended. Arnica must be considered a ***poisonous plant.***

Externally applied, as a ***TINCTURE,*** on the skin, it has **excellent vulnerary and anti-inflammatory** properties, being a traditional remedy for bumps, bruises, sprains, and hematomas **[❶]**. It is also used for **furuncles and abscess.**

ARNICA TINCTURE is prepared with 20 g of dry flowers and root, steeping them for 15 days into 100 ml of 90% ethyl alcohol to prepare an alcoholic cold extract. Cold extract can be also prepared with oil.

Description. *Herb of the Compositae family, growing from 30 to 50 cm high, with a composed flower, bright yellow in color, very exuberant. It can be easily mistaken with Inula (*Inula montana *L.), whose medicinal properties have not been exhaustively studied. Unlike these false arnicas, true arnica (*Arnica montana *L.) has only one or two pairs of leaves, which grow in opposite pairs.*

Parts used. *The flower and the root.*

Preparation and Use

EXTERNAL USE

❶ Tincture. Soak a compress with some drops of arnica tincture, ***dissolved*** in water, and then apply on the affected skin area. ***Pure (undissolved) tincture can irritate the skin.***

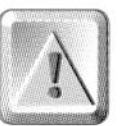
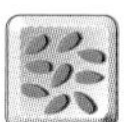
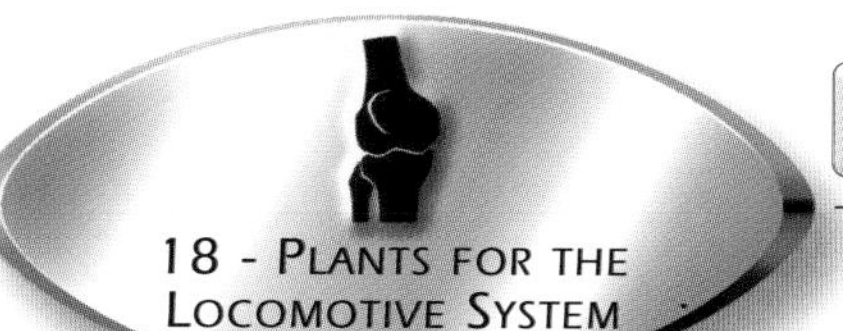

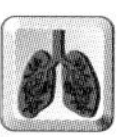
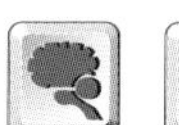
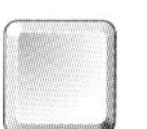

Black Mustard

The rubefacient plant par excellence

THE SMALL SEEDS of mustard, difficult to see just by looking at them, are a good example of the power of small things when we let them develop.

PROPERTIES AND INDICATIONS. The whole plant contains a glycoside (sinigrin), which by means of an enzyme, mironase, becomes a sulphur essential oil with strong revulsive properties. Its seeds also contain mucilage, with emollient (soothing) properties, which partially balance its strong revulsive properties.

Mustard ***FLOUR*** is mainly used in external applications. As a **revulsive** substance, it acts by attracting the blood towards the skin, thus reducing the congestion of internal organs and

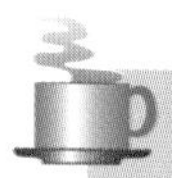

Preparation and Use

EXTERNAL USE

❶ **Poultices.** Mustard flour is applied as hot poultices, mixing it with linseed flour so as to be less irritant. These poultices are applied up to twice per day, for 10-15 minutes (a prolonged application can produce blisters).

Mustard poultices are called **sinapisms** (a word which comes from the Greek *sinapsis*, mustard: see one of its scientific names).

❷ **Foot baths.** Dissolve 1-2 spoonfuls of mustard flour into 2-3 liters of hot water. Take 2-3 baths daily, during 5-10 minutes each.

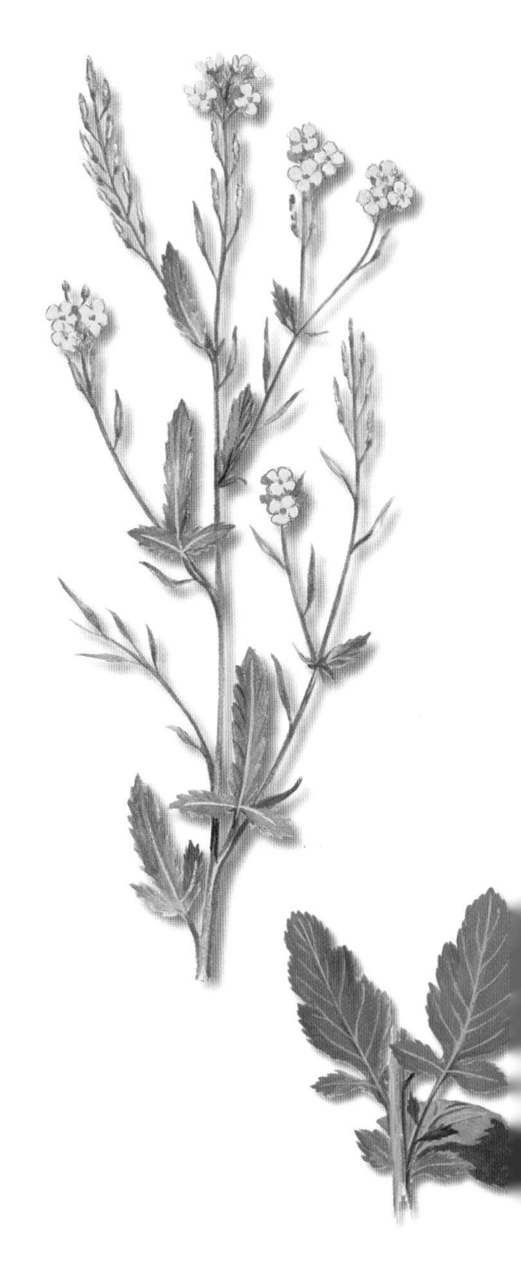

Description. *Annual plant of the Cruciferae family, growing from 0.2 to 1 m high, with yellow flowers gathering in terminal clusters, and round seeds of 1 mm in diameter.*

Parts used. *The seeds.*

Traditional foot baths with mustard flour are still a highly desirable remedy, because of their effectiveness, for headaches, especially when these are caused by colds, influenza, and sinusitis.

Foot baths are also useful for high blood pressure.

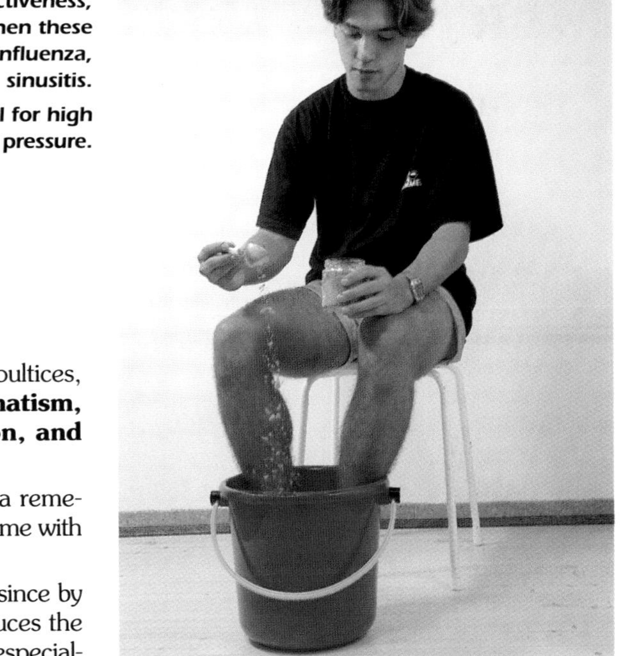

tissues. When applied in the form of poultices, it is ***very effective*** in treating **rheumatism, sciatic, neuralgia, lung congestion, and acute bronchitis [❶]**.

Foot baths with mustard flour are a remedy which has been used for a very long time with two main applications:

- **Headaches.** It alleviates headaches, since by attracting the blood towards feet it reduces the congestion of the head. Foot baths are especially recommended for cephalalgia caused by viral infection of upper respiratory airways (nasal catarrh, sinusitis, influenza) or by high blood pressure [❷].
- **High blood pressure.** Mustard produces a peripheral vasodilatation (a dilatation of the small arteries on the extremities), which makes blood pressure decrease [❷].

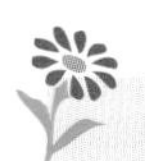

Other Mustard Species

Besides black mustard, there are two other species.

- **White mustard** (*Sinapis alba* L.) which produce bigger seeds, whitish in color, used to produce edible mustard (seasoning).
- **Wild mustard** (*Brassica kaber* Wheeler = *Brassica arvensis* Rabenh. = *Sinapis arvensis* L.), which has very small seeds.

Both mustard species have **similar properties** to those of black mustard, though less intense.

Warning

*Orally taken, mustard is an irritant **seasoning,** which is better to **avoid.** People suffering from **dyspepsia** or gastro-duodenal **ulcer** should **completely abstain** from mustard.*

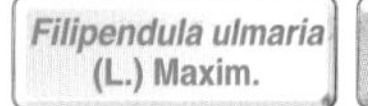
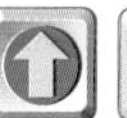
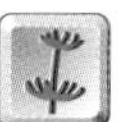
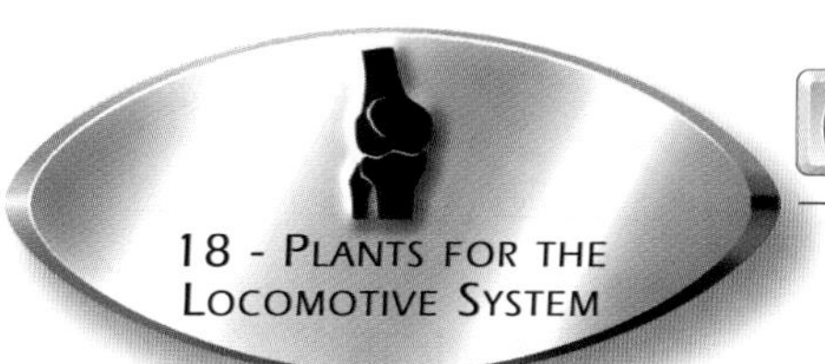
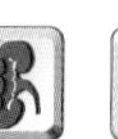
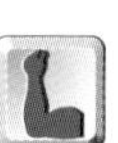
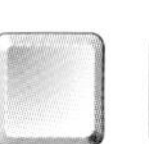
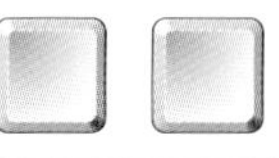

Meadow-Sweet

Antirrheumatic and depurative

THE LEAVES of this plant resemble those of the elm-tree, after which, in some Latin-rooted languages, the herb is named. It has been used from the seventeenth century onwards to treat rheumatic aches. Recently other virtues in this plant have been discovered.

PROPERTIES AND INDICATIONS. Its flowers, and in lesser proportion its leaves, contain a glycoside: monotropine, which by means of hydrolysis on the fresh plant becomes methyl salicylate, and once the herb is dried it turns into free salicylic acid and alkaline salicylates. All those salicylic compounds provide, like acetylsalicylic acid (aspirin), **anti-inflammatory**, **analgesic**, and **febrifuge** actions. The plant contains also flavonoid substances whose action is **diuretic**.

These are its applications:

• **Rheumatic aches**, produced by arthrosis,

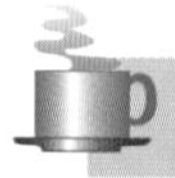

Preparation and Use

INTERNAL USE

❶ **Infusion (tea),** with 30-40 g of flowers per liter of water, drinking up to five cups daily.

EXTERNAL USE

❷ **Compresses** soaked in a more concentrated infusion than that made for internal use (up to 80 g) applied on the aching area, or cellulite-affected area, during 10 minutes, two or three times a day.

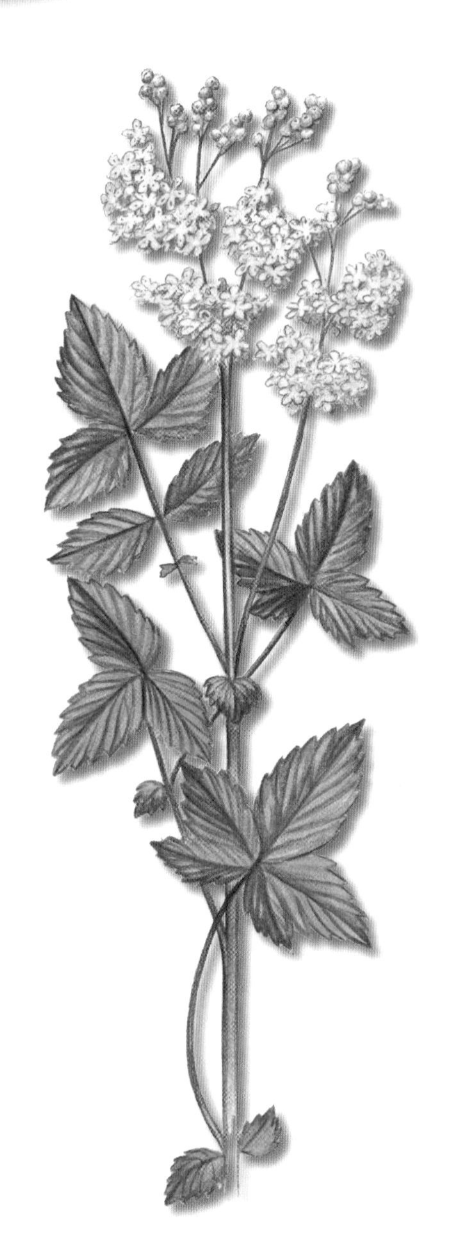

***Description**: Vivacious plant of the Rosaceae family, growing up to 1.5 m. high, with upright stems and silver-colored leaves on their underside, with small, aromatic white-cream colored flowers, gathering in terminal bouquets.*

***Parts used.** The flowers (bouquets).*

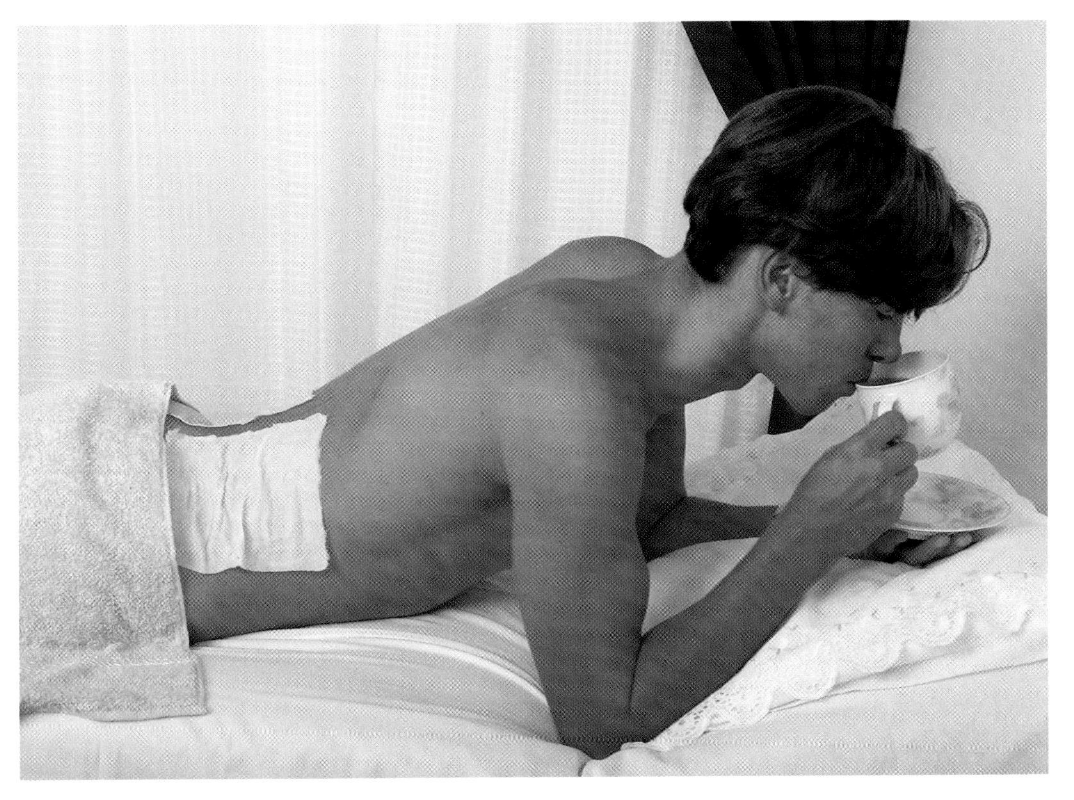

Meadowsweet, because its content includes a precursor of acetylsalicylic acid (aspirin), has anti-inflammatory and analgesic properties. It eases osteo-articular (bone and joint) aches, such as torticollis, lumbago and those widespread and nasty backaches, as well as neuralgic aches.

It should be used in external application of compresses, while drinking its infusion, to achieve better effectiveness.

polyarticular acute rheumatism, or uric arthritis (gout) (❶).

- **Different aches**. The plant also eases osteo-articular aches (lumbago, torticollis, backaches) and neuralgic aches (sciatica, headaches). This painkiller activity of meadowsweet is improved when, besides drinking an infusion (❶) of the plant, it is locally applied in compresses on the affected area (❷).

- **Diuretic**: Strong but not irritant, it is quite useful for **cellulite**, **edema** (retention of fluids) caused by heart failure, which usually appears in ankles and feet, and to diminish **ascitis** (retention of liquids in abdomen) of persons with liver disorders (❶).

- **Depurative**: Meadowsweet is a great eliminator of uric acid, as well as uric salts and other toxins, since it increases the excretion of these substances through kidneys (uricosuric action). The plant filters these gout-producing substances, which can also produce arthritis and many rheumatic aches, from the blood (❶). Thus, and also because of its anti-inflammatory and analgesic action, it is ***an ideal plant for people suffering from gout***.

- **Kidney stone solvent**: The plant is good for those people suffering from kidney stone and gravel, especially those formed by uric salts, since it promotes dissolution and elimination of these salts (❶).

- **General invigorating**: The plant increases appetite, has tonic heart effects and provokes a general sensation of well-being. Its use is recommended to treat cold and influenza, as well as for people recovering from dehabilitation diseases (❶).

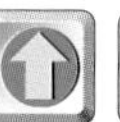
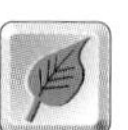
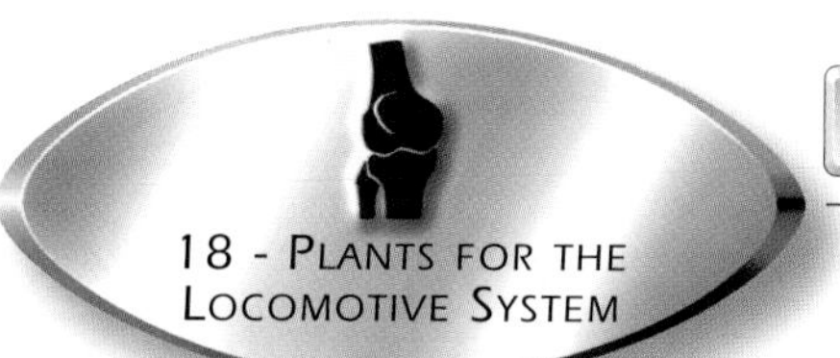

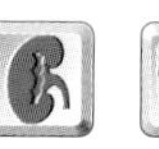
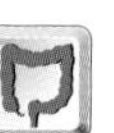
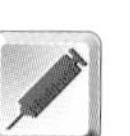
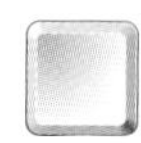

Common Ash Tree

A good remedy against arthritis

PROPERTIES AND INDICATIONS. Ash tree ***LEAVES*** contain flavonic glycosides (quercetin), coumarin, malic acid, copper, iron, and tannin. They have **diuretic, depurative, and laxative** properties, and are recommended for arthritis (rheumatism caused by an excess of uric acid), gout, and kidney stones (leaves promote the elimination of urate and oxalate crystals which form calculi), as well as to fight constipation [❶].

The ***BARK*** of the ash tree contains glycosides (fraxin), as well as diverse sugars and resins. It has **febrifuge and astringent** properties, and was used in former times as a substitute substance for quinine. It also has **appetizer and digestive** properties [❷].

The so-called ***MANA TEARS,*** or simply mana, are obtained from the solidified sap of two ash tree species growing in southern Italy and Sicily: *Fraxinus ornus* L., and *Fraxinus rotundifolia* Miller. Mana is a ***very effective and reliable*** **laxative** substance, with a pleasant flavor which makes it highly recommended for children.

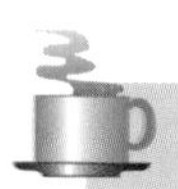

Preparation and Use

INTERNAL USE

❶ **Decoction or infusion of leaves,** with 30 g per liter of water. In order to enhance its effects, some lemon juice can be added to it. Drink three cups daily.

❷ **Bark decoction,** with 40 g per liter of water. Drink two or three cups a day.

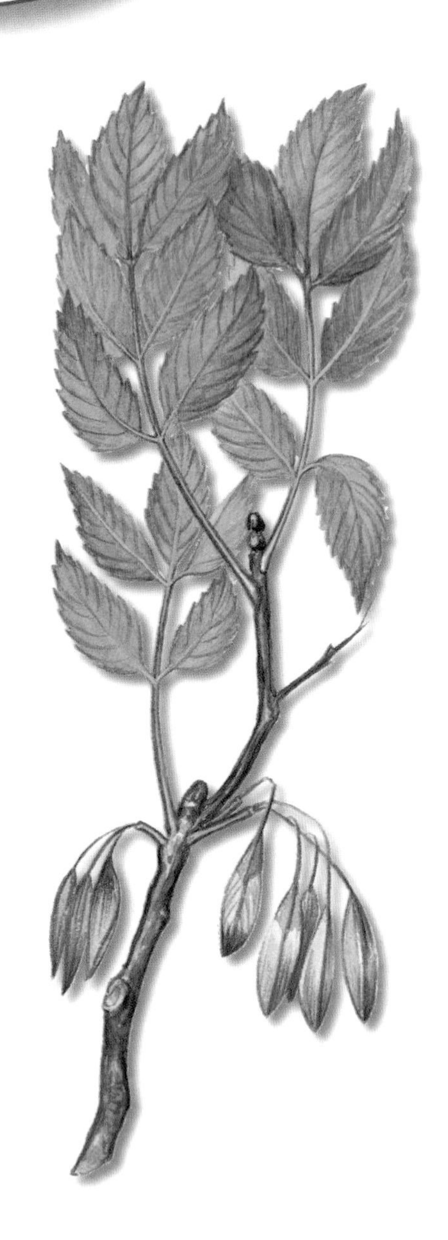

Description. *Deciduous tree of the Oleaceae family (the same family the olive tree belongs to), growing up to 20 m high, or even more. It has a smooth trunk, compound leaves, with an odd number of folioles (usually 9 or 11),and dry, winged fruit hanging in clusters.*

Parts used. *The leaves and the bark.*

Kidney Vetch

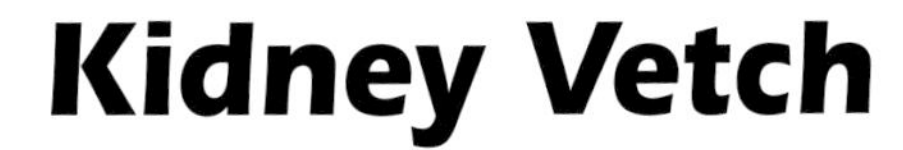

Heals wounds

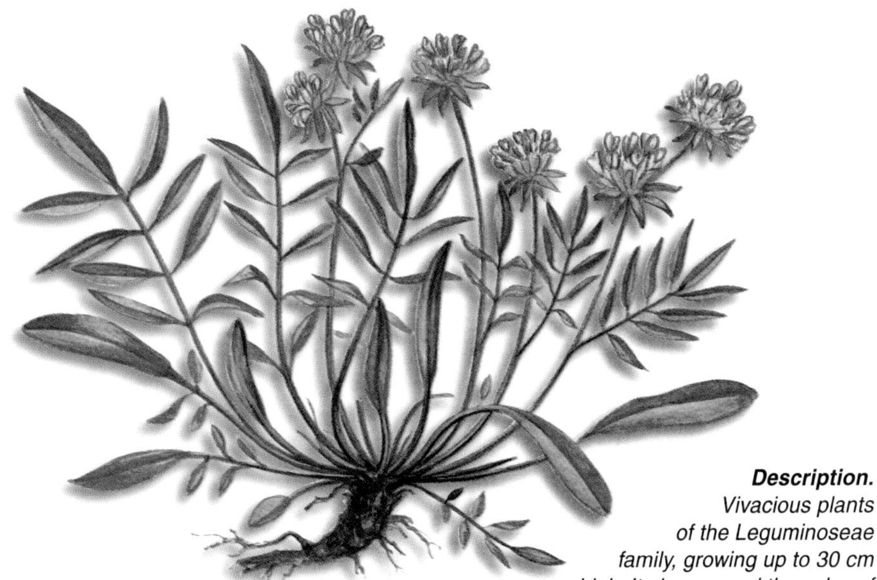

Description. *Vivacious plants of the Leguminoseae family, growing up to 30 cm high. Its leaves and the calyx of its flower heads are covered by a layer of fine hairs. The flowers are yellow, and gather in flower heads which grow at the tip of an upright stem.*

Parts used. *The whole plant.*

PHYTOTHERAPY regards as vulnerary all plants which have the capacity to heal and cicatrize wounds. The term vulnerary comes from the Latin word *vulnum* (wound). This plant has been regarded as the ***vulnerary plant par excellence*** from the Renaissance onwards, due to its notable healing properties.

Properties and indications. The whole plant contains saponins, tannin, and flavonoids. It is used as an infusion to wash **wounds,** either clean or infected, as well as **difficult healing sores and ulcerations, excoriations, and bruised areas.** It promotes the formation of a scar, and a quick epithelization (skin covering) of the injured areas [❷].

In Switzerland and other central European countries, it is taken in the form of infusion as blood **depurative,** and is part of the so-called "spring herbal teas" [❶].

Preparation and Use

Internal use

❶ **Infusion** with 10-20 g of plant per liter of water. Drink two or three cups daily.

External use

❷ **Cleansing** of the wounds with a decoction of 20-30 g of plant per liter of water, boiling for at least three minutes. Apply three or four washings daily.

Devil's Claw

Powerful antirrheumatic

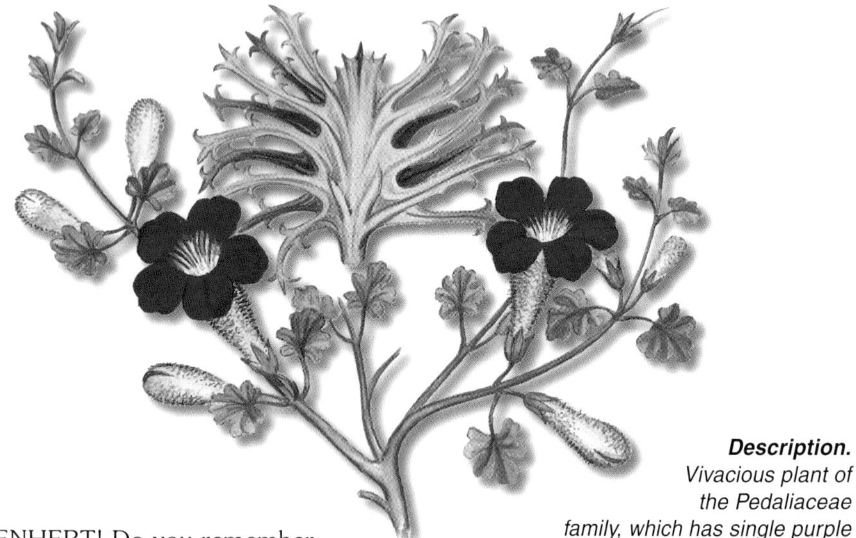

Description. *Vivacious plant of the Pedaliaceae family, which has single purple flowers similar to those of foxglove. The fruit grow at soil level, and are woody, with hooks. The primary root is a long tuber of which secondary roots, similar to peanuts, grow. These have a very sour flavor, and are the medicinal part of the plant.*

Parts used. *The secondary roots.*

"MR. MENHERT! Do you remember that severely wounded soldier who the German physicians said they could not cure?" the native asked his master.

"Of course I remember him. Poor boy, he has died for sure!"

"But no, Mr. Menhert! He was healed with a plant the medicine men applied to him!"

"Oh, yes? I have to know which plant that is!"

The location was South Africa, near the Kalahari Desert, north of the River Orange. It was 1904, and the Hottentot uprising against German colonization had just broken out. Menhert was a German settler who worked hard on his farm, and kept good relations with natives.

"I will ask the medicine men to show me that plant which is able to heal such severe wounds," Menhert thought. "I am sure it is unknown in Europe."

However, the Hottentot medicine men did not reveal to him their secret. Therefore, the settler managed to train a dog to follow the medicine men and locate the plant. Once Menhert gathered a certain amount of the plant's roots, which was later identified as *Harpagophytum procumbens*, he sent the roots to Germany for further analysis.

Since then, the prestige of this plant has been increasing. At present it is ***one of the most effective remedies*** phytotherapy has in order to treat **rheumatic afflictions.**

PROPERTIES AND INDICATIONS. Since the early twentieth century, the root of the devil's claw has been deeply analyzed in depth, mainly in German laboratories, being the object of much research. More than 40 active substances have been discovered in this root, among which the

Preparation and Use

INTERNAL USE

❶ **Infusion.** The usual dose is 15 g (a spoonful) of **root powder** per half a liter of water. Steep for half an hour to one hour. Drink three or four cups per day.

❷ **Capsules.** Due to its sour flavor, it is also available as capsules containing root powder. Three or four should be swallowed daily.

We recommend that you take infusions of pharmaceutical preparations of devil's claw before meals.

EXTERNAL USE

❸ **Compresses or fomentations** soaked in the infusion described for internal use, though it is better to prepare it more concentrated. Apply directly on the affected skin area, several times.

Antirrheumatic properties of devil's claw are produced both when it is taken orally [❶,❷] and when it is applied externally [❶,❷]. Best effects are achieved when simultaneaously combining internal and external applications of devil's claw [❸].

• **Depurative.** This plant promotes the elimination through urine of acid metabolic waste, like uric acid, which is the causative agent of **gout** and of many cases of **arthritis** (inflammation of the joints) [❶,❷].

• **Antispasmodic.** It has a relaxing effect on spasms or intestinal colic, irritable bowel, and biliary and renal colic [❶,❷].

• **Hypolipemic.** Devil's claw reduces the level of **cholesterol** in the blood, and regenerates the elastic fibers which make arterial walls, being thus essential for **arteriosclerosis** [❶,❷].

• **Cicatrizant.** When ***externally*** applied, this plant is an excellent cicatrizant (heals wounds) for all kind of wounds and skin sores [❸].

most outstanding are monoterpenic glycosides of the iridoid group (glycoiridoid), harpagine, harpagide, and procumbide. The plant owes to these substances its **analgesic, anti-inflammatory, and antispasmodic** properties. Devil's claw also has **wound healing** properties, and decreases the level of **cholesterol and uric acid** in the blood. Its indications are the following:

• **Anti-inflammatory and antirrheumatic.** Devil's claw is especially recommended for rheumatic aches caused by arthrosis. Very good results are obtained for cervical, lumbar, hip, and knee arthrosis. This has been confirmed by clinic research. After two or three months of treatment, articular motility improves significatively, and pain disappears. The plant has proven useful for all kinds of articular rheumatism [❶,❷].

Unlike many anti-inflammatory medicines, devil's claw root does not produce ***irritant effects*** on the ***digestive system.*** It completely lacks any side effect when taken in therapeutic doses.

Devil's claw is a successfully proven anti-inflammatory and antirrheumatic plant which, when taken in therapeutical doses, is completely free of undesirable side effects. Therefore, it is being used more and more all the time.

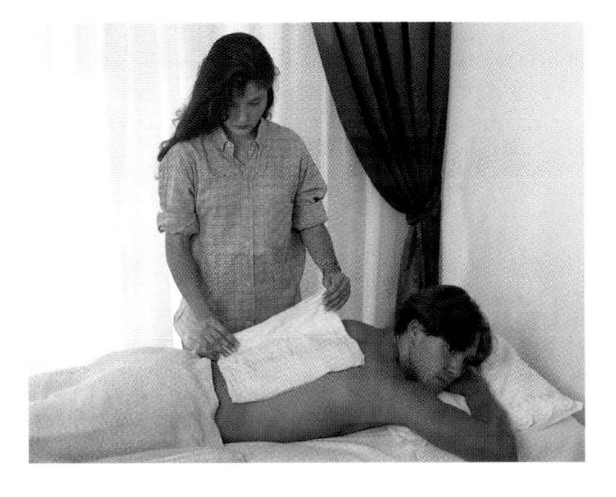

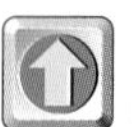

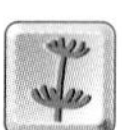

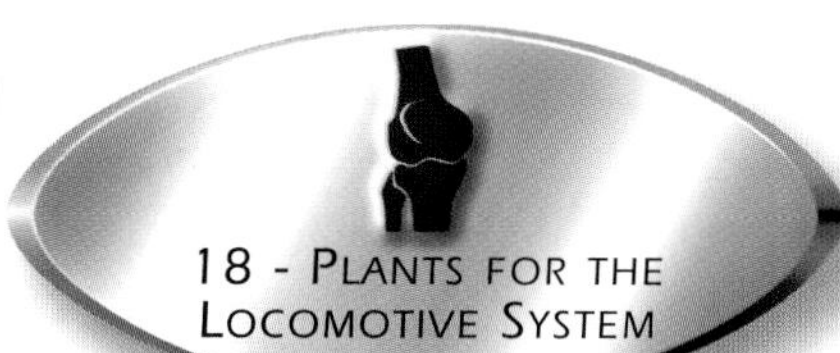

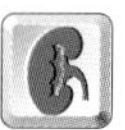

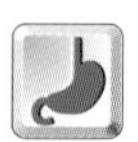

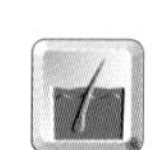

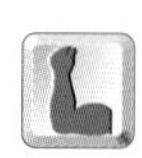

Rosemary

Revitalizes, invigorates, rejuvenates... and reduces inflammation

ROSEMARY is one of the most widely spread aromatic herbs, but it is fully effective. It is not easy to go to the countryside in Mediterranean countries without finding this noble shrub. In winter, it gives us its evergreen leaves, and in spring and summer, its cool fragrance.

Rosemary has been known for many centuries. Egyptian Pharaohs reportedly ordered a rosemary bouquet put on their tombs to perfume their trip to the world of death. In the fourteenth century, Queen Elizabeth of Hungary, who suffered from rheumatism, was cured by this plant, and even recovered her youth to the point that, at age 72, she was proposed to by the king of Poland. Since then, the "water of the Hungarian Queen" has been a reference point and one of the names of rosemary. Another famous woman who also suffered from rheumatism, Madame de Sevigné, even wrote that she was madly in love with rosemary, which to her became "alleviation for all sorrow."

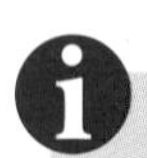

Rosemary Alcohol

To prepare rosemary alcohol, mash a handful of green rosemary leaves in a bowl. Once mashed, put them into a hermetic bottle with 100-150 ml of ethyl alcohol, steep for three days and strain.

Apply it in the form of massage on the aching area, with the help of a cotton cloth.

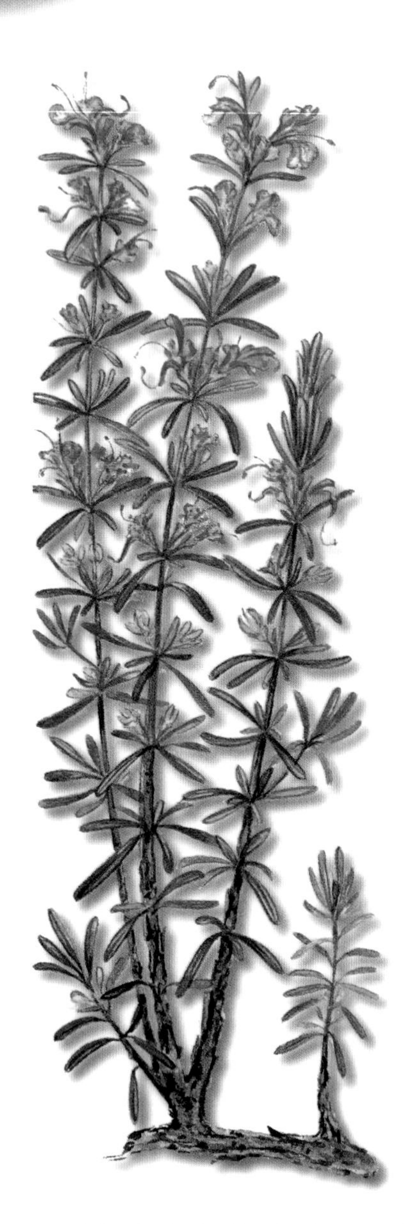

***Description.** Woody shrub of the Labiatae family, growing up to one meter high, with narrow, elongated leaves, dark green on their uppersides, and covered with a layer of silver fine hairs on their undersides. Its flowers are small, blue or light violet in color. The whole plant has a pleasant camphor aroma.*

***Parts used.** The leaves and the flower clusters.*

Preparation and Use

INTERNAL USE

❶ **Infusion or decoction** with 20-40 g of leaves or flower clusters per liter of water. Drink up to two or three cups daily.

❷ **Essence.** The recommended dose is 3-4 drops, three times a day.

EXTERNAL USE

❸ **Baths and cleansing** with a concentrated infusion or decoction made with 80-100 g per liter of water. Steep for 20 minutes and strain. This decoction can be applied directly on the inflamed area, or poured in the water of the bathtub to take an invigorating bath.

❹ **Gargles** with the aforementioned concentrated infusion.

❺ **Massage with rosemary alcohol.** See the method to prepare it in the box on this page.

❻ **Frictions with rosemary essence,** dissolved into alcohol or oil, in a proportion of 2-5 ml per 100 ml.

❼ **Fomentations and hot compresses** soaked into the concentrated infusion or into hot water, to which 15-20 drops of essence per each liter have been added.

PROPERTIES AND INDICATIONS. Rosemary contains an essence with terpenic derivatives, to which the plant owes most of its medicinal properties; phenolic acids with diuretic properties, and flavonoids with antispasmodic action.

Its properties are as follows:

• **Invigorating,** which is ***its most important effect.*** Convalescent people and those suffering from exhaustion, depression, and aged people will find rosemary infusions a stupendous invigorating which will bring them back their lost vitality, as they did to the Queen of Hungary **[❶,❷]**.

Baths with an infusion or decoction **[❸]**, and massage with alcohol **[❺]** or essence **[❻]** of rosemary, have a significant **stimulant** effect for low blood pressure or physical exhaustion.

• **Diuretic and antispasmodic.** It is recommended renal colic, when the expulsion of calculi is required **[❶,❷]**.

• **Digestive.** Its cholagogue properties (stimulant of the bile secretion), as well as its hepatic protective and regenerative, and carminative (eliminates intestinal gas) properties, make rosemary effective at easing digestion, when ingested after meals **[❶,❷]**.

However, perhaps its ***external applications*** are the most widely known of all, due to their ***great effectiveness.***

• **Vulnerary and antirrheumatic.** Rosemary has strong **anti-inflammatory** properties, which make it an ideal plant to perform massages on **sprains, edema, muscular, and rheumatic aches.** It is applied as massages **[❺,❻]** (with rosemary alcohol or essence), fomentations, or hot compresses **[❼]**. The latter are very effective to **relax** the muscles of the **back** and to ease pains on the cervical, back, or lumbar areas.

• **Healing and antiseptic.** Rosemary stimulates **wound,** skin **ulcerations,** and **eczema** healing **[❸]**. When applied as gargles **[❹]** it also heals mouth **aphthas** (mouth sores).

Rosemary is one of the most desirable plants in Mediterranean countries. And the plant deserves this reputation, since it has many medicinal properties. Baths with an infusion or decoction of rosemary are recommended because of their stimulant properties.

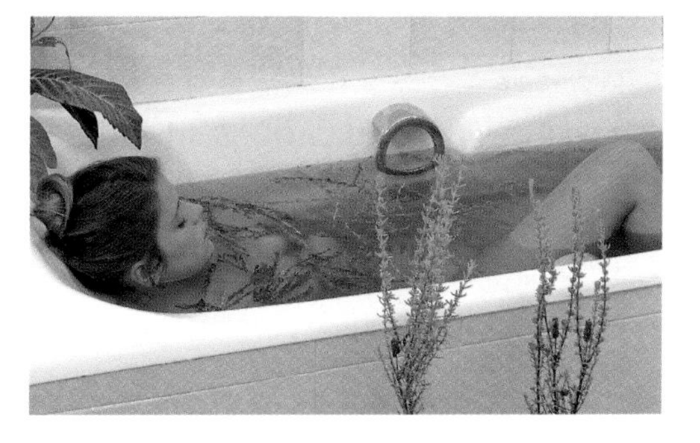

White Willow

Successfully fights pain and fever

WILLOW WAS one of the most widely used plant remedies in Assur and Babylon. From the time of Dioscorides, in the first century A.D., the supporters of the theory of signs have believed that, since willow is able to endure the "bad air" of the moist, marshy soils where it grows, it was likely to contain any effective substance to heal malaria (from the Italian: *mala aria*, which means "bad air"), as well as rheumatic aches, which are frequently suffered by the inhabitants of such places. Indeed, willow was successfully used as a febrifuge against malaria and other fevers, to the point that it was called "European quinine."

By the mid-nineteenth century, Felix Hoffmann, a chemist for the German Bayer laboratory, experimented with willow bark extracts. After several chemical processes, he obtained a derivative substance whose analgesic and antithermic properties were much more powerful than those of the original substance (willow bark).

Hoffmann gave this substance—acetylsalicylic acid—to his own father, who suffered from continuous rheumatic attacks. The success was so great that Bayer laboratories decided to sell the derivative from willow bark with the name ***aspirin.*** That humble substance, aspirin, is still the most commonly used medicine in the history of mankind. At present, some 40,000 tons of aspirin are consumed world-wide each year.

PROPERTIES AND INDICATIONS. The ***BARK,*** and in lesser amounts the leaves and flowers of the willow tree, contain tannin which give them astringent and invigorating properties, as well as mineral salts and coloring substances. However, their most important active component is a glycoside: salicin, which the flowers also have. By means of an enzyme called glycosidase, the

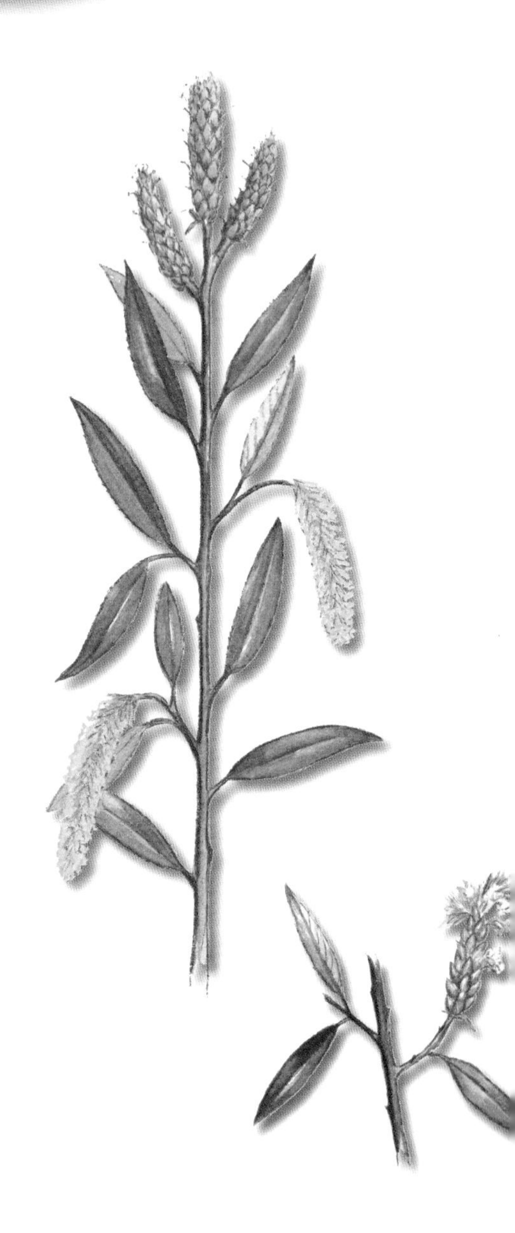

Description. *Tree or shrub of the Salicaceae family, growing from 4 to 20 m high, with a slim trunk, greyish bark and flexible branches. It has toothed, lanceolated, narrow leaves.*

Parts used. *The bark, the leaves, and the flowers.*

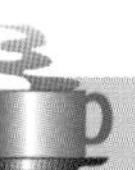

Preparation and Use

INTERNAL USE

❶ **Decoction** with 30 g of **bark** and/or leaves per liter of water, boiling for 15-20 minutes. Steep for another 15-20 minutes. Drink three or four cups daily, sweetened with honey if desired.

❷ **Powder.** It can be obtained by grinding the **bark** with an electric mill. Administer after dissolving it in water with honey, before each meal. The recommended dose is 3-5 g (a teaspoonful) per intake.

❸ **Infusion** with a spoonful of dry **flowers** per cup of water. Drink from two to four cups daily, especially before going to bed. This infusion has strong sedative properties.

EXTERNAL USE

❹ **Compresses** soaked in a decoction more concentrated than that used internally 70-100 g per liter of water.

❺ Skin **washings** with the aforementioned decoction.

❻ **Vaginal irrigations** with the liquid of the aforementioned decoction, once well strained.

salicin can turn into glucose and salygenine. The latter substance, by undergoing an oxidization process, becomes first salicylic aldehyde, and then salicylic acid. From salicylic acid, ***acetylsalicylic acid*** or aspirin is easily obtained.

Because of its salicin content, the willow tree has febrifuge, analgesic, anti-inflammatory, antirrheumatic, and mildly antispasmodic and sedative properties, which makes the tree useful in the following cases:

• **Diverse aches.** Due to its antispasmodic and sedative properties, it is ***highly effective*** in alleviating any kind of aches, especially those of **rheumatic** origin, as well as genital pain in women, caused by **dysmenorrhea** (painful menstruation) or **uterine spasms [❶,❷]**.

• **Fever.** As a febrifuge, it can be used in all kind of febrile afflictions **[❶,❷]**. It has the advantage of **invigorating the digestive system** (increases appetite, fights pyrosis and gastric hyperacidity, and stops diarrhea), because of its bark content of tannin.

• **Nervous excitation.** Due to its sedative properties, especially those of the ***FLOWERS,*** it is used for **nervousness, anxiety, and insomnia [❸]**. It has been used as an antiaphrodisiac for many centuries, following the thought that, if it decreases fever, it will also decrease an excessive love appetite.

• **Reduces the infection** of the skin and the mucosa. ***Externally applied,*** the willow tree is used to wash **wounds and sores** of the skin **[❹,❺]**, and as vaginal irrigations it can be used to treat **leukorrhea [❻]**.

Contrary to what one might think, discovery of acetylsalicylic acid has not ended the use of the willow tree. Though the synthetic derivative has a quicker and more powerful febrifuge and analgesic effect than the natural product, the willow tree has the advantage that it is ***not as irritant on the stomach*** as is aspirin, which easily causes acute gastritis, hemorrhages, and gastro-duodenal ulcers. The willow tree, on the other hand, **invigorates the digestive system.** In addition to the analgesic properties the willow tree has a mild sedative effect.

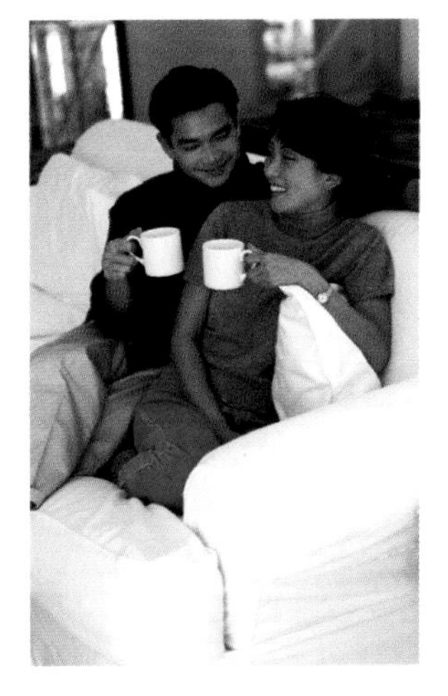

A decoction of willow tree bark is an excellent antirrheumatic substance, because of its content in salicin, a chemical precursor of aspirin.

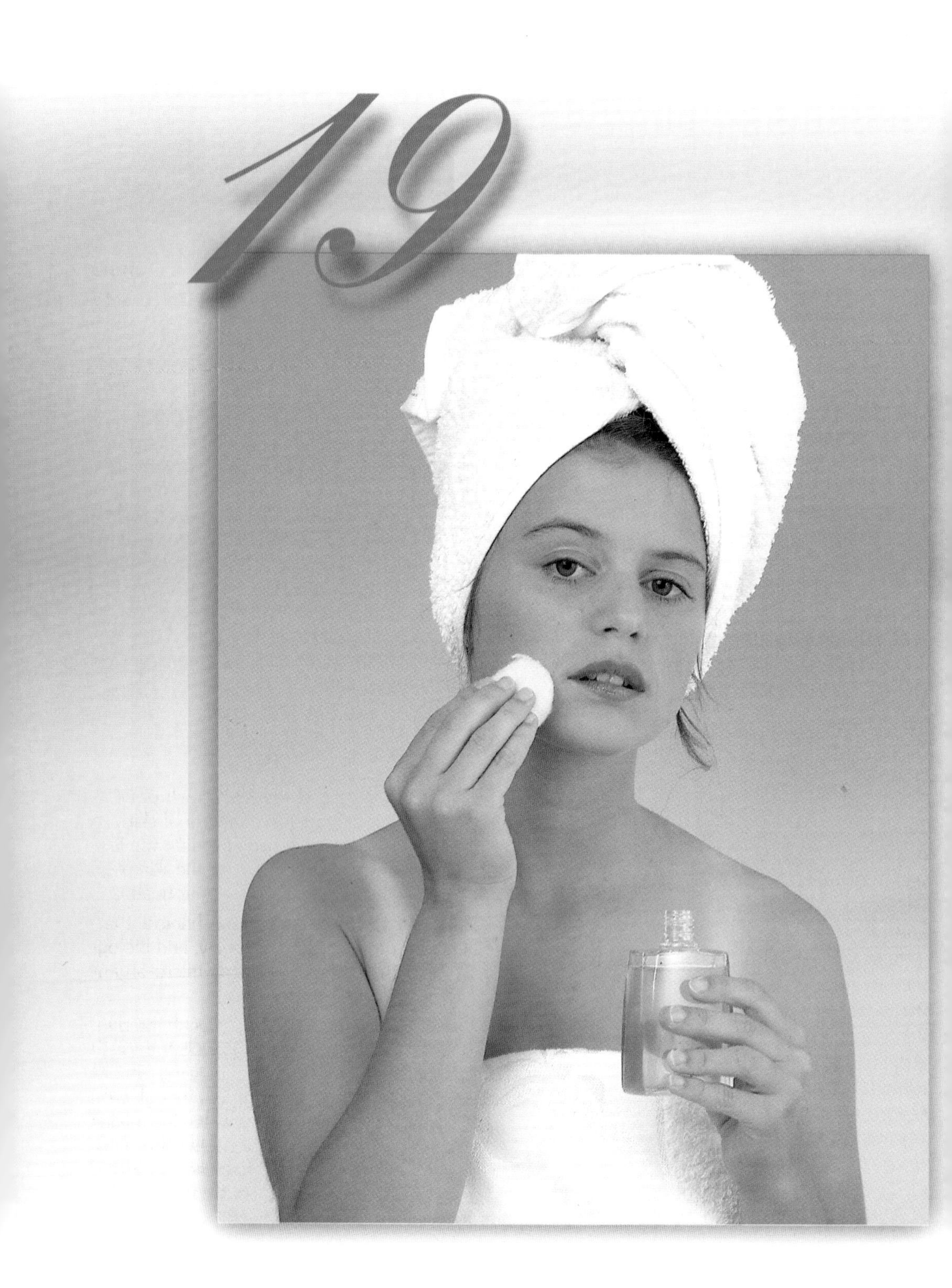
19

Plants for the Skin

DISEASES	PAGES
Abscesses	341
Acne	339
Beauty, skin	340
Callus	336
Cellulitis	339
Corns, see Callus	336
Cracks, skin	336
Dry skin	339
Eczema	338
Fungi, skin, see Skin mycosis	338
Furuncles and abscesses	341
Hair loss	340
Herpes	341
Irritation, skin	339
Loss of hair	340
Mycosis, skin	338
Nails, fragile	341
Perspiration, excessive	337
Psoriasis	340
Ringworm	341
Roughness, see Callus	336
Scabies	341
Skin beauty	340
Skin cracks	336
Skin dryness	339
Skin fungi, see Skin mycosis	338
Skin irritation	339
Skin mycosis	338
Skin sores	337
Skin stretch marks	338
Stretch marks, skin	338
Warts	336
Wounds and sores	337

PLANTS	PAGES
Aloe	344
Annatto tree	347
Burdock	346
Comfrey	354
Ground cherry	353
Horsetail	348
Prickly pear	352
Milfoil	342
St. Johnswort	350

THE BODY of an adult is wrapped in around two square meters of skin, to which we only pay attention for reasons of beauty. However, the skin plays many important roles in keeping our health.

- **Functions of protection:** mechanical, thermal (against temperature changes), and biological (it defends us from the many micro-organisms surrounding us).
- **Functions of elimination:** through the skin, water is continuously eliminated, whether through perspiration (unconscious) or by sweating. **Sweat** has a composition similar to urine, though with a lesser concentration: besides water, it contains sodium chlorine, urea, and many other substances. The skin has been defined as our ***"third kidney"*** because of its capacity to eliminate toxins and metabolic wastes.

• **Sensorial functions.** The skin has many nerve terminals, to the point of being called ***"the external brain."*** The condition of our nervous system is directly reflected in our skin health.

The skin's health and beauty strongly depend on the ***inner*** condition of our body. Applications of medicinal herbs, or any other direct treatment on the skin will not achieve great results if **the blood is "dirty"** (full of metabolic waste), if there are **nervous imbalances,** or if the **diet** is rich in proteins and fats of animal origin.

Therefore, in many cases, **eczema** and other dermatitis will be healed not only with **local applications** of medicinal herbs via compresses, lotions, or poultices, which are effective indeed, but also by administering:

• **Depurative** plants such as the white birch tree or the pansy, which promote the elimination of waste substances in the blood, which tend to form deposits on the skin, through urine and perspiration.

• Plants which **improve liver functions,** in which many processes eliminating toxic substances contained on the blood flowing are carried out.

• **Laxative** plants, which prevent internal toxicity for chronic constipation.

SKIN CRACKS

Definition

These are small **fissures** in the skin, generally painful, which affect the epidermis and the superficial part of the dermis. They are usually located on the palms of hand and feet. Their causes are not well-known, though they are related to **allergy** to certain chemical products, and to **lack** of vitamins and trace elements.

Treatment

Besides ***treating the causative factors,*** we recommend local applications of these plants in order to heal this ailment.

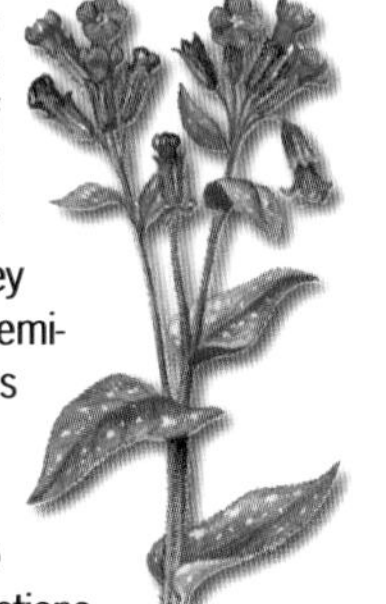

Lungwort

OAK TREE	Dries and heals skin, and reduces its inflammation
LUNGWORT	Astringent, heals skin cracks
PELLITORY OF THE WALL	Anti-inflammatory, emollient
ALOE	Revitalizes skin, giving it more resistance and beauty

CALLUS

Definition

Also called **corns.** These are roughenings of the skin caused by excessive friction or pressure, which appear mainly on the fingers or toes.

Phytotherapy

When locally applied, these medicinal plants ***soften*** callus, since they contain substances such as salicylic acid, able to ***breaking*** the ***corn layer*** of the skin.

CALENDULA	Corn remover, contains salicylic acid which makes corns and warts softer

WARTS

Definition

These are skin excrescencies caused by an **excessive growing** of certain skin cells. In many cases, they have a ***viral causative agent.***

Phytotherapy

When applied locally, these plants exert ***antimitotic*** (prevent mitosis, or cell division) ***and soothing*** actions on the skin.

CALENDULA	Corn remover, contains salicylic acid which makes corns and warts softer

WOUNDS AND SORES

Definition

A **wound** is a break in the continuity of the skin, caused by traumatic reasons.

An **ulceration** is also a break in the continuity of a skin or mucous layer, however it has the following features:

• There is a **necrosis** (destruction) of the affected tissue, either the skin or the mucosa, with loss of substance.

• **It does not tend** to heal spontaneously as in the case of wounds.

One of the more frequent classes of skin ulceration is that of **varicose ulceration,** which appears on the lower extremities and is related to disorders of the venous blood flow.

Phytotherapy

Phytotherapeutical treatment of both lesions is mainly based on plants with ***antiseptic and wound healing*** properties.

Clean wounds tend to heal spontaneously. What you have to do in this case is just, apart from making a suture, wash them with infusions or decoctions of ***cicatrizant and antiseptic*** plants.

St. Johnswort

When the case is that of **infected or open wounds** which have a slow healing process, application of poultices or compresses with these plants can be useful.

For skin **ulcerations,** cleansing, compresses, and poultices with ***cicatrizant and antiseptic*** plants can also be applied. We recommend also ***astringent*** plants, which eliminate the tissues suffering from necrosis and dry ulcers.

Some medicinal herbs are highly effective for skin care and hygiene.

STICKLEWORT	Wound healer, promotes healing of slow-healing ulcers and wounds
FOXGLOVE	Excellent wound healer
WATERCRESS	Promotes the formation of new skin
GERMAN CAMOMILE	Wound healer, emollient,antiseptic
WALNUT	Astringent, wound healer, antiseptic
CALENDULA	Wound healer, speeds up healing of skin wounds and ulcers
ROSEMARY	Wound healer, antiseptic, stimulates healing of wounds and ulcers
MILFOIL	Wound healer, antiseptic. Very effective to heal wounds and ulcers
ST. JOHNSWORT	Moderates inflammatory reaction on tissues surrounding bruises and wounds, stimulates epithelization
COMFREY	Very effective to speed up healing of slow-healing ulcers and sores
ECHINACEA	Anti-infectious, wound healer, regenerates tissues

EXCESSIVE PERSPIRATION

This can be caused by acute or chronic **infections,** nervous **weakness or imbalance,** and other reasons. ***Before*** taking this plant, ***the causes for perspiration have to be known.***

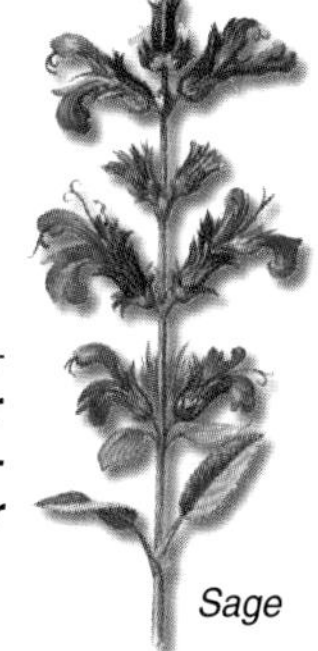
Sage

SAGE	Reduces excessive perspiration, especially at night

ECZEMA

Definition

The term eczema is a synonym for **dermatitis.** It comprises all **skin inflammations** with proper features, both from a clinical and from a histological (microscopic) point of view.

Causes

Many agents can lead to eczema; some are known, and some aren't. Besides the **aggressive local factors** which directly affect the skin, such as chemical products, radiation, bacteria, virus, fungi, and parasites, the presence of **toxins** in the blood can be also a causative agent of eczema, since they are eliminated through the skin, then irritating it. It is what is popularly called "dirty blood."

Licorice

Phytotherapy

Therefore, the phytotherapy of eczema and dermatitis demands:

- ***Local applications*** as lotions, compresses, and poultices.
- ***Internal treatment*** which consists of ***depurative*** plants such as pansy or the white birch tree, and with plants which ***promote liver functions*** such as dandelion and fumitory.

OAK TREE	Dries and heals the skin, reduces its inflammation
EVENING PRIMROSE	Nourishes skin, fights rashes
WATERCRESS	Regenerates skin
NETTLE	Soothing. Recommended in chronic skin afflictions
LICORICE	Enhances skin eczema
GERMAN CAMOMILE	Anti-inflammatory, antiseptic
FUMITORY	Avoids internal toxicity caused by intestinal putrefaction, and the consequent eczema and rashes
DANDELION	Laxative and depurative, avoids internal toxicity caused by constipation
PSYLLIUM	Protects irritated skin and reduces inflammation
WHITE BIRCH	Diuretic, cleanses the skin from impurities in the case of chronic eczema
MILFOIL	Cicatrizant, antiseptic, anti-inflammatory
ALOE	Cicatrizant, soothing, increases defenses Bittersweet nightshade

SKIN MYCOSIS

Definition

This is an infection caused by **fungi** and located on the skin. There are usually fungi on the skin and the mucosa, which under certain circumstances can become pathogenic and be very contagious.

Phytotherapy

These plants have ***antifungal*** properties, this is to say, they eliminate fungi.

BALM	Antifungal (eliminates fungi), antiseptic
PINE TREE	Regenerates the skin, emollient, eliminates fungi and skin parasites
ALOE	Regenerates the skin, fights athlete's foot and other mycosis

SKIN STRETCH MARKS

Definition

Skin stretch marks are caused by a break of its elastic fibers, caused by a degeneration of the connective tissue which forms them. They usually appear during pregnancy or as a consequence of **weight changes. Nervous stress and constipation** promote their appearance.

Phytotherapy

Local applications with these plants in help decisively the reduction or disappearing of stretching marks.

FUCUS	Soothing, anti-inflammatory. Useful for cellulitis, stretch marks, and flaccidity
ALOE	Revitalizes the skin, giving it resistance and beauty
HORSETAIL	Improves flaccid skin, giving it smoothness and elasticity

SKIN IRRITATION

Definition

This can be caused by **mechanical** (bruises), **chemical** (irritant substances), or **physical** (sunlight or other radiations) reasons.

Phytotherapy

Local applications of these plants with ***emollient*** (soothing) properties can help the skin recover its usual appearance and smoothness.

LINDEN	Skin anti-inflammatory and soothing
HIGH MALLOW	Alleviates skin and mucosa irritation
CALENDULA	Soothes the skin, recommended for dry or delicate skin
PRICKLY PEAR	Alleviates skin irritations
COMFREY	Emollient, healing, contains alantoin

ACNE

Definition

This ailment is characterized by **pustules** which form from the sebaceous glands of the skin.

Causes

Acne pustules are usually infected by anaerobic bacteria. The ***ultimate causative agent*** of acne is still ***unknown,*** though it is related to ***hormonal and genetic*** factors. A **diet** rich in fats, and **internal toxicity** caused by chronic constipation are some of the ***factors which make it more severe.***

Local applications of these medicinal herbs can dry the pustules and improve the skin's appearance.

EVENING PRIMROSE	Nourishes the skin, fights rashes
MILFOIL	Wound healer, antiseptic, cleanses skin
ALOE	Wound healer, soothing, increases defenses
BURDOCK	Antibiotic. Useful for acne and skin rashes
BLACK ELDER	Sudorific, depurative. Useful for eczema, furuncles, or acne

DRY SKIN

To keep the water soaking skin tissues from quickly evaporating, and the skin becoming dry and cracked, it is covered by a fine layer of waterproof fat.

The mentioned medicinal herbs here ***protect and balance*** the fat layer of the skin, thus stopping the evaporation process and enhancing hydration and beauty of the skin.

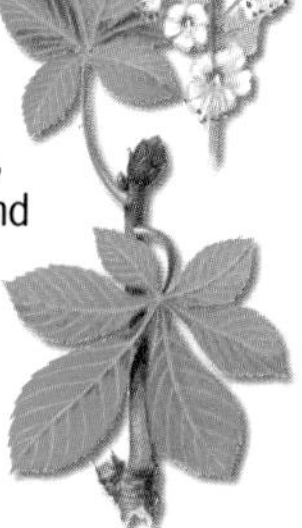

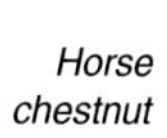

Horse chestnut

LINDEN	Opens pores, soothes and moisturizes the skin
EVENING PRIMROSE	Nourishes the skin, fights dryness and skin rashes
HORSE CHESTNUT	Soothes and protects the skin
SPEEDWELL	Soothes skin when dried by cold weather, cosmetic
FLAX	Soothes and moisturizes the skin
PSYLLIUM	Protects the skin, reduces its inflammation, cosmetic
CALENDULA	Soothes and moisturizes the skin. Useful for dry or delicate skin

CELLULITIS

Definition

This is an inflammatory process of subcutaneous conjunctive tissues, which is caused by the ***deposit of toxins*** and ***retention of water.***

Phytotherapy

Phytotherapy provides medicinal plants in ***local*** application, which ***cleanse*** skin impurities, as well as other plants that, when ***taken orally,*** eliminate any ***excess of liquids, and purify*** the blood.

DANDELION	Depurative, enhances liver function, prevents internal toxicity
WHITE BIRCH	Cleans skin impurities from cellulitis
FUCUS	Helps reducing the volume of fatty tissues

SKIN BEAUTY

External applications of these plants help clean and soothe the skin, in a natural way. However, skin beauty depends ***both*** on the conditions of **the interior and exterior** of our body. A ***healthy diet*** and ***"clean blood"*** are two ***required factors*** to maintain a skin in optimum conditions.

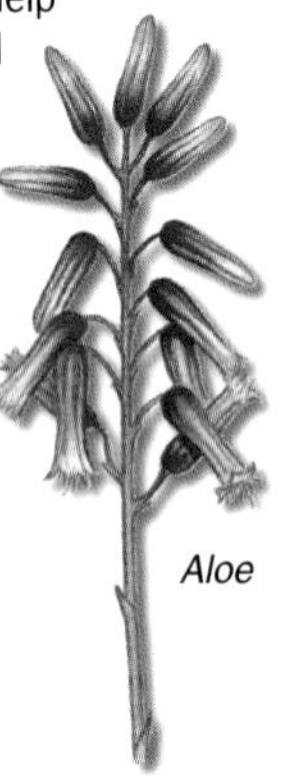

Aloe

CORNFLOWER	Gives a fresh, smooth appearance to tired eyelids
LINDEN	Opens pores and cleanses skin, fights the effects of cold and wind on the skin
WITCH HAZEL	Activates skin blood flow, cicatrizant, astringent
SPEEDWELL	Soothes dry skin, cosmetic
ROSE	Invigorates the skin, cleanses facial skin, fights wrinkles
ALOE	Revitalizes skin, giving it beauty and resistance

In the space between the toes there are usually mycosis, caused by pathogenic fungi.

Daily applications of the plants mentioned in the table, as shown in this picture, are a valuable alternative to treatment with antifungal medicines.

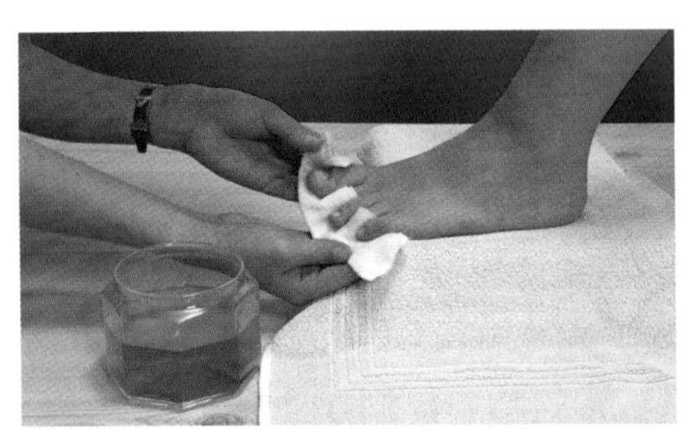

HAIR LOSS

Definition

Hair loss is also know as **alopecia.** Most cases occur in men, and are related to androgen production (male hormones).

Causes

Local treatment with medicinal plants stimulate and give strength to the hair follicles, from which hair grows.

Phytotherapy

In some cases, hair loss may be caused by **general reasons,** such as lack of nutrients, toxins, systemic ailments, or nervous tension.

WATERCRESS	Regenerates the skin, prevents hair loss
NETTLE	Prevents hair loss
CINCHONA	Hair invigorating
NASTURTIUM	Stimulates the hair root, revitalizes the hair

PSORIASIS

Definition

This is an ailment of unknown causes, in which the cells of certain epidermis areas reproduce themselves at higher rate than usual. This gives birth to the formation of thick scales, with reddening of the skin.

Treatment

Up to now, ***there has been no treatment*** able to heal psoriasis completely. These plants exert a beneficial action on the whole skin, and thus can positively influence the course of this ailment.

LICORICE	Enhances skin eczema
PINE TREE	Powerful skin emollient
RUE	Revulsive, useful for psoriasis
ALOE	Wound healer, soothing, increases defenses
GROUND CHERRY	Wound healer, anti-inflammatory, enhances psoriasis
ECHINACEA	Wound healer, regenerates tissues, stimulates defenses

FURUNCLES AND ABSCESSES

Definition

A **furuncle** is formed by the infection of a sebaceous hair gland (these are glands which produce fats, and are located at the root of every hair). The causative agent is usually a germ called staphylococcus, which turns fat into pus.

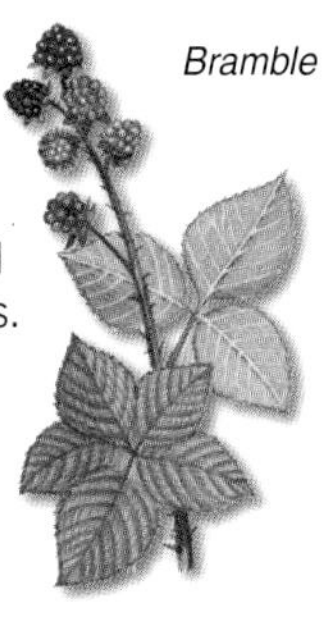

Bramble

Abscess is a more general term, for every accumulation of pus in a cavity formed by tissue disintegration. We could say that furuncles are specific types of abscesses.

Phytotherapy

Phytotherapy provides ***healing and antiseptic*** plants, able to ***ripen*** furuncles and abscesses, thus allowing pus to leave, and regenerate tissues.

FENUGREEK	Promotes skin cleaning
BRAMBLE	Heals skin furuncles and ulcers
MILFOIL	Cicatrizant, antiseptic. Effective in the treatment of skin furuncles and infections
ECHINACEA	Natural antibiotic, cicatrizant, regenerates tissues

FRAGILE NAILS

Definition

Nails are keratinized extensions of the skin. **Lack** of vitamins and minerals, especially iron and silicon, produce a softening of nails. In some cases, nail afflictions can be a ***symptom*** of a body disease.

Phytotherapy

Application of these plants, both ***internally*** and ***externally,*** can help ***harden*** nails.

EVENING PRIMROSE	Nourishes the skin, fights nail fragility
HORSETAIL	Promotes regeneration of tissues, especially those of the skin, nails, and hair

SCABIES

This is an infestation (an ailment caused by parasites) produced by the acarus *Sarcoptes scabiei*, which is difficult to see with the naked eye. This parasite introduces itself into the skin, where it causes intense **itching,** especially at night, after going to bed.

PINE TREE	Regenerates the skin, emollient, eliminates fungi and skin parasites
THYME	Powerful antiseptic, insecticide, antiparasite

RINGWORM

Definition

This is a **mycosis** (infection), which is very contagious, and affects the scalp, caused by dermatophyte fungi. It manifests itself with **hair loss** in localized areas, with **skin lesions and itching.**

Treatment

These plants ***eliminate fungi*** when used in ***local application.***

WALNUT	Astringent, cicatrizant, anti-inflammatory
ALOE	Regenerates the skin, fights athlete's foot and other mycosis

HERPES

Definition

This is an infection caused by the virus of the same name, which is recidivist (it repeats with certain frequency), can become very painful, and manifests itself by means of small vesicles on the skin.

Phytotherapy

These plants are very useful because of their ***antiviral and soothing*** properties on the skin.

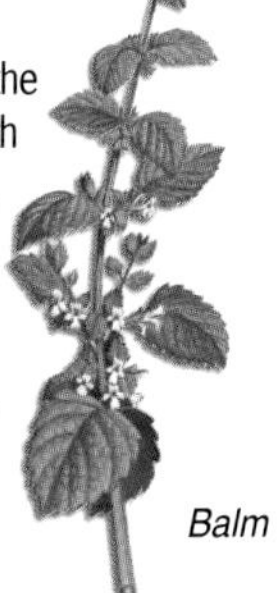

Balm

BALM	Antiseptic, destroys fungi and viruses

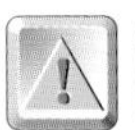

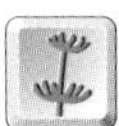

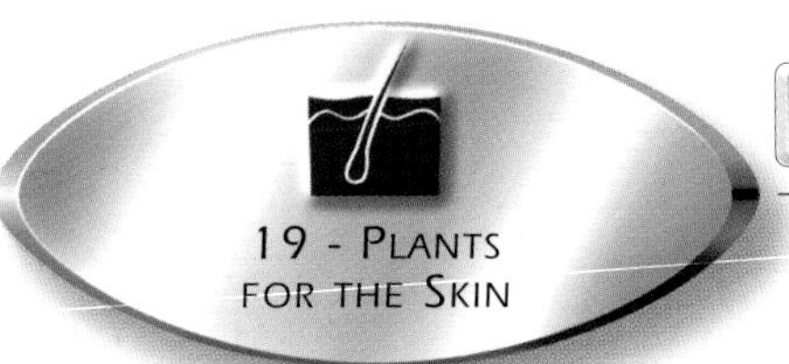

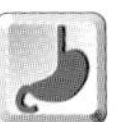

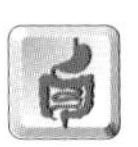

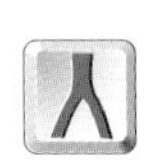

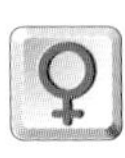

Milfoil

A mythical cicatrizant

AT THE TIME of the Trojan War, in ancient Greece, the great hero Achilles, symbol of strength and virility, was injured with a poisoned arrow which his enemy Paris had shot at him. The wound was deep, and bled constantly. According to the myth, the goddess Aphrodite washed the wounded ankle of the famous warrior with milfoil, which after this fact was named *achillea*, in honor of the hero.

Despite using the plant which has his name, Achilles died because of his ankle wound. However, milfoil or achillea became a beloved friend for soldiers and warriors, who tried to heal their wounds with it. The famous Spanish physician Andrés de Laguna said in the sixteenth century that "it is very useful to heal wounds in wars."

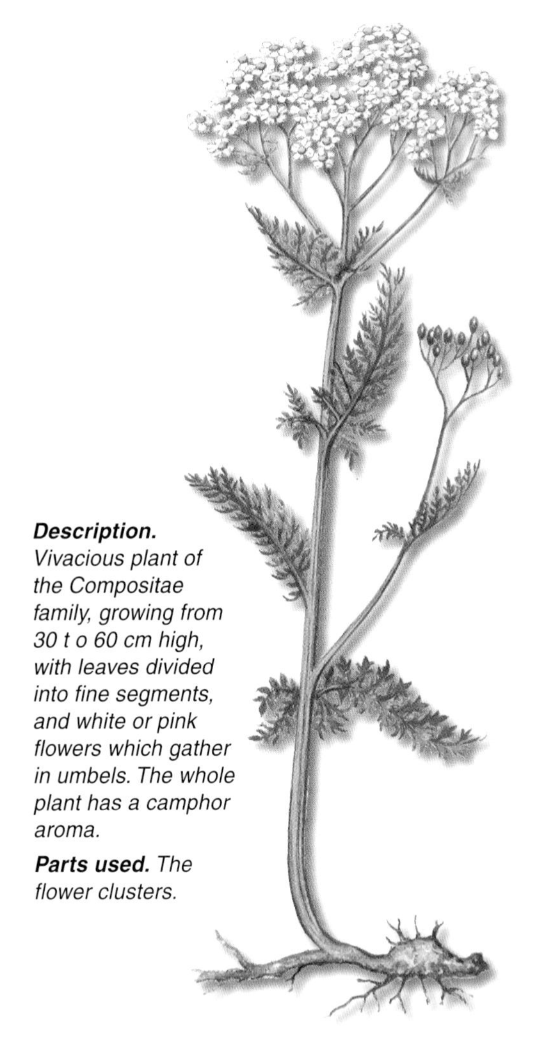

Description. *Vivacious plant of the Compositae family, growing from 30 t o 60 cm high, with leaves divided into fine segments, and white or pink flowers which gather in umbels. The whole plant has a camphor aroma.*

Parts used. *The flower clusters.*

PROPERTIES AND INDICATIONS. The whole plant contains up to 0.8% of essence rich in cineole and azulene, to which it is supposed to owe its **anti-inflammatory, cicatrizant, and vulnerary** properties, which are enhanced by the lack of tannin. It also contains a bitter component (achilleine) with **invigorating** properties on the digestive system, as well as flavonoids and other glycosides, which give the plant **antispasmodic** properties.

It has a diverse range of applications. Milfoil is highly effective both in internal and external use.

• **Digestive system.** Because of its bitter component, it acts as an invigorant of the digestive organs, increasing both their action and the secretion of juices, required for a good digestion. Its effects are stronger for the stomach (where it increases the production of gastric juice) and for the liver (increases bile secretion: **cholagogue** properties). Due to its **antiseptic** properties, it reduces intestinal fermentation. It is used with good results for chronic **gastritis, hypochloridria** (lack of juice), **dyspepsia** (heavy digestion), **liver** malfunction, digestive **spasms, and flatulence** (carminative properties) **[O]**. When taken before meals, it has **appetizer** properties.

• **Circulatory system.** Milfoil is a great blood depurative, which also makes blood more fluid (by decreasing its viscosity) and enhancing blood flow. It is very useful for treating **arteriosclerosis [O]**.

• **Female genital system.** Due to its emmenagogue properties, milfoil **regulates the menstrual cycle** when irregular, and **alleviates dysmenorrhea** (spasmodic aches which some-

Preparation and Use

INTERNAL USE

❶ **Infusion** with 20 g of flower clusters per liter of water. Drink three or four cups daily. It is better to prepare this infusion soon after harvesting it, since when it is prepared earlier, it becomes black in color and sour in taste.

EXTERNAL USE

❷ **Cleansing and baths** with an infusion made with 30-40 g of flower clusters per liter of water.

❸ **Nose packing** with a gauze soaked in the infusion or the fresh juice of this plant.

❹ **Lotions** with the **fresh juice** of the plant, directly applied on the affected skin area.

❺ **Poultices** with the plant, mashed, and heated in a pan.

❻ **Compresses** with a hot infusion.

times accompany menstruation). Due to its hemostatic properties, it helps stop **excessive menstruation** and uterine **hemorrhages** (bleeding) [❶].

• In ***external application,*** milfoil has notable **vulnerary** properties (heals wounds and bruises), as well as **antiseptic, cicatrizant, and hemostatic** (helps to stop bleeding). Dioscorides said that it is very useful "against blood effusion, and against recent sores." It is a **necessary** plant for treating **wounds, ulcers, sores, furuncles, chilblains, and cracks.** Messegué called it "the iodine tincture of the meadows and greenlands." It is therefore used in the following cases:

- **Epistaxis.** Gauzes soaked in milfoil infusion or fresh juice are packed into the nostrils to stop nose bleeds [❸].
- **Antisudorific and deodorant.** Foot baths with a milfoil infusion fight bad foot odor, and excess of perspiration [❷].
- **Hemorrhoids.** It is an excellent remedy against hemorrhoid inflammation. When hemorrhoids flare up and itch, it reduces their inflammation and volume [❷,❻].
- **Acne and eczema.** For these cases, good results are achieved when the plant is used in local applications [❹,❺], and it is taken in infusion [❶].
- **Beauty.** It promotes the elimination of toxins through the skin, cleansing it [❹,❻]. It also improves the appearance of the skin, and soothes it.

Compresses of milfoil, as well as infusions of the same plant, are good remedies to fight uncomfortable, unpleasant acne.

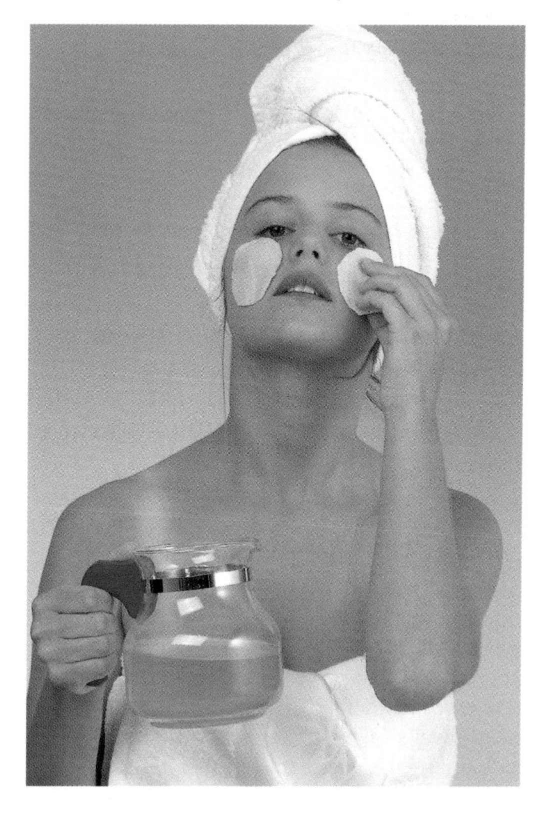

Aloe

Invigorates, soothes the skin, and heals wounds

AT PRESENT, we know that aloe belongs to the group of xeroid plants, which close the stomas of their leaves after any cut or wound in them. Thus, they avoid loss of moisture.

Indeed aloe has been used to heal the wounds of many people throughout history. Greek soldiers, Roman emperors, and warriors from many countries have been treated with this plant.

PROPERTIES AND INDICATIONS. From the fleshy leaves of aloe, two main products are obtained: bitter aloes, and aloe gel.

BITTER ALOES. When cutting the surface of the aloe leaves, no matter which aloe species, a viscous, yellow juice with bitter flavor flows out. It is concentrated under the sunlight or by evaporation, and becomes a shapeless mass of dark brown color and very bitter flavor, called bitter aloes.

Based on the daily dose, bitter aloes have diverse applications [❶].

- Up to 0.1 g it has **appetizer, stomachic, and cholagogue** properties, promoting digestion.
- From 0.1 g it has **laxative and emmenagogue** properties (increases menstrual flowing).
- With a dose of 0.5 g (the maximum per day) it has strong **purgative and oxytocic** properties (it provokes uterine contractions).

ALOE GEL or ***JUICE.*** It is obtained from the flesh of its leaves, which give an almost transparent sticky juice, with no flavor. This juice is responsible for the fame aloe gel has been acquiring for the last few years, especially because of its healing properties on the skin. It contains ***acemanan,*** an immunostimulating substance

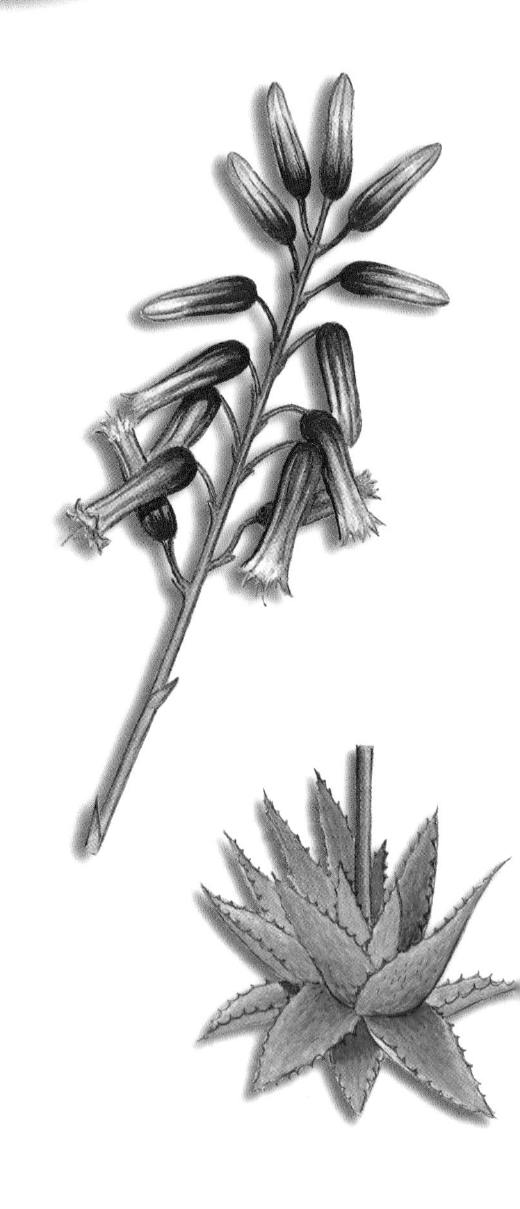

Description. *Plant of the Liliaceae family, growing up to three or four meters high, through growth of its central axis or stem. It has fleshy, lanceolated, spiked leaves, and red or yellow flowers according to its variety, which hang from a large stem.*

Parts used. *The juice of the leaves.*

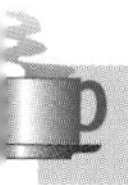

Preparation and Use

INTERNAL USE

❶ **Bitter aloes.** It is used as pills, and **pharmaceutically** made. As a laxative or purgative substance, bitter aloes act slowly, thus have to be administered at night to achieve effects the next day.

❷ **Aloe gel or juice.** Take 1-2 spoonfuls, three or four times a day, dissolved into water, fruit juice, or milk.

EXTERNAL USE

❸ **Compresses** with aloe juice. Keep them for the whole day, soaking them with juice every time they get dry. At night, olive oil or an hydrating cream can be applied, since aloe juice dries the skin.

❹ **Lotion** with aloe juice. Apply two or three times a day on the affected skin area. It is recommended that you combine its use with that of some emollient (soothing) such as olive oil.

❺ **Creams and ointments,** and other **pharmaceutical preparations** based in aloe. These usually include an emollient or hydrating substance.

which increases defenses. Unlike bitter aloes, aloe gel does not have laxative properties.

In ***local*** applications, aloe can exert beneficial effects in many cases. The most important are the following:

- **Wounds,** whether clean or infected. Aloe juice is applied as compresses {❸}, though the aloe flesh can be also put directly on the wound. It promotes the cleaning of the wound and accelerates its regeneration, while reducing the scar.
- **Burns.** Aloe gel or juice is applied as compresses for two days after the burn has taken place {❸}. For first degree burns, two or three days of treatment will suffice. In more severe cases, we recommend you ***consult the doctor.*** Aloe manages to accelerate skin regeneration in the burned area, as well as reduce scarring to a minimum.
- **Skin afflictions.** Aloe juice, applied from lotion, has a favorable effect on psoriasis and skin eczema, as well as on acne, athlete's foot (fungal infection), and herpes {❹}. We recommend you take aloe orally also to enhance its effects {❷}.
- **Skin beauty.** Aloe revitalizes skin, giving it better endurance, smoothness, and beauty. When applied to the skin, it improves the appearance of scars and cracks. It is also used for nail and hair care {❹,❺}.

When ***taken orally,*** aloe juice has **depurative and invigorating** properties. It is used as a **digestive,** and in the treatment of gastro-duodenal **ulcer** {❷}.

ACEMANAN contained in aloe juice has been scientifically proven to be able to **stimulate the defenses** of the body {❷}. Internally used, it activates the lymphocytes, a kind of cell whose main function is that of destroying cancer cells, as well as those which have been infected by the AIDS virus. Research is being conducted on using acemanan to treat both modern plagues; however without any definitive results up to now.

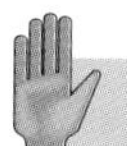

Warning

Aloe gel or juice *can produce* ***allergic reactions*** *when applied on the skin.*

Bitter aloes *must not be used by* ***pregnant women, nor during menstruation,*** *since it produces congestion of the pelvic organs and uterine contractions.* ***Never exceed the dose*** *of 0.5 grams per day.*

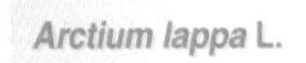

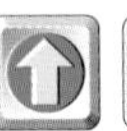
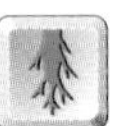
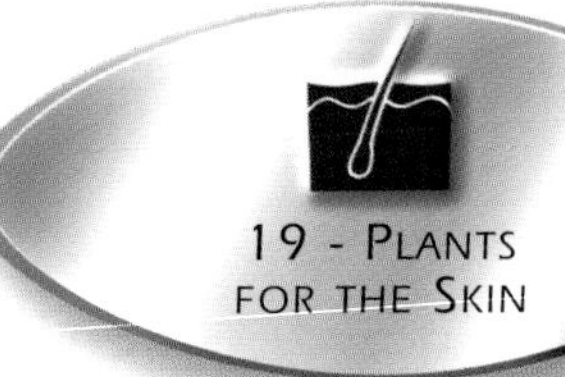

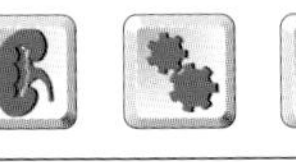
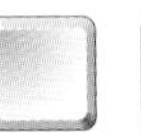
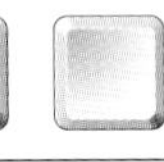

Burdock

Depurative and sudorific

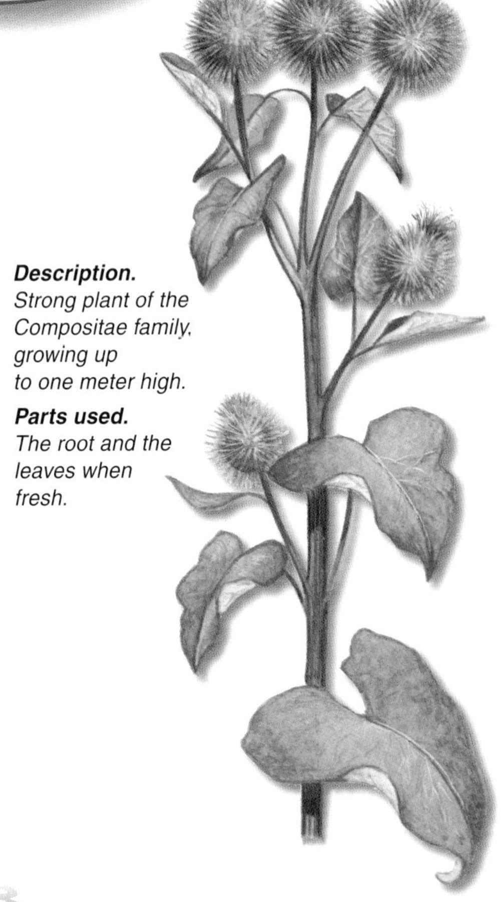

Description. *Strong plant of the Compositae family, growing up to one meter high.*

Parts used. *The root and the leaves when fresh.*

THIS PLANT DEMANDS attention because of its large leaves.

We do not know how the effects of this plant on the skin were discovered. Perhaps one of those actors had acne or furuncles, and after some plays the appearance of his skin improved.

PROPERTIES AND INDICATIONS. The root and leaves of burdock contain different active components which explain its properties:

- **Antibiotic.** Artiopicrine, mainly contained in the root is a plant antibiotic of the glycosidic type, which has been proven especially effective against staphylococcus, a germ which causes many skin infections.

Its use, both in external and internal applications, is recommended for **skin infections** caused by **staphylococcus,** such as abscesses, furuncles, gumboils, adenitis, and infected sebaceous cysts **[❶,❸]**.

It is also useful for **chronic eczema** and **acne,** as well as in **eruptive infectious diseases** (measles, chicken pox, scarlet fever, etc.) **[❶,❸]**.

The antibiotic properties of burdock also benefit the urinary system, since burdock is eliminated through the urine, and is thus recommended for **cystitis** and recidivist **urinary infections [❶,❷]**.

- **Depurative.** Because of its content in essential oil and mineral salts rich in potassium, burdock is an excellent sudorific and depurative plant. It promotes the elimination of waste substances through the skin. Thus, the skin, which is also an excreting organ, frees itself of impurities.

Preparation and Use

INTERNAL USE

❶ **Infusion** with 50 g of root per liter of water. Drink two or three daily cups.

❷ **Cold extract** of 20-30 g of ground root in a liter of water, steeping for six hours. Boil the resulting liquid for one minute. Drink two or three cups daily. This method enhances its depurative properties.

EXTERNAL USE

❸ **Compresses.** Made with the same infusion or decoction taken internally, but slightly more concentrated. Apply from two to six times a day, for 10-15 minutes.

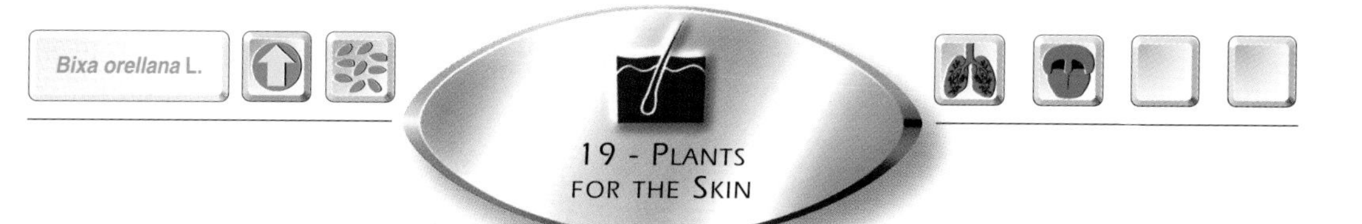

Annatto Tree

Remedy against burns, and expectorant

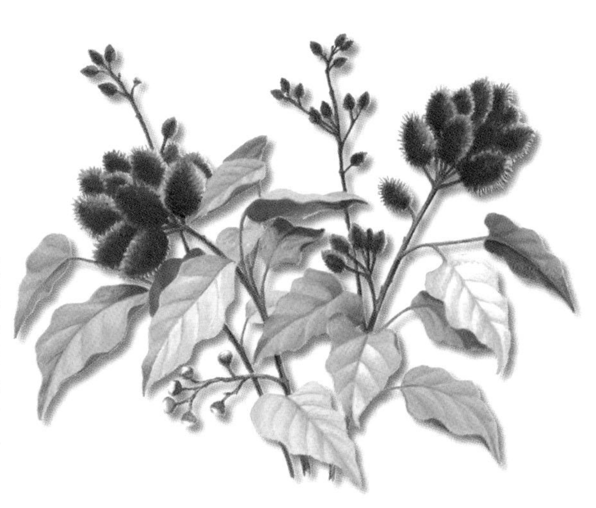

THE MAYANS and the Aztecs, who had notable phytotherapeutic knowledge, used the annatto tree to treat leprosy. At present, we know that this tree shares botanical and chemical similarities with the *Hydnocarpus kurzii* [King] Warb. (= *Taraktogenos kurzii* King), an Asian tree from which an oil is extracted, used today to treat leprosy.

PROPERTIES AND INDICATIONS. The ***LEAVES,*** because of their tannin content, have **astringent and cicatrizant** properties. With their infusion, as gargles, **mouth aphthas, pharyngitis, and tonsillitis** will improve [❷].

In ***external applications*** (baths and compresses), the infusion of annatto tree leaves has interesting **cicatrizant, emollient** (soothing), and **anti-inflammatory** properties. Its use is highly recommended for skin infections, rashes, mild burns, and cellulitis [❸].

The ***SEEDS*** contain bixin (a coloring substance) and resin. The infusion of seeds is used as an **expectorant** for bronchitis or asthma [❶]. The powder of seeds, dissolved into oil, has emollient properties, and ***externally* applied** it is an excellent remedy against **mild burns** [❹].

Description. *Tree of the Bixaceae family, growing up to five meters high.*
It has big red flowers. The fruit are oval-shaped capsules, about 4 cm in size, covered with soft thorns and containing several seeds.

Parts used. *The seeds and the leaves.*

Preparation and Use

INTERNAL USE

❶ **Infusion** with a spoonful of seeds per liter of water. Drink two or three cups daily.

EXTERNAL USE

❷ **Gargles** with an infusion made with 40-50 g of leaves per liter of water.

❸ **Baths compresses** with the same infusion, on the affected skin area.

❹ **Poultices** with the powder of the seeds.

The **seed powder** is obtained by cold extracting them for four hours, then mashing the seeds, and steeping under sunlight until the water evaporates. Mix a spoonful of powder with 100 ml of **olive oil,** and apply as fine poultice on the burn area.

Horsetail

Regenerates tissues

HORSETAIL is an original plant, from a botanical standpoint. It is criptogamous, and like ferns, it reproduces itself with spores. These spores are only found in the so-called fertile stem, which grows in spring, and is shaped like an asparagus.

At present, it is highly valued because of its content in silicon, a mineral which plays a role in the processes of tissue regeneration.

PROPERTIES AND INDICATIONS. The whole plant is rich in minerals, especially silicon and potassium. Moreover, it contains a saponin (echisetonine), flavonoids, to which it owes its diuretic properties, different organic acids, and resin. It has remineralizing, diuretic, depurative, hemostatic, and when externally applied, wound healing properties.

Best results are achieved when combining internal use (herbal teas) and external applications (on the skin). These are its main applications:

- **Degenerative processes of the skin, the conjunctive tissues, and the bones.** Latest research on the role played by ***silicon*** in our body has proven that this trace element is present on the skin, nails, cartilages, bones, and ligaments. In all these tissues, it stimulates the ***regeneration*** of ***collagen and elastin*** fibers which form them, which, with the ageing process, lose consistence and elasticity. Silicon promotes the "reconstruction" or regeneration of our tissues, since without it, the synthesis of collagen and elastin fibers cannot occur (catalyzer effect).

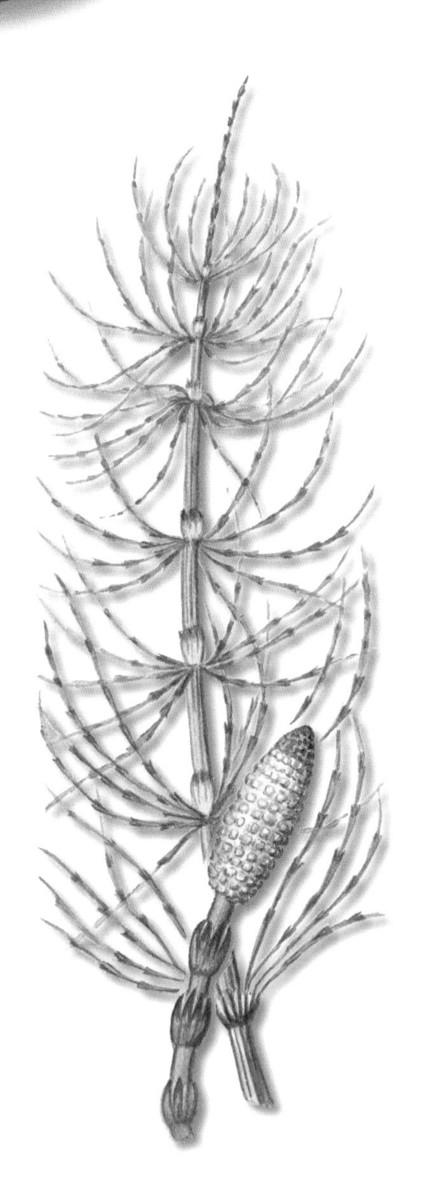

Description. *Vivacious, herbaceous plant, of the Echisetaceae family, growing from 10 to 30 cm high. It has two kind of stems: some are fertile, reddish in color, without branches. In their tips there is a spike with a spore: these stems appear first. The other ones are sterile, grow in late spring, and are formed by several articulated segments from which fine branches grow.*

Parts used. *The sterile stems and their branches.*

Preparation and Use

INTERNAL USE

❶ **Decoction** with 40-50 g of plant per liter of water. Boil in low heat for 10 minutes. Drink from three to five cups daily.

❷ **Fresh juice** of the plant. Three spoonfuls with every meal.

EXTERNAL USE

❸ **Compresses** soaked in a decoction similar to the aforementioned one, however slightly more concentrated (100-150 g of plant per liter of water). These compresses are directly applied on the affected area, such as breasts or anus.

❹ **Nose packing** with a gauze soaked in the aforementioned concentrated decoction.

Although silicon is also found in integral grains and beer yeast, horsetail is the ***plant with the highest proportion of organic silicon*** that is to say, combined with proteins (0.5-0.8 %). Isolated silicon, when chemically pure, cannot be absorbed and used by our bodies.

• **Skin wrinkles and stretch marks,** produced by ageing, obesity or sudden weight loss, pregnancy, muscular tension, etc. It improves skin appearance, and gives it a smooth, elastic appearance, both taken orally [❶,❷] and applied as compresses [❸].

• **Fragile nails** [❶,❷].

• **Breast flaccidity.** When applied as compresses on the breasts, it strengthens and tones up their tissues [❸]. This effect is improved when also taking a decoction [❶].

• **Varicose ulcerations, abscesses, infected wounds, eczema, conjunctivitis.** Horsetail renders good results, because of its wound healing properties, when applied as compresses.

• **Arthrosis** (degeneration of joint cartilage). Because of its content of silicon, and its depurative properties, horsetail is likely to be **one of the few back treatments** which at present can be used for this difficult ailment [❶].

• **Osteoporosis** (loss of bone consistency). Silicon stimulates osteoblasti and fiberblasti activity. These are the connective tissue cells which synthesize collagen fibers and form the matrix of the bones [❶].

• **Decalcification, bone breaking, rachitis.** Silicon eases the assimilation and fixing of calcium on the bones [❶].

• **Arteriosclerosis.** Recent research shows that lack of silicon is an important causative factor. Silicon has preventive effects, and perhaps also regenerative ones, on arterial degeneration, by stimulating the regeneration of elastic fibers on arterial walls [❶].

• **Edema** (retention of liquids), **kidney stones, urinary infections, gout,** excess of **uric acid,** and whenever a mild but effective diuretic and depurative effect is required [❶,❷].

• **Hemorrhages.** Horsetail has a significant hemostatic effect (stops bleeding), both in local applications and taken orally. For **epistaxis** (nose bleeds) apply a nose plug with a gauze soaked in a concentrated decoction [❹]. For **bleeding hemorrhoids** apply compresses soaked in this decoction on the anus [❸]. In both cases, the hemostatic effect is improved when also taking a decoction [❶].

For **hypermenorrhea** (excessive menstruation), **gastric hemorrhage** (caused, for instance, by gastro-duodenal ulcer), or **bronchial hemorrhages** (caused by tuberculosis, for instance), the use of a horsetail decoction helps heal bleeding tissues and stop hemorrhage [❶]. Of course, in any of these cases, ***a doctor must be consulted.***

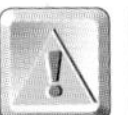
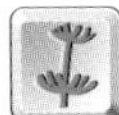
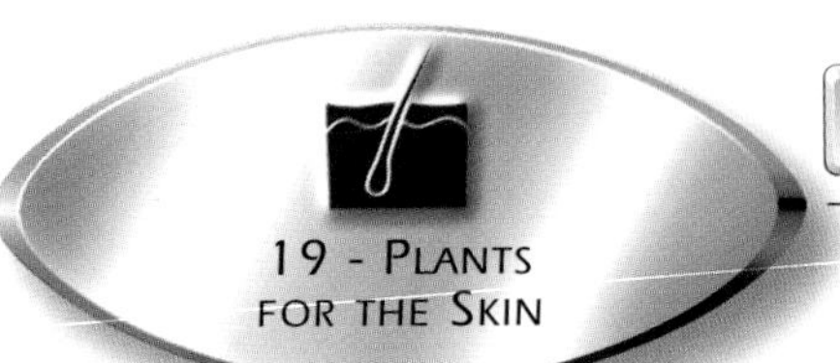

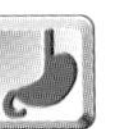
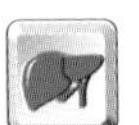
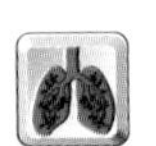
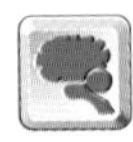

St. Johnswort

An excellent remedy for burns

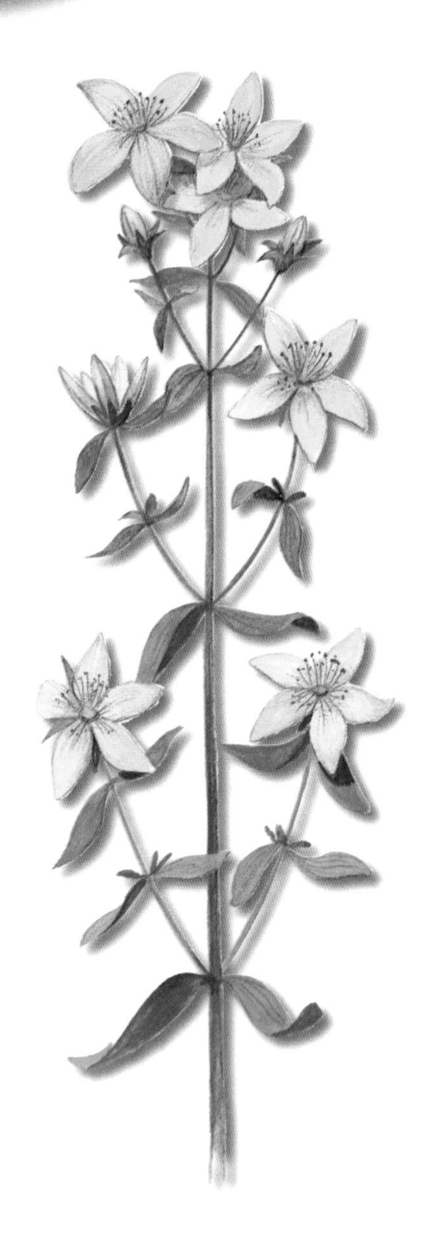

ST. JOHNSWORT is ***one of the medicinal herbs*** which was ***well known*** in ancient times, a fame which has not decreased with time. Dioscorides (first century A.D.) praised St. Johnswort. Its Latin name comes from the Greek word *hyper* (upon) and *eikon* (image), since this plant is above any other thing.

St. Johnswort leaves are covered with small secreting bags, visible against the light, which look like small holes. Thus the name *perforatum*. In the Renaissance, people supporting the theory of signs saw in its "perforated but cicatrized" leaves a sign that the plant should have cicatrizant (wound healing) properties. In the eighteenth century, this plant was known as the "military plant," because it was valued by soldiers.

Properties and indications. The leaves and flowers of St. Johnswort contain an essential oil, tannin, flavonoids, and a red coloring substance known as hypericin. St. Johnswort has the following properties:

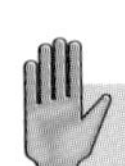

Warning

Avoid direct sunlight on the skin while taking or applying St. Johnswort. Hypericin produces ***photosensitization*** *which produces reddening of the skin after sunbathing.*

Description. *Vivacious plant of the Gutiferae family, growing from 30 to 60 cm high, with an upright stem, and leaves perforated by many holes, as if they were in rags. The flowers are yellow, with five petals each.*

Parts used. *The flower clusters (leaves and flowers), and their oil.*

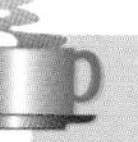

Preparation and Use

INTERNAL USE

❶ **Infusion** with 30-40 g of dry plant per liter of water. Drink a cup after every meal.

EXTERNAL USE

❷ **St. Johnswort oil.** There are several **pharmaceutical preparations** which currently contain this oil. It is applied using cotton on the burn or wounded skin, then covering with a gauze or a dressing.

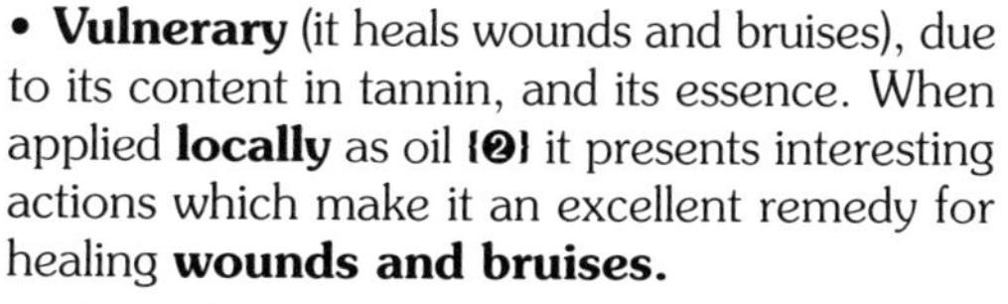

- **Vulnerary** (it heals wounds and bruises), due to its content in tannin, and its essence. When applied **locally** as oil [❷] it presents interesting actions which make it an excellent remedy for healing **wounds and bruises.**
  - It moderates the **inflammatory reaction** in the tissues surrounding the wound or bruise.
  - It has **local anesthetic** properties, thus easing pain in a gentle, but persistent manner.
  - It has **antiseptic** properties.
  - It stimulates **epithelization,** that is, the regeneration of skin on the lesion.

Hence, St. Johnswort has been used for more than 2000 years to heal any kind of wounds, sores, and mainly **burns.**

For first- and second-degree **burns**, it is ***more effective than most creams*** prepared from chemically synthesized products; for **major burns**, or **deep** ones, we always recommend that a ***doctor prescribe a treatment.***

Used internally, [❶] St. Johnswort has the following properties:

- **Balsamic and antispasmodic.** It is recommended for asthma, bronchial catarrh, and bronchitis.
- **Digestive, cholagogue, and choleretic.** It helps digestion, decreases stomach acidity, and promotes gall bladder functions.
- **Nervous system stabilizer and invigorator.** Hypericin has a balancing effect on the nervous system, and it has been proven to help those people suffering from **depression or neurosis.** It is used for **children's enuresis.**

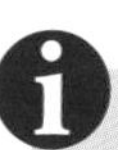

Preparation of St. Johnswort Oil

Those people wanting to follow traditional customs may prepare their own St. Johnswort oil in the following way, which is what the Spanish botanist Font Quer recommended:

*Put 100 g of flower clusters (the tips of the stems) recently gathered, but already dry, into a glass jar, and add 250 g of good **olive oil.** Steep in **cold extract** for 20 or 30 days, moving the bottle every day. After this time, strain the oil and bottle it in small containers which must be kept in a cool, shady place, **well closed.***

Every time one of these bottles is open, throw the unused oil away because it will lose its properties.

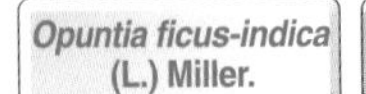

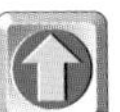
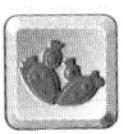
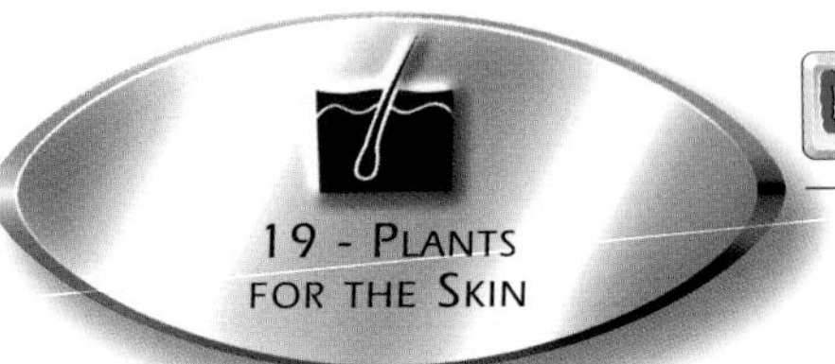

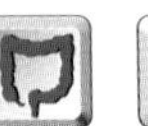
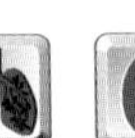
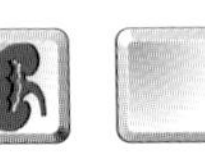

Prickly Pear

The leaves have emollient properties

ANCIENT Mexican natives used Indian fig leaves as poultices to heal wounds and bruises. Spanish colonists brought it to Europe, where it quickly spread all over the Mediterranean basin.

PROPERTIES AND INDICATIONS. The ***FRUIT*** has astringent properties, and render good results in stopping summer **diarrhea [❶]**. Their juice is used in Mexico as a syrup to calm coughs **[❷]**.

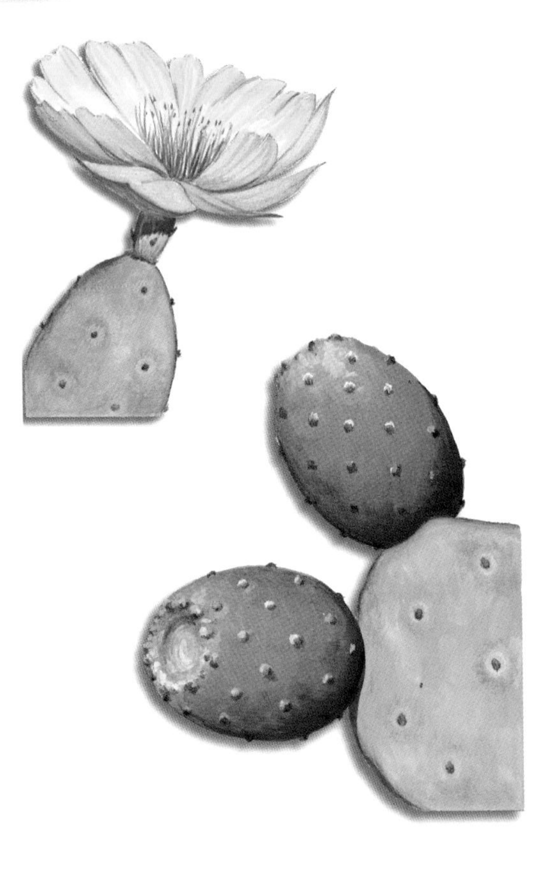

Description. Fleshy plant of the Cactaceae family, with fleshy leaves and stems, plenty of juice. It is formed by a series of oval-shaped leaves (fleshy), with prickles or thorns. The fruit is orange or red, and is covered by prickles.

Parts used. *The fruit (Indian figs), the flowers, and the leaves.*

The ***FLOWERS*** have diuretic and antispasmodic properties, being used in **oliguria** (lack of urine production), and **cystitis [❸]**.

The ***LEAVES*** contain high amounts of mucilage and cellulose, which gives them emollient properties. They are used as poultices to heal **wounds, bruises, and skin irritations [❹]**.

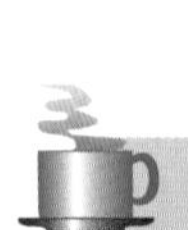

Preparation and Use

INTERNAL USE

❶ The **fruit** must be carefully rinsed so as not to touch them with bare fingers, because its many prickles are quite difficult to remove. Fruit can be eaten in **syrup** or **fresh.**

❷ **Syrup.** It is prepared by slicing the fruit and covering it with brown sugar. Steep for ten hours and then take the syrup (the resulting liquid), straining it to separate seeds. Drink it hot, by the spoonful.

❸ **Infusion** with 20-30 g of flowers per liter of water. Drink 3-4 cups per day.

EXTERNAL USE

❹ **Poultices.** The **leaves** are cut, then softly heated in an oven, and directly applied on the affected skin area.

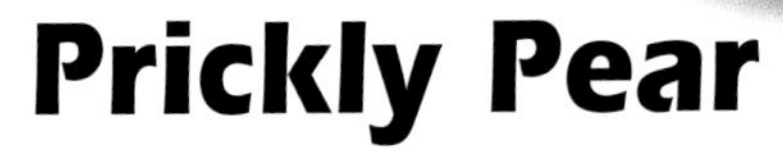

Ground Cherry

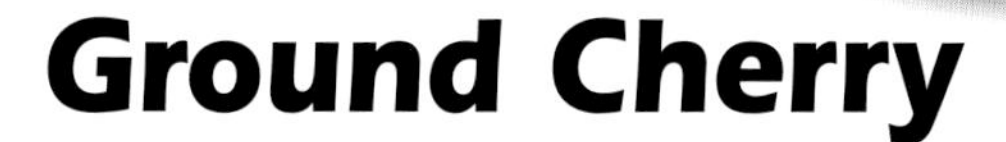

Heals and reduces skin inflammation

THIS SMALL plant grows in roadsides in Mexico and most areas of America. Its fruits are a pleasant gift for walkers.

PROPERTIES AND INDICATIONS. The ***FRUITS*** have **diuretic** and mildly laxative properties.

The ***STEMS*** and the ***LEAVES*** of the plant contain saponins and enzymes (peroxidase). As a decoction, they are ***externally*** used for skin rashes, because of its **cicatrizant and anti-inflammatory** properties **[❷]**. This plant has been successfully used for **psoriasis,** applying lotions with its decoction **[❸]**.

The aforementioned decoction of leaves and stems, when ***taken orally,*** has **expectorant and antitussive** properties **[❶]**.

Preparation and Use

INTERNAL USE

❶ **Decoction** with 30 g of stems and leaves per liter of water. Boil for 15 minutes. Drink two or three cups daily, which can be sweetened with honey.

EXTERNAL USE

❷ **Compresses** soaked in the liquid of the decoction internally used.

❸ **Lotions** on the affected skin area, with the aforementioned decoction.

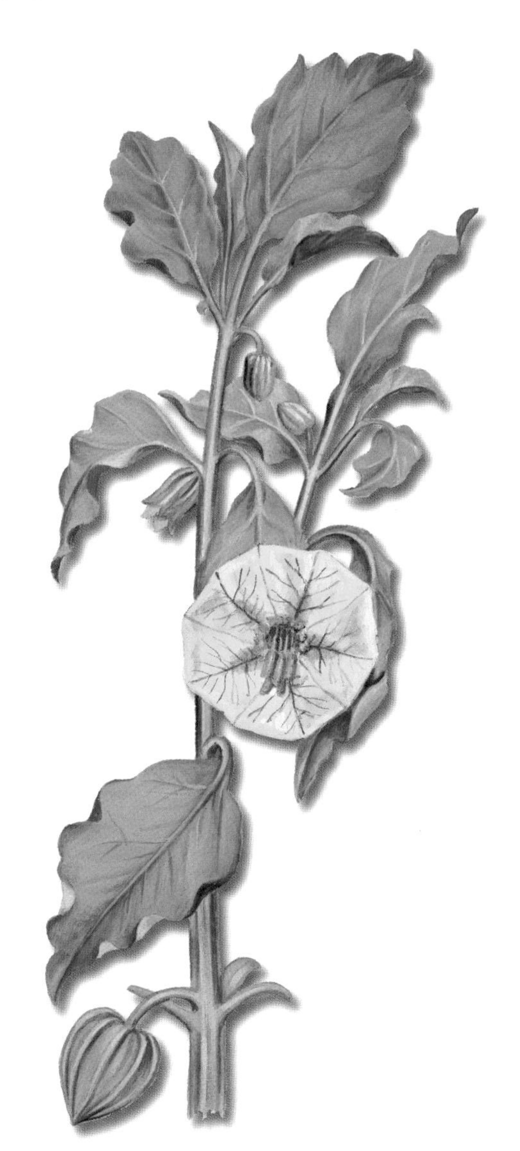

Description. *Plant of the Solanaceae family, growing from 30 to 50 cm high, with fruits of a cherry in size, yellow or red in color, edible, with a pleasant sweet-and-sour flavor.*

Parts used. *The fruits, the stems and the leaves.*

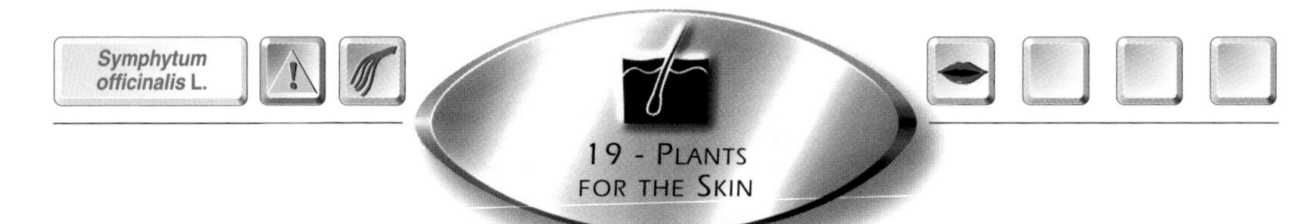

Comfrey

One of the most effective wound healers

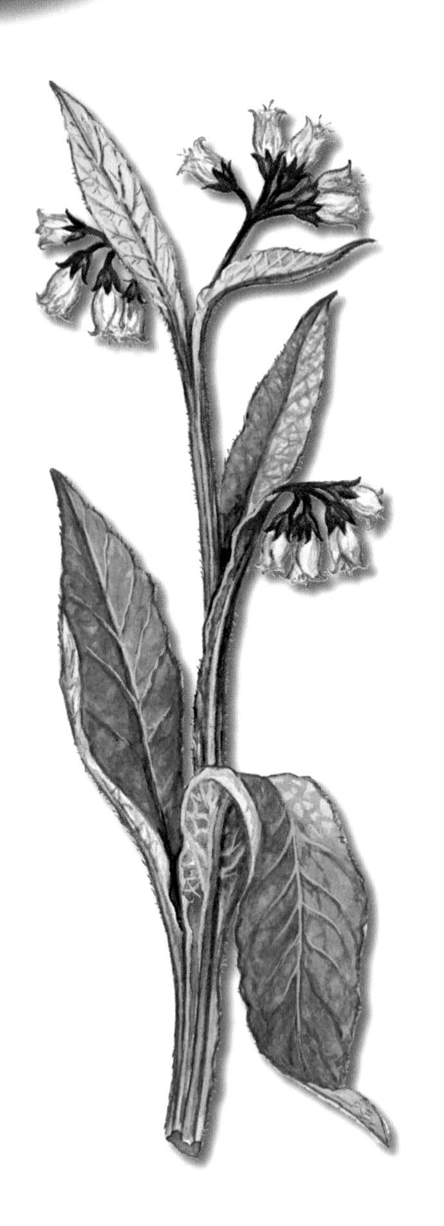

ANDRÉS DE LAGUNA, a Spanish physician of the sixteenth century, who translated and commented on the works of Dioscorides, said about comfrey that it "shows a great strength in fixing divorces of any parts or members."

According to the people who supported the theory of signs, the union between the leaves and the stem of comfrey is the sign that nature has bestowed on the plant, to let us know that it is able to close wounds and fix recent fractures. The truth is that some decades ago, in the root of comfrey a substance called ***alantoin*** was identified, which has a ***great healing power,*** and which at present is part of several ***pharmaceutical preparations.***

PROPERTIES AND INDICATIONS. The root of comfrey contains ***alantoin*** (1 %-1.5 %), as well as sugars (starch, saccharose, inulin), high amounts

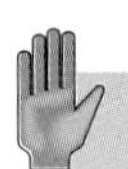

Warning

*The **root,** the **stem,** and the **leaves** of this plant are **toxic** when taken orally, since the alkaloid symphytine is present in them. This alkaloid has toxic effects on the liver. Another substance, the glycoside called consolidine, produces paralysis on the central nervous system, and when taken in high doses, respiratory failure, is also present in the plant.*

Description. *Vivacious plant of the Boraginaceae family, growing from 60 to 100 cm high. It has lanceolate, decurrent leaves (they grow directly from the stem, without petioles), which are covered by hairs. The flowers are pink, yellow, or violet in color.*

Parts used. *The rhizome (underground stem), and the root.*

Preparation and Use

EXTERNAL USE

Comfrey root is **only** applied **externally,** on wounds, ulcerations, bruises, and burns.

❶ **Compresses.** Prepare an infusion with 100 or 200 g of root per liter of water, steeping in cold extract for a couple of hours. Soak cotton or gauze compresses in this liquid, and apply them on the affected skin area, changing them two or three times per day.

❷ **Poultices** with comfrey root, fresh, ground or mashed. Change them as compresses, two or three times a day.

❸ **Mouth rinses** with the liquid of the cold extract, used for compresses.

of mucilage, glycosides, alkaloids, tannin, choline, and resin. It has the following properties:

• **Cicatrizant** (wound healing), due to its content in alantoin. It has been experimentally proven that this substance stimulates fibroblast proliferation. These are cells of the conjunctive tissues, which form the scar of wounds. Therefore, its use assists slow-healing wounds (**torpid wounds**), skin **sores and ulcers, burns,** and whenever stimulation of wounded or bruised tissues is required **{❶,❷}**.

Alantoin also acts on the periostium, a layer of tissue which surrounds the bones, and where the bone callus which closes any breakage is formed. However, it is ***not used in traumatology,*** perhaps because its application on the bone is quite difficult to perform. Moreover, there are other physical measures to close fractures, at present.

• **Emollient,** that is, it soothes inflamed skin and mucosa, due to its content in mucilage. It promotes the healing of **eczema and rashes,** as well as skin **irritations and inflammations {❶,❷}**.

• **Astringent,** due to its content in tannin. It dries the mucosa and clots capillary vessels. Mouth rinses with comfrey root are recommended for **stomatitis, gingivitis** (inflammation of the gums), and **pharyngitis {❸}**.

Internally applied, comfrey root has antidiarrheic and pectoral properties (eases cough), but it is better to use it ***only in external applications,*** since ***internally used*** it can be ***toxic.***

The content in alantoin of comfrey gives the plant a great cicatrizant power.

It has been scientifically proven that this plant is able to heal sores, ulcerations, and burns, as well as diverse types of wounds, especially those which are difficult to cure.

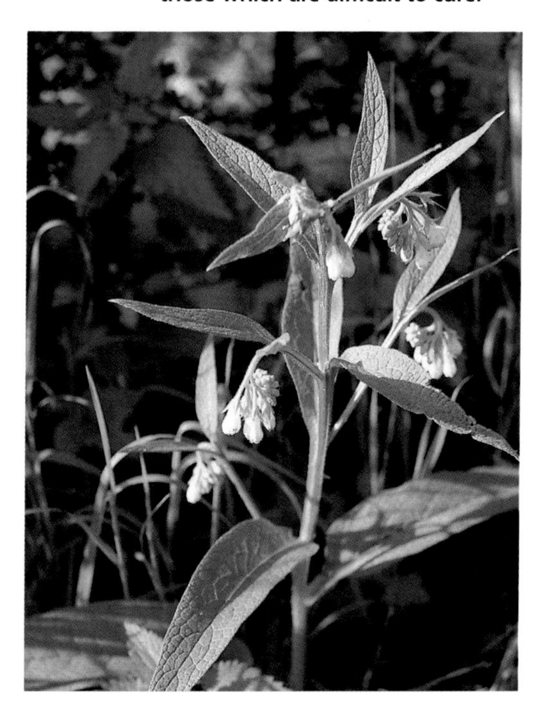

20

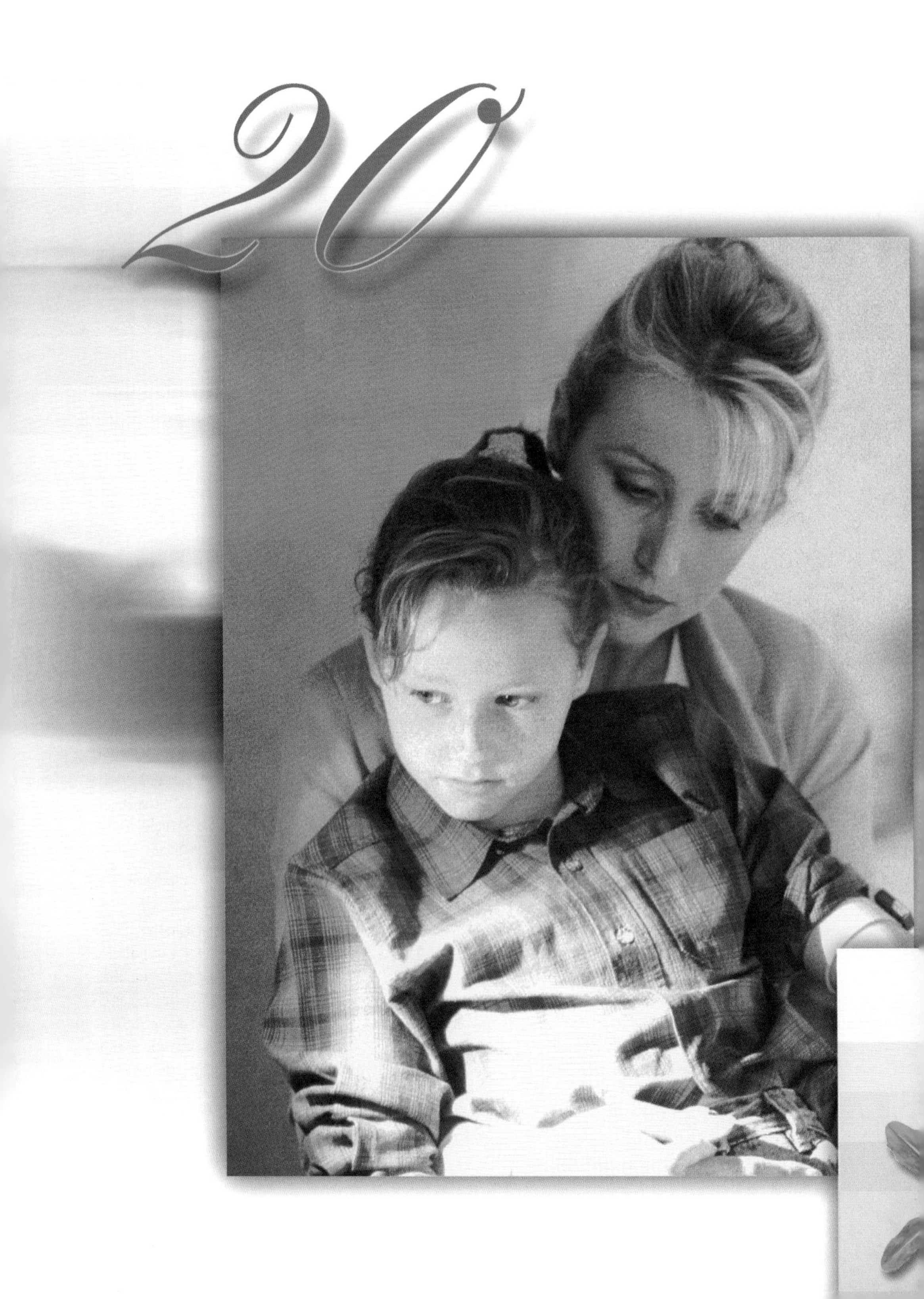

Plants for Infectious Diseases

DISEASES	PAGES
AIDS	361
Alimentary intoxication, see Salmonellosis	358
Amebiasis	360
Amebic dysentery, see Amebiasis	360
Cholera	359
Convalescence	359
Depression, immune system, see Low defenses	358
Diseases, febrile, see Febrile diseases	359
Febrile diseases	359
Fever	359
Fever, typhoid	359
Immune system depression, see Low defenses	358
Influenza	361
Low defenses	358
Malaria	360
Salmonellosis	358
Toxoinfection, alimentary, see Salmonellosis	358
Tuberculosis	360
Typhoid fever	359
Whooping cough	360

PLANTS	PAGES
Black elder	374
Brier hip	372
Cinchona tree	364
Echinacea	366
Nasturtium	378
Noni	368
Thyme	376
Wild daisy	362

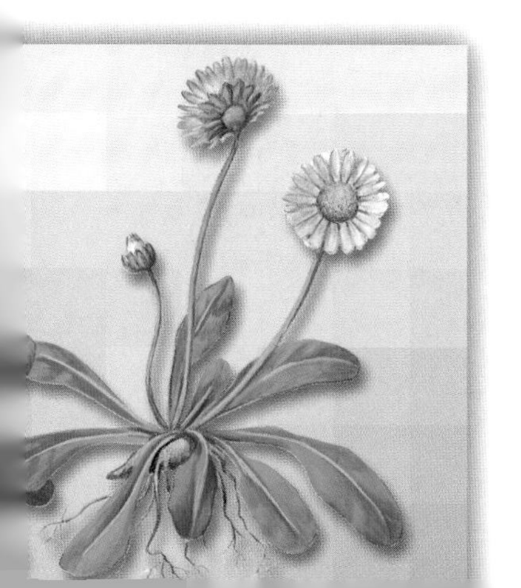

AT THIS POINT we leave the anatomical sequence of former chapters to talk about phytotherapy for diseases which affect not only a single body part or system, but the body as a whole.

Medicinal herbs help healing infectious diseases in three ways:

• **Antibiotic action.** Natural antibiotics contained in superior plants do not act as quickly and as effectively as chemically treated, purified antibiotics, contained in pharmaceutical products. However, they have the advantage of being ***much better tolerated,*** since as a rule they lack any side or toxic effects. Moreover, they do not depress natural defenses, as pharmaceutical antibiotics usually do. Plants also contain antiseptic substances which act on the skin or mucosal surface.

• **Depurative action.** Plants promote elimination through the kidneys, the skin, and the liver, of toxins which our bodies are continuously producing, even more so with infectious diseases.

• **Immunostimulant action.** Some plants are able to stimulate the immune system, which produces defenses against infections. These defenses are double: **cellular** (for instance, the leukocytes or white blood corpuscles) and **humoral** (antibodies). Both increase in number with phytotherapeutic remedies.

In the fight against infection, plants act mainly organically, improving their conditions to allow the body to confront the germs ***by itself.*** Bear in mind that the best antibiotic will fail if the defense mechanisms of the body do not act in an effective manner.

SALMONELLOSIS

This is a disease caused by bacteria of the genus *Salmonella*, which are present in **food in bad conditions.** It manifests itself as severe **gastroenteritis.** Besides these plants, those recommended for **gastroenteritis** are useful.

GARLIC	Antibiotic, respects normal saprophyte flora, increases defenses
THYME	Antibiotic, fights intestinal putrefaction

Herbal teas of medicinal plants complement the treatment infectious diseases, both during their acute phase and during convalescence.

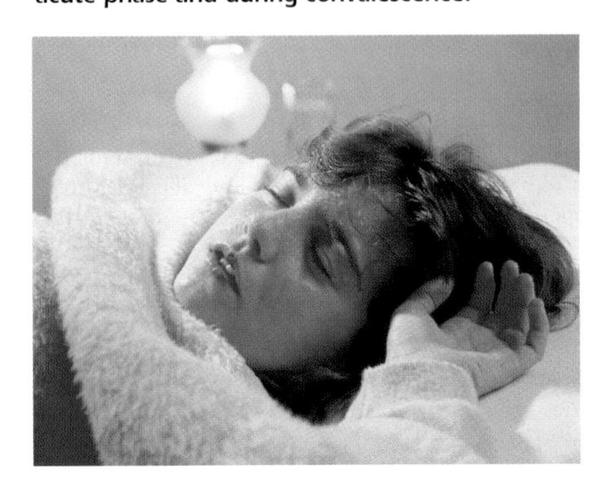

LOW DEFENSES

Definition

Unhealthy diet, lack of physical exercise, and abuse of antibiotics are some of the causes which can depress the immune system. In other cases, lack of defenses is caused by severe ailments such as AIDS or certain types of cancer.

Garlic

Theatment

Besides ***correcting the causative factors,*** whenever possible, the use of these plants has a ***notable immunostimulant effect.*** Their use is recommended in any case of severe infection, as well as when it occurs a depression in defenses against infections.

GARLIC	Increases the activity of defensive body cells, natural antibiotic
GENTIAN	Increases production of leukocytes (white blood cells)
ECHINACEA	Stimulates defenses against infections
BRIAR HIP	Stimulates defenses, recommended for all infectious diseases

CONVALESCENCE

Definition

This is an intermediate period between the conditions of illness and health, during which our body corrects the losses suffered, and normalizes the altered functions. The term is generally applied to the phase of recovering from any infectious disease.

Phytotherapy

Phytotherapy uses important plants to ***ease and make*** the convalescence process ***shorter.*** These plants ***complement*** other measures such as ***diet*** or ***physical rehabilitation***.

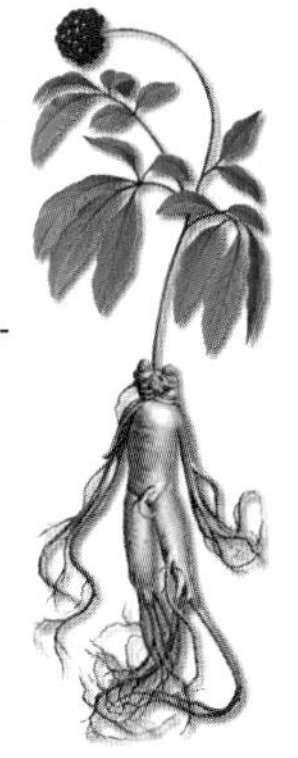

Ginseng

SPIRULINA	Nutritive, invigorating, general revitalizing of the body
GINSENG	General invigorating of the body
MEADOWSWEET	General invigorating, increases appetite
ROSEMARY	Invigorating, revitalizing
WILD DAISY	Perspirant, febrifuge, expectorant, promotes elimination of toxins
BRIER HIP	Stimulates defenses. Recommended in all infectious diseases

FEBRILE DISEASES

Causes

In any case of fever, ***the diagnosis of the causative disease*** is required, since there are many which can cause fever. Hence, a specific treatment could be applied.

Theatment

These medicinal herbs are a ***complement*** for treatment of the fever-causative disease. They not only produce a ***decrease*** in temperature, but also increase ***perspiration,*** promote elimination of toxins, ***refresh, and invigorate.*** Therefore, they are ***better*** than antipyretic ***medicines.***

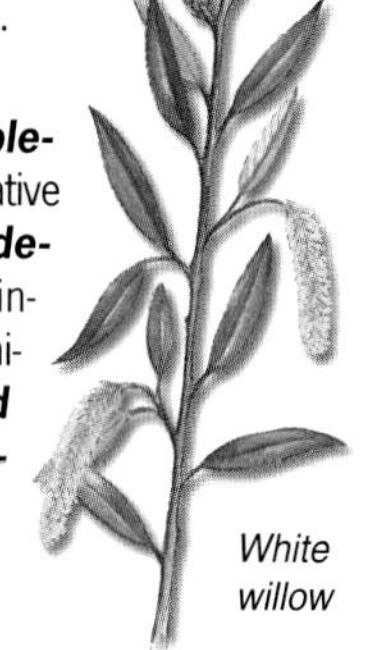

White willow

GERMAN CAMOMILE	Decreases fever, provokes perspiration
BARBERRY	Quenches thirst, refreshes, invigorates
BRAMBLE	Refreshing, invigorating
WITCH GRASS	Perspirant, diuretic, depurative
WHITE WILLOW	Decreases fever, invigorates the digestive system
WILD DAISY	Perspirant, febrifuge, expectorant, promotes elimination of toxins
CINCHONA	Decreases fever, eliminates toxines through sweat and urine
BLACK ELDER	Effective perspirant and depurative

TYPHOID FEVER

This disease is caused by the bacteria *Salmonella typhi,* which comes in infected water or foods, especially seafood. It appears as severe **diarrhea** and **intoxication.** These medicinal plants have a ***positive influence*** in the course of this disease.

ECHINACEA	Increases defenses against infections, stimulates processes of detoxification on the liver and kidneys

CHOLERA

A disease caused by choleric vibrion, which manifests itself as **vomiting,** liquid **diarrhea, and dehydration.** ***Besides the treatment with antibiotics,*** this plant ***helps*** with its healing. See also plants against **gastroenteritis**.

GARLIC	Antibiotic, respects normal saprophyte flora, increases defenses
NETTLE	Astringent. Effective for cholera and dysentery

MALARIA

Definition

This is an infection caused by protozoa (unicellular animals) of the genus *Plasmodium*, which are transmitted by a mosquito bite. According to the WHO, this is the ***disease*** which affects ***the highest amount of people*** worldwide.

Phytotherapy

Medicinal herbs have an important role in the treatment of malaria, since ***antimalarial medicines*** are all derivatives from ***quinine,*** a substance which is extracted from the bark of the cinchona tree, native to South America.

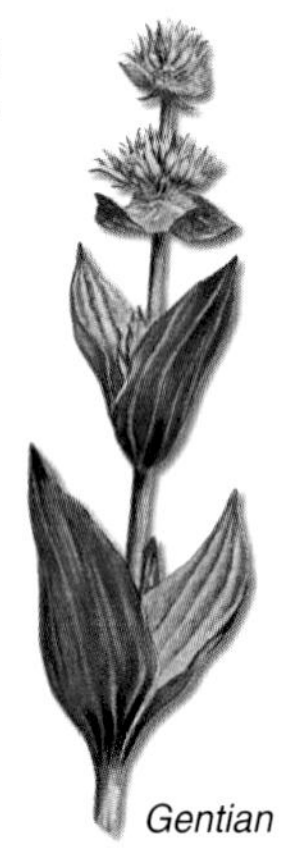

Gentian

GENTIAN	Febrifuge. Destroys the protozoa causing malaria
CINCHONA	Decreases fever. Antimalarial. Eliminates toxins from the blood through sweat and urine

AMEBIASIS

This is a disease caused by amoebae, which are protozoa (unicellular animals). They provoke severe **diarrhea** (amebic dysentery), and **hepatic afflictions.** With the extract of this tropical shrub, some ***pharmaceutical preparations*** are made.

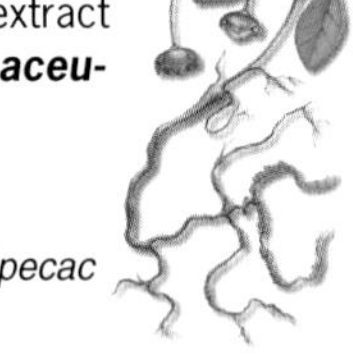

Ipecac

GARLIC	Destroys amebas, preserves normal flora
IPECAC	Destroys the amoebas causing dysentery, vomitive

WHOOPING COUGH

A disease caused by the micro-organism *Bacillus pertussis*, which manifests itself as crises of spasmodic cough, which repeat for several weeks. These plants are highly effective to ***ease cough and promote the healing*** of this disease. See also the plants recommended against **cough.**

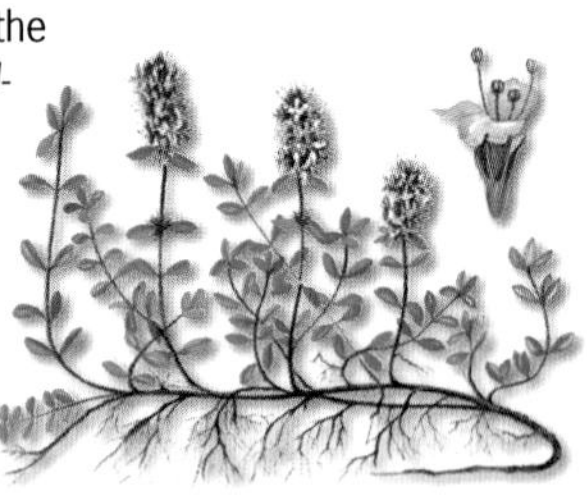

Mother of thyme

PRICKLY LETTUCE	Sedative, antitussive, calms irritative cough
MOTHER OF THYME	Antispasmodic, antiseptic, calms cough spasms
WILD MARJORAM	Expectorant, calms dry or irritative cough

TUBERCULOSIS

Definition

This is an infection caused by the Koch bacillus, called *Mycobacterium tuberculosis*. It is a disease with a slow progression, which mainly affects lungs, and manifests itself, or becomes more severe, when there is an **imbalanced diet,** or **unhealthy lifestyle.**

Theatment

These plants ***cannot heal*** this disease by themselves, but they ***promote*** the body healing mechanisms, which have a great influence in preventing and healing tuberculosis.

ICELAND MOSS	Pectoral, expectorant. Complement of antitubercular treatment
LICORICE	Expectorant, antibiotic, reduces inflammation of the respiratory ways
LUNGWORT	Emollient and anti-inflammatory on the respiratory system
ECHINACEA	Stimulates defenses against infections

INFLUENZA

Definition

This is an infectious disease caused by a virus, which manifests itself as **fever, muscular pain, respiratory catarrh,** and a trend toward bronchial and lung **complications.**

Theatment

There is no specific pharmacological treatment for influenza. The best one consists in helping the body to overcome the infection by itself, by ***enhancing*** its healing mechanisms.

Phytotherapy

Phytotherapy acts precisely in that way. These medicinal herbs increase ***perspiration*** and thus the elimination of toxins, as well as ***stimulating the defenses*** against infection. They also ***decrease the fever and alleviate the discomforts*** of the disease.

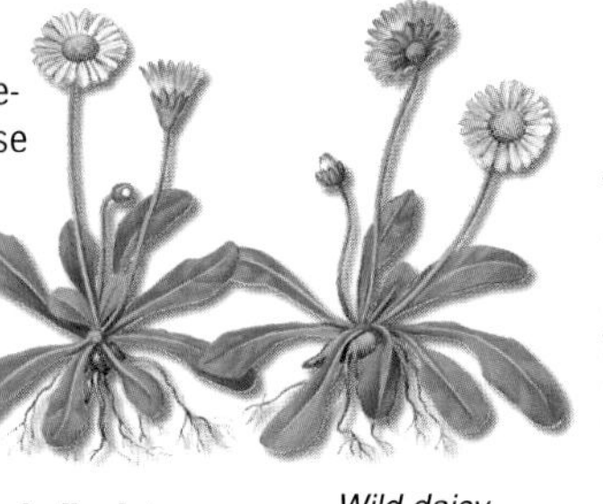

Wild daisy

LINDEN	Sedative, antispasmodic, alleviates headache
CYPRESS	Perspirant, decreases fever, balsamic
MEADOWSWEET	General invigorating of the body, diuretic, depurative, and appetizer
WILD DAISY	Perspirant, febrifuge, expectorant, promotes elimination of toxins
ECHINACEA	Stimulates defenses against infections
BRIAR HIP	Stimulates defenses, preventive for all infectious diseases
BLACK ELDER	Very effective perspirant and depurative
NASTURTIUM	Natural antibiotic, expectorant, invigorating

AIDS

We cannot say that the use of these plants can heal this terrible ailment, though some people have stated so. However, they can positively help its evolution, by stimulating the abilities of our body to fight against the disease.

Actually, the ***increase of the defensive ability*** of our body seems to be the ***best manner*** to heal AIDS, since up to now its virus has not been eliminated with medicines. These plants, along with a **healthy lifestyle,** can do their best to fight AIDS.

GARLIC	Increases the activity of defensive body cells, natural antibiotic
ECHINACEA	Increases antibody production, stimulates defense cells, reduces toxicity in the liver and kidneys
NONI	Immune booster, antioxidant

To achieve a healthy, infection-free body, fighting the micro-organisms which cause infections is not enough. Current medicine gives more and more importance to the body itself, in fighting infectious diseases.

Medicinal herbs do not act by destroying micro-organisms, but rather by giving strength to the body defenses. Their use, as well as the adoption of a healthier lifestyle, can help us more than the most powerful antibiotic.

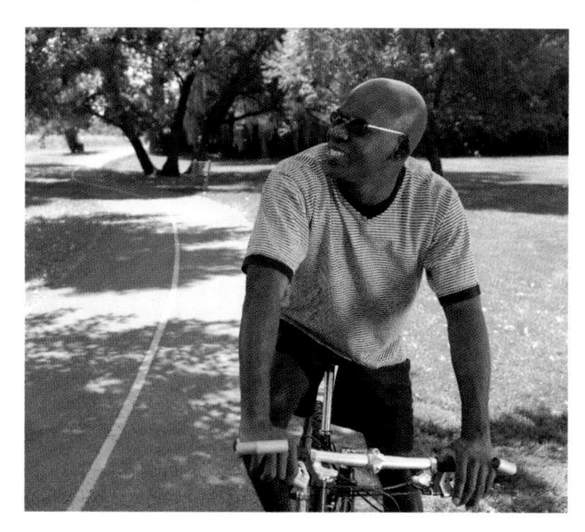

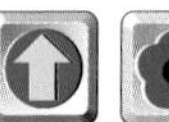

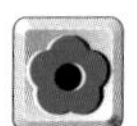

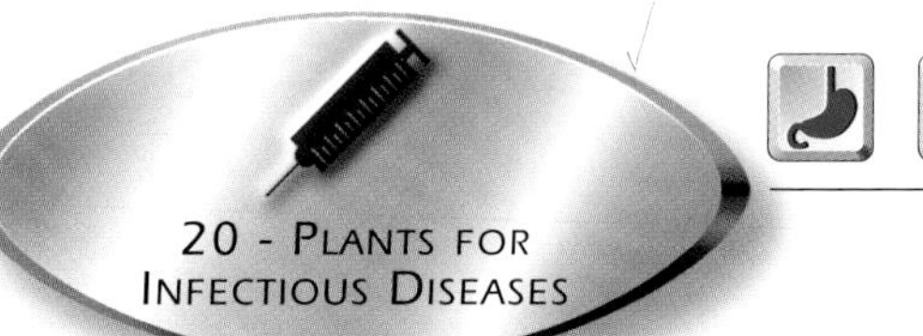

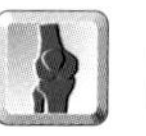

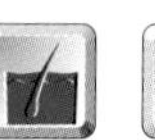

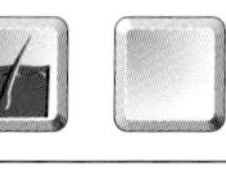

Wild Daisy

Invigorator and depurative for infectious diseases

HE LOVES ME, he loves me not....Who has never taken a wild daisy and asked a question of its petals?

This plant is pretty *(Bellis),* and vivacious *(perennis);* however it is tough and resilient as few plants are. When the weather is cold, when it rains, or when it snows, it bows down and closes itself. When the sun rises, wild daisy opens up and greets the sun, following it across the sky. Wild daisy is a type of daisy, smaller than the common one.

The Spring season invites us to eat tasty wild salads, which have depurative and invigorating properties. The ***LEAVES*** of wild daisy, somewhat sweet, are a perfect combination with those of sorrel (bitter), and the dandelion (bitter). A wonderful symphony of natural flavors! Next time you go to the countryside in springtime, enjoy it by serving yourself *a la carte* a tasty and healthy ***wild salad.***

Could anyone have told you that this humble plant made the German government go angry? German rulers demanded it be exterminated by the late eighteenth century, because they accused of being abortifacient. That accusation has never been proven.

PROPERTIES AND INDICATIONS. Its medicinal active components are most concentrated in the leaves, and especially in the flowers of wild daisy: saponins, tannin, organic acids (malic, tar-

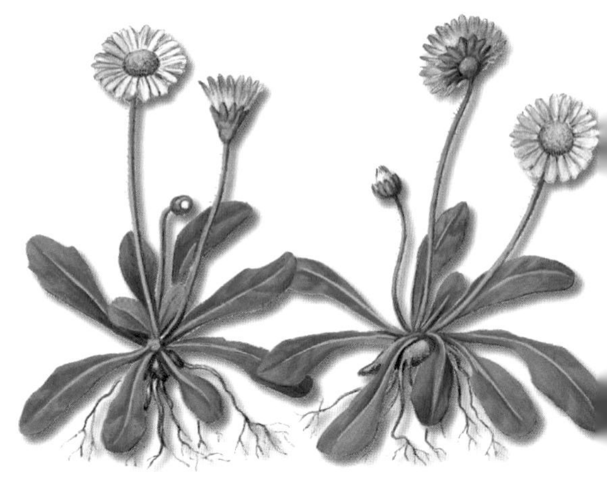

Description. *Plant of the Compositae family, usually growing between 10 and 15 cm high, with wide leaves forming a rose at the base of the plant. The flowers have a yellow disc, and white or pink petals.*

Parts used. *The flowers and the leaves.*

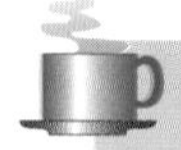

Preparation and Use

INTERNAL USE

❶ As a **vegetable,** especially raw, in salads and other dishes.

❷ **Infusion** with a large spoonful of flowers and/or leaves per cup of water. Drink two or three cups daily.

EXTERNAL USE

❸ **Compresses** soaked in a decoction made with 50-60 g of flowers and/or leaves per liter of water. Boil for two minutes, then steep for 15 minutes before straining. Apply the compresses on the affected skin area, changing them every hour.

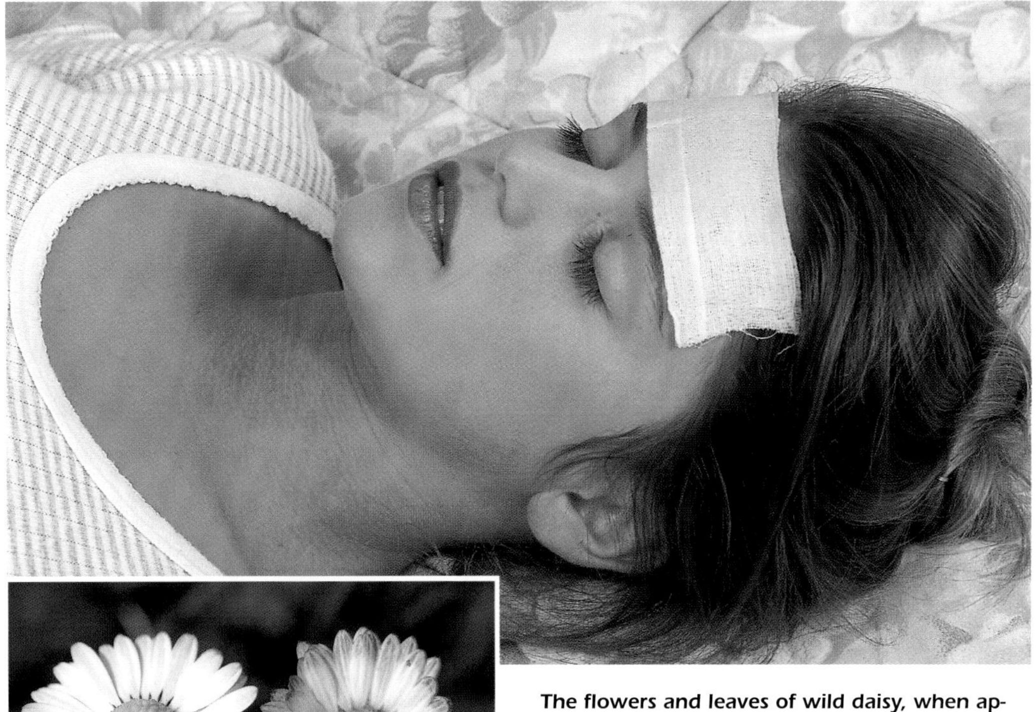

The flowers and leaves of wild daisy, when applied in compresses on the forehead, help lower fever. A herbal tea made with them is also recommended.

taric, acetic, oxalic, etc.), mineral salts, inuline, and an essential oil.

From the Renaissance onwards, many properties have been attributed to wild daisy, but according to its composition, the main ones are:

- **Depurative, laxative,** and mildly **diuretic.**
- **Sudorific, febrifuge** (decreases fever), and **expectorant.**
- **Invigorator and appetizer** (increases appetite).
- **Vulnerary** (heals wounds and heals bruises), when ***externally*** applied.

Its use is recommended in the following cases:

- **Fever and infectious diseases** (influenza, bronchitis, catarrh, measles, scarlet fever, parotiditis, etc.) **[❶,❷]**. It promotes the elimination of toxins and metabolic waste produced by infection (through the urine and sweat), as well as invigorates the body, cutting short its convalescence period. Moreover, it decreases fever and helps expectoration. For high fever we recommend putting compresses on the forehead with a decoction of flowers and/or leaves **[❸]**, in addition to taking it orally.
- Traumas, bruises, sprains, furuncles, sores, and as a rule, **any skin** or soft tissue **lesion** where an **anti-inflammatory and cicatrizant** (wound healing) action is required **[❸]**.

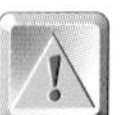

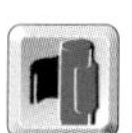

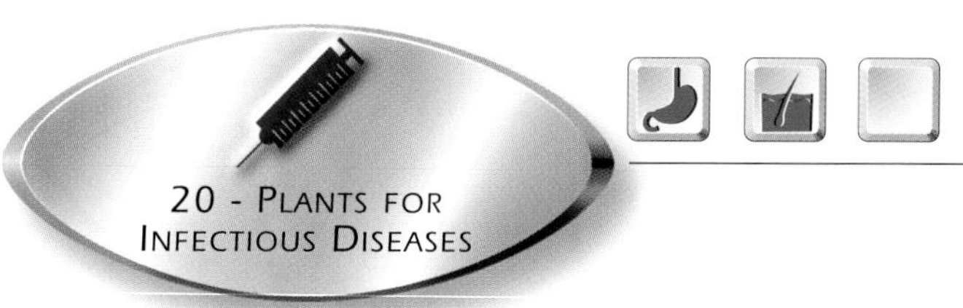

Cinchona Tree

The febrifuge and invigorator par excellence

THE CINCHONA tree is a true national wealth for Andean South American countries. It is said that the Incas had known of its extraordinary febrifuge properties for a long time, but kept the secret so that the Spanish conquistadors would become weakened by malarial fever.

The counts of Chinchón, who were viceroys of Peru, brought to Spain a huge pack of cinchona bark, in 1640. Because of its wonderful results in decreasing fever as well as an invigorator substance, its use quickly spread all over Europe, as powder, extract, and decoction. In 1920, the French pharmacists Pelletier and Caventou managed to isolate the active components of the cinchona bark: two alkaloids known as quinine and cinchonine, as well as some others.

Currently, millions of people take advantage of the cinchona tree and its derivatives, both for individual prophylaxis (prevention) and for malaria treatment.

Properties and indications. ***Cinchona*** tree bark contains more than 20 alkaloids, among which there are two pairs of isomers: quinine-quinidine, and cinchonine-cinchonidine.

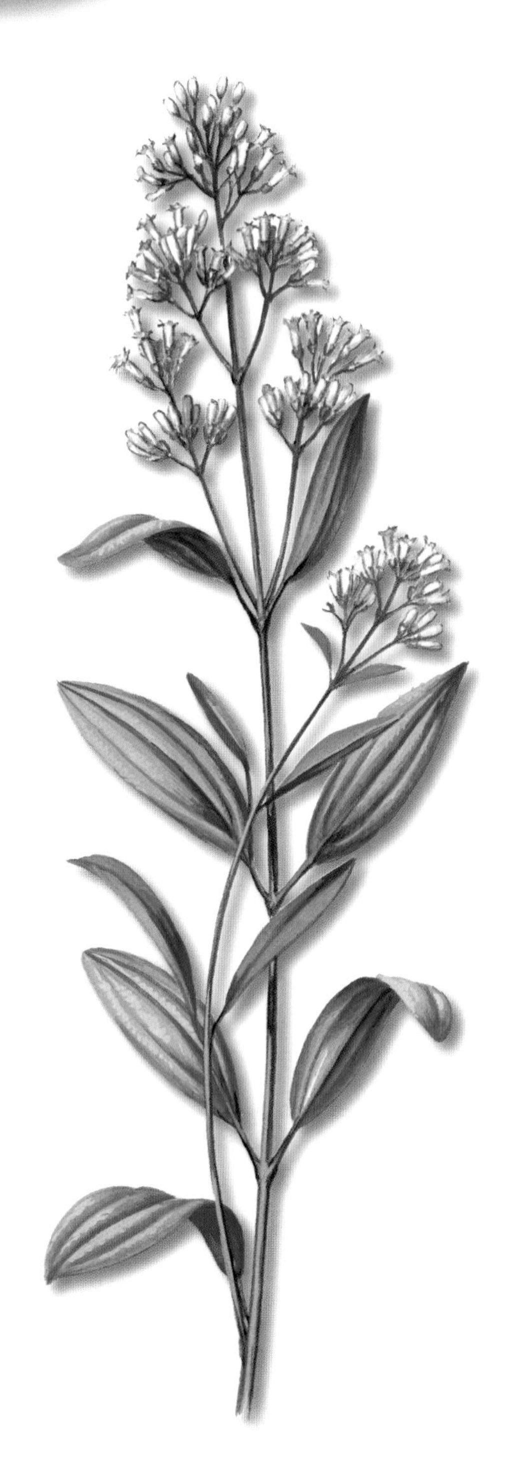

Description. *Shrub or tree of the Rubiaceae family, growing up to 30 m high. The bark of the trunk is reddish or ochre, and the top is formed by large green opposite leaves. It has white or pink flowers.*

Parts used. *The bark of the trunk and branches, especially, as well as that of the root, ground up.*

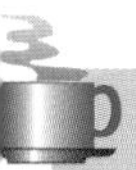

Preparation and Use

INTERNAL USE

❶ **Cold extract.** Steep 20-30 g of cinchona tree bark in one liter of water for one hour. Drink a cup before every meal.

❷ **Infusion** with half teaspoonful of ground cinchona tree bark per cup of water. Drink one cup before every meal, never exceeding four cups daily.

EXTERNAL USE

❸ **Compresses** with a decoction of 30-40 g of bark per liter of water. Boil for 10 minutes. With the resulting liquid, soak compresses and apply them on the scalp, for 10 minutes, three times per day.

❹ **Gargles and mouth rinses** with the aforementioned decoction.

These alkaloids give the plant **febrifuge, antimalarial, and invigorating** properties, as well as a bitter taste. Cinchona bark also contains catechic tannin, which make it **strongly astringent,** as well as essences, bitter components, and starch.

The most important applications of the bark are the following:

• **Malaria.** This is likely to be ***the disease affecting the largest number of people world-wide.*** It manifests itself as high fever and perspiration, as well as sleepiness, headaches, nausea, and anemia. The causative agents are diverse protozoa of the *Plasmodium* genus, which attack the red blood corpuscles after being injected by the anopheles mosquito bite.

The cinchona bark alkaloids are ***very useful*** to treat ***acute phases*** of the malaria attack. They decrease fever, alleviate headache and nausea, and eliminate the general discomfort this disease causes. Cinchona bark has been used with these aims since the times of the Incas [❶,❷].

Since the mid-twentieth century, pharmaceutical research has developed ***synthetic antimalarial medicines,*** such as chloroquine and primaquine, which also serve ***to prevent*** the disease.

However, the quinine obtained from cinchona bark is still successfully used, especially in rural areas of South America and Asia.

• **Febrile condition.** Cinchona bark decreases the fever caused by many other infectious diseases, besides malaria. Its beneficial effects are enhanced because it promotes the elimination of blood toxins, both through the skin and through the urine (**depurative** properties). Its use is recommended for influenza, viral infections, and any type of chronic infections [❶,❷].

• **Lack of appetite.** All cinchona bark, but especially that one obtained from the red cinchona tree, have a marked appetizer and invigorator effect. Moreover, they are **digestive** and successfully fight intestinal fermentation [❷].

• **Cicatrizant. *In external applications,*** quine is a good **antiseptic** and promotes healing. It is used for **stomatitis** (inflammation of the oral mucosa), **mouth sores, pyorrhea, and pharyngitis** [❹]. It is also applied as compresses on any kind of wounds [❸].

• **Hair invigorator.** When applied as compresses, it renders good results in certain types of hair loss [❸].

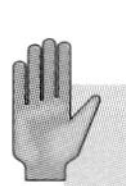

Warning

***Never exceed the** recommended **dose** in internal use, since it can provoke nausea and vomiting.*

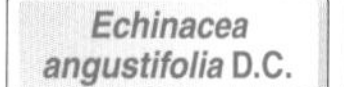

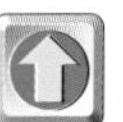

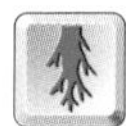

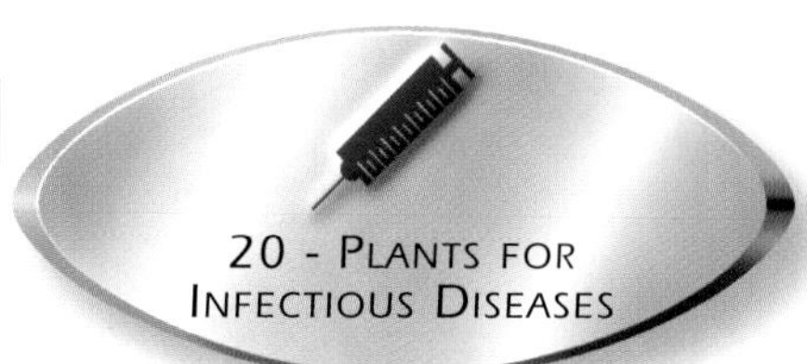

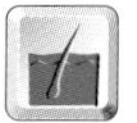

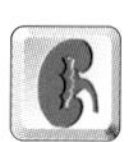

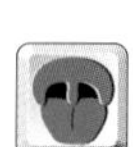

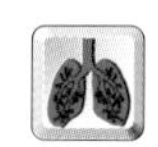

Echinacea

Heals and prevents by increasing defenses

THE NATIVES of the American states of Nebraska and Missouri used the root of echinacea to heal infected wounds and snake bites. By the late nineteenth century, Dr. Meyer, a medical researcher, discovered its properties while living among the Indians. From then onwards, echinacea has been the focus of many scientific studies, which revealed the many virtues of this plant, as well as its active mechanisms.

At present, echinacea is part of several ***pharmaceutical preparations,*** and it is one of the plants about which ***a higher number of scientific studies*** has been performed.

PROPERTIES AND INDICATIONS. The composition of the root of echinacea is highly complex. Many active substances have been identified, among these we can underline essential oil, responsible for the immune stimulation (incrase of defenses).

As frequently happens in phytotherapy, the extract of the plant (of its root, in this case) is much more active than any of its active components when isolated. This is due to the interaction among its components, when some of them enhance the action of others. Also there may be some unidentified active components.

The basic properties of echinacea are the following:

• **Immunostimulant.** It increases the defense mechanisms, with a general non-specific stimulation both in the humoral activity (antibody production, activation of the complementary system) and in the cell immunity (phagocytosis: destruction of micro-organisms by leukocytes). It produces an increase in the number of leukocytes in the blood.

• **Anti-inflammatory.** It prevents the progres-

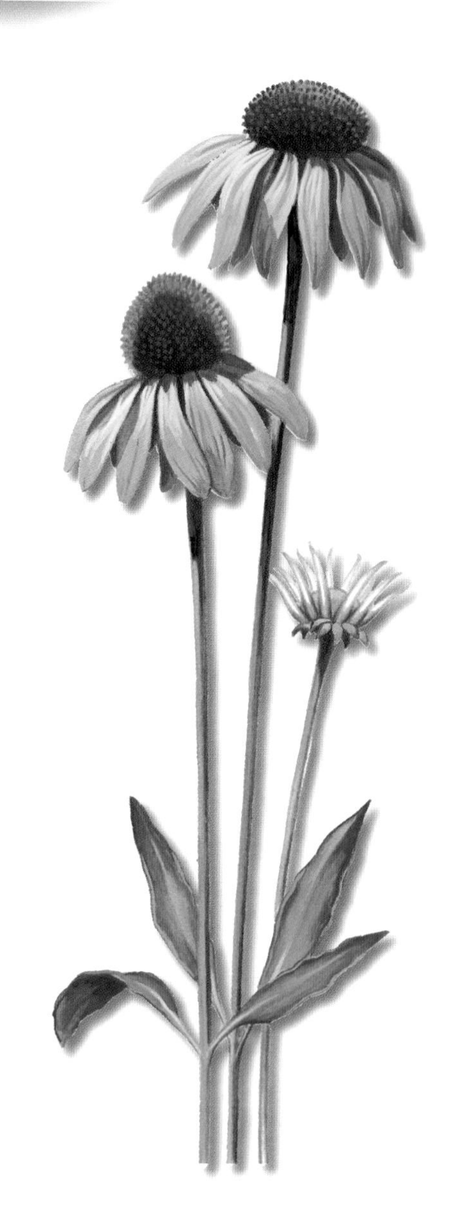

Description. *Plant of the Compositae family, whose hollow stems grow up to one meter high. It has elongated, hairy, narrow leaves, and mauve flowers which grow on the tip of the stems, and are quite exuberant.*

Parts used. *The root.*

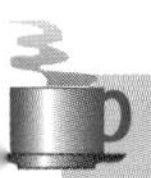

Preparation and Use

INTERNAL USE

❶ **Decoction** with 30-50 g of ground root per liter of water. Drink from three to five cups daily.

❷ **Pharmaceutical preparations.** Echinacea is usually presented in several forms: fluid extract, tincture, capsules, etc. In any case, carefully follow the instructions.

EXTERNAL USE

❸ **Compresses** with the same decoction used internally.

❹ **Lotions** with the liquid of the aforementioned decoction.

❺ **Pharmaceutical preparations:** creams, ointments, and other.

sion of infections, by inhibiting the enzyme hyaluronidase, produced by many bacteria species. It also promotes the growth of granulation tissue, which is responsible for wound healing; stimulates the reproduction of fiberblasts, which are basic cells of the connective tissue and are responsible for the regeneration of tissues and scar formation.

• **Antitoxic.** It stimulates the purifying process of the liver and kidneys, through which toxic and foreign substances flowing into the blood are neutralized and eliminated.

• **Antibiotic and antiviral.** This action has been experimentally proven *in vitro* (in a test tube). However, the property of stimulating defenses is more important *in vivo* (in the body).

• **Anticancerous.** It is able to destroy malignant cells (an effect which has been only proven *in vitro* up to now).

Hence, the clinical applications of this plant are **infectious diseases.** The best antibiotic will fail when our body's defenses do not cooperate in the fight against infection. Echinacea acts on the field, that is to say, on the body suffering from the infection, rather than destroying the causative agents. This means that its action is slower, and perhaps less spectacular than that of antibiotics; however in many cases it renders best results in the middle and long term. It has preventive and healing actions, and lacks the side effects antibiotics have.

It is recommended, among other cases, for **children's infectious diseases, influenza, sinusitis, tonsillitis, and** acute and chronic **respiratory infections,** especially when these are frequent (preventive effect); for **typhoid fever;** in all **septicemia** (blood infection) for any reason (gynecological, urinary, biliary, etc.) [❶,❷].

It has been applied in the treatment of ***AIDS,*** combined with other remedies, with promising results.

The best antibiotic treatment will fail if the defenses of the body do not cooperate to fight the infection.

Echinacea exerts a notable immunostimulant action (which increases defenses) by increasing the production and activity of antibodies and leukocytes (white blood cells) in the blood.

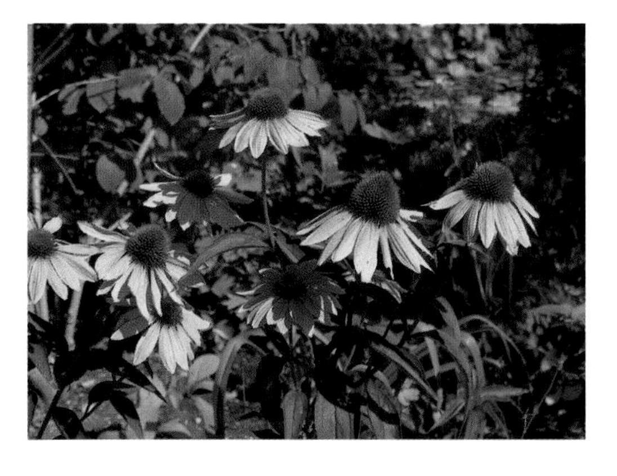

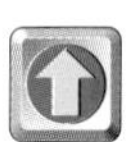

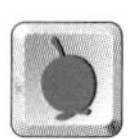

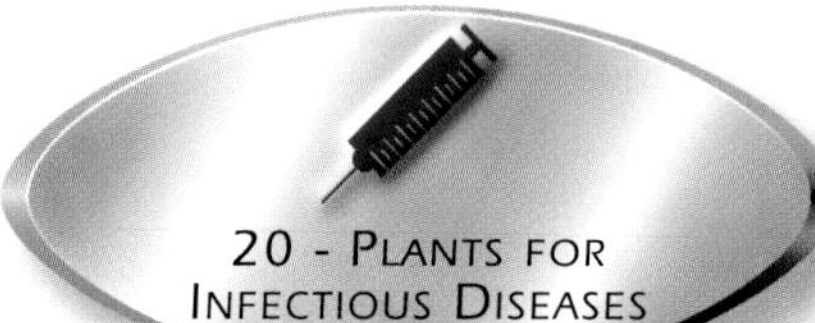

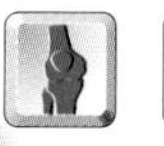

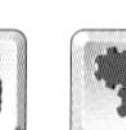

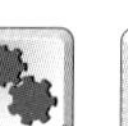

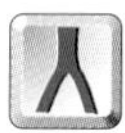

Noni

A true natural medication

NONI HAS BEEN used as a folk remedy for two millennia on the islands of Polynesia. However, only as recently as just over half a century ago did Western scientists become interested in this humble bush, so there was no data to confirm the healing properties attributed to it by the natives.

It is believed that the early settlers of the Polynesian islands took noni plants with them when they set off from Southeast Asia some two thousand years ago. Since then, they have been using the fruit, leaves and roots of this shrub as a folk remedy against numerous ailments.

Despite its somewhat unpleasant taste, noni fruit has also been used as food by the natives of Myanmar (former Burma) and other areas of Southeast Asia, India, Australia and the Pacific islands. World-famous Captain Cook of the British Navy left a record about the year 1700 that noni was already used in Tahiti. The earliest scientific research regarding noni was carried out about the middle of the 20th century.

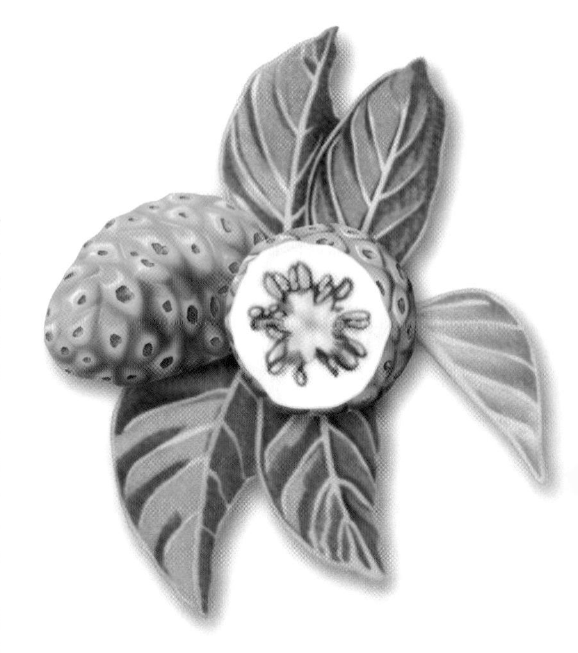

Description: *A small shrub of the Rubiaceae family, it is characterised by its narrow trunk, its big bright green, elliptic leaves and its tubular flowers.*

The ovoid fruit, yellowish or orange in colour, has a diameter of about 12 cm and its surface is full of small polyhedric-shaped lumps.

Used parts: *The fruit.*

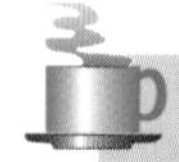

Preparation and Use

INTERNAL USE

❶ Noni juice:

– As a preventive medication, for the general upkeep of health: 2 spoonfuls (30 ml) every 24 or 12 hours.

– As a treatment of disease: 2 spoonfuls every 2, 3 or 4 hours, depending on the seriousness of the condition.

Doctors Levand, Heinicke and Solomon have distinguished themselves by their work about the composition and properties of noni.

COMPOSITION: More than 150 active substances have been identified in noni juice. Although the effects of them all are not known yet, significant advances have been made in the last few years. These are the best-known components in noni juice:

- **Alkaloids**: Ten alkaloids have been isolated in noni fruit. They all exert important pharmacological effects on the nervous, cardiovascular and immune systems, although they are present in very low concentrations.
- **Antraquinones**: These substances stand out because of their anti-carcinogenic and anti-inflammatory effect. One of the most widely studied is damnacanthal, which neutralises the effects carcinogens have on cells, thereby averting the development of tumours.
- **Escopoletin**: This is one of the most widely studied components because of its anti-infectious and immune system boost action.
- **Energising nutrients**: Just sugars such as fructose and glucose. It does not contain any fat or protein.
- **Vitamins**: Beta-carotene (provitamin A) and vitamins B, C and E.
- **Minerals, particularly potassium**.

PROPERTIES AND INDICATIONS: A few years ago, noni aroused a big deal of enthusiasm in the Western world, and some of its advocates recommended it to cure nearly any illness. Nowadays, several lines of scientific research have demonstrated the real healing properties of noni. They are certainly numerous, although perhaps not to the extent originally believed. These are the properties of noni that have been verified:

- **Anti-infectious**: Extracts of the ripe noni fruit have been proven effective in laboratory experiments against various types of micro-organisms:
  - Bacteria causing skin infections, such as Pseudomona aeruginosa.
  - Bacteria causing digestive infections, such as Escherichia coli, and others of the Salmonella and Shigella genera.
  - Mycobacterium tuberculosis, Koch's bacillus responsible for tuberculosis. Noni extract, particularly when it comes from its leaves, is almost as efficient 'in vitro' as the antibiotic Rifampicin in the destruction of the bacillus that causes tuberculosis.
  - Helicobacter pylori, responsible for gastritis and stomach ulcers: Noni juice has been shown to be efficient to inhibit the growth of this bacterium.
  - Viruses, including AIDS-causing HIV.

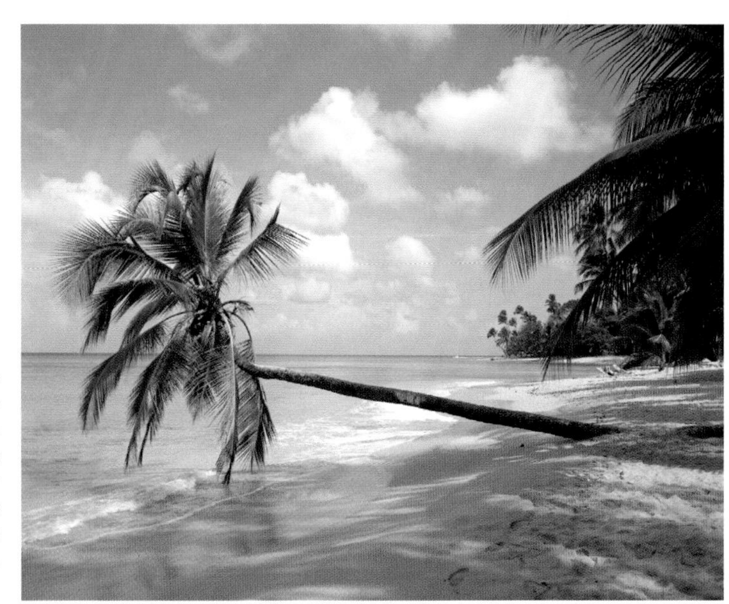

It is on the islands of the Tahiti archipelago that the best noni fruit is produced. Experts ascribe this to the high purity of air and water, and to the soil's wealth in micronutrients on those paradisiacal islands.

• **Analgesic and anti-inflammatory**: In test animals, noni juice soothes pain and produces a mild sedating effect. In a way similar to aspirin or indometacin, it inhibits COX-I enzymes responsible for swelling.[4]

• **Antihypertensive**: The extract of noni roots and, to a lesser extent, of the fruit produces some degree of vasodilation because it regulates the production of nitrous oxide, a substance that relaxes the walls of the arteries.

• **Immunestimulating**, Due to a polysaccharide found in noni fruit, it stimulates the production of antibodies and defensive 'T' cells. The volume of thymus, a gland closely connected with the defensive system, has been shown to increase by 70% after ingesting noni juice for 7 consecutive days.

• **Antioxidant**: Noni juice blocks the action of free radicals, aggressive chemical substances formed inside our body. This way, it protects against cancer, against arteriosclerosis and against the effects of cellular ageing.

• **Anti-cancer**: Noni is effective against cancer through several pathways:

- It protects DNA against the mutagenic effect of carcinogenic substances.
- It slows down the growth of tumours, favouring apoptosis (necrosis of tumour cells).
- It inhibits angiogenesis (formation of new capillaries and blood vessels) in the tumour, which hinders blood circulation in cancerous cells and slows down tumour development.
- It stimulates the immune system, particularly defensive 'T' cells that destroy tumour cells.

No clinical tests have been carried out yet to confirm in clinical practice all the healing properties of noni verified in laboratory experiments. However, there are enough signs to recommend the use of noni in these cases:

• **Skin infections**, applied directly on the affected area.

• **Infections of the digestive tract** (gastroenteritis and colitis).

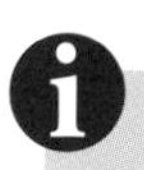

Noni and cancer

In 1992 a researcher at the University of Hawaii showed at the yearly meeting of the American Association for Cancer Research that the alcohol precipitate of noni juice, known as 'noni-ppt,' has an anti-carcinogenic activity. Approximately 75% of the mice with lung cancer that were administered noni juice extended their life span relative to the control group.

It has also been shown to be effective against cultured cells of leukemia, in which it induces apoptosis (cellular death), destroying them. Other experiments have shown it is also effective against cancerous cells of the pancreas and the colon.

This anti-carcinogenic effect is attributed to two glucosides present in noni juice. Experiments carried out recently with mice have shown that noni juice achieves the cure of 25 to 45% of the animals affected by sarcoma (a type of cancer).[8]

Noni has been shown to foster the effect of certain medications used in cancer chemotherapy, whereas it slows down the effect of others.

- Taking noni with the following chemotherapies is beneficial: Cisplatin, adriamycin, mitomycin-C, bleomycin, etoposide, 5-fluoracil, vincristine, camptothecin, Th-1 cytokine, imexon and interferon gamma. Anyone undergoing treatment with any of these medications can simultaneously have noni juice to obtain a larger anti-carcinogenic effect.[8]

- On the contrary, since it reduces their effect, noni should not be taken with the following medications: Th-2 cytokine, MVE-2 copolymer, interleukin-2, 4, 10 and 12.

- **Infections in general**, particularly those of viral type.
- **High blood pressure**, heart disease, arteriosclerosis, excess cholesterol.
- **Digestive disorders**, gastroduodenal ulcer.
- **Arthritis**, joint- or muscle-related rheumatic pain, inflammatory conditions resulting from various causes.
- **Diabetes**.
- **Depression**, senility, premature ageing.
- **AIDS**.
- **Cancer**.

TOXICITY AND SIDE EFFECTS: Noni juice has been proven to be well tolerated in animal trials up to a limit of 80 ml per kilo of weight per day (about 5 litres a day for an adult). This allows for a very large, safe therapeutic margin, since the customary effective dose is much smaller.

Adverse side effects are generally slight and infrequent. The following have been reported:

- **Slight burping** in 5% of the cases; it disappears when the dosage is diminished.
- **Skin allergy**, with a slight rash in the first two days after noni juice begins to be taken. It subsides spontaneously.
- **Hyperkaliemia** (excess potassium): Noni juice contains about 100 mg of potassium for every 100 ml, less than orange, apple or pineapple juice. Even so, this should be taken into account for patients suffering from kidney failure or uncompensated diabetes, in which high levels of potassium can cause heart alterations.
- A single case of toxic hepatitis with elevated liver transaminase enzymes has been reported after taking noni for 3 weeks.

Noni is not toxic for the foetus or the suckling. So, pregnant women and lactating mothers can also take it.

Noni is a true natural plant-based medication discovered a few decades ago on the beautiful islands of the Pacific Ocean. Noni is endowed with outstanding healing properties, and it is free of side effects. Undoubtedly, it is worth a try.

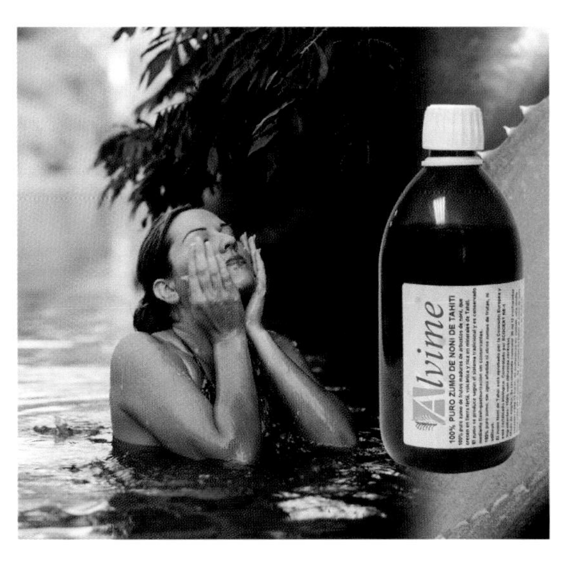

The usual preparation is noni juice bottled by specialised laboratories. It is recommended that it be pure, not coming from concentrate, and harvested from organic certified crops.

Just before drinking it, it can be mixed with water, or with blueberry or grape juice in order to mask its bad taste.

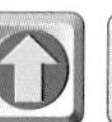
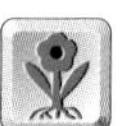
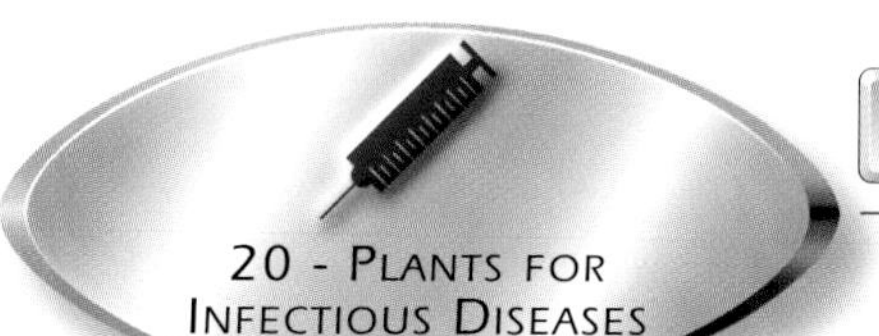

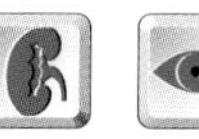
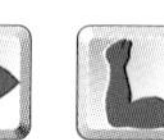
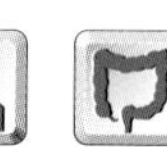

Brier Hip

A vitaminic concentration which is absolutely natural

THE INNER surface of the brier hip fruit is covered by a layer of blonde, rigid hair, popularly called "itch-scratch," about which Font Quer said that "provokes itching when introduced between the shirt and the skin. The same is felt around the anus when, after eating brier hip fruit, these hairs cross the whole digestive tract undamaged and leave their host."

PROPERTIES AND INDICATIONS. The ***FRUIT*** of brier hip contains diverse sugars and organic acids, as well as pectin, mineral salts, carotene (provitamin A), and vitamins B_1, B_2, C, E, and P (flavonoids). Its content in vitamin C reaches 600 mg per 100 g, and can be up to 800 mg, being superior to that of lemon, which only contains 50 mg. Therefore, brier hip is ***one of the richest plants in vitamin C,*** ranked over the currant (181 mg) and kiwi (98 mg). Brier hip is only second to the exceptional *Malpighia punicifolia* L., *Malpighia glabra* L. (Acerola), fruit which, when ripe, can reach 2500 mg of vitamin C per 100 g, and when green can reach 6000 mg.

The properties of the brier hip ***FRUIT*** are the following:

- **Invigorating and antiscorbutic.** They are useful for **physical exhaustion, asthenia** (Spring fatigue), **and convalescence** **[❶,❷]**. Brier hip fruits are a ***true concentrate of natural vitamins,*** especially vitamin C. Though scurvy (lack of vitamin C) is a rare ailment in developed countries, a high supply of this vitamin has an invigorating effect.
- **Immunostimulant.** The fruit of brier hip is used as defense stimulants, especially to ***prevent*** **influenza and colds.** It is recommended for all **infectious diseases,** especially in children **[❶,❷]**.

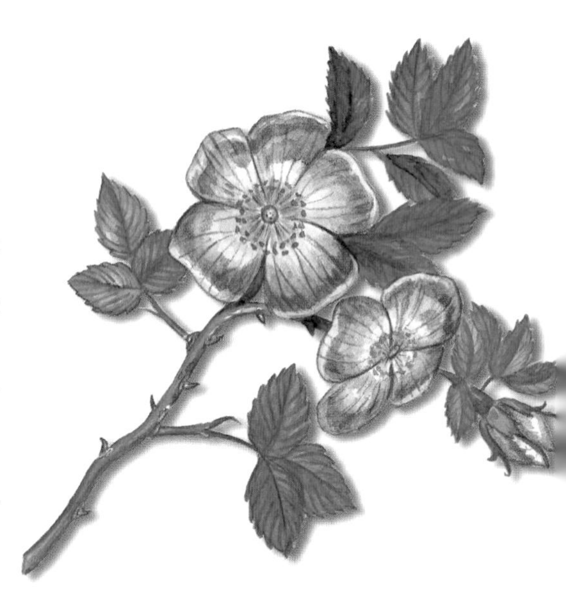

Description. *Shrub of the Rosaceae family, growing from one to three meters high, with prickly stems. The leaves are alternated, with 5-7 oval folioles, and toothed edges. The flowers have five pink or whitish petals. What is commonly known as fruit, red, and olive-shaped, is a pseudo-fruit, formed by the remains of the flower calyx.*

Parts used. *The fruits, the flowers, the leaves, and the root.*

- **Diuretic and depurative.** They are recommended for edema (retention of liquids), overload diet when it is rich in meat and animal products, gout and arthritis, and whenever the action of a mild diuretic with depurative properties is required **[❶,❷]**.

The ***FRUIT*** of brier hip has been used, eating it whole, against taeniae and other intestinal parasites, though with no scientific basis. Some people said that they were effective due to their itching hairs, which intestinal parasites could not endure.

Preparation and Use

INTERNAL USE

❶ **Fresh fruit.** This is the best way to take advantage of the vitaminic content of brier hip. Choose ripe fruit, open it, and wash under water, withdrawing all hairs and seeds. Eat a generous handful every day.

❷ **Fruit decoction,** with 50-60 g of fruit per liter of water. Drink four or five cups daily. Vitamin C is lost, but its diuretic, depurative, and mild astringent properties remain.

❸ **Decoction of root and leaves,** with 100 g of root and/of leaves of brier hip in one and a half liters of water. Boil until the liquid reduces to one liter. Drink several cups daily, as an antidiarrheic.

EXTERNAL USE

❹ **Water of roses.** Steep in cold extract a handful of brier hip petals in a glass of water. After 24 hours, wring them out and throw away the petals. **Wash the eyes** with the resulting liquid.

The ***PETALS*** of its flowers contain pectin, tannin, organic acids, and small amounts of essence. Like all rose petals they serve as an ingredient to prepare **rose water** from which good results are obtained when washing eyes suffering from **conjunctivitis or blepharitis** (inflammation of the eyelids) [❹].

The ***LEAVES*** and the ***ROOT*** contain tannic acid, and have astringent properties. They are used for simple **diarrhea** and **gastroenteritis** [❸].

The ***SEEDS*** of brier hip, very hard, not only lack any effect on urine calculi as it was formerly thought, but when ground, they liberate a **toxic essence** which affects the nervous system.

The fruit of brier hip, which is also known as wild brier and eglantine gall, is a true natural tonic, recommended for children and adults, for both healthy and unhealthy people.

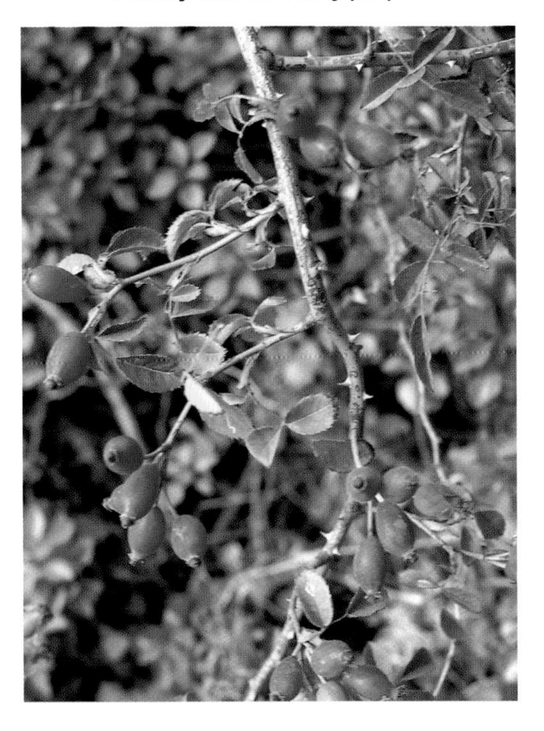

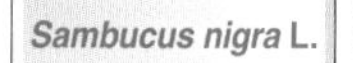
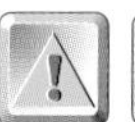
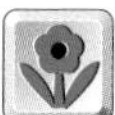
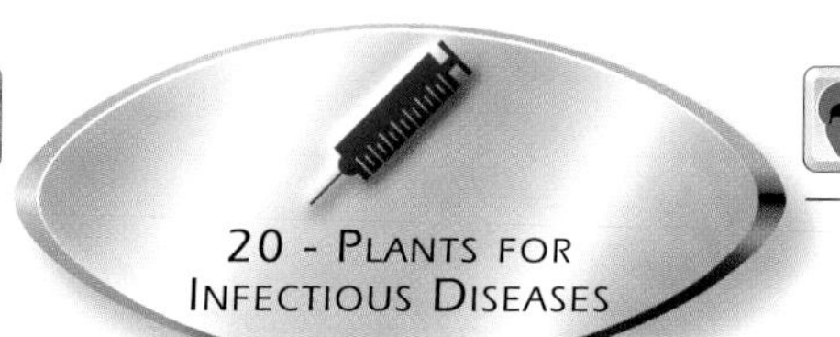

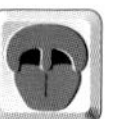
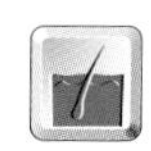
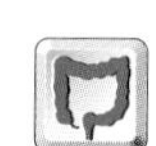
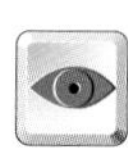

Black Elder

A good remedy for fever and colds

THE BERRIES of black elder have been a food for humans since ancient times, even though the smell of its leaves can be unpleasant. Black elder is worthy to be distinguished from another similar species, the dwarf elder (*Sambucus ebulus* L.) whose flowers and leaves have the same properties black elder, but whose fruits are poisonous. Here are some details which can help distinguish both species:

✓ **Black elder** is a shrub with **woody trunk and branches,** while the **dwarf elder** is a **herbaceous** (like an herb) plant.

✓ **Black elder** has **five or seven folioles** per leaf, while **dwarf elder** has **eleven or more.**

✓ The **fruits** of black elder **hang down** when ripe, while those of **dwarf elder keep** upright.

✓ The **smell** of black elder is **not as strong** and unpleasant as that of dwarf elder.

PROPERTIES AND INDICATIONS. The flowers, which are the part of black elder most often used in phytotherapy, contain mineral salts (especially potassium nitrate), flavonic glycosides (rhutin and quercetin), and organic acids, which give them **sudorific, diuretic, depurative,**

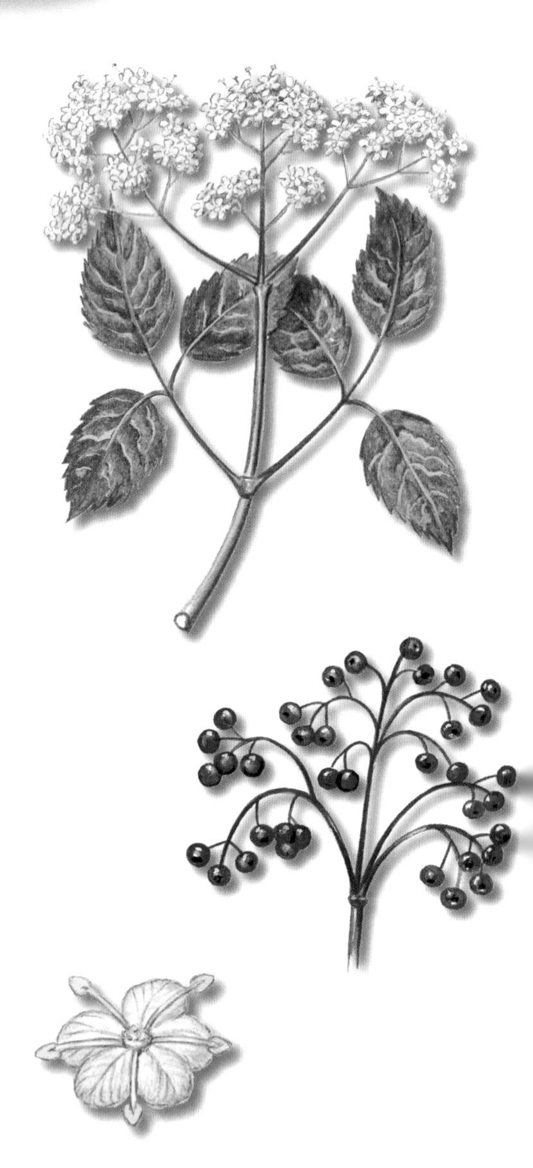

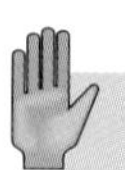

Warning

*Never eat **large amounts of berries** of the black elder, since they can provoke **nausea** and digestive **intolerance.***

***Description.** Shrub of the Caprifoliaceae family, growing from two to four meters high, with deciduous, large leaves, each one comprising five or seven lanceolated folioles, with toothed edges. The flowers are whitish and grow in umbels. The fruits are small berries, black or violet in color.*

***Parts used.** The flowers, the fruits, and the inner bark of the trunk and branches (liber).*

and anti-inflammatory properties. Due to their content in mucilage, they also have a mild laxative action.

The ***FLOWERS*** of the black elder are ***one of the most effective sudorific and depurative substances*** known, and are recommended in any kind of febrile states, especially the following ones.

- **Catarrh, colds, and influenza,** to provoke an abundant perspiration and depurative action as well as reducing congestion. They also ease **coughs** [❶].
- **Children's rash diseases.** For measles, chicken pox, and scarlet fever, with the perspiration provoked by black elder, waste substances (toxins) are eliminated, and fever decreases [❶].
- **Throat afflictions.** As rinses and gargles, the infusion of black elder flowers is recommended for pharyngitis, stomatitis, and tonsillitis [❼].
- **Skin afflictions.** For furuncles, eczema, acne, and other dermatosis, compresses and baths with an infusion of black elder leaves render good results [❺,❻].
- **Conjunctivitis.** Apply compresses on the eyes and/or eye baths with the infusion of black elder flowers [❺,❻].

The ***LEAVES*** of black elder have similar properties to those of the flowers, though their infusion is less pleasant due to their strong smell [❷].

The ***LIBER,*** that is to say, the inner bark of the trunk and branches (the one left after superficially scratching them) has **purgative and diuretic** properties. It has been used since ancient times for edema (retention of fluids) and dropsy (retention of fluids in the whole body), as well as ascitis (accumulation of fluids in the abdominal cavity) [❸].

The ***BERRIES*** of black elder contain organic acids, sugar, vitamin C, and a cyanogenic glycoside (sambunigrin), whose toxicity is uncertain, but when taken ***in moderate amounts is harmless.*** Due to their composition, they have **invigorating and laxative** properties [❹].

Preparation and Use

INTERNAL USE

❶ **Infusion of flowers,** with 20-30 g per liter of water. Drink from three to five hot cups daily.

❷ **Infusion of leaves,** with 10-15 g per liter of water. Drink from three to five cups daily.

❸ **Decoction,** with 70-100 g of liber (inner bark) per liter of water. Drink three cups a day.

❹ The **fruit** can be eaten fresh, or in the form of an extract known as **black elder rob**.

EXTERNAL USE

❺ **Compresses** soaked in a concentrated infusion of flowers (50-60 g per liter).

❻ **Cleansing** of the affected skin area or of the eyes, with the concentrated infusion.

❼ **Mouth rinses and gargles** with the aforementioned infusion.

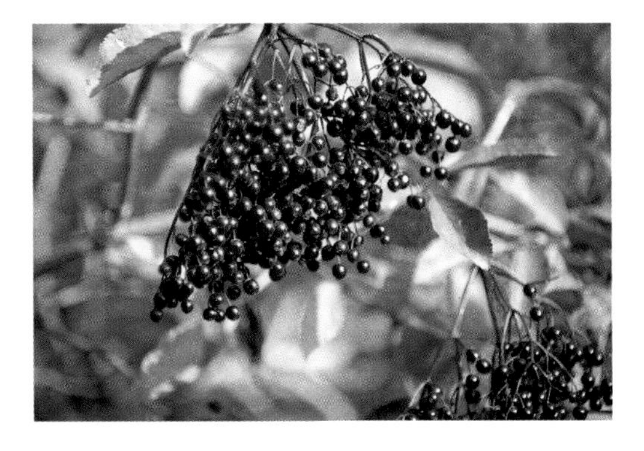

The fruit of the black elder has invigorating and laxative properties. And its flowers are one of the best sudorifics and depuratives, both for children and adults, for infectious diseases which occur accompanied by fever.

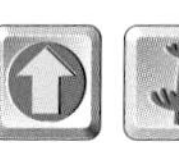

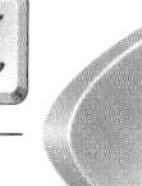

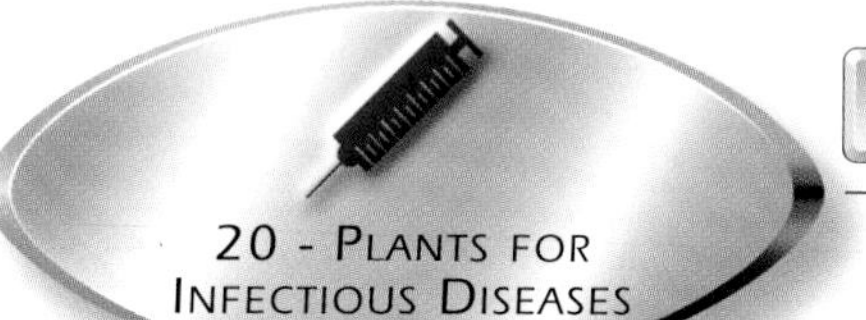

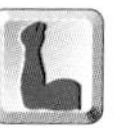

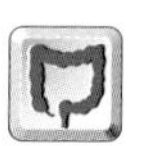

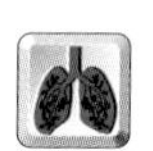

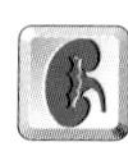

Thyme

Powerful antiseptic and natural stimulant

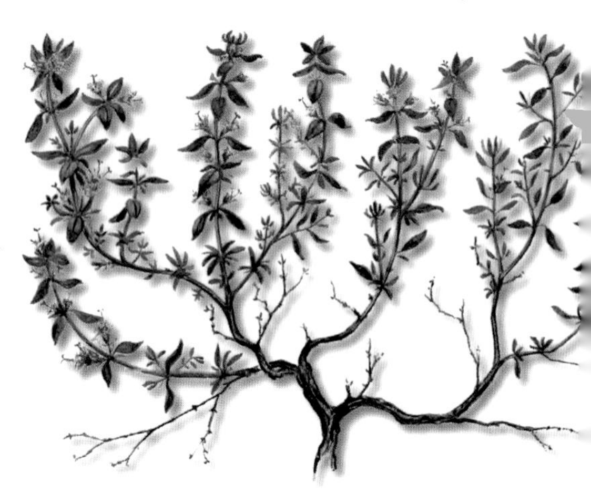

THE PLEASANT aroma of thyme already drew the attention of ancient Egyptians, who used it to make ointments for embalming. At present, we know that its ability to prevent putrefaction and bacteria reproduction is due to its content of thymol and carvacrol, two powerful antiseptic substances.

PROPERTIES AND INDICATIONS. The plant contains 1%-2% of essence rich in two isomers, thymol and carvacrol, as well as other monoterpenes such as p-cymene, borneol, and geraniol. Thyme owes most of its properties to this essence.

The use of thyme is adequate in the following cases:

• **Antiseptic.** The ***essence*** has an antiseptic power ***superior*** to that of ***phenol*** and ***peroxide.*** In the nineteenth century and the early twentieth century, when antibiotics were still not known, thyme was regarded as the "disinfectant of the poor."

Its antimicrobial action is enhanced by the capabilities of thyme to **stimulate leukocytosis** (increase of leukocytes in the blood), as it has been experimentally proven. Unlike antibiotics, which depress the **immune system** (defenses), thyme **stimulates** it, promoting the activity of leukocytes.

The use of thyme is thus recommended for all **infectious diseases,** and especially those with a bacterial cause affecting the **digestive, respiratory, genital, and urinary systems.**

• **Digestive system. Antispasmodic, eupeptic** (digestion invigorating), and **carminative** (prevents flatulence and gas formation). It increases appetite, promotes digestion, and combats intestinal putrefactions caused by imbalances in the colon flora.

__Description.__ Little shrub of the Labiatae family, growing up to 30 cm high, with winding woody stems, very branched. The leaves are small, oval-shaped, with edges turned downside, and lighter on their undersides. The flowers are small, terminal, pink or white in color, with the upper lip divided into three superficial teeth, and the lower one into two deep teeth.

__Parts used.__ The flower clusters (leaves and flowers).

It is recommended for gastroenteritis and colitis caused by bacteria of the genus *Salmonella*, responsible for many **infections caused by food** in bad condition, especially in Summer [❶,❷].

• **Vermifuge** (it expels intestinal parasites). Especially active with taeniae. It is also a good **insecticide** for lice and fleas [❶,❷].

• **Oral and pharyngeal afflictions.** As rinsings it combats **sores, pyorrhea, and stomatitis** (inflammation or irritation of the oral mucosa). As gargles it is very effective to treat **pharyngitis and tonsillitis** [❸].

• **Respiratory system.** Thyme has **expecto-**

Preparation and Use

INTERNAL USE

❶ **Infusion,** with 20-30 g of flower clusters per liter of water. Drink up to five cups daily. When **concentrated,** (50-60 g per liter), it achieves a **stimulant effect** similar to that of tea or coffee, but lacking any of their disadvantages.

❷ **Essence.** Do not exceed the dose of 2-3 drops, three times a day.

EXTERNAL USE

❸ **Mouth rinses and gargles** with a decoction made with 100-120 g of flower clusters per liter of water, boiling until the liquid reduces to a half.

❹ **Steam inhalations** with the essence.

❺ **Compresses and baths** with this decoction.

❻ **Lotions and massage** with the decoction or the essence.

❼ **Baths:** Infusion with 300-500 g of thyme in 2-3 liters of water, this can be added to the bathwater.

❽ **Poultices.** Wrap flowers and leaves of thyme, without branches, in a cotton cloth. Heat the cloth on an iron, or over a heater, and apply to the aching area.

rant, antitussive, and balsamic properties, which together with its **antiseptic** powers make it very useful for sinusitis, laryngitis, bronchial catarrh and bronchitis, asthma, spasmodic cough, and whooping cough. In these cases we recommend taking its infusion [❶] or essence [❷], and take inhalations [❹] as we describe in the box on this page.

We recommend its consumption during **influenza** epidemics, whether as infusion or in the more traditional thyme soup, as well as in salad dressing.

• **Genital and urinary system.** Due to its **diuretic and antiseptic** properties, it is recommended for urinary **infections** (cystitis and glomerulonephritis) [❶,❷].

When ***externally*** applied as cleansing, it acts favorably on infection on the **external genitalia** caused by lack of hygiene, diabetes, or other reasons, both in females (vaginitis, vulvitis with or without leukorrhea) and in males (balanitis, posthitis, infection of the glans and the foreskin) [❺].

When applied as hot poultice, it alleviates **colic renal pain** and that of **cystitis.**

• **Antirrheumatic.** ***Externally*** applied as a massage, baths, and poultices, it calms rheumatic aches caused by arthritis and gout [❻,❼,❽]. When ***orally taken*** [❶,❷] it also has **diuretic and sudorific** properties, eliminating from the blood any excess acid metabolic waste which causes arthritis and gout.

In ***external*** applications, thyme also alleviates pain caused by **stiff neck, lumbalgia, sciatica, arthrosis,** etc. [❻,❼,❽].

• **Skin infections.** As baths and compresses it is applied on infected or torpid wounds, sores, varicose ulcerations, chilblains, furuncles, abscesses, dermatitis, etc. [❺].

Due to its **antiparasite** properties, it is very useful for scabies and lice and flea infestation.

• **Hair invigorating.** Applied as a lotion or massage on the scalp, it gives strength to the hair and prevents its loss [❻].

Thyme is a medicinal herb with many well proven medicinal virtues. As hot poultices it alleviates cystitis aches and renal colic.

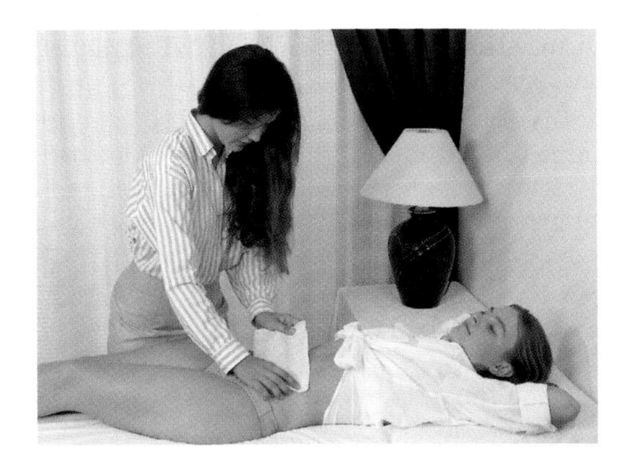

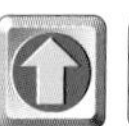
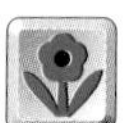
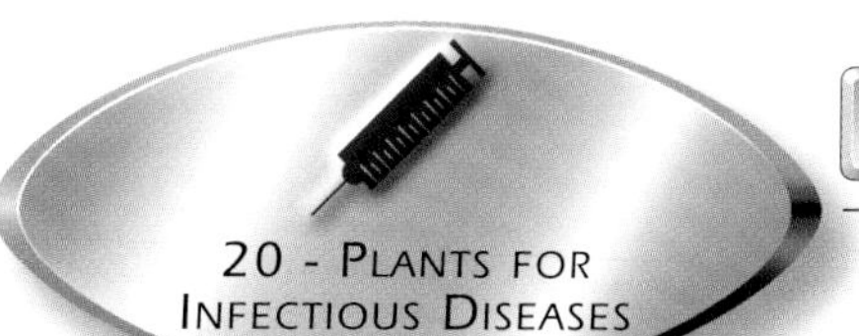

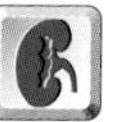
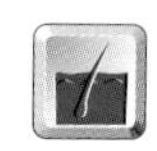
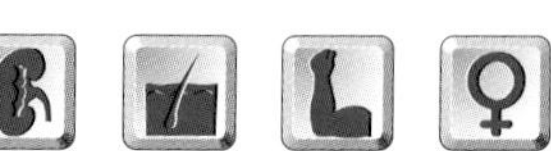
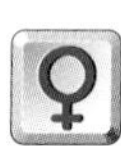

Nasturtium

A natural antibiotic of proven effectiveness

MANY ANTIBIOTICS used in therapeutics are produced by fungi and bacteria. Nasturtium is ***one of the few superior plants*** known ***to have the capability of producing a natural antibiotic substance,*** which presents the following advantages over conventional antibiotics.

✓ **It does not destroy the bacterial flora** usually living in the digestive conduct. Nasturtium does not produce diarrhea or intestinal decomposition, two frequent symptoms when taking orally other antibiotics.

✓ **It does not produce sensitivities or allergic reactions,** quite common when using other antibiotics.

✓ **Its application is easy and comfortable.** It requires neither injections, nor suppositories. It can be ingested in the form of a succulent salad vegetable, which has a pleasant flavor similar to that of mustard.

PROPERTIES AND INDICATIONS. All parts of the plant contain a sulphur glycoside, glucotropaeolin, which through the action of myrosine, an enzyme contained in the plant itself, and which is liberated when breaking or mashing the plant, produces, among other substances, a sulphur essential oil with ***powerful*** **antibiotic** properties. After taking the plant, this essential oil passes into the blood, and is eliminated through the respiratory and urinary systems. In these organs is where the oil reaches a higher concentration, produces its antimicrobial actions, preventing bacterial growth and reproduction. This means that the two most important applications of nasturtium are the following:

• **Infections of the respiratory system:** sinusitis, rhinitis, pharyngitis, and especially bron-

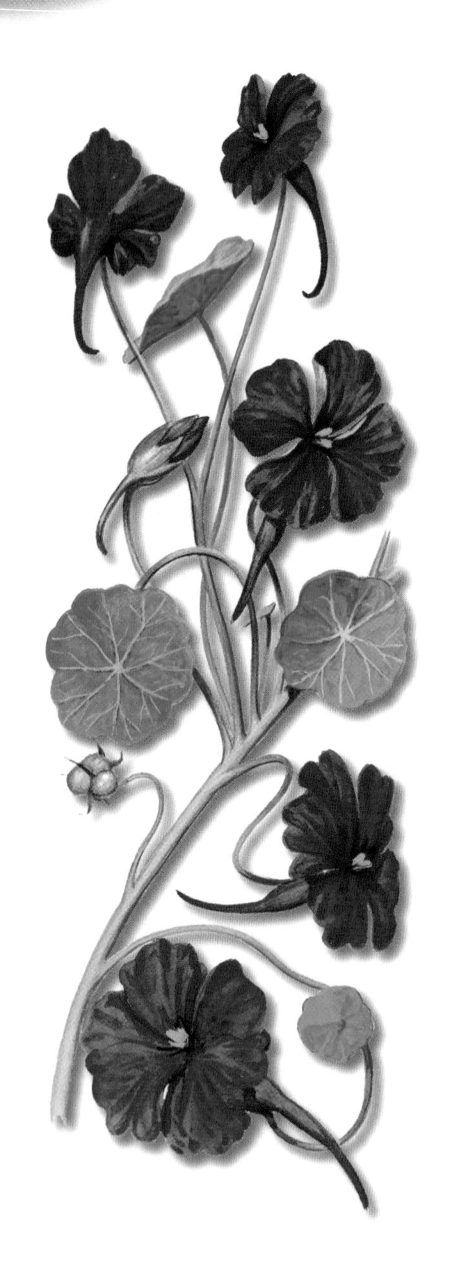

Description. *Herbaceous annual plant of the Tropaeolaceae family, which usually grows like a creeper. It has round leaves, with five groins, and exuberant orange flowers with five petals.*

Parts used. *The leaves, the flowers, and the fruit.*

Preparation and Use

INTERNAL USE

❶ **Salad** (as invigorating and appetizer). Use young flowers and leaves. It combines perfectly with lettuce.

❷ **Infusion or decoction.** Prepared with 30 g of flowers, leaves, and fruit, per liter of water. Drink a cup every four hours.

EXTERNAL USE

❸ **Sitz baths.** A handful of flowers or fruit per liter of water. The bath must be hot.

❹ **Lotions.** Grind two handfuls (20 g) of leaves, flowers, and fresh seeds of nasturtium. Then, steep in cold extract in half a liter of ethyl alcohol 96%, for two weeks. To this cold extract you can add ten leaves of nettle, five leaves of boxwood, and a spoonful of rosemary. Strain, and with the resulting liquid, energetically rub the scalp.

chitis, both acute and chronic. Dr. Leclerc, a famous French phytotherapist physician, stated that the use of nasturtium "gives expectoration of people suffering from bronchitis a greater fluidity, and from being mucopurulent it becomes simply mucus" (**mucolytic** action). It is also useful for influenza and colds, since its active component with antibiotic action impregnates the whole respiratory system, reducing the congestion of the bronchi and easing coughs [❶,❷].

• **Infections of the urinary system:** Pyelonephritis (renal pelvis and kidney) and cystitis (urinary bladder) [❶,❷]. Dr. Schneider wrote about experiences which prove that, nine hours after eating a nasturtium salad, its active principle with antibiotic action is still detected in the urine.

Besides its antibiotic properties, nasturtium has other properties.

• **It promotes skin functions,** because of its high content in sulphur. When ***locally applied*** it has **cicatrizant** effects on wounds and sores. It regenerates and gives smoothness to the dry skin, and stimulates the hair bulb (the root of hair), **revitalizing hair** and even making it grow again. Hence, nasturtium is ***one of the plants most used*** in **hair-loss** treatments. In order to enhance its effects, you should shave your head before applying it [❹].

• **Invigorating and tonic.** Perhaps due to its high content in vitamin C (285 mg per 100 g of fresh leaves, while lemon contains, for instance, only 50 mg per 100 g of flesh) [❶,❷].

• **Menstrual regulator.** According to Mességué, sitz baths with nasturtium flowers or fruits balance and normalize the menstrual cycle [❸].

• **Aphrodisiac.** Moreover, and perhaps with a certain base, nasturtium is said to have aphrodisiac effects [❶,❷]. It has been called the **"love flower".** Taste it!

Nasturtium has proven to be one of the more effective antibiotic plants in treating infections of the respiratory and urinary systems. Moreover, it is a basic component of diverse preparations and shampoos which revitalize hair.

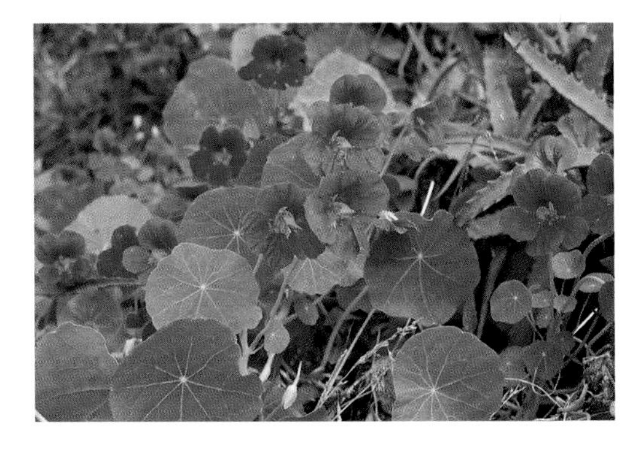

Index of Scientific Names

Abies alba (Silver Fir), 150
Abies balsamea (Canadian Fir Tree), 151
Achillea millefolium (Milfoil), 342
Aesculus hippocastanum (Horse Chestnut), 130
Agave americana (Agave), 272
Agrimonia eupatoria (Sticklework), 99
Agropyrum repens (Witch Grass), 273
Allium sativum (Garlic), 118
Aloe vera (Aloe), 344
Althaea officinalis (Althea), 94
Anethum graveolens (Dill), 173
Anthyllis vulneraria (Kidney Vetch), 327
Arctium lappa (Burdock), 346
Arctostaphylos uva-ursi (Bearberry), 274
Arnica montana (Arnica), 321
Artemisia vulgaris (Mugwort), 294
Arundo donax (Cane), 276

Barosma betulina (Buchu), 277
Bellis perennis (Wild Daisy), 362
Berberis vulgaris (Barberry), 194
Betula alba (White Birch), 278
Bixa orellana (Annatto Tree), 347
Brassica nigra (Black Mustard), 322

Calendula officinalis (Calendula), 296
Capsella bursa-pastoris (Shepherd's Purse), 298
Carum carvi (Caraway), 174
Cassia angustifolia (Tinnevelly Senna), 242
Cassia fistula (Purging Cassia), 244
Ceanothus americanus (New Jersey Tea), 95
Centaurea cyanus (Cornflower), 60
Cephaelis ipecacuana (Ipecac), 210
Ceratonia siliqua (Carob Tree), 245
Cereus gradiflorus (Cactus), 108
Cetraria islandica (Iceland Moss), 152
Chenopodium ambrosioides (Wormseed), 211
Chondrus crispus (Irish Moss), 153
Chrysophyllum caimito (Caimito), 154
Cichorium intybus (Chicory), 212
Cinchona officinalis (Cinchona Tree), 364
Cinnamomum aromaticum
(Chinese Cinnamon), 215
Cinnamomum camphora (Camphor Tree), 109
Cinnamomum zeylanicum (Cinnamon Tree), 214
Citrus aurantium (Orange Tree), 70
Copaifera officinalis (Copaiba), 280
Coriandrum sativum (Coriander), 216
Crataegus monogyna (Hawthorn), 110
Crocus sativus (Saffron), 217
Cuminum cyminum (Cumin), 218
Cupressus sempervirens (Cypress), 132
Curcuma longa (Turmeric), 219
Cynara scolymus (Artichoke), 197

Digitalis purpurea (Foxglove), 112

Echinacea angustifolia (Equinacea), 366
Ephedra distachya (Desert Tea), 155
Epilobium angustifolium (Willowherb), 246
Equisetum arvense (Horsetail), 348
Eryngium campestre (Eryngo), 281
Eucalyptus globulus (Eucalyptus), 156
Eugenia caryophyllata (Clove Tree), 96
Euphrasia officinalis (Red Eyebright), 62

Fagus silvatica (Beech Tree), 247
Filipendula ulmaria (Meadow-Sweet), 324
Foeniculum vulgare (Fennel), 175
Fraxinus excelsior (Common Ash Tree), 326
Fucus vesiculosus (Fucus), 312
Fumaria officinalis (Fumitory), 196

Gentiana lutea (Gentian), 220
Geranium robertianum
(Herb Robert), 63
Ginkgo biloba (Ginkgo), 122
Glycyrrhiza glabra (Licorice), 158

Hamamelis virginiana (Witch Hazel), 129
Harpagophytum procumbens (Devil's Claw), 328
Hedeoma pulegioides (American Pennyroyal), 227
Hibiscus abelmoschus (Abelmosk), 176
Hibiscus sabdariffa (Guinea Sorrel), 177
Humulus lupulus (Hops), 72
Hydrastis canadensis (Goldenseal), 100
Hypericum perforatum (St. Johnswort), 350

Illicium verum (Star Anise), 222

Jasonia glutinosa (Rock's Tea), 223
Juglans regia (Walnut Tree), 248
Juniperus communis (Juniper), 282

Krameria triandra (Rhatany), 97

Lactuca virosa (Prickly Lettuce), 73
Laminaria saccharina (Kelp), 314
Laurus nobilis (Laurel), 224
Lavandula angustifolia (Lavender), 74
Linum usitatissimum (Flax), 250
Lippia triphylla (Lemon Verbena), 225

Malva silvestris (High Mallow), 252
Matricaria chamomilla (German Camomile), 178
Medicago sativa (Alfalfa), 137
Melissa officinalis (Balm), 76
Mentha piperita (Peppermint), 180
Mentha pulegium (European Pennyroyal), 226
Morinda citrifolia (Noni), 368

Nasturtium officinalis (Watercress), 138
Nepeta cataria (Catnip), 181

Ocimum basilicum (Basil), 182
Oenothera biennis (Evening Primrose), 124
Opuntia ficus-indica (Prickly Pear), 352
Orchis mascula (Early Purple Orchid), 253
Origanum majorana (Marjoram), 183
Origanum vulgare (Wild Marjoram), 228
Ortosiphon stamineus (Javan Tea), 315

Panax ginseng (Ginseng), 300
Parietaria officinalis (Pellitory of the Wall), 283
Passiflora edulis (Purple Passion Flower), 79
Passiflora incarnata (Passion Flower), 78
Peumus boldus (Boldo), 198
Physalis viscosa (Ground Cherry), 353
Pimpinela anisum (Anise), 230
Pinus pinaster (Pine Tree), 160
Pistacia lentiscus (Mastic Tree), 98
Plantago major (Common Plantain), 162
Plantago psyllium (Psyllium), 254
Polygonum bistortum (Bistort), 93
Portulaca oleracea (Purslane), 256
Potentilla erecta (Tormentil), 257
Prunus spinosa (Blackthorn), 184
Pulmonaria officinalis (Lungwort), 164

Quassia amara (Quassia), 229
Quercus robur (Oak Tree), 102

Rhamnus frangula (Alder Buckthorn), 258
Rhamnus purshiana (Cascara Sagrada), 260
Rheum officinale Baillon (Rhubarb), 261
Ricinus communis (Castor Bean), 262
Robinia pseudoacacia (False Acacia), 232
Rosa canina (Brier Hip), 372
Rosa gallica (Rose), 302
Rosmarinus officinalis (Rosemary), 330
Rubia tinctorum (Madder), 284
Rubus fruticosus (Bramble), 264
Ruta graveolens (Rue), 303

Saccharum officinarum (Sugar Cane), 165
Salix alba (White Willow), 332
Salvia officinalis (Sage), 304
Sambucus nigra (Black Elder), 374
Santolina chamaecyparissus
(Lavender Cotton), 233
Satureja fruticosa (White Savory), 187
Satureja hortensis (Summer Savory), 187
Satureja montana (Winter Savory), 186
Satureja odorata (Tiny Savory), 187
Saxifraga granulata (Saxifrage), 285
Serenoa repens (Shrub Palmetto), 306
Silybum marianum (Milk Thistle), 200
Sisymbrium officinale (Hedge Mustard), 101
Solidago virga-aurea (Goldenrod), 286
Spirulina maxima (Spirulina), 140
Symphytum officinalis (Comfrey), 354

Tamarindus indica (Tamarind), 263
Taraxacum officinale (Dandelion), 202
Thymus serpyllum (Mother of Thyme), 166
Thymus vulgaris (Thyme), 376
Tilia europaea (Linden), 80
Trigonella foenum-graecum (Fenugreek), 234
Tropaeolum majus (Nasturtium), 378
Turnera diffusa (Damiana), 307

Urtica dioica (Nettle), 142

Valeriana officinalis (Valerian), 82
Vanilla planifolia Andrews (Vanilla), 188
Verbena hastata (Blue Vervain), 84
Verbena officinalis (Vervain), 84
Veronica officinalis (Speedwell), 235
Viola odorata (Garden Violet), 168

Zingiber officinale (Ginger), 189

Source of Illustrations

All **photographs,** except those being specified below according to their page, have been taken by:

Ludwig Werner,

Andrés Tejel,

George D. Pamplona-Roger,

Gunther Klenk.

Embassy of Chile in Spain, p. 199; Edouard Naenny, p. 92; Tourism Office of Switzerland, p. 54

Botanical **illustrations** have been drawn by **Angel S. Chicharro,** and are property, like all other ones appearing in this work, of Editorial Safeliz, S. L.

Units of Measure

cc: at present, cubic centimeters are no longer used as a liquid volume measure. One cubic centimeter equates to one milliliter (ml)

cl: symbol of centiliter, the hundredth part of a liter: 1 l = 100 cl

cm: symbol of centimeter, the hundredth part of a meter: 1 m = 100 cm

dl: symbol of deciliter, the tenth part of a liter: 1 l = 10 dl

g: symbol of gram, unit of weight measurement in the decimal measurement system. It is equal to the thousandth part of a kilogram: 1 g = 0.001 kg

kg: symbol of kilogram: 1 kg = 1,000 g

l: symbol of liter, unit of liquid measurement in the decimal measurement system: 1 l = 1,000 cc = 1,000 ml

m: symbol of meter, the universally accepted patron unit of the decimal measurement system: 1 m = 10 dm = 100 cm =
1,000 mm

I.U.: Abbreviation of International Units, which was the measure unit used when weight of some vitamins could not be exactly measured. It was a measure of the "biologic" effects of a substance on living beings. At present, with more exact measurement systems, the unit used is the microgram (µg). In the case of vitamin A: 1 µg = 3.33 I.U.

mg: symbol of milligram, the thousandth part of a gram: 1 g = 1,000 mg

ml: symbol of milliliter, the thousandth part of a liter: 1 l = 1,000 ml (1 ml = 1 cc)

µ: symbol of micron, the millionth parth of a meter: 1 m = 1,000,000 µ; 1 mm = 1,000 µ

µg: symbol of microgram, the millionth part of a gram: 1 g = 1,000,000 µg

Temperature: in this encyclopedia we use the Celsius, centesimal, or centigrade scale to measure temperature. In some countries and publications, Fahrenheit degrees are used. Zero Celsius degrees equate to 32° F, and 100° C are 212° F

In the measurement of normal or fever body temperature, the main equivalences are: 36° C = 96.8° F; 37° C = 98.6° F; 38° C = 100.4° F; 39° C = 102.2° F

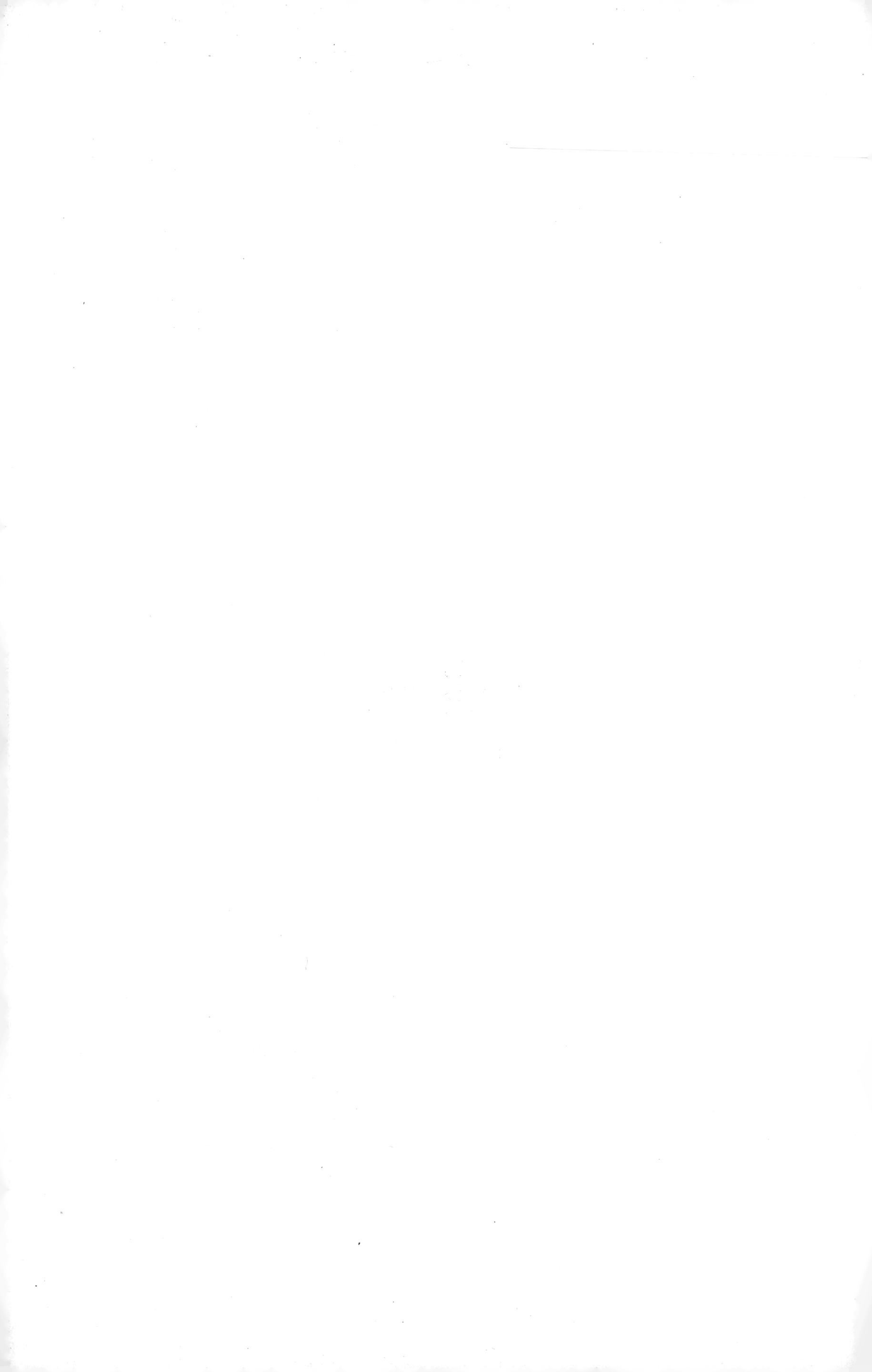